Infection Control in Clinical Practice

For Elsevier:

Senior Commissioning Editor: Steven Black
Development Editor: Mairi McCubbin
Project Manager: Jane Dingwall
Designer: George Ajayi
Illustrations Manager: Bruce Hogarth

Infection Control in Clinical Practice

Jennie Wilson BSc(Hons) MSc RGN DFPH
Senior Nurse Manager, Healthcare Associated Infection and Antimicrobial Resistance Department, Centre for Infections, Health Protection Agency; and Research Fellow, Richard Wells Research Centre, Thames Valley University, London, UK

Foreword by

Elizabeth A Jenner PhD MEd BSc(Hons) RGN HonDipHIC FRCN
Principal Lecturer, School of Nursing and Midwifery, University of Hertfordshire, Hatfield, UK

THIRD EDITION

Illustrations by
Oxford Illustrators

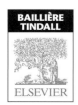

BAILLIÈRE TINDALL

ELSEVIER

EDINBURGH   LONDON   NEW YORK   OXFORD   PHILADELPHIA   ST LOUIS   SYDNEY   TORONTO   2006

BAILLIÈRE
TINDALL
ELSEVIER

First edition 1995
Second edition 2001
Third edition 2006
    Reprinted 2007 (twice)

ISBN 13: 978 0 7020 2761 1
ISBN 10: 0 7020 2761 8

BRITISH LIBRARY CATALOGUING IN PUBLICATION DATA
A catalogue record for this book is available from the British Library

LIBRARY OF CONGRESS CATALOGING IN PUBLICATION DATA
A catalog record for this book is available from the Library of Congress

Notice
Neither the Publisher nor the Author assumes any responsibility for any loss or
injury and/or damage to persons or property arising out of or related to any use of
the material contained in this book. It is the responsibility of the treating
practitioner, relying on independent expertise and knowledge of the patient, to
determine the best treatment and method of application for the patient.

The Publisher

Working together to grow
libraries in developing countries

www.elsevier.com | www.bookaid.org | www.sabre.org

ELSEVIER   BOOK AID International   Sabre Foundation

your source for books,
journals and multimedia
in the health sciences

www.elsevierhealth.com

The
publisher's
policy is to use
**paper manufactured
from sustainable forests**

Printed in China
C/03

Contents

List of colour plates

A colour plate section can be found between pages 132 and 133

Foreword

Since the last edition of this seminal textbook was produced, the problems of healthcare-associated infections have continued apace. Many, if not most, of these result from healthcare professionals' failure to decontaminate their hands at appropriate times to prevent infection and the use and abuse of antibiotics. For example, methicillin-resistant *Staphylococcus aureus*, which first caused epidemics of infection in the 1980s, is now endemic in most of our hospitals.

Glycopeptide-resistant enterococci and extended spectrum β-lactamases pose further challenges to therapeutic and control efforts as does multidrug-resistant tuberculosis (MDRTB). Multi-resistant *Acinetobacter* spp. pose an increasing threat to patients in Intensive Care Units. Frequent outbreaks of *Clostridium difficile* diarrhoea occur, especially in elderly care units. Not surprisingly, the increased use of antibiotics has contributed to a significant rise in the prevalence of fungal infections amongst hospitalized patients. Norovirus, which spreads rapidly from person to person, has become the main pathogen associated with outbreaks of gastrointestinal disease in hospitals in England and Wales.

However, poor hand hygiene and antibiotic-resistant micro-organisms are not the only causes for concern. Uncertainties about the transmissibility of variant Creutzfeldt–Jakob disease (vCJD) resulted in demands for improved standards for decontamination of medical equipment, both in hospitals and the community. The emergence of MDRTB and Sudden Acute Respiratory Syndrome (SARS) led to a review of the provision of properly ventilated isolation facilities and personal protective equipment. Now we prepare to face avian flu which will perhaps be the greatest challenge of all.

The third edition of this book has been updated to address all these issues. In particular, the role of handwashing in the prevention of infection is highlighted in most chapters. The chapter on antimicrobial chemotherapy has been considerably expanded to discuss this critically important aspect of the prevention, treatment and control of infection. Although only those nurses who have obtained the extended and supplementary prescribers' qualification may prescribe certain antibiotics, *all* nurses have a significant role to play in ensuring correct administration and teaching patients the importance of adhering to the prescribed regimen. The chapter on the epidemiology of infection has also been restructured. It emphasizes not only the size of the problem posed by healthcare-associated infections but also the socio-economic impact. The financial costs are considerable, but patient suffering should be reason enough for all healthcare professionals to reappraise their personal responsibility for the prevention of infection. The section on the surveillance of wound infection has been enriched by Jennie's first hand experience of the development and leadership of the surgical site infection module of the National Nosocomial Infection Surveillance System.

The fundamental format of the book is unchanged. The first section explains the principles of infection control whilst the second section explores the evidence base for various practices which cause the majority of healthcare-associated infections. As Jennie rightly points out, 'There is little evidence to suggest that the environment plays a major role in the transmission of healthcare-associated infection' (p. 41); whilst dirty hospitals are deplorable and unacceptable, they are not the root cause of the problem, despite what the tabloids would have us believe. As demonstrated by many observational studies, it is the suboptimal practice of healthcare professionals, particularly their failure to clean their hands, that is the main cause of cross-infection.

The key to reducing the prevalence of healthcare-associated infections lies in changing healthcare professionals' cognitions and behaviour regarding hand hygiene, in particular the way in which they risk assess the need for this basic hygiene measure (Jenner 2005). Rational beliefs, positive attitudes and a sound knowledge base are pre-requisites for behaviour change. By writing this book, Jennie has provided the sound knowledge base from which others can learn. There is a dearth of such books on the UK market and it is to be hoped that those who teach infection prevention and control will recommend that students of the health sciences read this book. It will certainly be classified as 'essential reading' on the infection control degree programme run by the University of Hertfordshire.

Jennie is to be thanked for the time and effort she has put into sharing her knowledge about the prevention and control of infection with us. A third edition of a book is testament to its success.

Hertfordshire, 2005   Elizabeth A Jenner

Reference

Jenner EA (2005) *Healthcare Professionals' Hand Hygiene: Predicting and Improving Practice*. Unpublished PhD, University of Hertfordshire.

Preface

In recent years healthcare-associated infection has become a high-profile problem. It now features regularly in the media and causes considerable political and public concern. Misinformation about both the causes of these infections and the most effective means of preventing them is widespread.

Whilst resources for infection control teams have generally improved in the UK, the main responsibility for preventing healthcare-associated infection lies with the staff directly involved in patient care. The purpose of this book is to provide a comprehensive guide to infection control practice that is both firmly grounded in the underpinning science and strongly evidence based.

This third edition has been thoroughly revised and updated to take account of new evidence and guidance. I have aimed to retain the accessible style, and many of the illustrations and tables have been updated and improved. In addition, the chapter on the epidemiology of infection has been reorganized and, in the light of the increasing concern about antimicrobial-resistant pathogens, the chapter on antimicrobial agents has been extensively updated and developed. The book has been divided into two sections. Section 1 contains chapters that cover the principles underpinning infection prevention and control such as microbiology, immunology and antimicrobial agents. Section 2 focuses on the practice of infection control, thoroughly reviewing the evidence and providing guidelines for best practice.

This book provides healthcare professionals with the knowledge they need to apply infection control practice confidently in their everyday work and will also act as a resource for infection control professionals, educators, those undertaking training and anyone wishing to learn more about the evidence base for infection prevention and control.

London, 2005   Jennie Wilson

Acknowledgements

I would like to thank the many people whose support has made the production of this book possible. In particular, Jill Swales for reviewing the entire text and providing many helpful suggestions; Elizabeth Jenner for her usual thoroughness and late night phone calls; Peter Hoffman and May Taylor for invaluable advice and comment; and Jacqui Prieto for the loan of her PhD thesis. Again I must also thank all those readers of the previous editions whose enthusiasm encouraged me to find the time, somehow, to complete this one, and my family Philip, Sarah, Josie and Claire for their love and forbearance.

SECTION 1

Principles

SECTION CONTENTS

Chapter 1

Introduction to microbiology

INTRODUCTION

Microbiology is the study of living organisms so small that they cannot be seen with the naked eye. This generally includes any organism of between 0.1 and 1 mm in diameter, which, although just visible, requires magnification for detail to be seen. Organisms of less than 0.1 mm cannot be seen at all without a microscope.

Investigation of the world of the microbe began in the 17th century with the invention of the microscope by a Dutch merchant, Antony van Leeuwenhoek, who, like many great scientists of his time, made astounding discoveries in his spare time. Although modern microscopes bear little resemblance to those designed by van Leeuwenhoek, they are based on broadly similar principles (Fig. 1.1).

Van Leeuwenhoek was the first to appreciate the variety and profusion of the microbial world, as he indicated in one of his letters to the Royal Society of London:

> I have had several gentlewomen in my house who were keen on seeing the little eels in vinegar; but some of them were so disgusted at the spectacle, that they vowed they'd never use vinegar again. But what if one should tell such people in future that there are more animals living in the scum on the teeth in a man's mouth, than there are men in a whole kingdom?

Microbes are found everywhere and can utilize almost any chemical substance as a source of energy. They are able to survive in almost every conceivable environment, even in conditions where other plants or animals cannot. Some can withstand temperatures of more than 95°C and live in hot water springs; others can grow at temperatures as low as −10°C.

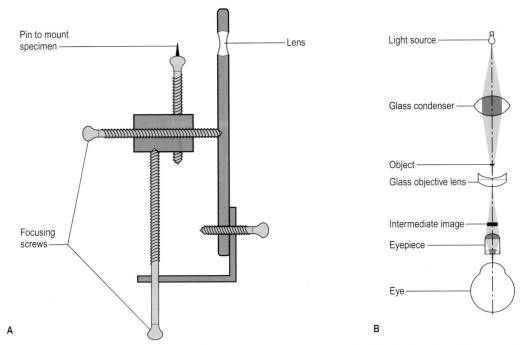

Figure 1.1 The principles of the light microscope. (A) van Leeuwenhoek's microscope. Magnification is achieved by means of a lens with a very short focal length which is capable of high magnification. The specimen is brought into focus by moving the position of the lens relative to the specimen. (B) A modern light microscope. Visible light is directed through the specimen and magnified by the lens and eyepiece. Several lenses are used to enable images to be magnified between 100 and 1000 times.

They perform many essential functions in the ecological cycle: they form the first link in the aquatic food chain (e.g. plankton, algae), fix atmospheric nitrogen into the soil so that it can be used by plants, and release nutrients for use by other living things by decomposing dead plants and other animals.

Many foods are produced by the activities of microbes, such as cheese, yoghurt, beer, wine, bread and vinegar, and microbes are also used to manufacture drugs, such as insulin and hepatitis B vaccine.

CLASSIFICATION

A system of identifying individual organisms and their relationship to one another has been gradually developed since the mid-18th century when Linnaeus established the first system of biological classification. Organisms are placed into groups according to similarities in their structure. Each is allocated two names; the first denotes the group or genus to which it belongs and the second gives it a specific name within that group, the species.

A particular species of bacteria can often be further distinguished into different 'strains', according to slightly different characteristics. This subdivision usually requires complex laboratory techniques called typing, based on the analysis of cellular characteristics, DNA or susceptibility to a range of bacterial viruses (bacteriophages). This may be important in outbreaks of infection to establish whether cases have been caused by the same organism.

In the early days, microbial science developed independently from other biological sciences and microbial cells were considered to be very different from plant or animal cells. By the mid-20th century it had become apparent that there were many similarities in the biochemistry of all living organisms and the study of microbes has considerably helped our understanding of how all cells work at a molecular level.

As our knowledge and laboratory techniques have improved, organisms previously categorized together are found to be unrelated or more closely related to another genus. These micro-organisms sometimes change their name and are reclassified (e.g. *Streptococcus faecium* has recently been renamed as an enterococcus). Some micro-organisms are very difficult to classify as they have features of more than one genus. For example,

Pneumocystis jiroveci (formerly *carinii*), although classified as a fungus, behaves more like a protozoon.

Modern molecular typing techniques have enabled scientists to determine how closely related organisms are by comparing DNA sequences. Commonly, the DNA that encodes ribosomal RNA is used for this purpose. The most widely accepted classification system is that developed by Carl Woese, an American molecular biologist, called the three domain system. This comprises two divisions of simple unicellular organisms, Bacteria and Archae, and a Eukaryotic division, which includes more complex micro-organisms such as protozoa with plants and animals (see Table 1.1).

THE STRUCTURE OF CELLS

A cell is the basic unit of living structures, consisting of a nucleus and cytoplasm enclosed in semipermeable membrane and, in some cases, an outer cell wall. The nucleus contains the genetic information unique to that cell. It is a code that, when translated, creates the specific proteins and enzymes necessary to build and operate the cell.

Although these basic mechanisms by which all cells function are broadly the same, two distinct types of cells can be identified (see Fig. 1.2). Plants, animals, protozoa, fungi and algae are all composed of eukaryotic cells. These have a complex structure, their DNA is surrounded by a nuclear membrane and they have many distinct organelles that carry out the functions of the cell. Plants and animals are composed of many cells, extensively differentiated so that groups of cells perform different tasks within the whole plant or animal. Protozoa and algae are much simpler organisms, consisting of single cells, while fungi can be unicellular or multicellular but without any differentiation between the cells.

Prokaryotic cells are far smaller and less complex; they do not have a nuclear membrane and they only form single-celled organisms. All bacteria are prokaryotic.

The cell wall

There are significant differences between the cell walls of prokaryotic and eukaryotic cells. Eukaryotic cells are usually enclosed by a membrane rather than a cell wall but if a cell wall is present then it is a simple structure composed of sugars or, in the case of algae and plant cells, cellulose. Prokaryotic cells have a rigid cell wall made of a network of carbohydrates and amino acids called peptidoglycan (see Fig. 1.3). This wall determines the shape of the cell and helps it to withstand high or low osmotic pressures outside the cell. The amount of peptidoglycan in the cell wall determines the staining properties of the bacterial cell (see Ch. 2) and provides a method for identifying and classifying bacteria.

Gram-positive bacteria have a cell wall made from a very thick mesh of peptidoglycan. Small molecules can pass into and out of the cell through this wall. The thick layer of peptidoglycan helps the cell to resist the immune system but it is vulnerable to attack by enzymes such as lysozyme. Gram-negative bacteria have more complicated walls. They have a thin layer of peptidoglycan surrounded by an outer membrane composed of protein, phospholipid and lipopolysaccharide (LPS). The LPS is toxic to animals, especially the lipid A component which causes fever and severe damage to the circulatory system. LPS is called an endotoxin because it is part of the structure of the cell rather than a secreted molecule. Although LPS is similar in all Gram-negative cells, the composition of the sugar side-chains (called O antigens) varies. Serological techniques are used to detect these differences and form an important means of identification and classification of Gram-negative bacteria. The outer membrane enables Gram-negative bacteria to resist penetration by many harmful substances (e.g. disinfectants) but with a much thinner layer of peptidoglycan they are more susceptible to desiccation in dry conditions; hence their preference for moist environments such as taps and sink outlets. Penicillin and many other antibiotics destroy bacteria by interfering with the synthesis of peptidoglycan. Eukaryotic cells do not contain peptidoglycan; therefore these drugs have no effect on the cells of the animal receiving treatment. Archaeans have cell walls but they do not contain peptidoglycan.

Table 1.1 Classification of organisms

Domain	Type of cell	Groups of organism
Bacteria	Prokaryotic Unicellular	Bacteria Mycoplasma Rickettsiae Chlamydia Cyanobacteria
Archaea	Prokaryotic Unicellular	Archaebacteria
Eucarya	Eukaryotic Unicellular Multicellular (undifferentiated) Multicellular (differentiated)	Algae Protozoa Fungi Plants Animals

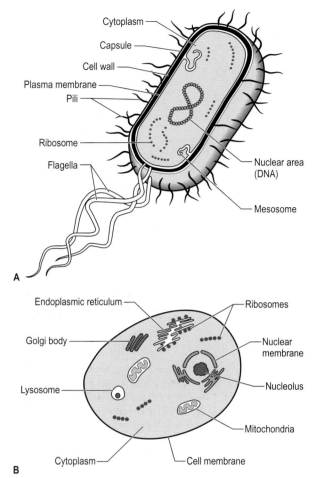

A

B

Figure 1.2 The structure of cells. (A) A bacterial cell. (B) A eukaryotic cell (reproduced with kind permission from Ackerman & Dunk-Richards 1991).

Capsules

Many bacteria produce a layer of gelatinous material outside the cell wall that adheres strongly to the cell to form a clearly defined capsule. Capsules play an important role in enabling some bacteria to cause infection by protecting them from white blood cells. Examples of important pathogens that have capsules are *Haemophilus influenzae* and *Streptococcus pneumoniae*. Some bacteria secrete a loose network of material called slime, which helps them to adhere to a range of surfaces, including teeth, plastic catheters and prosthetic devices.

Spores and cysts

These are resistant casings that form around the cell. They are made of a thick layer of peptidoglycan and a tough keratin-like protein, and are extremely difficult to destroy by heat or chemicals (see Ch. 13). Spores are made by some bacteria when they are exposed to adverse environmental conditions, e.g. lack of food source or moisture (see Fig. 1.4). When conditions improve the spores germinate – the spore cortex and coat disintegrates to reveal a single vegetative cell (outgrowth) which then starts to multiply. Most spore-forming bacteria live in soil and belong to the genera clostridia and bacillus. Spores can survive for very long periods; spores of *Bacillus anthrax* could still be recovered from the soil of an island off the Scottish coast used to test biological weapons many years after testing had ceased.

Some protozoa (e.g. toxoplasma and entamoeba) change into **cysts**, which enables them to survive for many months outside a host.

The cytoplasm and cytoplasmic membrane

The biochemical reactions that maintain the cell and enable it to reproduce all take place within the cytoplasm of the cell. The cytoplasm contains a variety

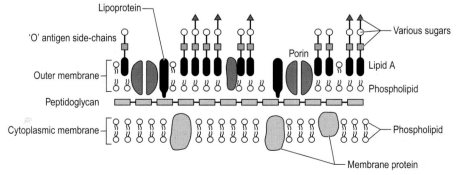

Figure 1.3 The structure of the cell wall of a Gram-negative bacterium. Both inner and outer membranes are made of phospholipid. The porins in the outer membrane enable substances to pass into the cell. The sugars and side-chains attached to the outer membrane are antigenic. The layer of peptidoglycan between the membranes is not as thick in Gram-positive cells (reproduced with kind permission from Ackerman & Dunk-Richards 1991).

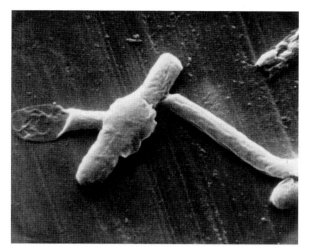

Figure 1.4 A clostridium cell showing a spore distending the middle of the rod (electron micrograph) (reproduced with kind permission from Ackerman & Dunk-Richards 1991).

Table 1.2 The function of organelles in eukaryotic cells

Organelle	Function
Endoplasmic reticulum	Makes lipids and directs movement of lipids and proteins through the cell
Ribosome	Translates RNA sequences into proteins. Found on the endoplasmic reticulum and free in the cytoplasm
Mitochondrion	Oxidizes glucose and fatty acids to make energy in the form of ATP (respiration)
Cytoskeleton	Internal framework of the cell that enables it to move and transport substances
Golgi apparatus	Modifies and sorts proteins and lipids
Lysosome	Contains enzymes that break down unwanted large molecules

of nutrients that are required for the activity of the cell and is surrounded by a cytoplasmic membrane. The cytoplasmic membrane is formed from two layers of lipid molecules interspersed with proteins. The lipids provide an impermeable barrier to most water-soluble molecules. Some of the protein molecules form pores that enable molecules to enter the cell; other proteins actively transport substances across the membrane.

In eukaryotic cells the cytoplasm contains a number of distinct structures called organelles, each containing its own set of enzymes and surrounded by a membrane. These organelles carry out the processes required by the cell (Table 1.2). Transport proteins carry substances between organelles and a network of small tubules called the cytoskeleton is involved in cell transport, movement and chromosome separation during cell division. The cytoskeleton is also thought to enable cells making up a tissue to communicate and work together (e.g. muscle fibres).

In prokaryotic cells the only structures in the cytoplasm are ribosomes, where proteins are synthesized, and inclusion bodies which are used to store lipids. Prokaryotic ribosomes are smaller than those in eukaryotic cells and are only found free in the cytoplasm. In prokaryotic cells, nutrients can be taken up easily from the environment because of the large surface area of cytoplasmic membrane available. Small molecules, such as sugars, pass through the cytoplasmic membrane of the cell by diffusion provided their concentration is higher outside the cell. If the concentration of required nutrients is lower outside the cell, the carrier proteins are used to take

them across the membrane. Large molecules cannot pass through the membrane and bacteria often excrete enzymes into their environment to break large molecules down into smaller compounds. Prokaryotic cells do not have complex transport systems and the cytoplasmic membrane also performs many of the functions of the cell, for example synthesis of cell wall components, respiration to form adenosine triphosphate (ATP) (see p. 9), secretion of enzymes and nutrient transport. Folded areas of membrane called mesosomes are thought to be involved in protein secretion and transport, in chromosome separation during cell division, and in some bacteria contain the enzymes required for respiration.

The nucleus

The structures within cells and the enzymes that regulate cellular activities are made of protein. The genetic information or genome of the cell determines what protein it can make. The genome is formed from molecules of deoxyribonucleic acid (DNA), each molecule arranged into a chromosome. The cells of higher animals have many chromosomes – for example human cells have 46 chromosomes – but prokaryotic cells have very few – *Escherichia coli* for example has only one chromosome. In eukaryotic cells the chromosomes are enclosed by a nuclear membrane; in prokaryotic cells they lie free in the cytoplasm.

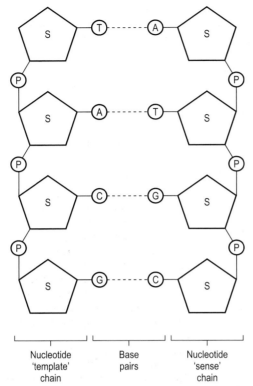

Figure 1.5   The structure of deoxyribonucleic acid (DNA). S, sugar molecule; P, phosphate molecule; C, cytosine; G, guanine; A, adenine; T, thymine; ..., hydrogen bond.

Table 1.3 The genetic code	
Sequence of bases on DNA	Equivalent amino acid
GCG	Alanine
TTC	Phenylalanine
CGC	Arginine
AAA	Lysine

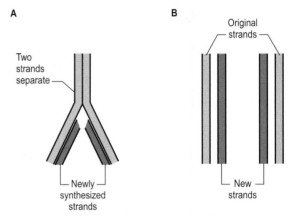

Figure 1.6   The copying of a chromosome. (A) The two strands of DNA are separated and a copy is made of each half. (B) The two identical chromosomes.

The genetic code

DNA is made of two complementary strands of nucleotides held together by hydrogen bonds and twisted together to form a double helix. In bacterial cells the helix is further coiled and, although it may be 1000 times the length of the cell, it takes up only 10% of the cytoplasm. Nucleotides consist of a sugar molecule, attached to a phosphate molecule and one of four bases: adenine, cytosine, guanine and thymine (see Fig. 1.5). A base is a molecule that can accept a hydrogen ion and can connect with another base by forming a weak association or hydrogen bond. Adenine always bonds or pairs with thymine, whilst guanine always pairs with cytosine. Two chains or strands of nucleotides are held together by hydrogen bonds between the pairs of bases and are therefore mirror images of each other.

The sequence of bases forms the code in which is stored all the information needed to make the constituent molecules of the cell. The code made by adenine, cytosine, guanine and thymine can be compared to making up three-letter 'words' with A, C, G and T. Each 'word' can be translated into one of the amino acids that are needed to make proteins (Table 1.3). Different series of amino acids can be made from the same length of DNA by changing the starting point of translation.

An average protein is composed of about 400 amino acids and corresponds to a sequence of 1200 bases along the nucleotide chain. Each section of DNA that codes for a protein is called a gene.

When cells divide, the chromosome of each new cell must contain both strands of DNA. To make an accurate copy of the DNA, the two strands are gradually separated and both then become a pattern against which a new strand is made. After replication, the two daughter chromosomes contain one strand from the parent and one new strand (see Fig. 1.6).

Plasmids

Many bacterial cells carry between one and six small circles of DNA called plasmids which are not incorporated into the main chromosome. Plasmid DNA can be replicated on its own and copied into each

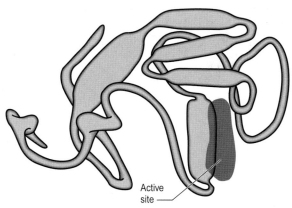

Active site

Figure 1.7 The structure of an enzyme. The complicated folded structure of enzymes is essential for their activity. The active site is where molecules combine with the enzyme (reproduced with kind permission from Ackerman & Dunk-Richards 1991).

daughter cell. Plasmids do not contain any genes essential for cell viability and can be lost without damaging the cell. They often contain genes that enable the cell to resist antibiotics, adhere to surfaces (e.g. fimbriae) or synthesize toxins, such as haemolysins that destroy red blood cells and diphtheria toxin.

THE PROPERTIES OF CELLS

The activities of all cells from the smallest bacterium to the largest mammal are controlled by proteins called enzymes (see Fig. 1.7). Enzymes catalyse or speed up a whole range of chemical reactions; they control energy-making reactions, enable the cell to synthesize complex materials from nutrients, and to grow and divide into new cells.

Cell metabolism

The chemical reactions that take place in all living cells are described as the metabolism of the cell. Anabolism is where new compounds are formed from simple molecules. Catabolism is where large and complicated compounds are broken down into their constituent molecules, releasing energy.

The protein structure of the cell and its enzymes is made up of amino acids and the main food reserves of the cell: carbohydrates and fats.

All living cells need energy to maintain the chemical and physical composition of their cytoplasm and to grow and replicate themselves. The original source of energy is solar energy from the sun. This is captured by plants and a few bacteria by a process called photosynthesis. Most bacteria and all animals then use plants as a source of nutrients and energy.

The biologically usable form of energy, which is present in all cells, is adenosine triphosphate (ATP). Glucose is broken down in the cell and its energy is captured in the form of ATP. There are 10 chemical reactions used to convert one molecule of glucose to carbon dioxide and water and during these reactions, 30 molecules of ATP are produced. ATP is then used by the cell to:

- make new cell components
- transport substances into the cell
- move the cell
- move the cell cytoplasm.

When this energy-forming process involves the use of oxygen, it is called respiration. Some cells use organic compounds instead of oxygen and produce alcohol as the end-product instead of water. This process is called fermentation and is characteristic of anaerobic bacteria. Some bacteria can switch from respiration to fermentation in the absence of oxygen and are called facultative anaerobes. These include many of the bacteria that both colonize and cause infection in humans, such as enterobacteria, streptococci and staphylococci. The by-products of fermentation are used in various commercial processes such as brewing and wine making. In eukaryotic cells, respiration occurs in the mitochondria. These have a highly folded internal membrane containing the enzymes that catalyse the energy-producing reactions.

Protein synthesis

The synthesis of a string of amino acids begins with the creation of a short length of ribonucleic acid (RNA) corresponding to the sequence of bases on the DNA strand. RNA has a similar structure to DNA except that it is a single chain, the sugar is ribose, not deoxyribose, and the thymine is replaced by a very similar base, uracil. This messenger RNA (mRNA) moves to the ribosomes where the code is read and the appropriate amino acids are assembled into a chain. Amino acids are collected from the cytoplasm by other RNA molecules called transfer RNA (tRNA). There is a specific tRNA for each type of amino acid (see Fig. 1.8).

Cell division

Prokaryotic cells multiply by dividing in two in a process called binary fission. When the cell has grown to a certain size, the single chromosome divides into two identical copies and the cell wall and membrane grow inwards, forming a new cell wall across the cell. Eventually the cell wall splits the cytoplasm into two cells, each with a chromosome (see Fig. 1.9). Often the two cells do not completely separate from each other but

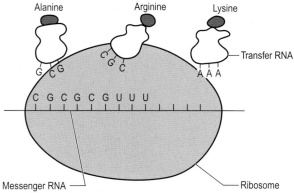

Figure 1.8 The synthesis of protein. A length of RNA is made from the DNA strand and moves to a ribosome. The amino acids corresponding to the code on the RNA are brought from the cytoplasm by transfer RNA and assembled into a protein.

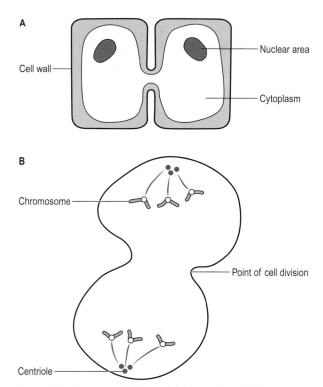

Figure 1.9 Simple cell division. (A) A bacterial cell. The chromosome replicates, a new cell wall forms and divides the original cell into two (binary fission). (B) A eukaryotic cell. The chromosome replicates, one set is distributed to each end of the cell which then divides into two (mitosis).

remain together as clumps (e.g. staphylococci), in chains (e.g. streptococci) or in pairs (e.g. pneumococci).

Eukaryotic cells can divide by simple division, or mitosis, in a similar way to prokaryotes. All the DNA is copied and each set enclosed in a nuclear membrane. The cytoplasm then divides to form two identical cells. This type of division will occur as the plant or animal makes new cells to grow or to repair damaged tissue.

Sexual reproduction

Sexual reproduction describes the process of mixing genetic information from more than one individual together and is a method of introducing variation into the population. Variation is important because it enables a species to adapt to its environment and gradually evolve.

Eukaryotes

In eukaryotic cells, sexual reproduction is achieved by fusing together two cells from different individuals. As this would result in one cell with double the usual number of chromosomes, a special type of cell division called meiosis is required. This creates daughter cells with half the usual number of chromosomes. At fertilization, two cells fuse together and the new cell will contain the full number of chromosomes.

Prokaryotes

Prokaryotic cells do not multiply by sexual reproduction. However, transfer of genetic material between bacterial cells occurs but always in one direction, from a donor cell to a recipient cell. Transfer happens in one of three ways (see Fig. 1.10).

Transformation Certain bacteria, e.g. *Streptococcus pneumoniae, Bacillus subtillis*, are able to take up fragments of DNA released from dead bacteria. These are absorbed through the cell wall and incorporated into the chromosome. Only DNA from closely related species will be expressed as proteins.

Transduction DNA from one bacterium is introduced into another cell by a bacterial virus or bacteriophage. Like other viruses, phages must incorporate into the host DNA in order to replicate. Sometimes some of the host's DNA is copied with the virus genome by mistake and is taken out of the cell with the phage. This is the method by which some bacteria acquire resistance to antibiotics.

Conjugation Plasmid DNA can transfer from one bacterial cell to another through a small tube or sex pilus which attaches to the sex pilus of the cell. The plasmid DNA then replicates and one copy enters the recipient cell. Plasmids commonly carry genes

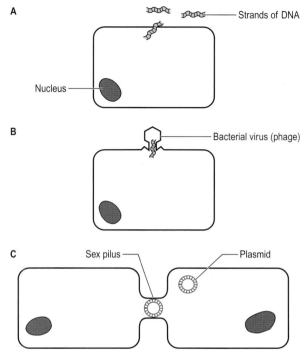

Figure 1.10   Methods used by bacteria to exchange genetic information. (A) Transformation. (B) Transduction. (C) Conjugation.

chromosome, and in the synthesis of substances useful in medicine and industry.

Nucleases, enzymes that cut the DNA strand, can be used to break strands of DNA into small fragments. Restriction endonucleases are special types of nuclease that recognize specific sequences of bases in DNA strands. As each enzyme will always recognize the same sequence, the same sections of DNA are always obtained from a particular chromosome. It is therefore possible to separate a single gene known to synthesize a particular chemical. If the same endonuclease is then used to cut a DNA plasmid, the gene cut from the chromosome can be inserted into the plasmid. Plasmids can be introduced into other bacteria by conjugation or into eukaryotic cells using specialized techniques. When the cells are cultured they then synthesize the substance coded for by the introduced gene.

This method has been used to manufacture substances used in the treatment of human disease by inserting genes from the human chromosome into bacteria. For example, the gene coding for human insulin has been inserted into a bacterium and human insulin can now be manufactured by the culture of these bacteria. Fragments of DNA from the hepatitis B virus have also been incorporated into a plasmid, which is inserted into a yeast. The viral proteins produced by the yeast as it multiplies are purified and made into a vaccine against hepatitis B virus. These recombinant DNA techniques are also used to provide rapid and specific tests for infections by detecting specific sequences of DNA.

Cell motility

Some bacteria are not capable of independent movement. Others, particularly bacilli and spirilli, have appendages called flagella which, by rotating like a propeller, enable them to swim (see Fig. 1.11). These motile bacteria swim towards chemicals such as nutrients, to which they are attracted, and swim away from toxic substances. Many Gram-negative bacteria such as *Escherichia coli* and pseudomonas have flagella and are motile. Some species have many flagella on one cell. Flagella are rarely found on cocci. Motile bacteria thrive in moist conditions where the ability to swim is an advantage, whilst non-motile bacteria are able to survive in dry environments.

Eukaryotic cells may also have flagella or cilia but with a much more complex structure.

Fimbriae or pili are hair-like appendages that are thinner and shorter than flagella. They are mostly found on Gram-negative cells and their purpose is to facilitate adherence to other cells. Variation in fimbriae affects the types of cell to which the bacteria can

conferring resistance to antibiotics or toxin production, so conjugation is of major importance in the spread of these characteristics between strains of bacteria. The genetic information required to make the sex pilus and DNA transfer proteins is carried on a plasmid. Only those bacteria with this plasmid can transfer DNA by conjugation.

Transposons are short sections of DNA that include genetic code for an enzyme called transposase. This enables the segment of DNA to be inserted into or taken out of other DNA sequences, from the DNA genome to a plasmid, from a plasmid to a genome or between plasmids. In addition to transposase, transposons can carry virulence genes, e.g. enterotoxin in *Escherichia coli*, or genes encoding resistance to one or more antibiotic. Methicillin resistance in *Staphylococcus aureus* is conferred by a set of genes called MecA that are carried on a transposon.

Recombinant DNA techniques

The study of bacterial genomes has enabled tremendous advances to be made both in our understanding of the genetic code, in particular the human

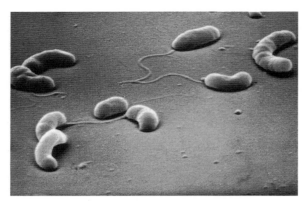

Figure 1.11   Flagella on a bacterial cell (reproduced by kind permission of Dr D Barrie, Charing Cross and Westminster Medical School, London).

adhere and determines their ability to cause disease. Sex pili are special types of fimbriae used in the exchange of genetic information between cells.

THE GROWTH AND MULTIPLICATION OF BACTERIA

Since bacteria live in a wide range of environments, it is not surprising that the nutrients they need vary widely from species to species. A bacterium such as *Escherichia coli*, supplied with all the nutrients it needs, will divide, on average, once every 15 minutes and will continue to grow at this rate until the supply of nutrients is exhausted. Some bacteria can synthesize a wide range of materials that they need to grow and multiply and can therefore survive in the presence of very few nutrients. Others need a source of specific molecules or amino acids and therefore have more exacting growth requirements. There are certain basic substances that are essential to support the growth of all bacteria.

Energy source

Energy is generally obtained from the breakdown of organic carbon-containing compounds, although some bacteria (e.g. cyanobacteria) are able to capture the energy of the sun using protein pigments similar to chlorophyll in plants.

Carbon source

Carbon is necessary to form the compounds that make up the structure of the cell. Most bacteria also use the breakdown of organic carbon compounds such as carbohydrates to obtain energy. However, bacteria can make use of almost any form of carbon including hydrocarbons, phenol, wood and atmospheric carbon dioxide.

Nitrogen source

Nitrogen is needed to make many of the cell structures, for example proteins and nucleic acids. Nitrogen can be obtained in the form of ammonia (NH_4) or nitrates (NO_3) and some microbes can use atmospheric nitrogen, e.g. cyanobacteria. Many pathogenic bacteria need a source of organic nitrogen such as amino acids.

Inorganic ions

Sodium, potassium, magnesium, chloride and sulphate are needed both to form the structure of the cell, for example to make amino acids, and to act as co-factors for enzymes. All organisms require phosphate to make lipids and nucleic acids and to store energy as ATP (see p. 9).

Some bacteria will grow in very simple media containing only these substances, although usually they grow very slowly. Most of the bacteria that cause disease in humans depend on the presence of additional 'growth factors' available in the host tissue. These are usually amino acids or vitamins that the bacteria cannot make themselves. Other chemicals, or trace elements such as iron or zinc, are required to make enzymes or other proteins.

We can help to prevent the multiplication of bacteria in the clinical environment by removing potential sources of nutrients. For example, body fluid spilt on to equipment, furniture or floors will support the growth of bacteria and should be removed as soon as possible; baths or washbowls that are not properly cleaned will retain a coating of skin scales and soap on their surface which provides a plentiful supply of nutrients for the growth of bacteria (Greaves 1985).

Environmental factors

Environmental conditions also have a very important effect on the growth of bacteria. Bacteria that cause disease usually grow most rapidly under the environmental conditions found in the human body.

Water

Water is an essential requirement for the growth of bacteria and most die rapidly in the absence of water. The moisture-loving Gram-negative bacteria, in particular, thrive in damp places. Since they have a relatively thin cell wall (see p. 5), they are particularly vulnerable to desiccation and will usually survive for only a short time on dry surfaces. The susceptibility of many bacteria to a lack of water provides us with a very useful infection control measure; we can prevent bacteria from multiplying by keeping surfaces clean and dry and by drying equipment thoroughly before it is stored. Equipment should not be immersed in liquids for prolonged periods as bacteria can grow even in disinfectants. Thermometers stored in disinfectant solutions or mops lingering in buckets of dirty water are therefore an infection hazard (Werry et al 1988). Equipment such as nebulizers or ventilator equipment that is in contact with water is particularly hazardous because bacteria can multiply rapidly in the moisture (Botman & de Krieger 1987, Cefai et al 1990).

Other bacteria are more resistant to drying out (e.g. staphylococci and mycobacteria) or are able to form spores (e.g. *Clostridium difficile*). They may be able to survive for hours or even months, recommencing multiplication if a supply of moisture is resumed. These organisms may survive in dust and thus preventing the accumulation of dust on surfaces and floors can be an important infection control measure (Cartmill et al 1994, Neely & Maley 2000).

Oxygen

To use respiration for energy production, bacteria must have an enzyme called catalase, which can degrade the toxic end-products of the process. Some bacteria do not have catalase and use fermentation rather than respiration to make energy (see p. 9). Many of these obligate anaerobes are rapidly killed when exposed to air and special laboratory techniques are required to culture them. Some bacteria can use either respiration or fermentation to make energy, changing the method according to the prevailing environmental conditions. These are called facultative anaerobes and include enteric bacteria and the staphylococci. Obligate aerobes such as pseudomonas and mycobacteria can use only respiration and therefore cannot survive without oxygen.

Anaerobes are found inside body cavities such as the intestines and vagina. Anaerobic bacteria such as *Clostridium perfringens* can cause serious infection in wounds where the tissue is extensively damaged or necrotic and poorly supplied with oxygen. Wounds that have a good blood supply will be well oxygenated and are unlikely to support the growth of anaerobic bacteria. *Bacteroides fragilis* is an anaerobe normally found in the intestine, which can cause intra-abdominal abscesses following surgery.

Temperature

Most bacteria grow within a wide range of temperatures but those that grow in association with humans multiply rapidly at around body temperature. Some bacteria are known for their ability to multiply even at very low temperatures. *Listeria monocytogenes*, for example, grows even at 5°C and can therefore spoil refrigerated food. Bacteria can adapt to almost any environment. Some species are even able to survive at temperatures of 100°C found in hot springs and volcanoes.

pH

The pH of a solution reflects the concentration of hydrogen ions. Most bacteria cannot maintain the neutral pH of their cytoplasm if the concentration of hydrogen ions outside the cell is too high or low, and prefer to live in approximately neutral solutions. A high pH is used to protect some body cavities from invasion by harmful bacteria; for example, the normally acidic stomach kills ingested pathogens. Lactobacilli that normally inhabit the vagina produce lactic acid, creating a local pH of 4.0 in which most pathogens are unable to survive.

Concentration of solution

Molecules that are dissolved in a solution are called solutes. The membrane surrounding the cell prevents the passage of solutes into the cell. If the cell is in a solution where the concentration of solutes is greater than in the cytoplasm of the cell, there is a tendency for water to diffuse out of the cell into the solution in order to equilibrate the concentrations. If the concentration of solutes in the cytoplasm is greater than outside the cell, the water will diffuse into the cell. This process is known as osmosis. Like all cells, bacteria have transport mechanisms operating at the membrane to make sure that the level of solutes in the cytoplasm remains at the desired concentration regardless of the concentration in their environment. In fact, the bacterial cell wall is able to withstand a wide range of very strong and dilute solutions.

The common practice of adding salt to a patient's bath to 'clean' wounds is of no actual value. The salt would need to be added in enormous quantities to achieve a final concentration in the bathwater sufficient to disrupt bacterial cells and simply adding a cupful of salt to a bath of water has no antibacterial effect at all (Austin 1988, Ayliffe et al 1975).

FUNGI

Fungi are a diverse group of eukaryotic organisms that include yeasts, moulds and mushrooms. They may be unicellular, e.g. yeasts, or grow as long branching tubes called filaments or hyphae. The cell walls of fungi contain a unique polysaccharide called chitin. Fungi are widely distributed in the environment. Many saprophytic fungi live in soil, where they decompose organic matter. They can be grown on agar media like bacteria but, because they can survive in relatively little moisture and in high osmolarity, they are often found growing on substances that will not support the growth of bacteria (e.g. jams and other preserved foods). Some species of fungi cause disease in plants and animals. In humans, they cause superficial infection of the skin such as ringworm, oral and vaginal candidiasis and more serious systemic infections in the immunocompromised (e.g. aspergillosis). Mycology is the term used to describe the study of fungi.

Growth

Most fungi are filamentous, their branching hyphae containing cytoplasm and many nuclei. These form a mass called a mycelium. The filaments of the mycelium act like roots, penetrating into the substance on which they are growing. In some species the filaments are separated into cells by transverse walls, although these are often perforated to allow the movement of cytoplasm and nuclei. A large mass of mycelium may become visible and some species (e.g. mushrooms) produce specialized spore-bearing structures above the surface. Some species of fungi have lost the mycelial form of growth, forming small single ovoid cells instead. These are called *yeasts* and this type of growth can be found in all the main groups of fungi. Sometimes one species can grow as either a yeast or a mycelium, depending on the temperature and availability of nutrients.

Yeast cells are between 20 and 100 times larger than a bacterial cell but can be seen only with the aid of a microscope. They can be grown on solid agar medium where, like bacteria, they appear as masses of cells or colonies (see Ch. 2). Most yeasts live in high concentrations of sugars, such as on the surface of fruit and flowers, which they ferment. Many species are extremely useful, for example in the fermentation of sugars to produce alcohol and carbon dioxide, a process used in brewing and bread making.

Reproduction

Fungi usually reproduce asexually by forming spores at the tips of the branched tubes. Each spore contains at least one nucleus. These are released to start a new mycelium elsewhere (Fig. 1.12). Sexual reproduction occurs by fusion of cells in the mycelium to form spores but the exact mechanism varies in each species. Yeasts multiply asexually by forming buds, where a new cell gradually grows out of the parent cell (Fig. 1.13). They reproduce sexually by meiotic division of a single cell, which then forms two daughter cells or ascospores. Later two ascospores will fuse to form a new cell.

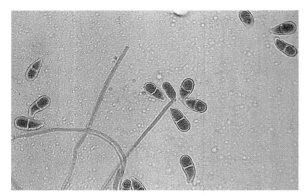

Figure 1.12   A filamentous fungus. Tubular hyphae with groups of spores. (Reproduced with kind permission from Ackerman V, Dunk-Richards G (1991) *Microbiology: An Introduction for the Health Sciences.* W B Saunders, London.)

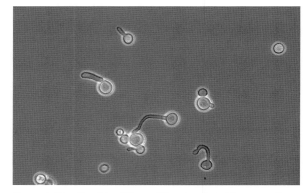

Figure 1.13   *Candida albicans.* When incubated in serum, the cells produce characteristic outgrowths called germ tubes. (Reproduced with kind permission from Ackerman V, Dunk-Richards G (1991) *Microbiology: An Introduction for the Health Sciences.* W B Saunders, London.)

ALGAE

These are photosynthetic eukaryotic organisms. They include microscopic unicellular organisms such as diatoms, dino flagellates and large multicellular seaweeds such as kelp. The main human disease associated with algae is phytotoxicosis, poisoning due to the ingestion of algal phytotoxins in shellfish or contaminated water.

PROTOZOA

These are relatively large, but still microscopic, eukaryotic cells (Fig. 1.14). They have a tough outer cell membrane instead of a cell wall, have mitochondria and can obtain nutrients by ingesting solid particles of food. These are then digested by enzymes into soluble compounds that can be transported into the

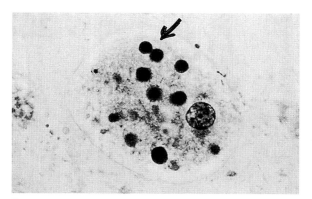

Figure 1.14   *Entamoeba histolytica.* These protozoa cause amoebic dysentery. The black dots are red blood cells which have been engulfed. The nucleus can be seen in the lower right of the cell. (Reproduced with kind permission from Ackerman V, Dunk-Richards G (1991) *Microbiology: An Introduction for the Health Sciences.* W B Saunders, London.)

cytoplasm. The cells multiply by dividing in two and some species differentiate between male and female cells. Many protozoa have complex life cycles; that is, a series of stages in their development (e.g. plasmodium species which cause malaria). They are motile in at least one of these stages and some form thick-walled, dormant cysts which are important in transmission (e.g. *Entamoeba histolytica*). Most protozoa are aquatic and some are animal parasites.

VIRUSES

Viruses are not cells; they are simply pieces of nucleic acid, which may be single or double stranded and either DNA or RNA, protected by a protein coat, called a capsid, made from many identical units of polypeptide. These are often formed into symmetrical shapes such as spheres or icosahedrons. In some viruses the capsid is surrounded by an envelope composed of lipids and glycoproteins, which is derived from the cell membranes of the host cell. Naked capsid viruses are able to withstand harsh environmental conditions and are generally resistant to drying and detergents, and can withstand the acid environment of the stomach. Many of these viruses are transmitted by the faecal–oral route. Enveloped viruses are more easily inactivated by detergents, acidic or dry conditions and since they prefer moist environments, are generally transmitted in respiratory secretions, blood and tissues.

Viruses contain none of the structures necessary to synthesize the proteins or enzymes encoded by their nucleic acid. The smallest viruses contain enough nucleic acid to make three or four proteins, the largest several hundred proteins (see Fig. 1.15).

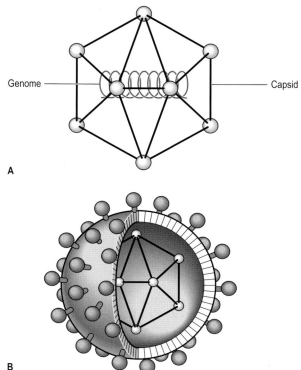

Figure 1.15   The structure of viruses. (A) Example of a naked capsid virus. The capsid is a rigid structure made of protein units that fit together symmetrically. The capsid protects the genome and its surface structures mediate the interaction with the target host cell. (B) The capsid of some viruses is enclosed by an envelope. The envelope is derived from host cell membranes and is composed of lipids and glycoproteins. It mediates the interaction with the target host cell.

Viruses are extremely small, ranging from 27 nm in diameter to about 200 nm, compared to an average bacterial cell of about 1000 nm in diameter, and are therefore too small to be seen with an ordinary light microscope. Instead, they can be seen with an electron microscope which uses a beam of electrons instead of light to create an image of an object on a photographic plate. Figure 1.16 shows an electron micrograph of adenovirus.

Viral replication

Viruses can only multiply inside living cells. Receptors on the protein coat recognize and attach to specific receptors on the surface of particular cells in the host. The presence of these specific receptors determines which cells are invaded by the virus. For example, the human immunodeficiency virus (HIV) attaches to a CD4 molecule found on the surface of some

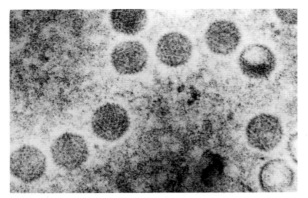

Figure 1.16   An electron micrograph of adenovirus (reproduced by kind permission of Dr D Barrie, Charing Cross and Westminster Medical School, London).

cytoplasm and new viruses are released from the cell either by budding out of the cell membrane or causing the cell to rupture (see Fig. 1.17). The host cells infected are usually destroyed by the virus but because cells are rapidly replaced, most viral illnesses are short and recovery is complete. However, some viral infections can cause permanent damage; for example, HIV depletes the T cells of the immune system to such an extent that the immune system becomes deficient.

Some viruses insert all or part of their nucleic acid into the host cell's DNA, where it remains and causes the cell to become malignant by coding for unlimited cell division. This has been suggested as the mechanism by which viruses such as herpes simplex type 2 virus and human papilloma virus could cause cancer of the cervix.

Viral growth requirements

As viruses depend on living cells for their replication, it is not possible to grow them in artificial media in the same way as bacteria. Instead, viruses are grown in cultures of living cells and require an environment that will maintain the cells, including salts, amino acids and vitamins. A few viruses, for example rotavirus, cannot even be grown in these artificial cell cultures and thus to experiment on them live animals must be used.

lymphocytes and macrophages. The viral nucleic acid then enters the nucleus of the host cell where it instructs the cell's own mechanism to copy the nucleic acids and translate its code into viral proteins. Many copies of the viral nucleic acid and proteins are made by the host cell in this way. Some RNA viruses can be translated directly as mRNA. Retroviruses have an enzyme called reverse transcriptase, which converts the RNA to DNA to enable viral proteins to be made. The virus components are then assembled in the

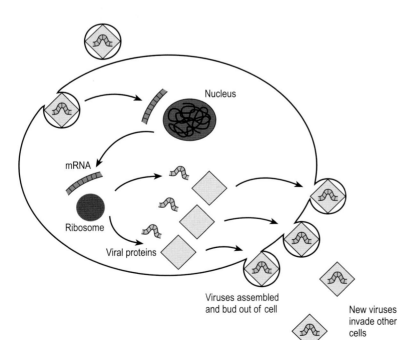

Nucleus

mRNA

Ribosome

Viral proteins

Viruses assembled and bud out of cell

New viruses invade other cells

Figure 1.17   Viral replication. The virus enters the host cell and its genome is released to the nucleus where it is copied and transcribed into mRNA. The mRNA is translated on the ribosomes of the host cell and many copies of the viral proteins are made. The genome and proteins are then assembled into new viruses and bud out of the cell membrane. Enveloped viruses acquire part of the membrane as they are released.

Most viruses are fragile and cannot survive outside a living cell for long. However, some viruses can survive for some time on surfaces or hands and from there are transmitted to a new host (Chadwick et al 2000). Viruses are fairly resistant to the activity of some disinfectants such as phenol or chlorhexidine which are unable to disrupt their protein coat or lipid membrane. Outbreaks of viral gastrointestinal or respiratory infection occur frequently in hospital. Preventing outbreaks of infection caused by viruses can be extremely difficult; they are very small, can be exhaled on small respiratory droplets or be excreted in high numbers in faeces. Transmission commonly occurs on hands and may occur on inadequately decontaminated equipment such as commodes or bedpans (Sattar et al 2002).

References

Ackerman V, Dunk-Richards G (1991) *Microbiology – An Introduction for the Health Sciences*. WB Saunders/Baillière Tindall, London.

Austin L (1988) The salt bath myth. *Nursing Times*, **84**(9): 79–83.

Ayliffe G, Babb JR, Collins BJ (1975) Disinfection of baths and bathwater. *Nursing Times*, **71**(37): 22–3.

Botman MJ, de Krieger RA (1987) Contamination of small-volume medication nebulizers and its association with oropharyngeal colonisation. *J. Hosp. Infect.*, **19**: 204–8.

Cartmill TDI, Parigrahi H, Worsley MA et al (1994) Management and control of a large outbreak of diarrhoea due to *Clostridium difficile*. *J. Hosp. Infect.*, **27**: 1–16.

Cefai C, Richards J, Gould FK et al (1990) An outbreak of *Acinetobacter* respiratory tract infection resulting from incomplete disinfection of ventilatory equipment. *J. Hosp. Infect.*, **15**: 177–82.

Chadwick PR, Beards G, Brown D et al (2000) Management of hospital outbreaks of gastro-enteritis due to small round structured viruses. *J. Hosp. Infect.*, **45**: 1–10.

Greaves A (1985) We'll just freshen you up, dear. *Nursing Times*, **Mar 6** (suppl.): 3–8.

Neely AN, Maley MP (2000) Survival of enterococci and staphylococci on hospital fabrics and plastics. *J. Clin. Microbiol.*, **38**(2): 724–6.

Sattar SA, Springthorpe VS, Tetro J et al (2002) Hygienic hand antiseptics: should they not have activity and label claims against viruses? *Am. J. Infect. Contr.*, **30**: 355–72

Werry C, Lawrence JM, Sanderson PJ (1988) Contamination of detergent cleaning solutions during hospital cleaning. *J. Hosp. Infect.*, **11**: 44–9.

Further Reading

Burton GRW, Englekirk PG (2004) *Microbiology for the Health Sciences*, 7th edn. Lippincott, Williams and Wilkins, Philadelphia.

Mims CA, Playfair JHL, Roitt IM et al (1998) *Medical Microbiology*, 2nd edn. Mosby, London.

Watson R (ed.) (1999) *Essential Science for Nursing Students. An Introductory Text*. Baillière Tindall, London.

Chapter 2

Understanding the microbiology laboratory

INTRODUCTION

In the modern age we rely extensively on antimicrobial agents to treat infection. It is easy to assume that at the first sign of fever we need only reach for an antibiotic to treat the infection and that identification and investigation of the causative organism are unnecessary. For minor infections it is reasonable to make an educated guess about the organism causing the infection; for example, skin infections such as boils or septic spots are invariably caused by organisms commonly found on the skin, such as *Staphylococcus aureus*, and are easily treated with flucloxacillin. However, the bacteria may be resistant to the antibiotic chosen, the bacteria may continue to multiply and the patient remains ill. Confirmation of the micro-organisms causing the infection, and the most appropriate method of treatment, requires the expertise of the microbiology laboratory.

The functions of the microbiology laboratory are to:

- assist in the diagnosis of infection
- identify the causative organism
- provide advice on the best antimicrobial agent to treat the infection
- provide epidemiological information that shows the changes in causative organisms and sensitivity to antibiotics.

The procedures used in the microbiology laboratory aim to reproduce the environmental conditions in which pathogenic micro-organisms grow and to identify the causative organism by separating out the different species present in the specimen.

Micro-organisms are found on every surface of the body as part of the normal flora (see Ch. 3) and they can therefore be isolated from almost any specimen. The microbiologist must be able to identify the organism that is causing infection amongst all the other micro-organisms that normally live at the site or that may have contaminated the specimen. The selection of appropriate tests and interpretation of the results rely on detailed, relevant information about the patient and the symptoms and signs. The specimen must be properly collected, transported and stored to ensure that the results of tests reliably detect the causative micro-organisms.

As well as helping to interpret the results of specimens, the laboratory can provide advice on how the infection should be treated, the type of antibiotic to use and for how long. This advice is provided by clinical microbiologists, doctors who, in addition to their medical qualification, have a specialist knowledge of microbiology. The infection control team can also provide a link between the laboratory and ward staff by helping to interpret results and advising on appropriate action.

Most acute hospitals have a microbiology laboratory on site. These laboratories may also provide a service to other local healthcare facilities such as clinics and nursing homes, as well as general practitioners. Specialist diagnostic and advisory services are provided by the Health Protection Agency in England, National Public Health Service in Wales and Health Protection – Scotland. These can assist in the identification of unusual organisms, bacteria present in food, water or other environmental samples, and advise on outbreaks of infection in hospitals or the community.

IDENTIFICATION OF BACTERIA

Microscopy

Examination of bacterial cells on glass slides under the microscope can reveal some important information about their structure, shape and arrangement. The two main shapes of bacterial cells are round (cocci) or oblong (bacilli or rods) but other bacteria forms include coccobacilli, curved rods (e.g. vibrios) or spirals (e.g. treponema). Some cocci congregate in clumps (staphylococci), whereas the cells of streptococci form into chains. Bacteria are not easy to see under a microscope as they appear colourless. In 1884 Christian Gram developed a method of colouring cells with dyes in a technique now known as the Gram stain. A Gram stain takes only a few minutes to carry out and is used to distinguish two main groups: Gram-positive and Gram-negative organisms. Gram-positive cells absorb a dark blue dye and appear blue under the microscope (Plate 1). Gram-negative cells do not absorb the blue dye but when counterstained with a red dye, they stain pink (Plate 2). Other, more specialized, staining techniques are used in the identification of some bacteria, for example the Ziehl-Neelsen (ZN) or auramine stain which is used to identify mycobacteria.

Microscopy and Gram staining can sometimes be used to provide a provisional identification, particularly where the infection is life threatening. For example, when meningitis is suspected, examination of cerebrospinal fluid under the microscope may enable a provisional diagnosis to be made and appropriate antibiotic therapy to be started immediately (see Plate 3). Fungi can also have a characteristic appearance under the microscope, for example the *Candida albicans* illustrated in Figure 1.13.

However, with some specimens, such as faeces, microscopy is of no value in identifying pathogens since many similar organisms will be present and it is not possible to distinguish between commensals and pathogens. For example, *Escherichia coli* (usually a commensal) and salmonella (a pathogen) are both Gram-negative bacilli.

Whilst the conventional light microscope can establish the shape of bacteria, it cannot distinguish internal structures of the cell. For this, an electron microscope, which uses a stream of electrons instead of light to magnify an image, is required.

Culture methods

Since bacteria cannot be reliably identified by their staining characteristics and morphology under the microscope alone, organisms are grown in a variety of special media and a range of tests are then used to identify them. Culture media commonly include meat or yeast extract, blood (usually horse), peptone, salt and water. Agar, a setting agent extracted from seaweed, is used to solidify the media. Specimens containing bacteria are spread out on an agar plate using a wire loop so that after incubation, single bacteria grow into isolated colonies that can then be selected for further testing (see Plates 4–8).

The concentration of chemicals in the medium can be altered to reflect more closely the environment in which the pathogens are growing or to prevent the growth of the normal flora, making pathogenic species easier to identify. For example, deoxycholate agar is used to isolate shigella from stool specimens as it inhibits the growth of normal faecal flora such as *Escherichia coli*. Bacteria can also be grown in a liquid medium called broth. This type of culture is used to grow large numbers of micro-organisms, especially from specimens such as blood where only a few micro-organisms may be present in the sample.

Bacteria that normally live on, or cause disease in, humans grow best in media that mimic the secretions or tissues of the human body. Some bacteria will grow in very simple media containing very few nutrients; others (fastidious organisms) require complex media to supply most of their growth requirements.

Incubation at around body temperature encourages most pathogenic bacteria to grow rapidly but it can still take between 24 and 48 h before there are enough cells present to enable further testing. Some specimens will be cultured in special oxygen-free cabinets if pathogens are likely to be **anaerobes**, for example swabs taken from infected wounds.

The appearance of colonies

When bacteria are grown on solid media, each bacterial cell will multiply many times and, after several hours, millions of bacteria will be present. The distinct group of cells appears as a colony and can be seen on the agar without a microscope. Their size, colour and shape vary quite markedly between different species of bacteria and an experienced microbiologist can identify some bacteria from the appearance of their colonies on different types of media. Some bacteria such as *Bacillus cereus* (Plate 4) produce characteristically large colonies, whilst others such as staphylococcus are smaller (Plate 5). Enzymes produced by certain bacteria lyse the red blood cells in blood agar, causing clear areas to form around the colonies (Plate 6). Other bacteria produce colonies of characteristic colour such as the green pigment of *Pseudomonas aeruginosa* (Plate 7) or red of *Serratia marcescens* (Plate 8).

Commonly, specimens contain a mixture of different bacteria and the skills of the microbiologist are needed to separate and identify each one (Plate 9). Single colonies are spread out over the surface of agar (Plates 5, 7, 8). They can then be picked off the agar and inoculated into broth to provide a pure culture. Care must be taken to ensure that micro-organisms from the air or environment do not contaminate the specimen and confuse the diagnosis.

Tests to identify the organism

Once the micro-organisms in a specimen have been cultured, further tests, for example their ability to metabolize certain substrates or to produce certain enzymes, e.g coagulase, may have to be conducted to establish the exact species present. On the basis of a Gram stain result, cell shape and sensitivity to oxygen bacteria can be divided into the following groups: Gram positive or negative, cocci or bacilli, and aerobic or anaerobic. This narrows the search for the exact species. Commercially prepared kits are available to further distinguish bacteria by their ability to break down a range of substances. These kits enable a quick and accurate identification to be made. They are

inoculated, incubated overnight and the subsequent colour change in each chamber is used to make the identification (see Plate 10).

Detection of antigens and antibodies

Molecules on the surface of micro-organisms, called antigens, are recognized by the immune system. Usually these are flagella, components of the cell wall or capsules. Specific antibodies will bind to a particular antigen and can be made into standard preparations, called antisera. This type of test can be applied to cerebrospinal fluid to give a rapid diagnosis for a patient with symptoms of meningitis. Laboratories use a range of these known antibody preparations that are specific to antigens on known species of micro-organism. The bacteria to be identified are mixed with the antisera. If they are of corresponding species, the specific antibody will bind to the bacterial cells and this reaction will be apparent as a clumping or agglutination of bacterial cells. Antisera can also be made to detect specific toxins, for example toxins produced by *Corynebacterium diphtheriae*.

Antibodies formed against a particular infecting organism can be detected to diagnose the infection. This can be done by agglutination tests, in which, if the blood contains the antibodies against a specific bacteria, it will cause visible aggregation of suspensions of the organism; immunofluorescence where antihuman globulin is labelled with a fluorescent dye and will attach to antibody recovered from the patient's blood; or enzyme-linked immunosorbent assay (ELISA) (see below).

Sensitivity to antibiotics

It is also important to establish whether different antibiotics have an effect on the organism to ensure that the right antibiotic is selected for treatment of the infection. Antibiotic sensitivity is tested by spreading the organism evenly over the surface of an agar plate, placing small circles of paper impregnated with different antibiotics on to the surface and incubating the plate overnight. The antibiotic diffuses from the paper into the agar and prevents sensitive bacteria from growing in the area around the paper. Bacteria that are not affected by an antibiotic will be able to grow right up to the impregnated paper and hence are resistant to the antibiotic (Fig. 2.1). The sensitivity of an organism to an antibiotic is assessed by comparing the size of the inhibitory zone around the disc with that from a control organism or by the correlation of the zone to the minimum inhibitory concentration (the lowest concentration of the antibiotic which prevents the growth of the micro-organism).

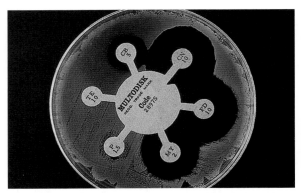

Figure 2.1   Antibiotic sensitivity testing. Antibiotics in each disc diffuse into the agar. Bacteria cannot grow around the discs unless they are resistant to the antibiotic in the disc. (Reproduced with kind permission of Dr D Barrie.)

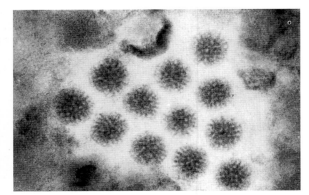

Figure 2.2   Electron micrograph of rotavirus (reproduced by kind permission of Dr D Barrie, Charing Cross and Westminster Medical School, London).

For some antibiotics, in particular vancomycin and aminoglycosides, the concentration of the drug in the blood must be regularly checked to ensure that the levels are therapeutic but not toxic.

Distinguishing microbial strains

Identification of different variants or strains of the same micro-organism can be important in the investigation of outbreaks of infection. The recovery of the same strain from more than one patient or member of staff is an indication that cross-infection has occurred. The tests required to 'type' strains are complex and usually carried out in specialist reference laboratories. A variety of techniques are used, for example susceptibility to bacterial viruses (bacteriophages), production of inhibitory substances or possession of specific antigens. More recently, molecular techniques that can be used directly to compare the nucleic acids of strains have been developed and are now in widespread use.

Identification of fungi and protozoa

The identification of fungi relies mostly on the morphology of colonies and characteristics of cells viewed under the microscope. As they tend to grow slowly, identification may take up to 2 weeks. Biochemical tests are used in the identification of some yeasts.

Protozoa are identified by means of their appearance under the microscope, particularly characteristic stages in their life cycle such as cysts.

IDENTIFICATION OF VIRUSES

There are two different approaches to the identification of viral infections. The first is the culture of virus or direct detection of virus particles by electron microscopy; the second is the detection of specific antibodies in blood by serological testing.

Virus culture

Unlike bacteria, viruses cannot be grown on artificial media but can be cultured only in living cells (i.e. tissue cultures). Sheets of cells are grown in nutrient medium on glass or plastic. Viruses present in clinical specimens grown in the culture will alter the appearance of the cells in a characteristic manner (e.g. herpes simplex). Not all viruses will grow in tissue culture. Some are diagnosed by special staining techniques or by electron microscopy. Provided sufficient viral particles are present, these very powerful microscopes can detect particles as small as $0.0001\ \mu m$ in size (Fig. 2.2). Detection of virus in samples of body fluid can resemble the search for a needle in a haystack and the absence of virus under the electron microscope should not be considered as conclusive evidence of the absence of infection.

Serological tests

Infection by a virus may be followed by the appearance of antibodies to the virus in the blood. The detection of these antibodies is the basis of serological testing and is used extensively to diagnose viral infections. There are several methods of diagnosing viral illnesses based on the same principle of detecting antibodies. The most widely used method is the enzyme-linked immunosorbent assay (ELISA). Antigen specific to the antibody to be detected is placed into small wells on special plates and incubated with serum from the patient. If an antibody specific to the antigen in the well is present in the blood, it will bind to it. Then an enzyme attached to an antibody that recognizes and

Table 2.1   Some methods of identifying viral infections

Infection	Specimen	Test	Viruses
Respiratory tract infection	Throat swab, nasopharyngeal washings	Culture	Influenza, para-influenza, RSV
	Paired sera	Serology	Influenza, para-influenza, RSV, adenovirus, mumps
Vesicular skin lesions	Fluid from lesion	Electron microscopy, culture, serology	Herpes simplex, varicella zoster
Erythematous skin rash	Paired sera	Serology	Measles, rubella
Hepatitis	Serum	Serology	Hepatitis B, hepatitis A
Eye infections	Conjunctival scrapings	Culture	Herpes simplex, adenovirus
Gastroenteritis	Faeces	Electron microscopy	Rotavirus, calicivirus, norovirus

Paired sera = serum from two samples of blood taken 10 days apart. RSV, respiratory syncytial virus.

binds to other antibodies is added and attaches to those wells containing the patient's antibody. This reaction is detected by a colour change caused by the enzyme.

Serum antibodies

Different types of antibody appear in the blood during the course of an infection (see Ch. 4). The type of antibody detected in the blood indicates whether the person has had the infection in the past or is recovering from the infection. This method is used to diagnose several viral infections including rubella and hepatitis. In the case of hepatitis B, identification of the types of antibody present is used to indicate whether infection has persisted and the patient is a chronic carrier of the virus (see Ch. 3). Relating symptoms of an infection to a particular virus is difficult if only one sample of the patient's blood is examined. Antibodies to the virus may already be present as the result of a previous infection. A second sample of blood, taken about 10 days after the first, can be examined to see whether the level of antibodies is greater than in the first sample. If a considerable increase in antibodies is found, this is evidence that the virus is causing the infection. This test is described as 'paired sera'. The different tests used to identify viral infections are summarized in Table 2.1.

Molecular techniques

Specialized techniques are now available which identify micro-organisms by detecting specific nucleotide sequences of DNA or RNA. These methods are sensitive and specific and because they do not require culture of the micro-organisms, they are also safe.

Molecular diagnosis is most valuable for the identification of some viruses. For example, tests that detect hepatitis B virus DNA can be used to determine the stage of infection and infectivity of an affected individual. However, these techniques are also increasingly used in diagnostic bacteriology and to distinguish strains of bacteria in outbreaks of infection (e.g. streptococci).

Electrophoresis

In this method the DNA of the micro-organism is cut into small fragments by restriction endonucleases, enzymes that recognize specific nucleic acid sequences and cleave the DNA at points where these sequences occur. The resulting fragments are separated out on a flat gel, using an electric current which attracts the charged particles and causes small and large fragments to move at different rates. The fragments are then made visible by staining and the pattern of spread is compared to identify related and unrelated strains (Fig. 2.3).

Genetic probes

Specific micro-organisms can be identified using gene probes. These are single-stranded molecules of nucleic acid that are known to correspond to a specific sequence of DNA in a particular organism. If the probe encounters the corresponding DNA sequence, it will bind (or hybridize) with it, indicating that the organism is present in the specimen. Hybridization reactions are detected by marking the gene probe with a radioactive isotope or a compound that gives a colour reaction.

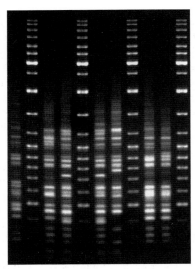

Figure 2.3 Example of an electrophoresis gel. Each column contains DNA from a micro-organism and each band represents a differently sized fragment of DNA. Similar patterns of fragments are used to identify strains or specific micro-organisms.

For example, specific gene probes can be used to detect enterotoxins produced by *Escherichia coli* and *Vibrio cholerae* in faeces or *Mycoplasma pneumoniae* in sputum, without the need to grow the organisms in culture.

Polymerase chain reaction

Gene probes are less likely to provide a reliable result if only a small number of organisms are present in the specimen. In these circumstances another technique, polymerase chain reaction (PCR), can be used. In PCR, two short single strands of nucleic acid (primers) recognize and hybridize with specific complementary sequences of DNA located close to each other on the genome, and then activate DNA polymerase enzymes. Within a few hours these enzymes will have made millions of copies of the specific segment of DNA between the two primers. These segments of DNA can then be detected using gene probes or electrophoresis. This type of amplification enables bacteria to be detected in a specimen when only a few cells are present and can be used to detect just one HIV proviral DNA sequence in a million cells.

Although employed mostly in research, PCR has been used to diagnose a range of infections including those caused by *Helicobacter pylori*, *Legionella pneumophila* and herpes and hepatitis B viruses but is now beginning to become available as a more routine diagnostic tool.

Molecular techniques of the future

The rapid evolution of molecular technologies coupled with a similar evolution in computing technology and mathematics (bioinformatics) will lead to a revolution in the way clinical microbiology laboratories work in the future.

Genomics is the study of an organism's genome, by employing (amongst other methods) nucleotide sequencing. It involves the study of individual genes (or sequences) and matching them to their function. For example, gene sequences that are genus specific and others that are species specific would form the basis of a molecular identification system. On the other hand, sequences that vary within a species would form the basis of a genotyping system; such methods are already very useful in looking at the epidemiology of some infections. An example of such a genotyping method is multiple locus sequence typing (MLST) which is employed in the typing of meningococci.

Other developments include 'microarrays'. This is a very powerful technique in which a number (can be hundreds) of specific gene probes (which may probe, for example, virulence factors, antimicrobial resistance genes, genus-specific and species-specific sequences, etc.) are placed on a single glass slide and can therefore be searched for simultaneously.

Such technology is likely to impact on clinical microbiology laboratories over the next 10–20 years.

THE COLLECTION OF SPECIMENS FOR MICROBIOLOGICAL INVESTIGATION

The quality of the specimen received in the laboratory can have a major impact on the subsequent microbiological diagnosis. The correct methods of collection, transport and storage are therefore an important part of the process. False results may occur if specimens are kept for prolonged periods before examination in the laboratory, as some species may outgrow others and other delicate organisms will not survive. Samples should be taken aseptically to avoid contamination of the material with micro-organisms not causing the infection. In addition, accurate information about the patient's illness and treatment is important for interpretation of the results. In most situations it is important to take specimens before antimicrobial therapy is started, otherwise the organisms causing the infection may be more difficult or impossible to grow. *Exceptions to this are patients with a severe tissue infection requiring immediate surgical debridement* or presumptive meningococcal meningitis.

The following section describes the important principles to be considered when collecting clinical specimens. The laboratory will be able to advise where there is doubt about the type of specimen or investigation required.

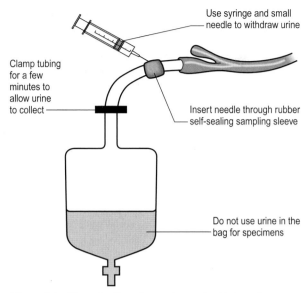

Use syringe and small needle to withdraw urine

Clamp tubing for a few minutes to allow urine to collect

Insert needle through rubber self-sealing sampling sleeve

Do not use urine in the bag for specimens

Figure 2.4   The collection of a specimen of catheter urine.

Urine

Bladder urine should be sterile but is easily contaminated during collection by bacteria that colonize the perineum or distal urethra. Contamination can be reduced by discarding the first few millilitres of urine and collecting the midstream of urine in a sterile container. Cleaning the perineum before the specimen is collected is of questionable value in reducing the risk of contamination (Holliday et al 1991, Pradoni et al 1996).

If the patient has a urinary catheter, the specimen must always be withdrawn from the designated sampling sleeve on the tubing with a sterile needle and syringe (Fig. 2.4). Urine obtained from the catheter bag will provide misleading results as bacteria may have multiplied in the stagnant urine (Bradley et al 1986). The bag must not be disconnected from the catheter to obtain a specimen, as this is likely to introduce bacteria into the system (Platt et al 1983). A urine sample of between 5 and 10 ml is usually sufficient for microbiological examination.

Urine specimens readily support the growth of bacteria and the multiplication of bacteria in specimens stored at room temperature can produce misleading results. The specimen should therefore be examined in the laboratory within 2 h but if refrigerated, can be stored for up to 24 h. The microbiologist investigates the number of white blood cells present in the specimen. Large numbers of white cells suggest that the body is mounting an immune response to infection and help to confirm that an organism present in the

urine is actually causing infection. The number of bacteria present in the urine is calculated by culturing a drop of urine on solid medium. If the patient has a urinary tract infection, the specimen will probably contain at least 100 000 bacterial cells per millilitre and several white cells will be visible on examination under the microscope. In patients with symptoms, e.g. dysuria, bacterial growth as low as 10^2 colony-forming units (cfu) per ml in women (10^3 cfu/ml in men) may be indicative of urinary tract infection (Health Protection Agency 2003a). In children, clean-catch specimens are more difficult to collect. Counts of 10^3 cfu/ml or more of a single species may be indicative of infection but higher counts and the same organism recovered from a repeat specimen are more conclusive. A positive bag urine sample from children may need to be confirmed by a more reliable method such as suprapubic aspirate (Health Protection Agency 2003a). Reagent strip tests are sometimes used to provide a rapid indication of possible infection by detecting blood protein and nitrite in the urine. However, their reliability in detecting infection is questionable (Tincello & Richmond 1998).

In the presence of a catheter, bacteria commonly colonize the bladder but do not necessarily invade the tissue to cause infection. Samples may reflect the organisms in the biofilm lining the catheter (see p. 217) and often several species of bacteria are present in catheter urine. Interpreting the significance of microorganisms grown from catheter urine is therefore difficult and antibiotic treatment is often unnecessary in the absence of clinical signs of infection such as pain or fever (Garibaldi 1993) (see Ch. 10).

Sputum

The lower part of the respiratory tract is normally sterile but the upper respiratory tract, mouth and nose are colonized by large numbers of different bacteria, some of which are able to cause pneumonia. A diagnosis of respiratory tract infection is therefore made by a combination of clinical examination, symptoms, history, chest radiography and microbiological examination of sputum to confirm the diagnosis and identify the causative organism.

Specimens of saliva are of no value, so it is important to ensure that the specimen is mucoid or mucopurulent. The physiotherapist may be able to help a patient who is having difficulty producing a specimen of sputum. Suctioning, using a sputum trap, may be required if the patient is unable to cough. For patients in intensive care units, bronchoscopy may be required to obtain an adequate specimen. Bronchoalveolar lavage (BAL) involves washing a segment of lung with sterile saline via a bronchoscope. This provides a reliable method of diagnosing pneumonia (Health Protection Agency 2003b). Washings can also be taken via the endotracheal tube using a suction catheter. Tracheal aspirate, like sputum, is prone to contamination and is not a reliable indication of pneumonia.

Sputum specimens should be sent to the laboratory immediately as respiratory pathogens will not survive for prolonged periods. If refrigerated for more than 2 h, *Haemophilus influenzae* and *Streptococcus pneumoniae* may die and Gram-negative species overgrow in the specimen (Health Protection Agency 2003c).

The range of micro-organisms causing pneumonia varies according to the patient's underlying condition. For example, Gram-negative bacteria or fungi are more likely pathogens in patients in intensive care or who are immunosuppressed. Adequate clinical details are therefore important to enable the laboratory to select the most appropriate media. The laboratory will examine the specimen for organisms likely to cause respiratory tract infection. If large numbers are present, identification can sometimes be assisted by Gram staining and viewing under the microscope prior to culture (Plate 11).

Tuberculosis

The organism that causes tuberculosis, *Mycobacterium tuberculosis*, grows extremely slowly. Colonies of the bacteria do not appear before a minimum of 1 week of incubation and can take up to 6 weeks. Microscopic examination of sputum is therefore used to make an initial tentative diagnosis of tuberculosis. The numbers of mycobacteria in the sputum may be quite low and to increase the chance of detection, three separate specimens, preferably collected in the early morning, should be examined (Plate 12). Gastric washings may be used to obtain these specimens in children.

Mycobacteria have particularly resistant cell walls; they are stained using a special dye (hot carbol fuchsin) which cannot be removed by acid or alcohol, leading to the term 'acid-fast bacilli' or AFB. This method was used to detect mycobacteria under the microscope but now auramine is commonly used. Atypical mycobacterial infections caused by other species, for example *Mycobacterium avium intracellulare* (MAI), cannot be distinguished from tuberculosis under the microscope and therefore several weeks of incubation are necessary before the species causing the infection can be identified. Commercial kits are now available that enable more rapid identification.

Faeces

There are normally 10^{14} micro-organisms in each gram of faeces. The detection of the bacteria or viruses responsible for diarrhoea or gastroenteritis is therefore not easy as pathogens need to be distinguished from normal flora before identification is possible. Faecal specimens can therefore take the laboratory 3–4 days to process and more than one specimen may be required to eliminate infection as a cause of symptoms.

For *Clostridium difficile,* tests are used to detect the toxin in faeces rather than grow the organism as only the presence of toxin-producing strains is indicative of the disease (see Ch 12).

Viruses that cause gastrointestinal infections cannot be cultured but are detected by examination of faeces under the electron microscope or by using PCR. Faecal specimens are often not automatically examined for viruses; therefore, if infection is suspected as the cause of diarrhoea, two specimens should be sent to the laboratory, one requesting examination for bacteria, the second for viruses.

A walnut-sized sample of faeces, or approximately 15 ml of a liquid stool, is sufficient for microbiological investigation. It should be examined within 12 h, unless faecal parasites are suspected when a fresh, warm stool is required.

Wound swabs

A wound infection is recognized by the presence of clinical signs of infection rather than just the isolation of bacteria from a wound swab. A wide range of bacteria able to cause infection may be grown from a wound swab but many of these organisms may be harmless colonizers of the wound or the surrounding skin. Bacteria isolated from a wound swab should not be considered as infecting the wound unless there is also evidence of an infection in the wound, for example pus, inflammation, erythema or fever. A swab should usually only be taken when the wound exhibits these signs of infection. This is particularly the case in chronic wounds such as pressure sores or ulcers, where wounds may be colonized by several different bacteria with no adverse effect (Gilchrist & Reed 1989).

The most accurate method of identifying micro-organisms causing infection in a wound is by aspiration using a fine needle or biopsy of the underlying tissues (Gilchrist 1996). In practice, these invasive methods are rarely used and the wound swab is the most common means of sampling. If possible, a sample of pus should be collected, either by drawing some up in a sterile syringe and transferring it to a sterile container or, if only a small amount is present, collecting on to a swab. A swab taken from the surface of the wound can also provide useful results but in wounds healing by secondary intention, the surface should first be cleaned with saline to remove traces of occlusive dressing or antibacterial agents (Health Protection Agency 2003d). The swab should be taken directly from the area of

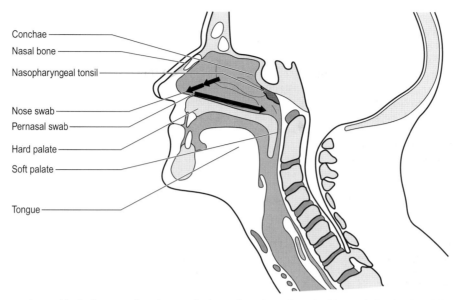

Figure 2.5 Areas to be swabbed when sampling the nose (redrawn from Ayton (1982) with permission of Mark Allen Publishing).

the wound suspected to be infected. Swabs taken from dry areas are unlikely to provide useful results. Most types of swab are accompanied by a tube of transport medium; this will prolong the survival of micro-organisms for several hours and should be refrigerated when immediate transport to the laboratory is not possible. In the laboratory, the swab is spread over an agar plate and the most likely cause of infection is assessed from the type and relative numbers of bacteria present.

It is extremely important to label the wound swab accurately, indicating the exact site from which it has been collected. This helps the laboratory predict the types of micro-organisms to expect in the swab and to identify the site of infection should the patient have more than one wound. However, the difficulty of distinguishing between bacteria infecting or colonizing the wound means that the results of wound swabs should be interpreted with caution (see Ch. 8).

Other swabs

Nose swabs are sometimes necessary to detect carriage of potentially pathogenic bacteria such as antibiotic-resistant strains of *Staphylococcus aureus*. A standard swab can be used but should first be moistened in the transport medium or some sterile saline and then rubbed inside the anterior nares. One swab can be used to sample both nostrils.

Pernasal swab of the nasopharynx is required when whooping cough is suspected and should be taken by

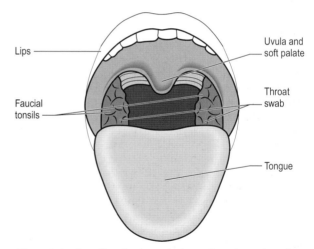

Figure 2.6 Sampling the throat (redrawn from Ayton (1982) with permission of Mark Allen Publishing).

a trained member of staff. The swab is fixed on to a long flexible wire and accompanied by charcoal transport medium (see Fig. 2.5).

Throat swabs should be taken by depressing the tongue and gently rubbing the swab over the pillars of the fauces, especially the inflamed area (see Fig. 2.6). Care should be taken to avoid touching other parts of the mouth which may contaminate the swab with other bacteria. The laboratory will examine the swabs for the presence of known pathogens such as streptococci and the bacilli causing diphtheria.

Swabbing exudate from the eye can be used to identify organisms responsible for 'sticky eye' in babies but conjunctival scrapings are preferred for other infections of the eye (e.g. chlamydia) and these are usually carried out in ophthalmology departments.

Infections of the outer ear can be swabbed carefully, ensuring that the swab is introduced gradually and is not inserted very far. If infection of the inner ear is suspected, a deeper swab is required which should be taken by medical staff using a speculum.

Vaginal swabs should be taken through a vaginal speculum and always sent to the laboratory in transport medium to protect the more fragile pathogens that could be present in the specimen. Investigation for some sexually transmitted diseases requires special transport media.

Occasionally swabs of skin (e.g. groin, axilla) are requested to look for antibiotic-resistant strains of bacteria which may colonize the skin, particularly methicillin-resistant *Staphylococcus aureus* (MRSA) (Ch. 5). Swabs should first be moistened in transport medium or sterile saline solution to improve the efficiency of sampling. MRSA can be isolated by growing the specimen on selective media containing antibiotics that will prevent the growth of sensitive strains of staphylococci. However, this method does not readily distinguish other organisms that are also able to grow on the media, e.g. coagulase-negative staphylococci. A more sensitive method of detecting MRSA is therefore to first place the specimen in nutrient broth for a few hours to increase the numbers of organisms present and then to plate the broth onto selective media. If swabs are being taken for screening to detect any MRSA carriage then several swabs from the same patient can be cultured in the same broth. This enrichment method is recommended for detecting MRSA but takes longer to provide a result (Health Protection Agency 2003e).

Viruses do not survive well on swabs or in samples. To detect viruses in skin lesions, special transport medium, obtained from the laboratory in advance, should be used. The swab should be broken off into the vial and taken to the laboratory as soon as possible.

Skin scrapings for the detection of fungal infections or scabies should be collected by a dermatologist or trained technician.

Blood cultures

Micro-organisms may enter the bloodstream from a focus of infection, e.g. pneumonia, urinary tract or wound infection, from an intravascular device or from the gastrointestinal tract. Transient bloodstream infections may occur in association with invasive procedures, e.g. surgery or urinary catheterization, or localized infections. If accompanied by symptoms such as fever, chills and hypotension, bloodstream infection is termed septicaemia.

Since the number of organisms circulating in the blood may be small (less than 1000 per ml) it is usual to take more than one set of blood samples to improve the chance of detecting a significant pathogen. Blood samples for culture must be taken very carefully to avoid contamination by skin flora and the skin must first be thoroughly cleaned with alcohol. Changing the needle before inoculating the bottles decreases the risk of contamination but increases the risk of needlestick injury (Health Protection Agency 2004a).

Blood is inoculated into two bottles, one which supports the growth of anaerobic bacteria, the other aerobic bacteria. The bottles must be transported to the laboratory rapidly where they will be incubated for at least 7 days but checked daily for signs of growth. Automated monitoring systems are now available. Since bacteria are not normally present in the blood, any growth from the bottle is usually significant. A Gram stain will be performed immediately to provide early evidence of the cause of infection. Some species (e.g. *Staphylococcus epidermidis*) are common skin contaminants but can infect the blood via intravenous devices, particularly in the immunocompromised. The diagnosis of catheter-related bloodstream infections is often difficult and based on specific criteria (see Ch. 9).

Cerebrospinal fluid (CSF)

In suspected meningitis, specimens should be collected by a spinal tap as aseptically as possible. The skin site should be disinfected with an antiseptic solution before the needle is inserted. The specimen should be transported to the laboratory immediately to increase the chance of growing meningococcus, which is extremely fragile. Viral transport medium is not necessary for CSF specimens. Specimens need to be cultured within 10 minutes of receipt by the laboratory as delay may affect the cell count.

The diagnosis of meningitis is based on a number of parameters, for example the differential leucocyte count (in meningitis there is usually a high polymorph to mononuclear leucocyte ratio), micro-organisms seen under Gram stain and organisms grown from culture (Health Protection Agency 2004b). Increased protein and decreased glucose concentrations are also indicative but these tests are usually performed by chemical pathology. PCR is available for the diagnosis of *Neisseria meningitidis*, *Haemophilus influenzae* and *Streptococcus pneumoniae* and can provide a result in 2 h. Since antimicrobial therapy prior to admission to hospital is recommended for suspected invasive meningitis, CSF specimens from patients with meningitis may be culture negative.

Sampling the environment

Bacteria are normally present in the environment on all types of surface and in the air, and usually present no risk to the patient. The results of sampling of the environment are difficult to interpret because the number of bacteria isolated is extremely variable and will depend on the exact area sampled. Little is known about what constitutes an unacceptably high level of contamination.

Routine sampling of equipment to demonstrate sterility is generally unnecessary; instead, the efficiency of the decontamination process itself should be monitored.

Environmental sampling may be of value in outbreaks of infection where an environmental reservoir of infection may be contributing to spread of the organism (Barrie et al 1992, Ravn et al 1991). Water and air quality samples may also be indicated in areas with very vulnerable patients who are susceptible to legionella and aspergillosis (Cooke 2004, Schulster & Chin 2003).

The air quality of operating theatres may sometimes need to be assessed, for example to test the efficacy of the ventilation in newly commissioned theatres. This requires the use of a microbiological air sampler which can measure the number of bacteria per cubic metre of air (Hoffman et al 2002).

BIOHAZARD LABELS

Laboratory staff regularly handle body fluid specimens containing pathogenic organisms and are therefore at particular risk of acquiring infection.

Although laboratories use standard precautions with all specimens, some procedures are particularly hazardous and special precautions that cannot be implemented routinely are therefore recommended where specimens are likely to contain dangerous pathogens. Biohazard labels should be used to indicate, both to staff who transport the specimens and to the laboratory, specimens that may contain particularly hazardous pathogens (Health Services Advisory Committee 1998) (Plate 13). The indication for use of biohazard labels may vary between hospitals but usually they should be applied to specimens known or suspected to contain bloodborne viruses or tuberculosis (Advisory Committee on Dangerous Pathogens 1994). If viral haemorrhagic fever is suspected, special precautions are required in the laboratory and the infection control team must be contacted before specimens are taken (Advisory Committee on Dangerous Pathogens 1996).

TRANSPORT OF SPECIMENS

Potentially infectious material presents a hazard when it is being transported and care must be taken to ensure that risk to other people is kept to a minimum. The Health Services Advisory Committee (1998) recommends procedures for the safe transport of specimens which include carriage in leak-proof boxes and a procedure for dealing with spillages. Specimens to be sent through the post must be specially packaged; advice should be sought from the microbiology laboratory.

The member of staff who collects the specimen has a responsibility to ensure the following:

- the specimen container is leak-proof and securely sealed
- all traces of body fluid have been removed from the outside of the container
- the specimen container is not overfilled
- biohazard labels are placed on the container and accompanying form where appropriate
- the specimen is accompanied by a fully completed request form in a separate pocket
- the container is sealed inside a plastic bag.

INFORMATION ON REQUEST FORMS

The request form provides a very important source of information for the clinical microbiology staff. It assists them in the identification of the causative organism and indicates factors that may influence the tests and methods to be used, and gives important clinical information that indicates the likely significance of micro-organisms grown. The request form should therefore always be completed accurately.

Of particular importance is an accurate indication of the site of the specimen. Some bacteria may form part of the normal flora in one site of the body and yet be pathogenic if isolated elsewhere. Anaerobes may be a likely cause of infection at some sites (e.g. pressure sores) and require special culture techniques. If the patient is receiving antibiotic therapy, antibiotic present in the specimen may inhibit the growth of bacteria in laboratory cultures and produce misleading results. The date and time of specimen collection indicate whether prolonged storage has occurred which may change the number of micro-organisms present. A relevant history, including symptoms of infection, suspected site of infection or recent travel abroad, can assist in the interpretation of the results and will direct the laboratory to perform a relevant range of tests. For example, information on the nature and frequency of vomiting and diarrhoea should accompany a specimen of faeces.

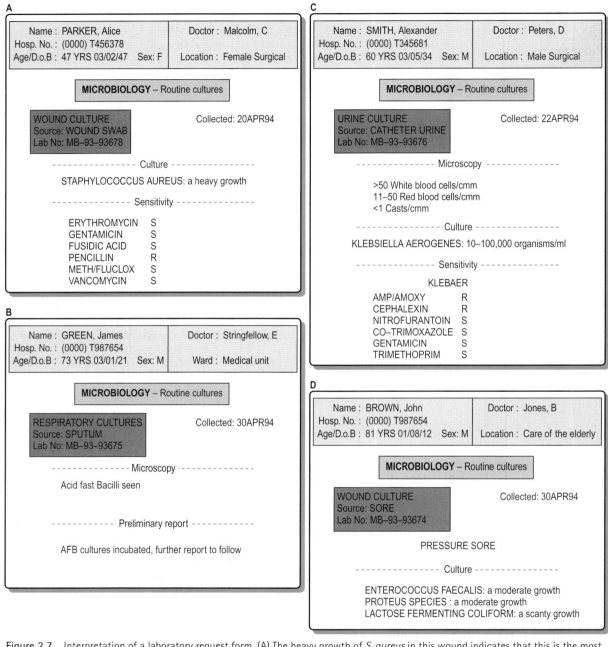

Figure 2.7   Interpretation of a laboratory request form. (A) The heavy growth of *S. aureus* in this wound indicates that this is the most likely cause of infection. In common with most hospital isolates of this organism, it is resistant to penicillin. The exact site of the wound has not been indicated on the request form and this may cause some confusion if the patient has more than one wound. (B) This patient has pulmonary tuberculosis and requires isolation to minimize the risk of cross-infection. Isolation can be discontinued after 2 weeks of treatment; repeat specimens of sputum are not usually necessary. The specimen will now be cultured to determine the species of mycobacterium and antibiotic sensitivities. (C) The presence of klebsiella and a large number of white cells in a specimen of catheter urine is not necessarily unusual. Treatment would be indicated if the patient had signs of infection, for example a pyrexia. The organism is resistant to ampicillin and cephalexin and these antibiotics should not be used to treat the infection. (D) It is not unusual to isolate several different species of bacteria from a chronic wound. Treatment for infection would be indicated only if clinical signs such as pus or inflammation were present.

INTERPRETATION OF LABORATORY REPORTS

The results of a microbiological examination must always be interpreted in combination with a clinical evaluation; without this the microbiological data are often meaningless, i.e. treat the *patient* rather than the results of microbiology tests. Some bacteria isolated from a specimen may be there as part of the normal flora and not be capable of causing infection (e.g. diphtheroids in a wound swab). Sometimes bacteria may be present in a specimen as a result of contamination during its collection but, in the absence of clinical signs of infection, antibiotic treatment is not indicated. For example, *Staphylococcus epidermidis* in a blood culture is often significant but in about 25% of cases organisms from the skin contaminate the blood culture bottle and if the patient is not pyrexial, treatment would not be indicated. Where treatment is indicated, the laboratory report provides information on suitable antibiotics to prescribe. Some examples of laboratory report forms are shown in Figure 2.7.

Advice and information about the interpretation of microbiology laboratory forms can be obtained from the consultant microbiologist.

References

Advisory Committee on Dangerous Pathogens (1994) *Categorisation of Biological Agents According to Hazard and Categories of Containment*, 4th edn. HSE Books, Sudbury.

Advisory Committee on Dangerous Pathogens (1996) *The Management and Control of Viral Haemorrhagic Fevers*. Stationery Office, London.

Barrie D, Wilson JA, Hoffman PN et al (1992) Bacillus cereus, meningitis in two neurosurgical patients: an investigation into the source of the organism. *J. Infect.*, **25**: 291–7.

Bradley C, Babb J, Davies J et al (1986) Taking precautions. *Nursing Times*, **5 March**: 70–3.

Cooke RDP (2004) Hazards of water. *J. Hosp. Infect.*, **57**: 290–3.

Garibaldi RA (1993) Hospital-acquired urinary tract infections. In: Wenzel RP (ed.) *Prevention and Control of Nosocomial Infections*, 2nd edn. Williams and Wilkins, Baltimore.

Gilchrist B (1996) Wound infection. *J. Wound Care*, **5**(8): 386–92.

Gilchrist B, Reed C (1989) The bacteriology of leg ulcers under hydrocolloid dressings. *Br. J. Dermatol.*, **121**: 337–44.

Health Protection Agency (2003a) *Standard Operating Procedure for the Investigation of Urine*. BSOP 41i4. Standards Unit, Evaluations and Standards Laboratory. Health Protection Agency, London. Available online at: www.evaluations-standards.org.uk.

Health Protection Agency (2003b) *Standard Operating Procedure for the Investigation of Bronchoalveolar Lavage and Associated Specimens*. BSOP 3i5.1 Standards Unit, Evaluations and Standards Laboratory. Health Protection Agency, London. Available online at: www.evaluations-standards.org.uk.

Health Protection Agency (2003c) *Standard Operating Procedure for the Investigation of Sputum*. BSOP 8i5.1 Standards Unit, Evaluations and Standards Laboratory. Health Protection Agency, London. Available online at: www.evaluations-standards.org.uk.

Health Protection Agency (2003d) *Investigation of Skin and Superficial Wound Swabs*. BSOP 11i3.1. Standards Unit, Evaluations and Standards Laboratory. Health Protection Agency, London. Available online at: www.evaluations-standards.org.uk.

Health Protection Agency (2003e) *Investigation of Specimens for Screening for MRSA*. BSOP 29i4.1 Standards Unit, Evaluations and Standards Laboratory. Health Protection Agency, London. Available online at: www.evaluations-standards.org.uk.

Health Protection Agency (2004a) *Standard Operating Procedure for the Investigation of Blood Cultures*. BSOP 37i4. Standards Unit, Evaluations and Standards Laboratory. Health Protection Agency, London. Available online at: www.evaluations-standards.org.uk.

Health Protection Agency (2004b) *Standard Operating Procedure for the Investigation of Cerebrospinal Fluid*. BSOP 27i4. Standards Unit, Evaluations and Standards Laboratory. Health Protection Agency, London. Available online at: www.evaluations-standards.org.uk.

Health Services Advisory Committee (1998) *Safe Working and Prevention of Infection in Clinical Laboratories*. Stationery Office, London.

Hoffman PN, Williams J, Stacey A et al (2002) Microbiological commissioning and monitoring of operating theatre suites. A report of a working party of the Hospital Infection Society. *J. Hosp. Infect.*, **52**: 1–28.

Holliday G, Strike PW, Masterton RG (1991) Perineal cleansing and midstream urine specimens in ambulatory women. *J. Hosp. Infect.*, **18**: 71–6.

Platt R, Polk BF, Murdock B, Rosner B (1983) Reduction of mortality associated with nosocomial urinary tract infection. *Lancet*, **i**: 893–7.

Pradoni RNC, Boone MH, Larson E et al (1996) Assessment of urine collection techniques for microbial culture. *Am. J. Infect. Contr.*, **24**: 219–21.

Ravn P, Lundgren JD, Kjaeldgaard et al (1991) Nosocomial outbreak of cryptosporidiosis in AIDS patients. *BMJ*, **302**: 277–80.

Schulster L, Chin RYW (2003) Guidelines for environmental control in healthcare facilities. Recommendations of CDC and the Healthcare Infection Control Practices Advisory Committee. *MMWR*, **52**: RR10.

Tincello DG, Richmond DH (1998) Evaluation of reagent strips in detecting asymptomatic bacteriuria in early pregnancy: prospective case series. *BMJ*, **316**: 435–7.

Further Reading

Mims CA, Playfair JHL, Roitt IM et al (1998) *Medical Microbiology*, 2nd edn. Mosby-Year Book, London.

Chapter 3

The epidemiology of infection and strategies for prevention

INTRODUCTION

The term epidemiology, derived from the Greek, means the study of things that happen to people. It is used to describe the study of disease and ill health in human populations and is particularly concerned with the frequency with which they occur and the factors that influence their distribution.

The interaction between humans and microbes has changed considerably through history. The microbes responsible for the great epidemics of the past have largely been controlled through improvements in living conditions, immunization and chemotherapy. However, many parts of the world have yet to benefit from our ability to understand and control infectious disease, whilst the re-emergence of old diseases such as tuberculosis and the appearance of new diseases such as acquired immune deficiency syndrome (AIDS), variant Creutzfeldt–Jakob disease and severe acute respiratory syndrome (SARS) present new challenges. In terms of infection, knowledge of potential sources of micro-organisms, an understanding of how they spread and what factors determine who may be susceptible to them enables appropriate measures to be taken to minimize the risk of transmission.

This chapter reviews how epidemiology has informed the development of public health services in the UK. It then goes on to explore how micro-organisms are spread from person to person, focusing on epidemiology of healthcare-associated infection: the frequency, distribution and determinants of infections that occur in healthcare settings. Subsequent chapters review the epidemiology of specific healthcare-associated infections in more detail.

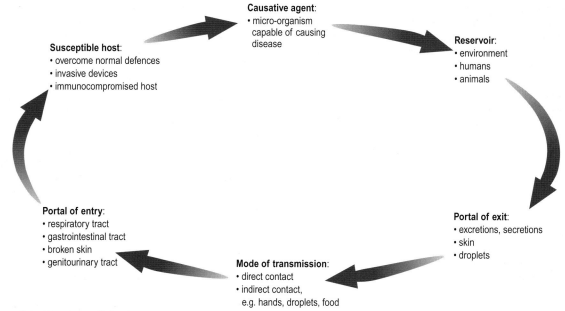

Figure 3.1 The chain of infection.

THE INTERACTION BETWEEN MICROBES AND THEIR HOSTS

The relationship between ourselves and microbes is complex and does not always result in infection. Whether an infection occurs depends on a series of events often referred to as the chain of infection. Micro-organisms capable of causing disease must have a means to transfer from where they are living (their reservoir) and find a route past the normal defences of a susceptible host (Fig. 3.1). A number of factors influence this chain of events. Action to prevent infection is targeted at breaking one or more of the links in the chain.

The surface of the body is densely populated by a wide variety of micro-organisms which use it as their habitat. These micro-organisms are commensals; they live on the host without causing harm and are referred to as the 'normal flora' of the body. The species present at different sites on the body vary according to the local conditions, in particular the availability of nutrients and oxygen and the temperature, pH, and humidity (Table 3.1). In many circumstances, the relationship between micro-organisms and their human host is symbiotic; that is, they both gain advantage from it. The key benefit to the host is that the presence of the normal flora prevents other harmful micro-organisms from occupying the surface. This is particularly important in the intestine. In ruminants, bacteria and protozoa

Table 3.1 The normal flora of body surfaces

Site of body	Common commensal micro–organisms
Skin	*Staphylococcus epidermidis*, streptococci, corynebacterium (diphtheroids), candida
Throat	*Streptococcus viridans*, diphtheroids
Mouth	*Streptococcus viridans*, *Moraxella catarrhalis*, actinomyces, spirochaetes
Respiratory tract	*Streptococcus viridans*, moraxella, diphtheroids, micrococci
Vagina	Lactobacilli, diphtheroids, streptococci, yeasts
Intestines	Bacteroides, anaerobic streptococci, *Clostridium perfringens*, escherichia, klebsiella, proteus, enterococci

living in the stomach are also actively involved in the digestion of cellulose.

Some micro-organisms have a parasitic relationship with their host; they not only use their host as a habitat but actively cause it harm. These harmful effects are recognized as a disease and micro-organisms able to cause disease are known as pathogens. Some pathogens cause a specific and characteristic disease, for example shigella, which causes an acute diarrhoeal illness called dysentery. Other pathogens can cause a wide variety of infections; for example, *Staphylococcus aureus* can infect the skin, causing abscesses, impetigo and wound infection but also causes osteomyelitis, pneumonia and gastroenteritis.

Pathogens account for only a small proportion of the microbial population but are often difficult to define because many species are neither always harmful nor always harmless. Bacteroides, which helps to digest cellulose in ruminants, acts as a harmless commensal in the human gut but can cause infection if it enters damaged tissues following surgery on the bowel. The commensals that make up the normal flora of the body are harmless in their usual habitat but may cause disease if transferred to a different part of the body; for example, *Escherichia coli* from the intestines causes urinary tract infection if it enters the bladder. Disruption of the host's normal barriers against infection, for example the insertion of an invasive device through the skin or a urinary catheter into the bladder, enables micro-organisms to gain access to the body more easily.

Viruses are the ultimate example of a parasite as they are totally dependent on the host for their replication but can also exist in a latent colonizing form. For example, varicella zoster virus remains dormant in nerve ganglia following chickenpox infection and can be reactivated to cause a local disease along the nerve (shingles).

Pathogens may not usually be a commensal of the host but may still inhabit part of the body without causing adverse effects or symptoms of infection. This is described as colonization and the colonized individual is called a carrier. The carriage may be short-lived or may continue indefinitely. In some situations the carrier spreads infection to others. Patients in hospital who are colonized with antibiotic-resistant bacteria provide a source from which the organisms may spread easily to other patients (see p. 106). In extreme examples a carrier can spread infection to many other people; in the late 19th century 'Typhoid Mary', a carrier of *Salmonella typhi*, infected 54 people over a period of 10 years through her employment as a cook.

Host susceptibility

The ability of a pathogen to cause disease is also affected by the susceptibility of the host. To establish infection, the micro-organisms must first be able to resist the defences of the host, such as the gastric acid in the stomach. The susceptibility of the host to infection varies; some individuals may acquire infection through exposure to a smaller dose of the same organisms than others. The number of micro-organisms introduced can also have an important effect on the outcome of the invasion. A few micro-organisms may be easily overpowered by the host defences or may not be able to compete against the normal commensal population, and therefore will be unable to establish infection. Some micro-organisms are able to produce disease even when the infective dose is very low. For example, the ingestion of only a few hundred campylobacter can cause disease as this micro-organism multiplies readily in the gastrointestinal tract. Other gastrointestinal pathogens must be present in high concentration (more than 10^5 per g) in the ingested food to cause infection (e.g. *Clostridium perfringens*). People with impaired immune defences are particularly vulnerable to infection (see Ch. 4). Even commensal micro-organisms may cause infection in people with an impaired immune response. These are known as opportunistic pathogens; an example is *Pneumocystis jiroveci* (formerly *carinii*), a fungus that is a common commensal of the respiratory tract but which causes a severe pneumonia in an immunocompromised host.

Virulence of microbes

The ability of an organism to cause disease is described as virulence. Virulence may depend on a number of factors that assist micro-organisms to invade, multiply and cause damage to tissues. These include fimbriae or slime production, which assist adhesion to surfaces or host cells; extracellular enzymes, which facilitate invasion; capsules that confer protection against the immune system; and toxins that cause tissue damage. Viruses are able to penetrate cells by recognizing and binding to specific molecules on their surface. The genetic information determining these traits may not be carried by all members of a particular species; some strains will therefore be more virulent than others. For example, only strains of *Corynebacterium diphtheriae* able to produce the diphtheria toxin can cause the neurological and cardiac effects associated with the disease.

Signs and symptoms of infection

The adverse effects caused by pathogens invading and multiplying in tissues are recognized as signs and symptoms of infection. These will vary according to the affected site (Table 3.2). If the invading micro-organisms overcome the local immune defences, systemic symptoms such as fever and malaise may develop.

Some pathogens cause a local infection only at the site of invasion, others may spread to more tissues or invade the bloodstream and be carried to other parts

Table 3.2   Symptoms of some common infections

System of the body	Symptoms of infection
Skin	Inflammation Pain Swelling Heat
Respiratory tract	Increased respiratory secretions Cough
Urinary tract	Pain (cystitis) Frequency Urgency
Central nervous system	Confusion Drowsiness Stiff neck Headache
Gastrointestinal tract	Abdominal pain Vomiting Diarrhoea

Box 3.1   Bacterial toxins

Exotoxins

These are proteins secreted by bacteria at the site of infection that may cause adverse effects at other sites if transported in the bloodstream. Some intestinal pathogens release exotoxins called enterotoxins which irritate the mucosal cells, causing profuse diarrhoea. *Clostridium botulinum* produces a powerful neurotoxin which, if ingested even in minute amounts, causes paralysis within hours.

Endotoxins

These are lipopolysaccharides (LPS) which form part of the structure of the outer membrane of Gram-negative bacteria. They are released when the cell is destroyed and can cause serious systemic effects such as high fever, hypotension and coagulation defects. These effects, called septic or endotoxic shock, are associated with bloodstream infections caused by Gram-negative bacteria and often result in the death of the patient.

of the body. For example, infection by *Salmonella typhi* begins with symptoms of gastrointestinal infection but may progress to a systemic illness, associated with high fever, when the bacteria invade the bloodstream. Polio virus enters via the gastrointestinal tract but causes paralysis by infecting and destroying motor neuron cells.

Invading micro-organisms may damage cells through the release of enzymes (e.g. proteases or collagenases) or toxins, substances that have specific adverse effects on tissues (Box 3.1). The toxin may damage tissue at a site remote from the infection. For example, in diphtheria, the infection remains localized in the upper respiratory tract but the toxin released by the organism circulates in the bloodstream and causes serious damage to the heart, nerves and kidneys. The immune response mounted against the infection can also result in damage to the host's own cells, with the affected area becoming inflamed and swollen, and invaded cells being destroyed by phagocytes (see Ch. 4).

SOURCES AND RESERVOIRS OF MICRO-ORGANISMS

Micro-organisms have a reservoir where they live, grow and multiply; this may be in the environment, animals or people (Table 3.3). Viruses, which cannot replicate outside living cells, rely on human or animal reservoirs and survive by passing from one to another. The human body is also the reservoir for many

Table 3.3   Examples of reservoirs of human pathogens

Reservoir	Micro-organism	Disease
Environment		
Soil	*Clostridium tetani*	Tetanus
Water	*Legionella pneumophila*	Legionnaires' disease
Animals		
Cow	*Escherichia coli* (toxigenic strains)	Gastroenteritis
Poultry	Salmonella spp.	Gastroenteritis
Humans		
Respiratory tract	Rhinovirus	Common cold
Gut	Rotavirus	Gastroenteritis

bacteria and fungi that colonize the bowel, skin and respiratory tract. Other micro-organisms, for example clostridium and legionella, normally inhabit the environment in soil, dust or water.

A microbial reservoir can become a source of infection when the micro-organisms have a means of transferring into a susceptible host (see Box 3.2). In clinical settings, environmental reservoirs of micro-organisms are most likely to occur where moisture is present. However, a reservoir does not necessarily become a source of infection. For example, vases of flowers probably contain a variety of potentially pathogenic Gram-negative bacteria but since these bacteria are unlikely to find a way out of the vase and into the patient, the vase is an improbable source of infection. Similarly, the outlet pipes and overflows of washbasins are a reservoir of many micro-organisms, particularly Gram-negative bacilli, but these are usually of low pathogenicity, not readily transferred to susceptible sites on patients, and therefore an unlikely source of infection (Orsi et al 1994).

The most common reservoir and source of micro-organisms in clinical areas are patients themselves, particularly their excretions, secretions and skin lesions. A patient does not need to have an overt infection to act as a source. Transmission may occur during the incubation period before symptoms develop. Even once symptoms have resolved, micro-organisms may continue to be excreted or secreted. Sometimes a person becomes a long-term carrier of the disease. Approximately 10% of people infected by the hepatitis B virus do not completely clear the infection and continue to carry the virus in their blood asymptomatically. *Salmonella typhi* may remain in the gallbladder or kidneys following a gastrointestinal infection and be excreted intermittently in the faeces or urine for months.

Sometimes a person who acquires a micro-organism does not develop infection themselves but acts as a source of infection to other susceptible individuals. This is a common feature of meningococcal disease. Many people carry *Neisseria meningitidis* asymptomatically in their respiratory tract but if it is transferred to a susceptible person, it can invade the tissues and cause meningococcal meningitis or septicaemia. Reservoirs of colonized patients are also an important factor in the spread of infection caused by antibiotic-resistant micro-organisms such as MRSA and glycopeptide-resistant enterococci (see Ch. 5).

If the micro-organisms causing an infection are acquired from another person or the environment, this is described as an exogenous source and the transmission is referred to as cross-infection. For example, streptococcus infecting a leg ulcer may be transferred by the hands of staff to the wound of another patient.

Endogenous or self-infection occurs when a micro-organism colonizing a site on the host enters another site and establishes infection. For example, the Gram-negative bacilli of the intestine are a common cause of wound infection following abdominal surgery or of urinary tract infections in catheterized patients. In practice, it can often be very difficult to determine whether an infection has been acquired endogenously or exogenously.

Identification of the source of a micro-organism can be important during the investigation and control of outbreaks of infection. Once a source has been found, action can be taken to prevent further transmission (see Box 3.3).

ROUTES OF MICROBIAL TRANSMISSION

Some micro-organisms are transmitted readily from person to person and the infections they cause are termed infectious or contagious diseases. The capacity to spread easily may relate to the whole species (for example varicella zoster virus causes an extremely contagious infection) or may be strain specific. For example, some strains of methicillin-resistant *Staphylococcus aureus* (MRSA) have a greater capacity to spread than others, although the reasons for these differences are unclear (Boyce 2002).

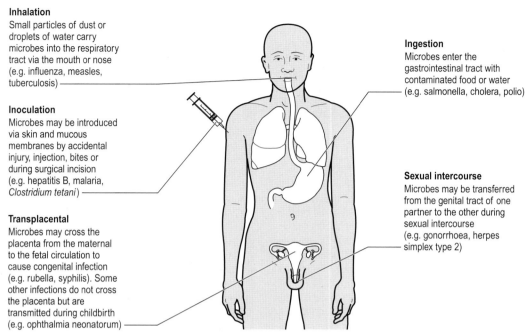

Inhalation
Small particles of dust or droplets of water carry microbes into the respiratory tract via the mouth or nose (e.g. influenza, measles, tuberculosis)

Inoculation
Microbes may be introduced via skin and mucous membranes by accidental injury, injection, bites or during surgical incision (e.g. hepatitis B, malaria, *Clostridium tetani*)

Transplacental
Microbes may cross the placenta from the maternal to the fetal circulation to cause congenital infection (e.g. rubella, syphilis). Some other infections do not cross the placenta but are transmitted during childbirth (e.g. ophthalmia neonatorum)

Ingestion
Microbes enter the gastrointestinal tract with contaminated food or water (e.g. salmonella, cholera, polio)

Sexual intercourse
Microbes may be transferred from the genital tract of one partner to the other during sexual intercourse (e.g. gonorrhoea, herpes simplex type 2)

Figure 3.2   Portals of entry into a human host.

To cause disease, a pathogen must have a way to enter the body – a portal of entry. Once a micro-organism has gained access to the body, it may spread to other tissues and then be expelled by the same or different route – a portal of exit. To transmit to another host, it must be able to leave the body. For example, enteric infections enter via the mouth and leave in the faeces, while micro-organisms that cause respiratory tract infection both enter and are expelled via the mouth and nose (Fig. 3.2). As pathogens leave the body in excretions and secretions, these are important sources of infection.

Micro-organisms use a range of different mechanisms to find new hosts and a particular microbe may be able to spread by using more than one method. For example, chickenpox may be acquired through inhalation of respiratory droplets or contact with fluid from the lesions. However, micro-organisms cannot move themselves from one host to another. They cannot fly or jump but transmit either as a result of direct physical contact or indirectly using another person, animal or inanimate object (fomite). Establishing the source and route of transmission of a particular micro-organism is clearly important if the appropriate control measures are to be instituted. For example, pulmonary tuberculosis is known to be transmitted from an infected person through the inhalation of airborne droplet nuclei expelled from the respiratory

tract. Effective control therefore depends on placing the patient in a well-ventilated room, so that the droplet nuclei are diluted, and prompt treatment of the infection to reduce the number of droplet nuclei expelled from the respiratory tract. Fomites, such as equipment and surfaces, play no part in the transmission of this micro-organism and therefore do not require special control measures.

Transmission by direct contact

Micro-organisms may spread to a susceptible host as a result of direct contact with body surfaces or fluids of an infected individual. There are several examples of this type of transmission. They include infections transmitted from mother to baby in utero (e.g. rubella), sexually transmitted diseases such as *Neisseria gonorrhoeae*, and infections transmitted by direct contact with respiratory secretions, for example by kissing (e.g. glandular fever and respiratory viruses). Some infections, such as *Clostridium tetani*, may be acquired directly from the environment if contaminated material is inoculated through the skin.

Transmission by indirect contact

Many micro-organisms are transferred from their reservoirs to a new host indirectly on people, animals or inanimate objects. In clinical settings, indirect transmission may involve vehicles such as hands, equipment, food and water, or airborne particles. Common-source transmission is where the same infection is acquired by several people following exposure to the same contaminated item, such as food, water or equipment. Indirect transmission by vectors (insects or animals) also occurs but is an unusual mode of transmission in hospitals.

Hands

The first clear indication of the important role that hands play in the transmission of infection emanated from the work of Semmelweis in the 1850s. Semmelweis noticed that puerperal fever was more common on the maternity ward where the medical students worked than on the ward where midwives provided care. He thought that the medical students might be transferring the disease on their hands from cadavers they were dissecting and ordered that they must wash their hands in chlorinated lime after dissection and before examining patients. This simple measure resulted in a dramatic reduction in the rates of infection and mortality. Later, he ordered that hands should be washed between examinations of all patients to prevent cross-infection within wards (Newsom 1993).

Unfortunately, until the late 1960s, the significance of hands as vectors of hospital-acquired infection was not fully appreciated and airborne transmission was considered more important. This view was changed by a study published in 1966 (Mortimer et al 1966) in which babies in the same nursery were divided into two groups attended by different staff. Although both groups occupied the same room, transmission of staphylococci occurred mostly between babies in the same group. When hands were not washed after handling the babies, the rate of transmission was even greater. The results strongly implicated hands as the main vector of infection whilst illustrating that air was not a significant route of transmission.

Microbes acquired on hands through contact with excretions, secretions or infected lesions are readily transferred to another host by touch (Mackintosh & Hoffman 1984). This type of contact is probably responsible for the transmission of a large number of infections, particularly among hospital patients where healthcare workers have frequent and intimate contact with secretions and excretions of patients (Larson 1988, Pittet et al 1999, Reybrouck 1983, Sanderson & Weissler 1992). Most micro-organisms acquired on the hands are not able to survive for long and are usually transferred rapidly to the next object or patient that is touched. However, some species including antibiotic-resistant bacteria have been found to survive for

prolonged periods, providing plenty of opportunity for them to be transferred to another patient (Musa et al 1990). See Chapter 7 for more information about interrupting the spread of infection via hands.

Food or water

Some bacteria, viruses and protozoa may be transmitted by food or water. Many foods are contaminated by pathogens in their raw state and, if these are not destroyed by thorough cooking, will cause infection when the food is eaten. Food may also be indirectly contaminated by hands in what is described as a faecal–oral route of transmission. The microbe is ingested, causes gastrointestinal infection and is excreted in faeces. Transmission to another host occurs when the infected person contaminates his or her hands with micro-organisms in their faeces, and the hands transfer the organism to food which is then ingested by someone else. Food that is cooked, handled prior to ingestion and then eaten cold, such as cold meats, desserts, sandwiches, salads, etc., may easily be contaminated by a food-handler with poor hand hygiene and could then transmit infection as the organism will not be destroyed by further cooking. Food that is cooked after handling is less likely to transmit infection because the organisms will be destroyed unless the inoculum is extremely large and the food not cooked thoroughly.

Water may be readily contaminated by faecal pathogens and must be filtered and treated with chemicals to ensure that it does not transmit infection. Common waterborne infections include *Vibrio cholerae* (the bacterium that causes cholera), giardia and cryptosporidium. Gastrointestinal viruses such as norovirus can contaminate shellfish grown near to sewage outlets.

In hospitals, hydrotherapy pools or other treatment baths may transmit infection if water filtration or chlorination is inadequate. The presence of agitation channels that are difficult to disinfect is a particular hazard (Hollyoak et al 1995). The risk is particularly great where patients using the pool are faecally incontinent or have infected wounds, as the warm water will encourage the growth of micro-organisms contaminating the water.

Airborne particles

Contrary to popular belief, microbes cannot travel through the air on their own but may be carried on airborne particles, such as dust, water or respiratory droplets.

Dust   Dust is largely composed of skin squames and lint fibres released from clothing and other fabrics. Skin squames are flat flakes of dead skin about 10–20 µm in diameter, which are shed from the surface of the skin into the air at a rate of about 300 million per day. The rate of release is particularly high during movement, when 10^4 skin squames may be shed from one person in a minute (Hambraeus 1988). About 10% of these squames carry micro-organisms. The larger particles of dust settle within a few minutes onto exposed horizontal surfaces such as the floor, furniture and equipment (see below). Small particles may remain airborne for several hours and microbes carried on them may be inhaled into the respiratory tract or settle into wounds.

Some species of fungus release spores into the air, which can remain airborne for prolonged periods and gain access to buildings from the outside. Whilst most of these fungal spores are not harmful to humans, aspergillus can cause serious infection if inhaled by immunocompromised patients (Manuel & Kibbler 1998) (see pp. 51,133).

The main significance of airborne dust particles is in the operating department where there is a strong correlation between the numbers of airborne particles and the number of personnel in the operating room. Pathogens carried on these particles may settle into the wound or onto surgical instruments and subsequently cause wound infection (Howarth 1985, Whyte et al 1982). Barrie et al (1992) reported an outbreak of surgical wound infection caused by *Bacillus cereus*, where this spore-forming bacterium probably entered surgical wounds on airborne lint particles released from contaminated scrub-suits. In wards, activities such as bed making can increase the number of bacteria carried in the air, although they will settle rapidly onto surfaces (Overton 1988).

Respiratory droplets   Droplets of saliva are expelled from the respiratory tract by coughing, sneezing and talking. These droplets may contain a small number of pathogenic organisms from the respiratory tract. The large droplets (more than 0.1 mm in diameter) fall to the ground within a few seconds and are not inhaled. Small droplets (less than 0.1 mm in diameter) evaporate rapidly to a size of between 1 and 10 µm in diameter. These very small particles, called droplet nuclei, can remain airborne for hours and be inhaled in the same way as small dust particles and carried deep into the alveoli of the lungs.

Although some infections are transmitted by respiratory particles in the air, most notably *Mycobacterium tuberculosis* (Riley et al 1959), the probability of inhaling particles carrying pathogenic organisms is quite low. Many respiratory infections are more commonly transmitted through contact with respiratory secretions, for example on tissues, handkerchiefs and hands (Goldmann 2000). Pathogens in droplets expelled onto the hand that covers the sneezer's mouth will be readily passed on to others unless they are removed by handwashing.

Water droplets   The inhalation of aerosols of contaminated water may also transmit infection. The bacterium *Legionella pneumophila* commonly colonizes static water and is responsible for the respiratory infection Legionnaires' disease (see pp. 130, 238). Infection is acquired through inhalation of aerosols generated from contaminated water sources by fountains, whirlpools, showers or air-conditioning systems (Bartlett et al 1986).

Inanimate objects and the environment

Inanimate objects that become contaminated with pathogenic bacteria and then spread infection to others are often referred to as fomites. These objects include beds, curtains, bedclothes, toys, bedpans and sphygmomanometers. Most micro-organisms are not able to survive in the absence of moisture, warmth and nutrients and unless they are able to multiply on the fomite, the numbers present are unlikely to be sufficient to transmit infection in most situations (Devine et al 2001).

Provided that equipment is kept clean and dry, bacteria will not be able to multiply and their presence on surfaces will be transitory. Occasionally, outbreaks of infection associated with inadequate decontamination of fomites, such as linen, have been reported (Barrie et al 1994). Hands may acquire micro-organisms when handling heavily contaminated fomites, for example during bed making or through handling used linen or equipment in the sluice (Sanderson & Weissler 1992).

Most outbreaks of infection associated with inanimate objects are caused by items that should be sterile but have been inadequately decontaminated. Instruments that enter sterile parts of the body or are in close contact with mucous membranes present particular cross-infection hazards.

Wet environments present a particular hazard. Some bacteria, particularly pseudomonas, acinetobacter and other Gram-negative bacilli, are able to survive and multiply easily in moisture, which may become a source of infection (see Box 3.4). Equipment that is filled with fluid, for example humidifiers, bowls of disinfectant or wash bowls, is particularly prone to contamination (Gormon et al 1993, Greaves 1985). Again it is important to distinguish between sources and reservoirs. Many bacteria may be found in a washbasin but are unlikely to be transferred to a patient, whereas bacteria contaminating a nebulizer chamber

Box 3.4 The problem with mattresses ...

Despite strict isolation precautions, infections caused by an antibiotic-resistant strain of acinetobacter continued to colonize and infect patients on the burns and intensive care units. Whilst investigating the source of this organism, it was noticed that one patient's bedlinen was wet, yet she was not incontinent or perspiring and there was no leakage from her burns. When the linen was removed, a badly stained mattress cover was revealed and inside it the mattress was found to be wet. Further investigation found 23 mattresses with stained covers and all stained parts were no longer impermeable to fluid. Bacteria were isolated from inside 15 mattresses and the resistant strain of acinetobacter was found in nine. The damage to the mattress covers may have been related to the use of phenolic disinfectants to clean the mattress cover and silver nitrate applied to burns. No further cases of the resistant acinetobacter occurred once the stained mattresses had been replaced, a regular system of mattress inspection implemented and the use of phenolic agents to clean mattresses discontinued (Loomes 1988).

are highly likely to be inhaled into the respiratory tract of the patient.

There is little evidence to suggest that the environment plays a major role in the transmission of healthcare-associated infection. Maki et al (1982) studied the effect of transferring a whole hospital into a new facility. Despite much lower levels of microbial contamination on surfaces in the new building, the incidence of hospital-acquired infection remained unchanged.

Some micro-organisms do persist for prolonged periods on surfaces and a heavily contaminated environment may contribute to the spread of infection when they are acquired on the hands of staff (Boyce et al 1997). If dust that settles onto horizontal surfaces is allowed to accumulate, it can harbour micro-organisms and this may contribute to their spread between patients (Rampling et al 2001). Bacteria that form spores may survive for many months. The spores of *Clostridium difficile* are released from the faeces of infected patients who have diarrhoea and can contaminate surfaces or equipment such as commodes. However, although correlation between environmental contamination and cases of *Clostridium difficile* has been reported, it is difficult to establish whether this is a cause of, or an effect of, the infection (National *Clostridium difficile* Standards Group 2004).

In outbreaks of infection it is usually difficult to establish if micro-organisms recovered from the environment have played a role in transmission or are there as a result of contamination from the affected patients. Although outbreaks are commonly reported to have been terminated in association with extensive decontamination of the environment, usually this occurs as part of a range of other measures and the specific role of the environment cannot be determined. An important exception are some respiratory and gastrointestinal viruses, where contamination of the environment has been strongly implicated in transmission and may occur as a result of touching the mouth or nose after handling contaminated objects (Green et al 1998).

Animal and insect vectors

Some micro-organisms are spread by animal or insect vectors. Cockroaches, ants, rats or mice are often blamed for transmission of infection by carrying pathogens on the surface of their bodies but there is little evidence to substantiate such claims. The main significance of these pests is in food preparation areas where severe infestation may result in the contamination of food with enteric pathogens.

Other animals and insects act as a reservoir for human pathogens and transmit disease by bites. For example, rickettsia, which causes typhus, is carried by lice (human and rat lice) and transmitted by their bites. Malaria (a protozoon) and yellow fever (a virus) are transmitted by the bite of mosquitoes. In some cases humans act as a host for part of the life cycle of an animal (e.g. parasitic worms).

EPIDEMIC AND ENDEMIC INFECTION

Within a population, a disease can be *endemic* (i.e. it is always present at a static level) or *epidemic* (i.e. a definite increase in the incidence of the disease above its normal or endemic level). The rapidity and extent to which a particular disease spreads are dependent on its transmissibility. This is often described as a 'reproductive number'; that is, the average number of secondary cases of infection generated by one primary case. A reproductive number that is greater than 1 means that each primary case will generate at least one secondary case and an epidemic may result. Highly transmissible organisms will have a large reproductive number. In healthcare settings, the reproductive number of a particular pathogen will be affected by both its ability to transmit and the frequency with which transmission opportunities occur, for example the number of contacts between staff and patients (Bonten et al 2001).

A typical epidemic curve shows a gradual increase in the number of infections until all the susceptible individuals have become infected, followed by a fairly rapid decline in new cases of infection (Fig. 3.3A). Some epidemics occur every few years, for example whooping cough and measles. Children who are not immune through previous exposure or vaccination may acquire the infection. When all susceptible children have been infected, the number of new cases falls. Three to five years later there will be another increase in infections among the new population of non-immune children.

Other infections are associated with seasonal epidemics, for example influenza, rotavirus and chickenpox (Fig. 3.3B). Infections that induce long-term immunity usually cause epidemics amongst the very young or elderly who have either not been previously exposed or have a diminished immunity.

Epidemics of infection associated with a single exposure to infection (e.g. food poisoning) present with a sudden rise in the number of infections followed by a rapid fall. If the infection can be transmitted to others from infected individuals during the incubation period, then a second epidemic due to cross-infection may follow shortly after the first (Fig. 3.3C).

Measuring the occurrence of disease

Two measures are commonly used to represent the occurrence of a disease within a population. A prevalence rate measures the number of infections present in a particular population at a particular time; for example, 'the number of patients who have an infection on a particular ward on a specific day expressed as a percentage of the total number of patients on the ward on that day'. An incidence rate measures the number of new infections that occur in a particular population over a specified period of time; for example, 'the number of patients who develop surgical wound infections during the year expressed as a percentage of the total number of operations performed during the same time'. Sometimes it is necessary to take account of the period of exposure to a particular risk. For example, the rate of bloodstream infections associated with intravenous devices may be expressed as the number of infections per 100 days of device use (see Box 3.5).

INFECTION PREVENTION AND CONTROL – A HISTORICAL PERSPECTIVE

The principles of epidemiology were first recognized in the time of Hippocrates, 300 BC. In Britain, the first form of record keeping began in the early 16th century with the introduction of 'Bills of Mortality' which provided information on deaths and disease. Epidemics of disease such as plague, typhus, smallpox

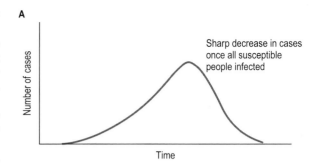

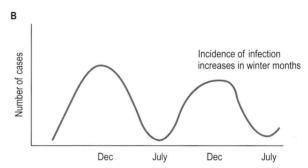

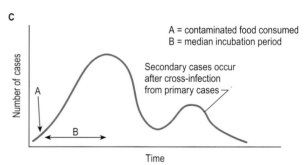

Figure 3.3 Epidemic curves. (A) Classic epidemic curve. (B) Seasonal epidemic. (C) Single-point epidemic of food poisoning with secondary spread by cross-infection.

and syphilis were commonplace in the Middle Ages and although attempts were made to control spread through quarantine, the widespread belief that diseases were punishment from God prevailed for hundreds of years.

Giralamo Fracastoro, who published *De Contagione* in 1546, realized that disease could be transmitted by contact with sick people, their bedding and excreta or through the air. The connection between contagious disease and the bacteria first seen under van Leeuwenhoek's microscope was not universally accepted until Louis Pasteur and Robert Koch began the study of micro-organisms in the late 19th century. These two scientists had to overturn the widespread

Box 3.5   Prevalence and incidence of infection

Prevalence rate
This measures the number of people in a population who have the disease or infection at a given time.

Incidence rate
This measures the number of new cases of a disease or infection that occur in a population over a specified period of time. It can be expressed as a risk (the proportion of people who develop one or more infections) or a ratio (the number of infections that occur within the given population). The ratio takes into account the fact that the same person may develop the infection more than once.

Relationship between prevalence and incidence
The prevalence rate depends on the incidence of the disease and duration of illness. Chronic diseases are more likely to be detected at a given point in time and their prevalence will therefore be relatively larger than the incidence within a given population.

and strongly held belief in 'evil humours' released by decomposing matter and dirt as the cause of disease.

Pasteur was able to prove that fermentation was initiated by microbes and that cultures of anthrax bacillus would cause the disease in sheep. Koch demonstrated that microbes were responsible for anthrax and tuberculosis. He isolated the microbes from infected tissue, cultured them outside the body, reinfected another animal with the culture and finally recovered the same microbes from the animal. Once the link between micro-organisms and human disease was established, other workers studied immunization as a method of protection against infection and the use of antimicrobial drugs to kill microbes without harming the host.

The public health reform acts

The progress made in the understanding of microbiology had an enormous effect on the control of infectious disease but of parallel importance was the revolution in public health that took place in the second half of the 19th century. The Industrial Revolution of the 1800s brought with it rapid development of towns, which were built with no provision for water supply or sewage drainage. These newly industrialized towns, with overcrowded, squalid conditions and sewage and rotting carcasses filling the streets, were associated with frequent epidemics of disease, particularly typhus, typhoid fever, cholera, smallpox, scarlet fever and

measles. Infant mortality of 200 deaths per 1000 births was recorded in some places.

The cholera epidemic of 1831, which killed 60 000 people in Britain, mostly those living in poor and densely populated areas, resulted in demands for action to improve the living conditions of the poor. The Poor Law Commission was established in 1832 to consider how the Poor Laws should be amended. Edwin Chadwick, a barrister, was appointed Secretary to the Poor Law Commissioners. His report in 1842 on 'The sanitary condition of the labouring population of Great Britain' highlighted the problems of inadequate sewage disposal, pointed to contaminated water as a cause of disease and suggested that a network of earthenware pipes, flushed with running water, should be used to drain sewage away. It also recommended the removal of refuse, improvement of water supplies and street cleansing. This report had an immense impact, although it was some years before the Act for Promoting Public Health was passed in 1848, in response. This Act established the role of district medical officers responsible for initiating sanitary improvements and inspectors to monitor their implementation.

Unfortunately, the provisions in this first Public Health Act were not obligatory and it was not until Gladstone became Prime Minister that a national public health service was created by parliamentary Acts in 1872 and 1875. These Acts resulted in the appointment of medical officers for health (MOH) in each local authority. The MOH was responsible for all aspects of public health including sewage disposal, water supply, food hygiene, infectious disease control, child welfare, maternity and venereal disease clinics, the school medical service and, until the formation of the National Health Service (NHS) in 1948, the municipal hospitals.

The compulsory registration of births and deaths, enacted in 1836, enabled accurate data to be produced on which decisions about public health issues could be made. Between 1840 and 1900, the death rate in Britain fell from 25 to 15 per 1000 and life expectancy increased from 40 to 50 years. By the end of the 19th century the combined effects of improved standards of hygiene, nutrition, drinking water supply and sewage control virtually eliminated the threat of epidemic disease in developed countries.

Today, vaccination is widely used to control the spread of many infectious diseases but different challenges in disease control develop as a result of changes in lifestyles. For example, the increase in sexual freedom has been associated with a rise in sexually transmitted diseases and the emergence of human immunodeficiency virus. The course of the epidemic of severe acute respiratory syndrome (SARS) in the spring of 2003 was strongly influenced by patterns of international travel (WHO 2003).

The public health service of today

In the 1970s, the NHS was restructured and many of the community health services previously under the control of the local authority moved to the newly formed district health authorities (DHAs). Monitoring of environmental services such as water and sewage supply, food hygiene and housing remained with the local authorities within environmental health departments. The old public health inspectors became environmental health officers (EHOs). The EHOs also retained responsibility for the control of communicable disease and food poisoning within the community. The office of MOH was replaced by a medical officer for environmental health (MOEH) employed by the health authorities. The medical specialty of community medicine was established to train doctors in all aspects of public health and the planning of health services.

In 1988, the monitoring of disease and the investigation of outbreaks of infection became the responsibility of the health authorities (health boards in Scotland). Health authorities appointed directors of public health (DPH) to advise them, the local authority and the general public on issues related to public health. The DPH would also be closely involved in drawing up health improvement programmes for local communities and in the planning and development of local services. These developments reflected the increasing realization that the social and physical environment in which people live powerfully influences health. Measures to prevent disease, including the spread of infectious disease, therefore need to address the wider determinants of health (Acheson 1998).

In practice, while responsibility for the prevention and control of infectious disease lay with the HA, the day-to-day management was undertaken by a consultant in communicable disease control (CCDC) (consultant in public health medicine, communicable disease and environmental health in Scotland). The CCDC liaises between the EHOs of the local authority, who have responsibility for food hygiene and pollution control within the local area, and the health authority. They are also designated as 'the Proper Officer' to whom cases of infectious disease must be notified (NHS Management Executive 1993).

In 2001, the organization of local and regional NHS structures changed (DoH 2001). The responsibility for developing and commissioning NHS services moved from the DHAs to primary care trusts (PCTs). The old NHS regional offices and health authorities were replaced by strategic health authorities (SHAs) with responsibility for supporting and monitoring local services. Leadership for public health is now located with DPHs at both PCT and SHA level.

The CCDCs, although mostly based in PCTs, have now become part of the Local and Regional Services (LARS) division of the Health Protection Agency and have a remit that includes protection of the public against a range of environmental hazards, e.g. radiological, chemical, and not just communicable diseases (DoH 2002).

Notification of infectious disease

A system of recording cases of infectious disease was recognized as an essential part of the control of epidemics in the early 1900s. Local authorities have a statutory responsibility to control infectious diseases within their boundaries and to facilitate this, some diseases must be notified to the Proper Officer, usually by the doctor who makes the diagnosis. Box 3.6 shows the infectious diseases that are notifiable in England and Wales, and in Scotland.

There are several reasons why notifications of infectious disease are necessary. First, close family or other contacts may have been exposed to the infection and require treatment or monitoring for signs of infection (e.g. tuberculosis, meningococcal meningitis). Second, the infection may have been acquired from contaminated food or water which necessitates investigation to identify the source of infection (e.g. food poisoning). Finally, the information is analysed and used at both local and national level to monitor fluctuations in the levels of infection and the effect of vaccination programmes, to detect epidemics at an early stage and to inform the planning of preventive programmes.

The Health Protection Agency

This organization was formed in April 2004, subsuming the functions of the Public Health Laboratory Service, Centre for Applied Microbiology and Research (CAMR), the National Radiological Protection Board (NRPB), the National Poisons Information Service and the National Focus for Chemical Incidents. It operates in England and Wales, although it also provides some specialist services for Scotland and Northern Ireland and some other services are provided independently in these countries. Its role is to provide key services and support to the NHS and other organizations to protect people's health from infectious diseases and other environmental hazards such as radiation or chemicals. It operates at a local, regional and national

Box 3.6   Notifiable diseases

Public Health (Control of Diseases) Act 1984
Cholera
Food poisoning
Plague
Relapsing fever
Smallpox
Typhus

Public Health (Infectious Diseases) Regulations 1988

Acute encephalitis	Ophthalmia neonatorum
Acute poliomyelitis	Paratyphoid fever
Anthrax	Rabies
Diphtheria	Rubella
Dysentery	Scarlet fever
Leprosy	Tetanus
Leptospirosis	Tuberculosis
Malaria	Typhoid fever
Measles	Viral haemorrhagic fever
Meningitis	Viral hepatitis
Meningococcal	Whooping cough
septicaemia	Yellow fever
Mumps	

Additional diseases notifiable in Scotland

Chickenpox	*Foodborne infections*
Erysipelas	Botulism
Legionellosis	Brucellosis
Lyme disease	Campylobacter
Membranous croup	Cryptosporidiosis
Puerperal fever	*Escherichia coli* 0157
Toxoplasmosis	Giardiasis
	Listeriosis
	Q fever
	Rotavirus
	Salmonellosis
	Yersiniosis

Local authorities have the power to add to, or subtract from, this list in order to prevent the spread of infectious diseases. AIDS is not a notifiable disease but doctors are asked to report cases to a voluntary, confidential scheme at the Health Protection Agency. Sexually transmitted diseases are reported anonymously by genitourinary clinics to the Department of Health.

level, providing advice and information to the public, professionals and government.

Local services are provided by CCDCs and their teams who develop policy in relation to disease control and respond to outbreaks of infection in the community. At a regional level there are epidemiology units and regional microbiologists. A regional microbiology laboratory supports the CCDCs and undertakes specialist public health work, for example processing food, water or other environmental specimens. At a national level, the Centre for Infections in London includes reference laboratories, which undertake specialist testing of micro-organisms to identify and type them, and epidemiological services which establish and manage surveillance systems for a range of infections, and analyse and disseminate data on communicable diseases. Data on the incidence of infectious diseases are published weekly in the *Communicable Disease Report*. Advice and information about infectious diseases are available from the Health Protection Agency website: www.hpa.org.uk.

In Scotland, a new organization, Health Protection Scotland (HPS), was formed in November 2004. HPS's aim is 'to work in partnership with others to protect the Scottish public from being exposed to hazards which damage their health and to limit any impact on health when such exposures cannot be avoided'. HPS was formed from the established Scottish Centre for Infection and Environmental Health (SCIEH). HPS's functions include co-ordinating national health protection activity, monitoring the quality and effectiveness of health protection services and publishing data on the incidence of infection. Information about HPS is available on the website: www.hps.scot.nhs.uk.

In Wales, microbiology and infectious disease surveillance services for public health are provided by the National Public Health Service (NPHS) – Wales. Further information is available on the website: www.wales.nhs.uk.

INFECTION ASSOCIATED WITH HEALTHCARE

A nosocomial or healthcare-associated infection (HCAI) is any infection that develops as a result of healthcare, from which the patient was not suffering or incubating at the time of admission to hospital. Rather than the infectious diseases commonly encountered in the community, most HCAI are caused by pathogens that take advantage of vulnerable patients whose normal defences against infection have been breached.

The risks of infection associated with hospitalization have been recognized for thousands of years. Before the development of effective antimicrobial agents, the mortality rate due to infection following surgical intervention was extremely high. Advances in technology have enabled many patients with previously fatal conditions to be treated but the use of invasive devices and immunosuppressive therapy increases their vulnerability to infection. At the same time, an increasing number of healthcare interventions can now be provided in the community rather than in hospitals, e.g. dialysis, intravenous nutritional support, and early discharge from hospital is now the norm. This means that hospitals contain a higher proportion of seriously ill patients who are most at risk of acquiring infection and some patients receiving healthcare in their own home are also vulnerable to infections previously only associated with hospitalization.

In addition, strains of bacteria highly resistant to antimicrobial agents are encouraged to emerge in a hospital environment where there is heavy use of antimicrobials. The infections they cause can be extremely difficult to treat and preventing their transmission is of paramount importance. Occasionally epidemics of HCAI occur as a result of a breakdown of infection control procedures or spread from a patient with an infectious disease.

Preventing infections in vulnerable patients and controlling their spread therefore presents particular challenges for healthcare workers.

Historical perspective of healthcare–associated infection

Hospitals for the sick existed in the civilized world as early as 500 BC, in particular in Asia, Egypt, Palestine and Greece. The standards of hygiene in these early hospitals were based on religious rituals and were far superior to those found in the hospitals of later centuries. Patients were generally housed in separate beds or rooms, good ventilation was considered essential and many of the rudiments of infection control were practised, such as not touching wounds, isolation of infected patients and use of cleaning and hot ovens to 'sterilize' instruments (Selwyn 1991).

Unfortunately, after the fall of the Roman Empire, standards deteriorated because of the influence of Christianity, which was associated with an aversion to washing and an absence of laws on hygiene. Severe overcrowding, with several patients sharing one bed, and poor ventilation were features of hospitals until the late 19th century and it is therefore not surprising that the mortality rate due to infection was extremely high and death rates from postoperative infection of more than 50% were frequently reported.

John Simpson, Professor of Medicine and Midwifery at Edinburgh University and an early advocate of infection control measures, made a detailed study of the epidemiology and prevention of 'surgical fever'. He observed a significantly higher rate of infection amongst patients operated on in hospital than in those operated on by a country surgeon (Simpson 1869).

Various attempts over the centuries to implement simple infection control measures met with considerable opposition. Many doctors recommended cleanliness of clothes, hands and dressings but surgeons preferred to blame 'intrinsic defects' in the patient or the 'atmosphere'. An increasing understanding of bacteria, asepsis and transmission of disease, combined with improvements in hospital conditions introduced by Florence Nightingale, finally brought HCAI under some control by the end of the 19th century (Nightingale 1863). In the 1940s, further reductions in the incidence of HCAI were associated with the emergence of antimicrobial drugs as effective treatments for infection.

In the early 20th century, streptococcus was the main problem of cross-infection. Later, in the 1950s, this was replaced by staphylococci, already resistant to a number of antibiotics. The HCAI problems of today reflect the nature of the hospital population: highly susceptible patients who in the past would have died from their illness and extensive use of invasive procedures, each with an attendant risk of infection.

The development of an organized structure within hospitals to prevent and control infection began in the 1940s with the appointment of part-time control of infection officers and the formation of infection control committees. In 1959 the first infection control nurse was appointed to provide a full-time infection control service. The increasing complexity of medical care, the cost of HCAI and the adverse effects of outbreaks (Fig. 3.4) have established infection control as an essential hospital service (National Audit Office 2000, 2004b).

In recent years there has been increased public and political interest in the problem of HCAI, in particular antibiotic-resistant organisms such as methicillin-resistant *Staphylococcus aureus* (MRSA). In England, the Chief Medical Officer has published a strategy for combatting infectious disease that highlighted both HCAI and antimicrobial resistance (DoH 2002). The action plan for tackling HCAI was subsequently published in 2003 (DoH 2003). This emphasized the need for infection control to be a core part of a clinical governance programme, with leadership at a senior level, high standards of infection control practice in clinical areas and increased surveillance to provide information about HCAI and antimicrobial resistance.

In Scotland a task force on HCAI led by the Chief Medical Officer was established by the Ministry of Health in 2003. Its work has included a Code of Practice (Healthcare Associated Infection Task Force 2004) and NHS Scotland national cleaning service specifications. An education programme (The Cleanliness Champions) accessible to all healthcare workers is also in place and

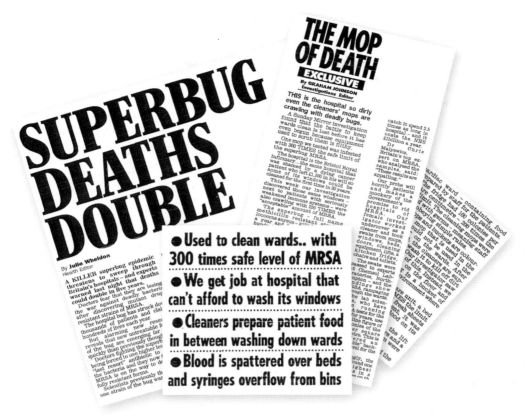

Figure 3.4   Hospital-acquired infection can cause considerable alarm.

aims to have a cleanliness champion in each clinical area. Standards in infection control have been devised and are monitored by Quality Improvement Scotland, previously the Clinical Standards Board (Clinical Standards Board for Scotland 2001).

Factors that affect the risk of acquiring infection in hospital

Healthcare exposes patients to an increased risk of infection. This risk is particularly high when care is provided in a hospital setting, where contact with healthcare staff and equipment occurs frequently and other patients may act as a source of infection. However, although patients in hospital are likely to be exposed to more factors that increase their risk of infection, the boundaries between hospital and community care are no longer clearcut. Day-case procedures now account for a significant proportion of surgery and even where an inpatient stay is required, the length of time spent in hospital after operation has reduced markedly. In 1974

the average postoperative stay was 9 days, compared with 4.5 days in 1997. Similarly, patients in elderly care now spend an average of 19 days in hospital, compared with 100 days in 1974 (Appleby 1997).

It may be difficult to distinguish between infections acquired in hospital and those acquired in the community. Patients with invasive devices such as urinary catheters or central vascular catheters may be cared for in their own homes and others receive treatment at home for chronic illnesses such as renal disease or cystic fibrosis. The principles of infection prevention and control are therefore applicable in both hospital and community settings, although adaptation for local circumstances may be necessary.

There are a number of factors associated with healthcare that make patients particularly vulnerable to infection.

Underlying disease

The ability of the immune system to respond to infection may be affected by underlying diseases, such as carcinoma or leukaemia, and immunosuppressive therapy. Some conditions (e.g. diabetes or vascular disease) affect the perfusion of the skin, leading to poor wound healing or tissue necrosis and increased susceptibility to infection. Symptoms of the disease process may also increase the risk of infection; for example, faecal incontinence increases the risk of urinary tract infection.

Extremes of age

The immature immune system of neonates and young children increases their susceptibility to infection. Immunity may also gradually be lost with increasing age, so that the elderly are likely to be susceptible to infections such as rotavirus, first encountered in childhood, and reactivation of chronic infection such as varicella zoster or tuberculosis.

Breach of defence mechanisms

The natural defences of the body, which protect us against invasion by micro-organisms, are frequently damaged or breached as a result of hospital treatment. The integrity of the skin may be interrupted by surgery, intravascular or other invasive devices, or decubitus ulceration. Intubation or respiratory ventilation may bypass the activity of cilia in the upper respiratory tract and normally sterile organs may be exposed to contamination by invasive procedures such as urinary catheterization and endoscopy. Antibiotic therapy may destroy bacteria that normally colonize and protect mucosal surfaces, enabling harmful micro-organisms to establish infection.

Exposure to infection

Places where many people are in close proximity with one another facilitate the spread of disease. However, the problem is exacerbated in hospitals because of the regular and intimate contact that occurs between patients and healthcare workers and which enables micro-organisms to transfer from person to person. A patient may have contact with many different healthcare workers, for example nurses, doctors, physiotherapists, occupational therapists, social workers and porters.

Hospital pathogens

Antimicrobial therapy is a common feature of hospital care, both for treatment and for prevention of infection. Types of micro-organisms intrinsically resistant to commonly used antimicrobial agents (e.g. enterococci, pseudomonads) and strains that have acquired genetic determinants of resistance (e.g. MRSA) are favoured in this environment. Patients admitted to hospital, particularly those who are critically ill, rapidly change

their normal bacterial flora for these more resistant organisms (Noone et al 1983). A patient previously treated with antimicrobial therapy may be more likely to develop infection with resistant micro-organisms, such as glycopeptide-resistant enterococci, *Clostridium difficile*. Once infection or colonization has established, the organisms may be transferred to other patients in close proximity (Chang & Nelson 2000).

Patients who are critically ill are also more vulnerable to a range of pathogens that are unlikely to cause infection in the healthy. For example, *Staphylococcus epidermidis* causes 15% of bacteraemia in hospital patients, normally in association with intravenous devices (Health Protection Agency 2003a). Candida takes advantage of a normal flora altered by antimicrobial therapy and is an increasingly common cause of systemic infection in the immunocompromised (Kibbler et al 2003).

Assessing a patient's susceptibility to infection

Some patients are at greater risk of acquiring infection than others. Figure 3.5 illustrates many of the factors that increase the risk. By identifying patients at risk of infection, actions required to manage or prevent infection can be incorporated into the planning of care (Kingsley 1992), for example the safe management of an intravenous infusion or urinary catheter, measures to improve nutrition or hydration. Integrated care pathways for invasive devices have been proposed as a means of ensuring that the risk of infection is minimized. Logan (2003) describes such a pathway for indwelling catheters that guides assessment of the need for catheterization, selection of an appropriate catheter and drainage system and the cycle for regular review.

THE SIZE OF THE PROBLEM

It is difficult to obtain precise figures for the number of infections acquired as a result of healthcare. The presence of infection is often not accurately recorded in medical or nursing notes and few hospitals have systems in place to routinely collect and analyse information about infections. A national prevalence study undertaken in 157 hospitals in the UK and Ireland found that, on average, nine of every 100 patients had a HCAI at the time of the survey. However, there were marked differences between hospitals, with the prevalence ranging from 2% to 29% and a higher rate of HCAI in teaching hospitals (11.2%) than in nonteaching hospitals (8.4%) (Emmerson et al 1996). Infections of the urinary tract, lower respiratory tract, surgical wounds and bloodstream accounted for about 60% of all HCAI identified in the survey (Fig. 3.6).

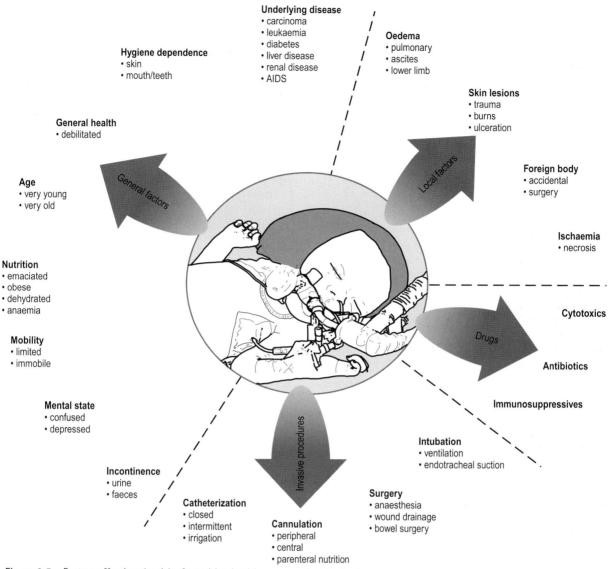

Underlying disease
• carcinoma
• leukaemia
• diabetes
• liver disease
• renal disease
• AIDS

Oedema
• pulmonary
• ascites
• lower limb

Hygiene dependence
• skin
• mouth/teeth

Skin lesions
• trauma
• burns
• ulceration

General health
• debilitated

Foreign body
• accidental
• surgery

Age
• very young
• very old

Ischaemia
• necrosis

Nutrition
• emaciated
• obese
• dehydrated
• anaemia

Cytotoxics

Antibiotics

Mobility
• limited
• immobile

Immunosuppressives

Mental state
• confused
• depressed

Intubation
• ventilation
• endotracheal suction

Incontinence
• urine
• faeces

Catheterization
• closed
• intermittent
• irrigation

Cannulation
• peripheral
• central
• parenteral nutrition

Surgery
• anaesthesia
• wound drainage
• bowel surgery

General factors

Local factors

Drugs

Invasive procedures

Figure 3.5 Factors affecting the risk of acquiring healthcare-associated infection.

Most of these infections are associated with invasive devices or procedures. Factors that predispose to them are summarized in Box 3.7 and described in more detail in subsequent chapters.

Prevalence surveys tend to overestimate the true level of infection because patients who develop an infection are more likely to stay in hospital for longer and will therefore account for a disproportionate number of hospital inpatients at a single point in time. A more accurate estimate is provided by incidence studies which measure how many patients acquire infection during hospitalization or after exposure to a specific event. These suggest that around 8% of patients admitted to hospital acquire an infection during their stay (Glenister et al 1992, Plowman et al 1999).

The risk of acquiring a HCAI has probably increased over recent decades as a result of more complex medical care and more acutely ill patients. However, such changes are difficult to measure, as the trend towards early discharge or treatment outside hospital means that many infections are not likely to be detected

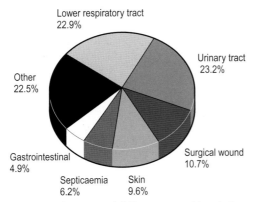

Figure 3.6 The frequency of different types of hospital-acquired infection (compiled using data from Emmerson et al 1996).

while the patient is in hospital. The study by Plowman et al (1999) estimated that at least a further 19% of patients developed an infection after discharge from hospital.

Some patients in hospital may be infected or colonized with micro-organisms that have a particular propensity to spread to others and may do so easily in hospital or other healthcare environments. These include infectious diseases such as chickenpox or tuberculosis or hospital pathogens such as MRSA. Isolation procedures are used to prevent the spread of these pathogens but occasionally transmission does occur. The main causes of outbreaks of infection in hospitals are listed in Box 3.8. Whilst outbreaks of infection are uncommon, probably accounting for less than 4% of all HCAI (Haley et al 1985a, Wenzel et al 1983), considerable resources may be required to control them. Barnass et al (1989) calculated the costs of an outbreak of salmonella, in which 17 patients and two staff were affected, to be over £21 000. Preventing the spread of MRSA can be particularly expensive as it may require staff and patients to be swabbed to detect carriage, treatment of those affected with topical creams or expensive antibiotics, ward or bed closures and additional staff to manage isolation precautions (Cox et al 1995).

Costs of healthcare-associated infections

Infections acquired as a result of healthcare cause considerable morbidity and mortality. Plowman et al (1999) assessed the general health of patients following hospitalization using a health status questionnaire that measured aspects of physical, social, emotional and mental health. They found that patients who acquired a HCAI had significantly lower health status

---

Box 3.7 Epidemiology of common hospital-acquired infections

Urinary tract infections

These are some of the most common infections associated with healthcare, accounting for 23% of HCAI. Most are related to urethral catheterization as this device facilitates the entry of bacteria into the bladder, either along the outside of the tube or through its lumen. Once in the bladder, micro-organisms may spread to the kidneys or invade the bloodstream. Urinary tract infection occurs most commonly in patients likely to be catheterized, such as those treated in urology, gynaecology and orthopaedic units (Glynn et al 1997).

Lower respiratory tract infections

These infections account for 23% of HCAI. Infection is acquired through aspiration of micro-organisms from the oropharynx or inhalation of airborne particles. The risk is increased by devices that bypass the normal defences (e.g. endotracheal and nasogastric tubes) and by reduced levels of consciousness (e.g. sedation). Opportunistic pathogens such as aspergillus may cause pneumonia in the immunocompromised.

Surgical wound infections

These account for nearly 11% of HCAI, although the risk of infection is highest for procedures more likely to encounter microbial contamination (e.g. operation on the bowel). Prolonged procedures, damaged tissue and the skills of the surgeon are important risk factors in the development of surgical wound infection.

Bloodstream infections

These account for approximately 6% of HCAI but are responsible for considerable morbidity and mortality. Some 38% are directly related to intravenous therapy, particularly central vascular devices, and are commonly caused by skin commensals such as *Staphylococcus epidermidis* (Health Protection Agency 2003a). Other bloodstream infections develop from another focus of infection (e.g. urinary or respiratory tract). Those caused by Gram-negative bacteria are particularly difficult to treat because these organisms produce a range of toxins that have severe systemic effects.

---

scores, particularly if they had symptoms of infection after discharge from hospital. Return to employment and normal activities was delayed in patients who developed a HCAI in hospital, by 6 and 12 days respectively.

Some infections may be serious enough to cause the death of the patient. It has been estimated that

---

Box 3.8   Detecting epidemiologically significant infections amongst hospital patients

Early detection of infections likely to transmit readily in a hospital setting is achieved by monitoring laboratory specimens and identifying patients with signs or symptoms suggestive of infection. Examples of these 'alert organisms' and 'alert conditions' are given below.

'Alert organisms'

Infection control precautions should be initiated when these micro-organisms are identified, either from a laboratory specimen or as a result of a clinical diagnosis to prevent their spread to other patients.

Clostridium difficile

Antibiotic-resistant organisms, e.g. MRSA, vancomycin-resistant enterococci (VRE), penicillin-resistant pneumococci

Salmonella, shigella or other gastrointestinal pathogens

Group A streptococci

Mycobacterium tuberculosis

Gastrointestinal viruses, e.g. rotavirus, norovirus

Respiratory viruses, e.g. influenza, respiratory syncytial virus

Chickenpox

'Alert conditions'

Infection control precautions should be taken when a patient develops any of the following signs or symptoms until an infectious cause has been excluded.

Diarrhoea

Vomiting

Symptoms of respiratory tract infection, e.g. cough, sputum

Fever of unknown origin

Skin rash

---

approximately 10% of patients who acquire an infection in hospital die (Haley 1986, Plowman et al 1999). Many of these patients would have died despite the infection; however, in one-third of cases the infection is likely to be a major contributory factor to death and in an estimated 10% of cases, infection is the main cause of death (Haley 1986).

In addition to the effect that HCAIs may have on the patient and the outcome of care, they have important resource implications for hospitals, community health-care services and society as a whole. In hospital, patients who acquire an infection incur nearly three times more costs than those who do not. These additional costs include specialist care, antimicrobial and other drug therapy, tests and treatments, and the costs associated with extra days spent in hospital (Plowman et al 1999). Overall, patients who acquire a HCAI spend nearly three times longer in hospital (Table 3.4). These extra costs vary according to the specific site of infection. Multiple infections (where a patient acquires more than one HCAI affecting different sites) are the most expensive to treat but occur infrequently, affecting only 1.4% of patients. Urinary tract infections incur greater costs because, although they are inexpensive to treat, they occur more commonly, affecting 2.7% of patients (Plowman et al 1999).

Many infections acquired as a result of care in hospital are not detected until after the patient has been discharged. The costs of consultation, drug therapy and treatment fall to the general practitioner and community nursing services, although these costs are much lower than those incurred by hospitals (Elliston et al 1994, Plowman et al 1999). There are also costs to society in terms of loss of earnings, productivity and social security payments, which may impinge on both the patients and their carers (Plowman et al 1997, 1999).

The effect that HCAIs have on the resources of the NHS is considerable. In 1993 Coello et al estimated that the cost of HCAI in surgical patients in England was over £170 million. Plowman et al (1999) extrapolated the data on the costs of HCAI at a single district general hospital and estimated that these infections cost the NHS in England £985 million annually, £930 million incurred during hospitalization and £55 million post discharge. The hospital costs represent 9% of the national budget for acute, elderly care and obstetric services.

These figures point to the value of measures to prevent HCAI. In an average hospital £300 000 of additional resources would be released by preventing 10% of HCAIs. A considerable proportion of these

Table 3.4 Additional costs and days spent in hospital by patients who develop a hospital-acquired infection

Site of infection	Additional costs (£ per patient)	Ratio of costs (compared to non-infected)	Additional days in hospital (per patient)	Incidence of HAI (%)
Urinary tract	1122	1.7	5	2.7
Lower respiratory tract	2080	2.3	8	1.2
Surgical wound	1594	2.0	7	1.0
Bloodstream	6209	4.3	4*	0.1
Skin	1615	2.0	11	0.6
Other	2465	2.5	12	0.8
Multiple	8631	6.3	29	1.4
Any infection	3154	2.8	11	7.8

*Two patients died. Estimates derived by regression modelling to control for confounding variables (e.g. age, sex, diagnosis, number of co-morbidities) that could have contributed to the increased costs. Data from Plowman et al (1999).

resources would be the release of additional bed-days for the treatment of other patients. The costs of establishing an infection control programme and employing sufficient specialist staff to maintain it are likely to be outweighed by the savings made through the prevention of HCAI and the elimination of costly and ineffective practices (National Audit Office 2004a, Plowman et al 2001).

Implications for service quality

The acquisition of infection as a result of hospital or other healthcare treatment has important implications both for the patients affected and the organizations concerned. HCAIs are seen as important quality indicators and as such, their prevention is key to ensuring that services provided by the NHS are of a high quality (Box 3.9) (National Audit Office 2004b, Quality Indicator Study Group 1995).

'Clinical governance' describes systems which ensure that the quality of services is continuously improved, high standards of care are safeguarded and an environment that fosters clinical excellence is created. Clinical governance requires organizations to have accountability for quality at corporate level, clear lines of responsibility and mechanisms in place to establish and monitor the quality of services (DoH 1998) (see Box 3.10).

Infection prevention and control are integral to providing a high-quality healthcare service in several ways. For example, identifying and managing risks related to infection, monitoring the outcome of care (e.g. by measuring the incidence of infection) and ensuring that appropriate procedures to prevent and control infection are in place, are evidence based and regularly audited (Pratt et al 2002).

Box 3.9   What is a quality indicator?

'A quantitative measure that can be used to monitor and evaluate the quality of important governance, management, clinical and support functions that affect patient outcomes' (Joint Commission on the Accreditation of Healthcare Organisations 1989).

Box 3.10   Clinical governance framework

Corporate accountability
Chief Executive accountable
Clear lines of responsibility

Internal mechanisms
Individual accountability
Professional regulation
Professional development

Core principles
Clinical audit
Evidence-based practice
Clinical effectiveness
Risk management
Risk reduction programmes
Monitoring outcomes of care
Learning lessons from complaints
Dissemination of good practice

In England, the quality of service that healthcare organizations are expected to deliver is defined in Healthcare Standards. These include, as part of a core Safety Standard, a requirement for systems to minimize the risk of infection, and infection control is also

Box 3.11   Risk analysis: a structured approach to the reduction of risk

1. **Risk assessment**
   Identify hazards and conditions under which they occur. Quantify the risk related to each hazard and make a formal record

2. **Risk management**
   Decide on and implement the actions required to eliminate or minimize the risk

3. **Risk communication**
   Inform and train staff about risks and risk management and control measures

4. **Risk monitoring**
   Assess the effectiveness of control measures

a component of several other standards (DoH 2004). NHS trusts therefore need to ensure that staff are trained in infection prevention and control, that protocols and other guidance on infection control are complied with and that infection risks associated with buildings, equipment and waste are identified and managed appropriately.

The Healthcare Commission is responsible for assessing the performance of healthcare organizations and the Healthcare Standards are used as a framework against which service quality and performance are measured.

Risk management and infection control

Infection presents a danger (a 'hazard') to both patients and staff involved in healthcare. A risk refers to the potential for a hazard to result in actual harm. Managing risk requires hazards to be identified and assessed in terms of their likely severity and frequency and the use of appropriate measures to either eliminate them or minimize their effect (Farrington & Pascoe 2001). Risk assessment should take account of risks to both patients and staff. Structures and policies should be in place to ensure that information about risks and their control can be clearly communicated (Box 3.11).

Risk management is a central component of the Healthcare Standards framework and to work effectively, it requires formal structures within NHS trusts, including a risk management committee at board level. Infection control has a key part to play in this risk management agenda. Risks related to infection are relevant to almost every aspect of the clinical environment; food delivery, water supply, building ventilation systems, decontamination of equipment and the appropriate use of hand hygiene and protective clothing in direct patient care. Mechanisms for making baseline assessment of risks, reporting arrangements where hazards are identified and developing plans for eliminating or minimizing risks are all essential parts of an effective risk management strategy. For example, needlestick injuries to staff are known to carry a significant risk of transmission of bloodborne viruses. Effective management of this risk requires a clearly stated policy on the safe disposal of used needles, training of staff who handle them, the provision of sufficient disposal containers and a system for reporting and monitoring injuries. Chapter 7 examines in more detail how these principles of risk management should be applied to basic standards of infection control in the care of all patients.

There are financial benefits associated with risk reduction systems since they will minimize the exposure of NHS organizations to litigation. This has taken on increasing importance since the removal of Crown Immunity in the late 1980s and early 1990s, which in the past exempted hospitals from prosecution and prevented enforcement of some legislation, for example food safety. Trusts can insure themselves against claims of negligence using the Clinical Negligence Scheme for Trusts (CNST). The level of contribution is determined by the extent to which the trust meets the risk management standards and these include activities to prevent and control infection. Contributions to the non-clinical risk pooling scheme are also affected by the trust's compliance with quality standards (NHS Litigation Authority 2003).

An important component of risk management is learning from things that go wrong and incorporating the lessons into future practice to minimize the risk of the same event recurring (DoH 2000a). For example, the analysis of causes of needlestick injuries can inform policies directed at preventing them.

PROGRAMMES FOR THE PREVENTION AND CONTROL OF HEALTHCARE-ASSOCIATED INFECTION

It may not be possible to prevent all HCAIs as many patients in hospital have compromised immune systems and are highly vulnerable to infection. However, the value of an effective HCAI prevention programme was demonstrated by a major American study carried out in the 1980s, called the Study of the Efficacy of Nosocomial Infection Control (SENIC). It evaluated the infection control activity in 338 hospitals and, through the review of clinical records, measured how the rate of HCAI changed in the 5-year period after infection control programmes were established. Those hospitals with the most comprehensive infection control programmes,

Box 3.12   Components of an infection control programme (SENIC)

Infection control personnel co-ordinating the programme
Trained infection control doctor
One infection control nurse to every 250 beds

Control activities
Detect, investigate and control outbreaks of infection
Produce, implement and monitor policies
Educate staff

Surveillance activities
Identify infections
Analyse data
Disseminate results

Source: Haley et al (1985b), by permission of Oxford University Press.

featuring all the components described in Box 3.12, were able to reduce the rate of HCAI by 32% during this period. In hospitals with a poor or non-existent infection control programme, the rate of HCAI increased by 18% over the same period.

The results of this study have important implications for clinical practice. They suggest that a significant proportion of HCAI can be prevented and that the quality of the infection control programme makes a difference. The study also highlighted the combination of activities that were important for an effective infection control programme, identifying surveillance of HCAI as a key component and the important role of specialist staff – the infection control nurse and infection control doctor. Although there have since been considerable changes in the provision of healthcare, a recent study in England reported that the majority of acute NHS trusts considered that there was scope to reduce HCAI by at least 15% (National Audit Office 2000). Data collected on the incidence of HCAI in several hospitals indicated significant differences between them. For example, the incidence of urinary tract infection in gynaecological patients varied from 1.4 to 3.3 infections per 1000 catheter-days (Glynn et al 1997).

Harbarth et al (2003), in a systematic review of 30 studies, found evidence for reductions in infection rates of between 10% and 70% depending on the baseline rates of infection, type of infection and study setting. Most studies used a combination of different interventions, together with active surveillance and feedback of rates of HCAI.

The Chief Executive of each NHS trust is responsible for ensuring that effective arrangements for infection control are in place and a planned programme has been defined and is regularly reviewed. In England, leadership at a senior level is provided by a director of infection prevention and control (DoH 2000b, 2003). The programme should define the focus of infection control activity, identify policies for development or review and include targets and objectives for surveillance, audit and education. Planning and implementing an infection control programme requires the expertise of specialist staff and all hospitals are recommended to employ a trained infection control nurse and infection control doctor to take on this role (DoH 1995, Scottish Office 1998). These staff work as a team, liaising with each other regularly, to ensure that measures required by the programme are implemented. The infection control team (ICT) is supported by an infection control committee with representation from clinical departments, pharmacy, occupational health and senior management.

Infection control nurse (ICN)   The ICN is usually the only full-time member of the infection control team (ICT) and carries the main responsibility for ensuring that the infection control programme is carried out, liaising with a wide range of departments and groups of staff within the trust. Every NHS trust should employ an ICN; many employ more than one but few have the ratio of one ICN for every 250 beds found in those SENIC hospitals with the most effective infection control programmes (Haley et al 1985b, National Audit Office 2000).

The ICN is usually a registered nurse with specialist training to degree or Master's level, who operates as a clinical nurse specialist, the characteristics of which have been defined by Hamric (1989) (Box 3.13). The ICN is required to act as an expert practitioner, interpreting laboratory and other relevant data and providing advice to clinical staff, patients and their families (Prieto 1994).

Many ICNs also work in PCTs, where they provide an advisory service and contribute to the infection control programme for community healthcare staff, nursing homes, general practitioners and practice nurses, or health protection units where they advise on infection prevention strategies for the community and the control of outbreaks of infection (Loveday et al 2003).

Infection control doctor (ICD)   The ICD is usually a consultant microbiologist based in an acute hospital with access to microbiology laboratory facilities. The ICD does not usually work full time in the role and is often unable to devote the recommended amount of time to it (National Audit Office 2000). ICDs should have specialist training in infection control and play a key part in developing the infection control programme, influencing the prescribing of antimicrobial agents, the treatment of HCAI and the training of medical students and qualified doctors.

Infection control committee (ICC)   Every hospital should have an infection control committee (DoH 1995). In addition to the ICT, the committee will draw its membership from the chief executive (or a senior member of the management team), director of nursing, CCDC, occupational health physician or nurse, senior clinical medical staff, pharmacy and sterile services supplies. The role of the committee is to endorse infection control policies, advise the ICT and act as a forum through which key groups can be consulted. The ICC will also approve the infection control programme and monitor progress in its implementation.

Director of infection prevention and control (DIPC)
The DIPC is responsible for the infection control team and oversees infection control policies and their implementation. The DIPC is an integral part of the clinical governance structures within the organization and reports directly to the chief executive and the trust board (DoH 2003).

Other key personnel
Consultant in communicable disease control (CCDC)
The CCDC is responsible for co-ordinating the surveil-

lance, prevention and control of all communicable diseases in a health district, together with systems for managing other environmental hazards to health such as chemicals and radiation. They are usually a member of the ICC and liaise with the hospital's ICT to co-ordinate the infection prevention and control activities between hospital and community. CCDCs have an important role in ensuring the effective management of outbreaks of infection. Many CCDCs now work directly with ICNs in health protection units as part of the Health Protection Agency.

Infection control link nurses (ICLNs)   Many hospitals use ICLNs to improve awareness of infection control in clinical areas. These staff receive some basic training in the principles of infection control and then help to provide information to other staff, undertake surveillance and audit, and report on infection control problems in their own area of practice (Dawson 2003).

Occupational health department (OHD)   Close liaison between the ICT and OHD is essential to ensure the health and safety of staff and the protection of patients from healthcare workers with infection. The OHD will undertake health surveillance for infectious diseases that may affect fitness to work (e.g. tuberculosis), health surveillance in relation to hazards (e.g. glutaraldehyde) and the ergonomic design of workplaces. They will also play an important role in formulating and implementing infection control policies (e.g. management of sharps injuries) and in monitoring their effectiveness (e.g. analysing sharps injury statistics). The OHD will be closely involved in outbreaks of infection, monitoring staff and ensuring that they remain off work whilst suffering from an illness that may affect patients. OHD staff should also be available to provide advice and support to staff who have been exposed to infection, such as those concerned about acquiring a bloodborne virus following a needlestick injury, and those who may be particularly susceptible to infection themselves, such as staff infected with HIV.

Key components of an infection control programme

The ICT has a key role to play in educating staff and ensuring appropriate systems are in place to encourage infection prevention and control as part of routine practice. Harbarth et al (2003) demonstrated that there is potential to reduce rates of HCAI but that multifaceted approaches are more likely to be effective, for example a combination of education, policies, engineering controls, and that the active surveillance and feedback of rates of HCAI to relevant clinical staff was an essential component.

Whilst all clinical staff are responsible for ensuring that they minimize the risk of transmitting infection to patients or themselves, a comprehensive programme of activities is required to ensure that high standards of infection prevention and control are maintained by all staff in all clinical areas. The programme should be developed by the ICT and reviewed annually by the ICC to define the focus of activity, identify policies that require development or revision and plan audit, surveillance and educational targets. There are several key areas of activity, as described below.

Advisory service

The ICT provides advice on a wide range of issues related to infection control such as the management of patients with infection, purchase and decontamination of equipment, cleaning, catering and waste management. Members of the ICT will also be required to attend various committees (e.g. health and safety, waste management, supplies and laundry users).

Education and training

A basic knowledge of microbiology underpins the practice of infection control and several workers have pointed to the lack of this knowledge amongst nurses and doctors (Courtenay 1998, Emmerson & Ridgway 1980). The fears and misunderstandings that surrounded the first patients diagnosed with AIDS demonstrate how important education is if such problems are to be avoided (Välimäki et al 1998). Concepts of infection control practice are often difficult to understand because germs are not visible and the consequence of transmitting them between patients is not immediately apparent (Jenner et al 1999). Deficits in knowledge and understanding of these basic principles can therefore affect the ability of staff to apply infection control precautions appropriately (Prieto 2003).

An important role of the ICN is therefore to educate and inform staff, helping them to apply the principles of infection control to clinical practice. This can take place informally, for example discussing the management of a particular patient whilst visiting a ward or clinic, during feedback sessions following audits or more formally as lectures and study days. Infection control should also form part of the basic training and continuous professional development of all groups of healthcare professionals and support staff such as domestics and porters.

There is a close relationship between health and safety and many aspects of infection control. The health and safety legislation recognizes the importance of training as a means of ensuring that staff understand procedures and know what is expected of them. Staff who join a healthcare organization should be made aware of local infection control policies and the ICT should be involved in their orientation programmes.

Staff who have received education are more able to educate others, both patients and other staff, and, as in the case of infection control link nurses, can provide a valuable adjunct to the ICT. Ching & Seto (1990) have used ICLNs to support the teaching activity of the ICN and were able to demonstrate significant improvements in adherence to an infection control policy when ICLNs were providing tutorials on the ward.

Surveillance of hospital-acquired infection

Surveillance is the systematic monitoring of the occurrence of disease in a population. The importance of surveillance in the control of infectious diseases was recognized at the beginning of the 20th century and there is now a statutory requirement for doctors to notify cases of infectious disease. Surveillance in a hospital setting has, until recently, been focused on detecting cases of infectious disease that have the potential to cause outbreaks of infection (see Box 3.8). Now, many more hospitals are recognizing HCAI as an important quality indicator and are using surveillance to assess the quality of care as part of the clinical audit process (Fig. 3.7) (Gaynes & Solomon 1996). However, surveillance data need to be interpreted

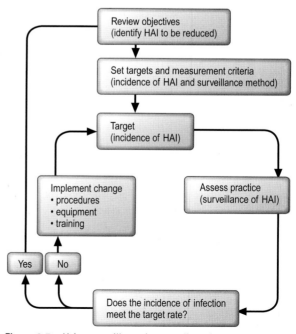

Figure 3.7 Using surveillance in an audit cycle.

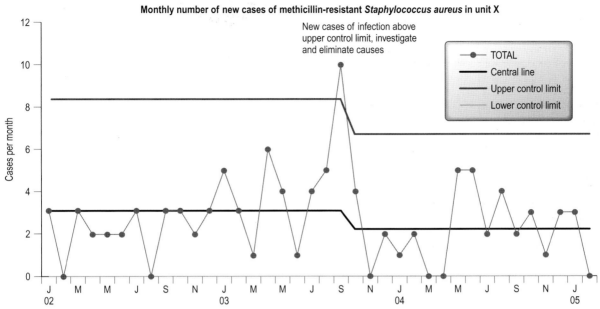

Figure 3.8 Example of a statistical process control (SPC) chart for monitoring new cases of hospital-acquired infection (reproduced with permission from Curran et al 2002).

with care because differences in methods of data collection, criteria for defining infections and the mix of patients can all affect the results and need to be considered when comparing data from different hospitals or from the same hospital over time (Wilson 1995). Active methods of surveillance that use designated, trained staff to identify cases of infection are more reliable, with a sensitivity of approximately 80%, compared to passive methods that rely on other staff to report cases of infection, which are associated with a sensitivity of less than 30% (Perl 1997). Reliable, high-quality data are essential if the information is to be used as a basis for assessing and reviewing practice (Gaynes et al 2001).

Although surveillance can consume considerable resources many would argue that its benefits in contributing to the prevention of healthcare-associated infection outweigh these costs (Haley 1985, Harbarth et al 2003, Wilson et al 2002). There is clear evidence for its value in motivating staff to identify problems with infection control and adhere to practice guidelines. Just as importantly, it can provide evidence for the efficacy of infection control and acknowledge and support good practice. Curran et al (2002) describe the use of a simple surveillance system that provides visual information to staff about the number of patients acquiring MRSA on their ward. These charts can be used to identify significant changes in infection

rates and target re-evaluation of infection control practices (Fig. 3.8).

The Health Protection Agency co-ordinates a programme to help hospitals in England to collect data on specific HCAIs using standard methodology and definitions, and to make national data on their incidence available for comparison. The scheme currently co-ordinates surveillance on surgical site infections associated with several different categories of surgical procedure. Hospitals participating in this scheme can compare their incidence of infections with other participating hospitals and, if their rates are found to be high, initiate an investigation of underlying causes and identify any changes of practice that may be indicated (Health Protection Agency 2003b). Such national comparative data can be particularly useful for benchmarking, providing confirmation of high standards of practice or pointing out where problems need to be addressed (Wilson et al 2002). Similar schemes are operated by Health Protection Scotland and the National Public Health Service for Wales, and many other European countries (Wilson et al 2005).

Monitoring clinical practice

Routine visits to clinical areas provide the ICN with the opportunity to monitor aspects of clinical practice and detect potential problems. However, in some situations a formal audit can be used to provide a

TOPIC:	Isolation room cleaning			
CARE OUTCOME:	The isolation room is clean and safe to use by another patient			
STATEMENT	**AUDIT CRITERIA**	**YES**	**NO**	**N/A**
The isolation room is effectively and appropriately decontaminated following the discontinuation of isolation precautions Target (%) _____ Actual (%) _____ Variance (%) _____	1. All contaminated materials have been removed as per local guidelines (including clinical waste, laundry, soft furnishings) 2. Cleaning has been completed to leave all surfaces within the room, including furniture and fittings, free from dust, debris and soilage 3. Disinfection procedures have been undertaken in accordance with local infection control guidance for the specific infection 4. Treatment-related equipment including commodes/drip stands, etc. have been cleaned as per local infection control guidance 5. The responsibilities of the nursing and domestic staff with regard to isolation room cleaning are clearly identified in local guidance			
Formula for calculating actual performance: Number of 'yes' responses/number of 'applicable' responses x 100 = % actual performance	**Action plan (including timescales)** 1. 2. 3.			

Signature of auditor: **Location of audit**

Date of audit: **Date of follow-up audit**

Figure 3.9 Example of an audit tool (reproduced with permission from Standards for Environmental Cleanliness in Hospitals 1999).

systematic measurement of the quality of care and to identify where improvements could be made (Millward et al 1993, 1995). This involves marking observed practice against predefined criteria and feeding back the score generated from the process to the clinical staff in the department concerned (Fig. 3.9). An effective audit process must be based on clearly defined standards of what constitutes good care or practice, evidence must be collected systematically and objectively, while reports of the results must be relevant and able to influence clinical practice (Baker

1997). Audit can help to uncover deficiencies in practice and identify where information about infection control policies, additional equipment or in-service education may be required; any problems identified should be discussed during the feedback session, solutions agreed and action monitored (Friedman et al 1984).

The Infection Control Nurses' Association has recently published a set of audit tools for monitoring a range of basic infection control standards (Infection Control Nurses Association 2004).

Detection, investigation and control of outbreaks of infection

Outbreaks or epidemics of infection can occur in any community but are a particular problem in institutions where many people live in close proximity (e.g. schools, universities, residential homes and military barracks). The risks are even greater in hospital settings, where many patients have underlying illnesses that increase their susceptibility to infection. An outbreak may develop rapidly and be related to an event that exposed many people to the pathogen (e.g. food poisoning) or may develop gradually over many days or weeks as the pathogen is spread from person to person (e.g. viral gastroenteritis).

When an outbreak of infection occurs within a hospital, the ICT will investigate the source of infection, identify people who have been in contact with the infection, advise on the control measures required and monitor their implementation. The ICT may establish an outbreak control group, involving clinicians and senior nurses from affected departments, the CCDC, occupational health physician and other staff whose help may be required to ensure that the outbreak is controlled effectively (DoH 1995).

Policies and procedures to prevent and control infection

Written information in the form of policies, guidelines or procedures is required to define routine practices and standards of care expected by the organization and to provide guidance when members of the ICT are not available. These policies and procedures are a key component of effective risk management. Infection control policies may refer to specific areas of practice, for example isolation of infectious patients, management of equipment, the environment and waste materials, use of protective clothing. Others may contain aspects of infection control practice within a broader practice guideline, for example recommended practices for the insertion and management of invasive devices such as nasogastric tubes, intravenous cannulae or urinary catheters. The ICT, in conjunction with other staff, is responsible for developing many of these policies. The ICC will decide on the priorities for policy development and revision and approve them when completed. In some situations staff will develop their own policies but seek the advice of the ICT on recommended practice.

There are often conflicting views about what constitutes best practice in terms of infection control. An analysis by Glynn et al (1997) demonstrated considerable variation in practices recommended for the prevention of infection in a range of policies from 19 hospitals across England and Wales. The publication of some simple clinical guidelines for preventing infection associated with a range of commonly used invasive devices may help to focus on those practices that have been most clearly demonstrated to reduce the risk of infection (Pratt et al 2001, Ward et al 1997).

EPIC project   The Department of Health in England has commissioned the development of national evidence-based guidelines on some key aspects of infection control practice, for example indwelling urethral catheters, intravenous catheters and general principles of infection control. These guidelines contain the broad principles of good practice, derived from research evidence and expert review, and are intended to inform the development of more detailed operational policies at a local level. Evidence has been gathered by systematically reviewing the literature and then critically appraising the study design, methodology, analysis and relevance to practice. Relevant evidence has then been graded into three categories:

- Category 1: generally consistent findings in a range of evidence derived from well-designed experimental studies
- Category 2: evidence based on a single acceptable study, or a weak or inconsistent finding in some multiple acceptable studies
- Category 3: limited scientific evidence that does not meet all the criteria of 'acceptable studies' or an absence of directly applicable studies of good quality. This includes published or unpublished expert opinion (Pratt et al 2001).

The National Institute for Clinical Excellence has also published similar, evidence-based guidelines on key aspects of infection control in the community (Pellowe et al 2003).

Dissemination and implementation of policies

National guidelines can help to ensure consistent evidence-based practice but more detailed policies and guidelines should be developed that take account of local practices and attitudes. Written policies alone may not be sufficient to ensure effective practice if staff are not aware of them or do not understand their content. There must, therefore, also be a system for implementation and dissemination, to ensure that the relevant staff know about the policy and understand its contents and the rationale for recommended practice (Cheater & Closs 1997). However, there are many barriers to translating policy into practice and a range of strategies, in addition to manuals or protocols, may be necessary if evidence-based practice is to be adopted. These include using local opinion leaders such as ward sisters, senior medical staff or link nurses, the audit or observation of practice, surveillance of infection with feedback of results to relevant clinical staff, and formal or informal training where the rules within the policy are made explicit (Jenner et al 1999, Pittet et al 2000, Richardson 1999, Seto et al 1991).

Sustaining compliance with infection prevention and control procedures

Understanding and applying theories of behaviour is essential if adherence to infection control precautions is to be established and sustained. Kretzer & Larson (1998) reviewed the major behavioural theories and suggest that there is a complex interaction between individual and institutional factors in motivating or inhibiting particular actions. Individuals may be motivated by the perceived risk to themselves, their personal attitudes (for example, to hygiene), social norms that pervade the area in which they work, their perception of their personal ability to carry out an act (for example, is there time?, is the necessary equipment readily available?), and their expectation that a particular consequence will follow from their action. The organization itself can affect the attitude of staff to infection control practice; for example, the explicit support and reinforcement of expectations by senior management has been shown to impact on the frequency of handwashing (Larson et al 2000).

All these factors should be taken into account when designing programmes to improve adherence to infection control practice. The complexity of factors that influence behaviours means that a single approach is unlikely to be successful. Several studies have demonstrated the value of a multi-focus approach, for example education, routine observation and feedback of practice, engineering controls, reminders in the workplace, administrative sanctions or rewards and securing support at both individual and institutional level (Harbarth et al 2003, Pittet et al 1999).

References

Acheson D (1998) *Great Britain Independent Inquiry into Inequalities in Health.* Stationery Office, London.

Appleby J (1997) The English patient. *Health Services J.,* **10 April**: 36–40.

Baker O (1997) Process surveillance: an epidemiologic challenge for all health care organisations. *Am. J. Infect. Contr.,* **25**: 96–101.

Barrie D, Wilson J, Hoffman PN et al (1992) *Bacillus cereus* meningitis in two neurosurgical patients: an investigation into the source of the organism. *J. Infect.,* **25**: 291–7.

Barrie D, Hoffman PN, Wilson JA, Kramer JM (1994) Contamination of hospital linen by *Bacillus cereus. Epidemiol. Infect.,* **113**: 297–306.

Barnass S, O'Mahony M, Socket PN et al (1989) The tangible cost implications of multiply-resistant salmonella. *Epidemiol. Infect.,* **103**: 227–34.

Bartlett CLR, Macrae AD, Macfarlane JD (1986) *Legionella Infections.* Edward Arnold, London.

Bonten MJM, Austin DJ, Lipsitch J (2001) Understanding the spread of antibiotic resistant pathogens in hospitals: mathematical models as tools for control. *Health. Epidemiol.,* **33**:1739–46.

Boyce JM (2002) Understanding and controlling methicillin-resistant *Staphylococcus aureus* infections. *Infect. Contr. Hosp. Epidemiol.,* **23**(9): 485–7.

Boyce JM, Potter-Bynoe G, Chenevert C et al (1997) Environmental contamination due to methicillin-resistant *Staphylococcus aureus*: possible infection control implications. *Infect. Contr. Hosp. Epidemiol.,* **21**: 442–8.

Chang VT, Nelson K (2000) The role of physical proximity in nosocomial diarrhoea. *Clin. Infect. Dis.,* **31**: 717–22.

Cheater FM, Closs SJ (1997) The effectiveness of methods of dissemination and implementation of clinical guidelines for nursing practice: a selective review. *Clin. Effect. Nurs.,* **1**: 4–15.

Ching TY, Seto WH (1990) Evaluating the efficacy of the infection control liaison nurse in the hospital. *J. Adv. Nurs.,* **15**: 1128–31.

Clinical Standards Board for Scotland (2001) *Infection Control Standards.* Scottish Executive Health Department: Edinburgh. Available online at: www.scotland.gov.uk.

Coello R, Glenister H, Fereres J et al (1993) The cost of infection in surgical patients: a case control study. *J. Hosp. Infect.,* **25**: 239–50.

Courtenay M (1998) The teaching, learning, and use of infection control knowledge in nursing. *NT Res.,* **3**(2): 118–30.

Cox RA, Conquest C, Mallghan C et al (1995) A major outbreak of methicillin-resistant *Staphylococcus aureus* caused by a new phage type (EMRSA 16). *J. Hosp. Infect.,* **29**: 87–106.

Curran ET, Benneyan JC, Hood J (2002) Controlling methicillin-resistant *Staphylococcus aureus*: a feedback approach using annotated statistical process control charts. *Infect. Contr. Hosp. Epidemiol.,* **23**(1): 13–18.

Dawson SJ (2003) The role of the infection control link nurse. *J. Hosp. Infect.,* **54**(4): 251–7.

Department of Health (1995) *Hospital Infection Control – Guidance on the Control of Infection in Hospitals.* DH/PHLS/ Hospital Infection Working Group. HMSO, London.

Department of Health (1998) *A First Class Service in the New NHS.* Department of Health, London.

Department of Health (2000a) *An Organisation with a Memory – Report of an Expert Group on Learning from*

Adverse Events in the NHS. Department of Health, London.

Department of Health (2000b) *The Management and Control of Hospital Infection*. HSC 2000/002. Department of Health, London.

Department of Health (2001) *Shifting the Balance of Power*. Department of Health, London.

Department of Health (2002) *Getting Ahead of the Curve: a Strategy for Combating Infectious Diseases and Other Aspects of Health Protection. A report by the Chief Medical Officer*. Department of Health, London.

Department of Health (2003) *Winning Ways. Working Together to Reduce Healthcare Associated Infection in England. A report from the Chief Medical Officer*. Department of Health, London.

Department of Health (2004) *Standards for Better Health*. Department of Health, London.

Devine J, Cooke RPD, Wright EP (2001) Is methicillin-resistant *Staphylococcus aureus* (MRSA) contamination of ward-based computer terminals a surrogate marker for nosocomial MRSA transmission and handwashing compliance? *J. Hosp. Infect.*, **48**: 72–5.

Elliston PRA, Slack RCB, Humphreys H et al (1994) The cost of postoperative wound infections. *J. Hosp. Infect.*, **28**(3): 241–2.

Emmerson AM, Ridgway GL (1980) Teaching asepsis to medical students. *J. Hosp. Infect.*, **1**: 289–92.

Emmerson AM, Enstone JE, Griffin M et al (1996) The second national prevalence survey of infection in hospitals – overview of the results. *J. Hosp. Infect.*, **32**: 175–90.

Farrington M, Pascoe G (2001) Risk management and infection control – time to get our priorities right in the United Kingdom. *J. Hosp. Infect.*, **47**: 19–24.

Friedman C, Richter D, Skylis T et al (1984) Process surveillance: auditing infection control policies and procedures. *Am. J. Infect. Contr.*, **12**: 228–32.

Gaynes RP, Solomon S (1996) Improving hospital-acquired infection rates: the CDC experience. *Joint Comm. J. Qual. Impr.*, **22**(7): 457–67.

Gaynes RP, Richards C, Edwards J et al (2001) Feeding back surveillance data to prevent hospital-acquired infections. *Emerg. Infect. Dis.*, **7**(2): 295–301.

Glenister HM, Taylor LJ, Cooke EM et al (1992) *A Study of Surveillance Methods for Detecting Hospital Infection*. PHLS, London.

Glynn A, Ward V, Wilson J et al (1997) *Hospital Acquired Infection: Surveillance Policies and Practice*. PHLS, London.

Goldmann DA (2000) Transmission of viral respiratory infections in the home. *Paedr. Infect. Dis. J.*, **19**: S97–102.

Gormon LJ, Sanai L, Notman W et al (1993) Cross-infection in an intensive care unit by *Klebsiella pneumoniae* from ventilator condensate. *J. Hosp. Infect.*, **23**: 17–26.

Greaves A (1985) We'll just freshen you up, dear. *Nursing Times*, **Mar 6** (suppl.): 3–8.

Green J, Wright PA, Gallimore CI et al (1998) The role of environmental contamination with small round structured viruses in a hospital outbreak investigated by reverse-transcriptase polymerase chain reaction assay. *J. Hosp. Infect.*, **39**: 39-46.

Haley RW (1985) Surveillance-by-objectives: a new priority-directed approach to the control of nosocomial infections. *Am. J. Infect. Contr.*, **13**: 78–89.

Haley RW (1986) *Managing Hospital Infection Control for Cost Effectiveness. A Strategy for Reducing Infectious Complications*. American Hospital Publishing, Chicago.

Haley RW, Tenney JH, Lindsay JO et al (1985a) How frequent are outbreaks of nosocomial infection in community hospitals? *Infect. Contr.*, **6**: 233–6.

Haley RW, Culver DH, White JW et al (1985b) The efficacy of infection surveillance and control programs in preventing nosocomial infections in US hospitals (SENIC Study). *Am. J. Epidemiol.*, **121**: 182–205.

Hambraeus A (1988) Aerobiology in the operating room – a review. *J. Hosp. Infect.*, **11** (suppl. A): 68–76.

Hamric AB (1989) History and overview of the CNS role. In: Hamric AB, Spross JA (eds) *The Clinical Nurse Specialist in Theory and Practice*, 2nd edn. WB Saunders, Philadelphia.

Harbarth S, Sax H, Gastemeier P (2003) The preventable proportion of nosocomial infections: an overview of published reports. *J. Hosp. Infect.*, **54**(4): 258–66.

Healthcare Associated Infection Task Force (2004) *The NHS Scotland Code of Practice for the Local Management of Hygiene and Healthcare Associated Infection*. NHS Scotland. Available online at: www.scotland.gov.uk.

Health Protection Agency (2003a) *Hospital-acquired Bacteraemia. Analysis of Surveillance in English Hospitals 1997–2002*. Health Protection Agency, London.

Health Protection Agency (2003b) *Surgical Site Infection. Analysis of Surveillance in English Hospitals, 1997–2002*. Health Protection Agency, London.

Hollyoak V, Allison D, Summers J (1995) *Pseudomonas aeruginosa*, wound infection associated with a nursing home's whirlpool bath. *CDR*, **5**(7): R100–2.

Howarth FH (1985) Prevention of airborne infection during surgery. *Lancet*, **i**: 386–8.

Infection Control Nurses Association/Department of Health (2004) *Audit Tools for Monitoring Infection Control Standards*. ICNA. Available online at: info.fitwise.co.uk.

Jenner EA, Mackintosh C, Scott GM (1999) Infection control – evidence into practice. *J. Hosp. Infect.*, **42**: 91–104.

Joint Commission on the Accreditation of Healthcare Organisations (1989) Characteristics of clinical indicators. *Qual. Rev. Bull.*, **15**: 330–9.

Kibbler CC, Seaton S, Barnes RA et al (2003) Management and outcome of bloodstream infection due to Candida species in England and Wales. *J. Hosp. Infect.*, **54**: 18–24.

Kingsley A (1992) First step towards a desired outcome. Preventing infection by risk recognition. *Prof. Nurse*, **7**(11): 725–9.

Kretzer EK, Larson EL (1998) Behavioral interventions to improve infection control practices. *Am. J. Infect. Contr.*, **26**: 245–53.

Larson EL (1988) A causal link between handwashing and risk of infection? Examination of the evidence. *Infect. Contr. Hosp. Epidemiol.*, **9**: 28–36.

Larson EL, Early E, Cloonan P et al (2000) An organisational climate intervention associated with increased handwashing and decreased nosocomial infections. *Behav. Med.*, **26**(1): 14–22.

Logan K (2003) Indwelling catheters: developing an integrated care pathway package. *Nursing Times,* **99**(44): 49–51.

Loomes S (1988) Is it safe to lie down in hospital? *Nursing Times*, **84**(49): 63–5.

Loveday HP, Harper PJ, Mulhall A et al (2003) Informing the future: 2. Developing the role of the community Infection Control nurse practitioner. *Prof. Nurse*, **18**(6): 327–31.

Mackintosh CA, Hoffman PN (1984) An extended model for the transfer of micro-organisms via the hands: differences between organisms and the effect of alcohol disinfection. *J. Hyg.*, **92**: 345–55.

Maki DG, Alvarado CJ, Hassemer CA et al (1982) Relation of the inanimate environment to evidence of nosocomial infection. *N. Engl. J. Med.,* **307**: 1562–6.

Manuel RJ, Kibbler CC (1998) The epidemiology and prevention of invasive aspergillosis. *J. Hosp. Infect.*, **39**: 95–109.

Millward S, Barnett J, Thomlinson D (1993) A clinical infection control audit programme: evaluation of an audit tool used by infection control nurses to monitor standard and assess effective staff training. *J. Hosp. Infect.*, **24**: 219–32.

Millward S, Barnett J, Thomlinson D (1995) Evaluation of the objectivity of an infection control audit tool. *J. Hosp. Infect.*, **31**: 229–33.

Mortimer EA, Wolinsky E, Gonzaga AJ et al (1966) Role of hands in the transmission of staphylococcal infections. *BMJ*, **1**: 319–22.

Musa FK, Desai N, Casewell MW et al (1990) The survival of *Acinetobacter calcoaceticus* inoculated on fingertips and formica. *J. Hosp. Infect.*, **15**: 219–28.

National Audit Office (2000) *The Management and Control of Hospital Acquired Infection in Acute NHS Trusts in England.* Report by the Comptroller and Auditor General. Stationery Office, London.

National Audit Office (2004a) *Improving Patient Care by Reducing the Risk of Hospital-Acquired Infection: A Progress Report.* Report by the Comptroller and Auditor General. Stationery Office, London.

National Audit Office (2004b) *The Management and Control of Hospital Acquired Infection in Acute NHS Trusts in England (update).* Report by the Comptroller and Auditor General. Stationery Office, London.

National *Clostridium difficile* Standards Group (2004) Report to the Department of Health. *J. Hosp. Infect.*, **56** (suppl. 1).

Newsom SWB (1993) Ignaz Philip P Semmelweis. *J. Hosp. Infect.*, **23**: 175–88.

NHS Litigation Authority (2003) *Risk Pooling Schemes for Trust Risk Management Standard.* NHS Litigation Authority, London.

NHS Management Executive (1993) *Public Health: Responsibilities of the NHS and Roles of Others.* Department of Health Publication Unit, Heywood, Lancs.

Nightingale F (1863) *Notes on Nursing.* Longman, London.

Noone MR, Pitt TL, Bedder M et al (1983) *Pseudomonas aeruginosa* in an intensive therapy unit: role of cross infection and host factors. *BMJ*, **286**: 341–4.

Orsi GB, Mansi A, Tomao P et al (1994) Lack of association between clinical and environmental isolates of *Pseudomonas aeruginosa* in hospital wards. *J. Hosp. Infect.*, **27**(1): 49–60.

Overton E (1988) Bed making and bacteria. *Nursing Times*, **84**(9): 69–71.

Pellowe CM, Pratt RJ, Harper P et al (2003) Evidence-based guidelines for preventing healthcare-associated infections in primary and community care in England. *J. Hosp. Infect.*, **55** (suppl. 2): S1–S27.

Perl T (1997) Surveillance, reporting and the use of computers. In: Wenzel RP (ed.) *Prevention and Control of Nosocomial Infections*, 3rd edn. Lippincott, Williams and Wilkins, Philadelphia.

Pittet D, Dharan S, Toureneau S et al (1999) Bacterial contamination of the hands of hospital staff during routine patient care. *Arch. Intern. Med.*, **159**: 821–6.

Pittet D, Hugonnet S, Harbarth S et al (2000) Effectiveness of a hospital-wide programme to improve compliance with hand hygiene. *Lancet*, **356**: 1307–12.

Plowman RM, Graves N, Roberts JA (1997) *Hospital-acquired Infection.* Office of Health Economics, London.

Plowman R, Graves N, Griffin M et al (1999) *The Socio-economic Burden of Hospital-acquired Infection.* PHLS, London.

Plowman R, Graves N, Griffin M et al (2001) The rate and cost of hospital-acquired infections occurring in patients admitted to selected specialties of a district general hospital in England and the national burden imposed. *J. Hosp. Infect.*, **47**: 198-209.

Pratt RA, Pellowe CM, Loveday HP et al (2001) The Epic project: developing national evidence-based guidelines for preventing healthcare associated infections. *J. Hosp. Infect.*, **47** (suppl. A).

Pratt R, Morgan S, Hughes J et al (2002) Healthcare governance and the modernisation of the NHS: infection prevention and control. *Br. J. Infect. Contr.*, **3**(5): 16–25.

Prieto J (1994) The specialist role of the ICN. *Nursing Times*, **90**(38): 63–6.

Prieto JA (2003) Influencing infection control practice: assessing the impact of supportive intervention for nurses. PhD thesis, University of Southampton.

Quality Indicator Study Group (1995) An approach to the evaluation of quality indicators of the outcome of care in hospitalised patients, with a focus on nosocomial infection indicators. *Infect. Contr. Hosp. Epidemiol.*, **16**: 308–16.

Rampling A, Wiseman S, Davis L et al (2001) Evidence that hospital hygiene is important in the control of methicillin-resistant *Staphylococcus aureus*. *J. Hosp. Infect.*, **49**: 109–16.

Reybrouck G (1983) Role of hands in the spread of nosocomial infections 1. *J. Hosp. Infect.*, **4**: 103–10.

Richardson R (1999) Implementing evidence-based practice. *Prof. Nurse*, **15**(2): 101–4.

Riley RL, Mills CC, Nyka W et al (1959) Aerial dissemination of pulmonary tuberculosis: a two year study of contagion in a tuberculosis ward. *Am. J. Hyg.*, **70**: 185.

Sanderson PJ, Weissler S (1992) Recovery of coliforms from

the hands of nurses and patients: activities leading to contamination. *J. Hosp. Infect.*, **21**: 85–93.

Scottish Office (1998) *Scottish Infection Manual. Guidance on Core Standards for the Control of Infection in Hospitals, Healthcare Premises and at the Community Interface.* Advisory Group on Infection, Scottish Office, Edinburgh.

Selwyn S (1991) Hospital infection: the first 2500 years. *J. Hosp. Infect.*, **18** (suppl. A): 5–65.

Seto WH, Ching RN, Yuen KY et al (1991) The enhancement of infection control in-service education by ward opinion leaders. *Am. J. Infect. Contr.*, **19**: 86–91.

Simpson JY (1869) Some propositions on hospitalism. *Lancet*, **Oct 16**: 535–8.

Välimäki M, Suominen T, Peate I (1998) Attitudes of professionals, students and the general public to HIV/AIDS and people with HIV/AIDS: a review of the research. *J. Adv. Nurs.*, **27**: 752–9.

Van der Berg RWA, Claahsen HL, Niessen M et al (1999) *Enterobacter cloacae* outbreak in the NICU related to disinfected thermometers. *J. Hosp. Infect.*, **45**: 29–34.

Ward V, Wilson J, Taylor L et al (1997) *Preventing Hospital-acquired Infection. Clinical Guidelines.* PHLS, London.

Wenzel RP, Thompson RL, Landry SM et al (1983) Hospital-acquired infections in intensive care unit patients: an overview with emphasis on epidemics. *Infect. Contr.*, **4**: 371.

Whyte W, Hodgson R, Tinkler J (1982) The importance of airborne bacterial contamination of wounds. *J. Hosp. Infect.*, **3**: 123–35.

Wilson J (1995) Infection control: surveying the risks. *Nursing Standard*, **9** (15 suppl. NU): 3–8.

Wilson J, Ward V, Coello R et al (2002) A user evaluation of the National Nosocomial Infection Surveillance System: surgical site infection module. *J. Hosp. Infect.*, **52**: 114–21.

Wilson J , Suetens C, De Laet C et al (2005) Hospitals in Europe Link for Infection Control Through Surveillance (HELICS). Intercountry comparison of rates of surgical site infection: opportunities and limitations. Society of Hospital Epidemiologists of America, 15th Annual Conference.

World Health Organization (2003) *Consensus Document on the Epidemiology of Severe Acute Respiratory Syndrome (SARS).* WHO, Geneva.

Further Reading

Ayliffe GAJ, English MP (2003) *Hospital Infection: from Miasmas to MRSA.* Cambridge University Press, Cambridge.

Haley RW (1998) A cost benefit analysis of infection control programs. In: Bennett JV, Brachman PS (eds) *Hospital Infections*, 4th edn. Little, Brown, Boston.

Jenner EA, Wilson JA (2000) Educating the infection control team – past, present and future. A British perspective. *J. Hosp. Infect.*, **46**: 96–105.

Larson EL, Early E, Cloonan P et al (2000) An organizational climate intervention associated with increased hand washing and decreased nosocomial infections. *Behav. Med.*, **26**(1): 14–21.

Rhame FS (1998) The inanimate environment. In: Bennett JV, Brachman PS (eds) *Hospital Infections*, 4th edn. Little, Brown, Boston.

Chapter **4**

The immune system and the immunocompromised patient

INTRODUCTION

Molecules recognized by the immune system as 'non-self' are called antigens. Single molecules, complex proteins and carbohydrates, and whole micro-organisms can all be antigenic.

The body possesses several different mechanisms that protect it against foreign material or invasion by micro-organisms. These begin with physical and biochemical barriers such as the skin and acid in the stomach, which protect vulnerable points of the body from invasion. The second level of defence comprises a set of phagocytic cells, enzymes and proteins that attack all types of invading micro-organisms. Since these defences are already in place in the body, they are able to respond immediately to the invasion and are referred to as the 'innate' immune system. The final component is the 'adaptive' immune system. This provides a targeted attack against specific antigens. This specific response is made by two types of white blood cell: the B lymphocytes, which produce antibodies, and the T lymphocytes, which attack cells that have been invaded by micro-organisms and co-ordinate the activity of different components of the response. The lymphocytes retain a 'memory' of micro-organisms or other antigens that have previously invaded so that when encountered again, a very rapid response can be mounted which prevents the micro-organism from causing disease. The innate and adaptive immune systems work synergistically to prevent the replication and spread of invading micro-organisms.

PHYSICAL BARRIERS TO INFECTION

The first line of defence against micro-organisms and other antigens is a series of physical barriers which protect potential points of entry into the body (Fig. 4.1).

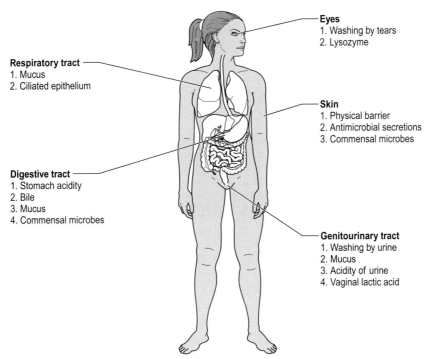

Eyes
1. Washing by tears
2. Lysozyme

Respiratory tract
1. Mucus
2. Ciliated epithelium

Skin
1. Physical barrier
2. Antimicrobial secretions
3. Commensal microbes

Digestive tract
1. Stomach acidity
2. Bile
3. Mucus
4. Commensal microbes

Genitourinary tract
1. Washing by urine
2. Mucus
3. Acidity of urine
4. Vaginal lactic acid

Figure 4.1 External defences against infection.

Skin

Intact skin provides the body with a tough outer layer that cannot be penetrated by microbes. Lactic acid and fatty acids secreted by sebaceous glands create a low pH which, together with an arid environment, prevent the growth of most micro-organisms. Some bacteria, for example diphtheroids and staphylococci, thrive on the surface of the skin and their presence discourages colonization by other species. Whilst this normal flora is usually harmless, some species (e.g. *Staphylococcus epidermidis*) may invade the bloodstream via invasive devices such as intravenous catheters (see Ch. 9). In hospital, the normal skin flora of patients may be replaced by strains of hospital bacteria that are more resistant to antibiotics and which can cause serious infections if they enter the body, for example methicillin-resistant *Staphylococcus aureus* (MRSA), klebsiella and acinetobacter species.

Skin that is damaged (e.g. burns, abrasions) or penetrated by invasive devices can be invaded by pathogens. Tetanus spores present in contaminated soil may be accidentally introduced through injured skin; human immunodeficiency virus (HIV) and hepatitis B virus by contact with infected blood or body fluids. Infection may also be introduced when skin is incised during surgical procedures or injured (e.g. stab wounds). Some micro-organisms are injected through the skin by the bites of insects (e.g. malaria, typhus and yellow fever).

Respiratory tract

Most micro-organisms are prevented from entering the bronchial tree by hairs in the nose, which filter particles, and the cough reflex, which prevents their aspiration. The membrane that lines the tract secretes mucus. This both traps particles that enter the airway and prevents micro-organisms from adhering to the tissues. Mucus is constantly moved by small hairs called cilia, which propel it upwards towards the mouth, where it is swallowed. This mechanism is called the ciliary escalator.

Lysozyme

This is an enzyme present in tears, nasal secretions and saliva, which breaks down bacterial cell walls and is especially active against Gram-positive bacteria.

Gastrointestinal tract

Gastric juices are highly acidic and a pH of between 2 and 3 destroys most ingested bacteria. Bile in the small intestine also inhibits bacterial growth. The large intestine contains many bacteria that discourage the growth of pathogens by competing for nutrients and producing inhibitory substances. Antimicrobial therapy may destroy some of the normal flora and enable other pathogenic species to establish, for example *Clostridium difficile* (see p. 257).

Genitourinary tract

These surfaces are protected by a mucous lining which prevents micro-organisms from adhering to the surface. In the urinary tract, the constant flow of urine flushes out bacteria. In the vagina, commensal lactobacilli produce lactic acid as a byproduct of their metabolism and the consequently low pH (between 4 and 5) prevents other species from establishing.

THE INNATE IMMUNE RESPONSE

When micro-organisms or other antigens penetrate the external defences of the body, the immune system starts to take action. A range of non-specific (innate) mechanisms effective against any antigen work in concert with the specific (adaptive) response discussed in the next section. The components of the innate defences are described below and summarized in Table 4.1.

Phagocytic cells

There are two types of phagocytic cell: polymorpho-nuclear granulocytes (neutrophils) and mononuclear macrophages (Plate 14). They are white blood cells that engulf foreign substances and destroy them with enzymes and other chemicals (e.g. hydroxyl radicals) by a process known as phagocytosis (Fig. 4.2).

Neutrophils are formed in the bone marrow (Fig. 4.3) and are the main white cell circulating in the blood. They are short-lived, circulating for only 6–8 h, and have receptors on their surface for complement proteins

Table 4.1   Components of the innate immune response

Component	Action
Phagocytic cells	Circulate through blood and tissues engulfing and destroying infectious agents
Complement system	A series of enzymes that attracts and activates phagocytic cells and increases the flow of blood to the affected area
Mast cells	Release factors that increase vascular permeability and attract phagocytic cells
Extracellular killer cells	Destroy virus–infected cells or large parasites by releasing enzymes onto them
Extracellular antimicrobial factors	Include lysozyme, lactoferrin and interferon

and antibodies. Large granules inside the cell contain enzymes such as lysozyme (which splits peptidoglycan walls) and lactoferrin (which prevents bacterial growth by depriving the cells of iron). These are used to destroy ingested micro-organisms.

Macrophages are also formed in the bone marrow (see Fig. 4.3). They are released into the blood as monocytes, maturing into macrophages which are long-lived and mostly concentrated in the tissues. In the spleen and lymph nodes, they filter out foreign material circulating through the lymph system. They pass into tissues by secreting enzymes that increase the permeability of blood vessels. Ingested micro-organisms are processed by enzymes and antigenic components of the micro-organism are then displayed

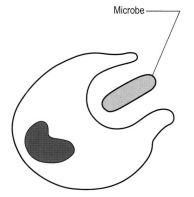 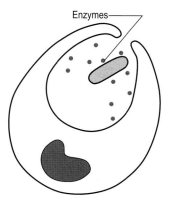

Figure 4.2   Phagocytosis.

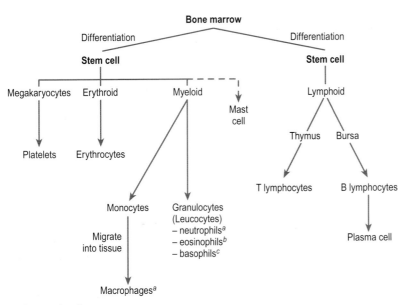

Figure 4.3   Differentiation of blood cells.

a Phagocytic cells
b Active against parasites, important in allergic reactions
c Circulating mast cells

on the surface of the macrophage for recognition by T and B lymphocytes (see p. 72).

Macrophages play an important role in attacking micro-organisms living inside host cells and in fighting chronic infections. *Mycobacterium tuberculosis* is ingested by macrophages but, by preventing the release of enzymes, is able to live and multiply in the white cell. Infected macrophages congregate and become surrounded by connective tissue to form a tubercle.

For phagocytosis to occur, the microbe (or other foreign substance) must first attach to a surface of the phagocytic cell. Recognition of foreign substances by phagocytes is not specific but greatly enhanced by complement proteins that coat the surface of the microbe. Phagocytes are attracted to the site of infection by damaged tissues, the products from bacterial cells, antibody complexes and complement proteins.

Extracellular killer cells

Eosinophils

These are polymorphonuclear cells, similar to neutrophils. They are activated by complement proteins to attack large invaders such as parasitic protozoa and helminths. These parasites are too large to be phagocytosed and instead are destroyed by enzymes and cationic proteins released on to them.

Natural killer cells

These are large granular lymphocytes that recognize and attach to virus-infected cells. They then release a protein, perforin, onto the target cell. This creates pores in the membrane, which allow other proteins into the cell to trigger its death.

Extracellular antimicrobial factors

Interferons

This is one of a family of chemical messenger molecules called cytokines (Table 4.2). They are synthesized and excreted by cells infected with a virus. They bind to specific receptors on non-infected cells and induce the production of enzymes, which degrade viral mRNA and inhibit protein synthesis. Interferon-α and -β are produced by all cells within 24 h of infection and play an important role in preventing the spread of viruses through tissues. Interferon is also produced by T lymphocytes when intracellular pathogens are encountered, acting to switch off antibody production and promote the activity of macrophages, causing them to degrade ingested micro-organisms and display their antigens on their surface for recognition by T lymphocytes.

Interferons are also known to be involved in mobilization of the immune response against tumour cells and are used to treat some cancers. Their value in therapy is limited by severe side-effects such as flu-

Table 4.2   Cytokines: chemical messengers of the immune system

Factor	Source	Activity
Interleukin 1	Macrophages	Vascular permeability
Interleukin 2, 7	T cells	T & B cell proliferation
Interleukin 4	T cells	T & B cell proliferation, activation of macrophages
Interleukin 6	T cells	B cell differentiation
Interleukin 8	T cells	Neutrophil activation
Interleukin 9	T cells	Growth of mast cells
Interleukin 10	T cells, B cells, macrophages	Inhibits T helper cell cytokine production
Interleukin 11	Bone marrow	Induces acute-phase proteins
Interleukin 12	Macrophages	Induces T helper cells
Interferon-α	All cells	Antiviral
Interferon-β	All cells	Antiviral
Interferon-γ	T cells, NK cells	Antiviral, activates macrophages, inhibits T helper cells
Tumour necrosis factor	Macrophages, T cells	Cytotoxicity, fever

like symptoms and bone marrow suppression but these problems may be overcome by using them in combination with other drugs.

Lactoferrin
This circulates in the blood, forming complexes of iron to prevent it being available for microbial growth.

Acute-phase proteins
These are proteins that appear in the plasma in response to infection. They include C-reactive protein, which triggers complement and opsonizes micro-organisms, fibrinogen, which causes coagulation, and fibronectin, which is involved in cell attachment.

Endotoxic shock occurs when microbial cells die and lipopolysaccharides (LPS) released from their cell walls strongly stimulate the immune response, in particular the cytokines interleukin-1 and tumour necrosis factor, causing high fever and vascular collapse (shock). Endotoxic shock is especially associated with infections caused by Gram-negative pathogens.

Complement proteins

These are a series of proteins that, when activated, have several important effects, essential for phagocytosis to take place:

- increase blood vessel permeability
- attract phagocytes (chemotaxis)
- increase efficiency of phagocytosis (opsonization)
- destroy foreign cells by puncturing their membrane.

The complement system is similar to blood clotting in that, once the first protein in the series is triggered, the product of each reaction is an enzyme that catalyses the next stage (Fig. 4.4). The series of reactions can be triggered in two ways. The classic pathway is initiated by the presence of antibody–antigen complexes; the alternative pathway is triggered by the attachment of the C3 convertase protein to molecules on the surface of micro-organisms. The subsequent reaction produces large amounts of C3b, which acts as an 'opsonin'; that is, it coats the surface of a particle, making it more susceptible to phagocytosis. Other complement proteins, such as C5a and C3a, trigger the release of mediators from mast cells (see below). Another component, C5b, binds to the bacterial membrane and, with several other proteins, causes a C9 protein to be inserted into the membrane. This allows water and electrolytes to flood in, causing lysis of the cell.

Mast cells

The mast cells are found in tissues and similar cells, basophils, circulate in the blood. When triggered by tissue injury or by complement proteins C3a, and C5a, they degranulate, releasing a range of vascular permeability mediators such as histamine, leukotrienes and prostaglandin, and chemotactic factors that attract phagocytic cells. The permeability mediators increase the permeability of capillaries so that more plasma fluid and proteins are brought into the area.

The acute inflammatory response

The capillary dilation and fluid exudation brought about by the activity of complement and mast cell mediators are visible as erythema and oedema. Together with the accumulation of phagocytes, this effect is called the acute inflammatory response. It provides a highly effective mechanism of repelling micro-organisms by directing phagocytic cells toward the primed, complement-coated, infectious agents. Increased body temperature, fever, is a systemic effect of the acute inflammatory response (Box 4.1).

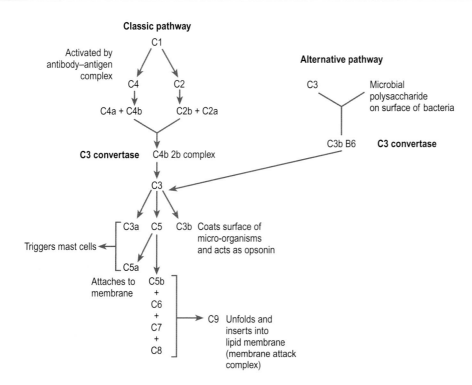

Figure 4.4   The complement system.

THE ADAPTIVE IMMUNE RESPONSE

Some microbes are able to evade the innate immune defences; they may not be readily ingested by phagocytic cells or recognized for attack by complement. The body therefore needs other mechanisms that can recognize specific micro-organisms and prevent them evading the innate defences. These mechanisms are provided by the lymphocytes and are called the adaptive immune response. Lymphocytes interact with specific antigens; they are able to remember a previous encounter with an antigen thus providing a very rapid response the next time the same antigen enters the body.

There are two types of lymphocytes, B and T, both of which recognize and bind to receptors on specific antigens. B lymphocytes produce antibodies against the specific antigen and are referred to as the humoral immune system. Humoral means 'of the body fluids' and is used to describe antibodies because they operate outside the cells in the blood and tissue fluids. T lymphocytes destroy abnormal or tumour cells and cells infected with viruses or other microbes. T lymphocytes are referred to as the cellular or cell-mediated immune system. The T lymphocytes also produce messenger molecules called cytokines (e.g. interferon) that activate other lymphocytes and macrophages.

The lymphocytes do not operate independently but act collectively to destroy the invading antigen. They interact with one another, with phagocytic cells and the complement system. The differentiation of blood cells into red cells, lymphocytes, leucocytes and macrophages is illustrated in Figure 4.3. The interaction between the different parts of the immune response is illustrated in Figure 4.5.

B lymphocytes

B lymphocytes originate from stem cells in the bone marrow. They are referred to as B cells because in birds they mature in a structure called the 'bursa of Fabricius'. B lymphocytes are responsible for the production of antibodies.

Structure of antibodies

Antibodies are Y-shaped proteins called globulins or immunoglobulins. The two arms of the Y vary in structure and are the parts of the molecule that enable the antibody to recognize or fit around different molecules on the surface of an antigen (Fig. 4.6). The antibody–antigen complex triggers the 'classic'

Box 4.1   Fever

The temperature of the body is maintained by a centre in the hypothalamus of the brain. Increased body temperature is a characteristic sign of infection, induced by pyrogens. These may be micro-organisms or their toxins or may be endogenous pyrogens such as interleukin or tumour necrosis factors released by macrophages and prostaglandins released by mast cells. These substances stimulate the hypothalamus and produce a rise in body temperature. Aspirin inhibits prostaglandins and is used to reduce fever in adults. Pyrexia is assumed to confer some advantage on the host, although the exact benefit is uncertain. High temperature increases the metabolic rate of the body and this may speed tissue repair and potentiate the immune response (Mackowiak et al 1997). Most pathogenic microbes prefer a temperature of around 37°C and therefore an increase in body temperature may help the body to destroy them. The effect of fever on the patient can be exhausting; the heart and respiratory rates increase and violent shivering or rigors may occur in severe fever. This increased activity may cause depletion of the glycogen energy reserves in the body and so protein may need to be broken down as a source of energy, the patient becomes debilitated and tissue repair is delayed. Children have immature temperature control and may experience febrile convulsions if the pyrexia develops rapidly. Although the convulsions are usually transient with no long-term effects, they may lead to aspiration of secretions and asphyxia.

pathway of the complement system (see Fig. 4.4) by activating C1, culminating in the formation of the membrane attack complex (MAC), which may destroy the micro-organisms, and the opsonization of the cell for engulfment by phagocytes. The stem of the antibody is also able to activate phagocytosis.

There are five different types of immunoglobulin, distinguishable by their structure and number of amino acid chains (Table 4.3). The same B lymphocytes produce all types of immunoglobulin and each recognizes the same antigen.

Synthesis of antibodies

Thousands of B lymphocytes are produced and circulate around the body. Each B lymphocyte displays a different antibody on its surface. These attach to a specific antigen that has a complementary shape, like a lock and key. When a lymphocyte encounters an antigen that fits the antibody it is carrying, it binds to the antigen and is triggered to convert into a plasma cell. This cell synthesizes large quantities of the particular antibody carried by the lymphocyte. The plasma cells then divide rapidly to produce a large number of identical cells or clones, all of which carry the same antibody. This mechanism enables a large amount of specific antibody to be produced when required. T lymphocytes influence the division and maturation of the plasma cells with messenger proteins (cytokines) which bind to receptors on the surface of the B lymphocyte.

The first type of immunoglobulin to be synthesized by the plasma cell is IgM. After a few days, T lymphocytes trigger a switch in production to IgG (see Table 4.3). Production of IgG can continue for up to 1 year. As IgG is the only class of immunoglobulin that can cross the placenta, newborn infants acquire only IgG from their mother. This disappears after approximately 6 months and the child begins to synthesize its own IgM. Levels of IgG and IgA remain below those of an adult until the child is 7 and 12 years old, respectively. IgE is a specialized antibody whose stem binds to the surface of mast cells. When its variable region binds to an antigen, it triggers the mast cell to release its vascular permeability and phagocyte chemotactic factors.

One micro-organism may have several receptor sites recognized by different antibodies. Antibodies can also bind to virus antigens, preventing them from binding to and entering host cells, or to bacterial toxins, preventing them from damaging host cells.

T lymphocytes

These lymphocytes are formed in the bone marrow but mature in a gland called the thymus that is situated behind the sternum. The thymus is prominent in children, continuing to grow until puberty. It then gradually diminishes in size, although it is still active in old age.

T lymphocytes provide a defence against micro-organisms that live inside cells and are therefore shielded from attack by antibodies. They also play a key role in co-ordinating the immune response through the release of cytokines (see Table 4.2).

There are two types of T lymphocyte: cytotoxic T cells, which destroy infected cells and tumour cells, and T helper cells, which regulate the activity of other cells, co-ordinating the attack by the immune system.

Recognition of infected cells

T lymphocytes are particularly important for the control of intracellular parasites such as mycobacteria, fungi, viruses and protozoa. Antibodies can attack

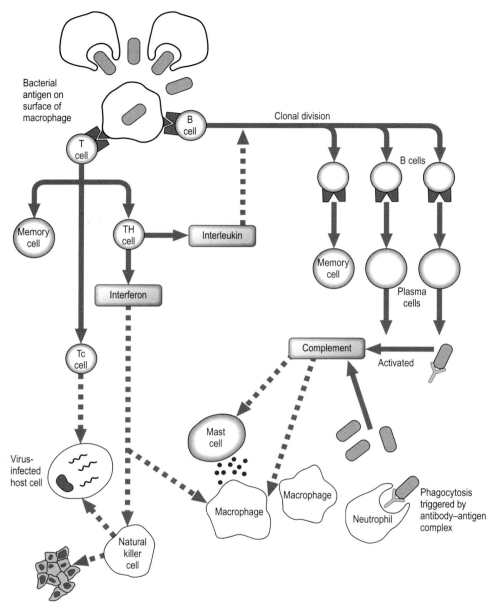

Figure 4.5 The specific immune response. The B cells, T cells and macrophages all interact to fend off the attack from invading micro-organisms.

these microbes while they are in the blood or tissue fluid but not if they are inside a host cell. Many micro-organisms can multiply inside phagocytes that engulf them. To attack these pathogens, the T lymphocyte must be able to identify infected cells. They do this by recognizing 'non-self' antigens on the surface of an infected cell. All cells constantly degrade proteins into small fragments which bind to a molecule called the major histocompatibility complex (MHC) and are carried to the surface of the cell. Fragments from the host cell proteins are ignored by circulating T lymphocytes but when a 'non-self' fragment from a micro-organism infecting the cell is displayed, a T lymphocyte with the appropriately shaped receptor

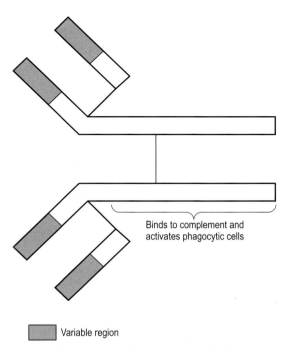

Variable region

Figure 4.6 The structure of immunoglobulin G. IgG is made of two long and two short peptide chains. The variable regions determine the specificity of the antibody.

Binds to complement and activates phagocytic cells

Immunoglobulin	Activity
IgG	The most abundant; diffuses from blood vessels into tissue fluids. Coats bacteria to facilitate phagocytosis and neutralize bacterial toxins. Crosses the placenta in the last 3 months of pregnancy
IgM	A large molecule made up of five short and five long chains of amino acids. Is the first to appear in an attack against an antigen but is confined to blood. Assists phagocytosis by coating the antigen and binds efficiently with complement
IgA	Acts as the early defence against microbial invasion of mucous membranes. Found in the secretions of reproductive, respiratory and gastrointestinal tract, where it coats micro-organisms and prevents them from adhering to epithelial cells
IgE	Mainly attached to mast cells where it causes the release of vasodilatory and chemotactic mediators if it encounters an antigen. Associated with allergic response (e.g. hay fever) but also thought to be involved in the destruction of parasites
IgD	Maximum levels are detected during childhood but function is unknown

Table 4.3 Different classes of immunoglobulin (antibody)

locks on to the combination of MHC and microbial fragment (Fig. 4.7). Like B lymphocytes, T lymphocytes are programmed at the time they are made with a unique surface receptor. Each T lymphocyte will therefore recognize a specific antigen which best fits the shape of this receptor.

Destruction of intracellular pathogens

Once the T lymphocyte has bound on to the MHC and microbial fragment, it is triggered to divide rapidly, producing a large number of T lymphocytes all carrying the same surface receptor. Some of these cells produce cytokines, others have cytotoxic activity. Cytotoxic T cells recognize viral fragments combined with the MHC and attack the infected cell with enzymes before new virus can be released. T helper lymphocytes recognize microbial fragments on an infected macrophage and release interferon-γ, which activates the suppressed macrophage to destroy the micro-organism.

T helper cells also produce a range of interleukins. These are cytokines, soluble factors that act on other cells in the immune system and co-ordinate the response to the invasion (see Table 4.2). They play a key role in the activity of B lymphocytes, promoting antibody production in response to bacterial invasion and suppressing it in favour of T lymphocyte activity in response to intracellular pathogens.

Memory cells

Following exposure to a particular antigen, both B and T lymphocytes produce memory cells to protect against subsequent infections (see Fig. 4.5). These are primed to respond if the same antigen is encountered again, enabling the production of a large number of specific lymphocytes. A second exposure to a previously encountered antigen therefore results in the appearance of specific antibody at 10–15 times the concentration of the first response within 3 days. These memory cells enable immunity to specific infections to develop and form the basis of active immunization to prevent the acquisition of infection.

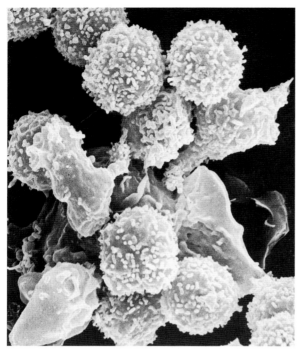

Figure 4.7 T cells recognize an antigen on the surface of a macrophage. The T cells are the small spherical objects, the macrophage the larger, flat object (reproduced with kind permission from Ackerman & Dunk-Richards 1991).

Monoclonal antibodies

A large amount of a single antibody can be manufactured artificially by fusing a cell producing specific antibodies with a cell from a B lymphocyte tumour. The fused cells survive and multiply indefinitely in tissue culture and produce many copies of the single specific antibody. These monoclonal antibodies are used in research on infectious diseases and the immune system and for the identification of some micro-organisms (e.g. legionella, chlamydia, viruses). They can provide very specific and sensitive tests enabling particular proteins to be isolated from complex mixtures.

The recognition of self and non-self

Defence against an invader is possible only if the immune system is able to distinguish between the cells of the host (self) and those of the invader (non-self). At birth the immune system is immature and does not respond to self and non-self antigens that it encounters, possibly because neonatal macrophages are unable to present antigens or because all the self-reacting B and T lymphocytes are inactivated. T lymphocytes are particularly important in the recognition and destruction of 'non-self' cells. They undergo a process of differentiation in the thymus that results in the elimination of any lymphocytes that might recognize self markers. The final set of T lymphocytes therefore recognizes only 'non-self' markers.

Each cell of the body also carries on its surface a distinct marker of 'selfness' called the major histo-compatibility complex (MHC), which not only differs between species but between individuals of the same species. The segment of chromosome that codes for these 'self-marking' molecules is called the human leucocyte antigen (HLA) system.

The MHC markers enable the immune system to recognize and destroy tissue grafted into the body from another person. Grafted material is less likely to be attacked by the immune system if the MHC proteins of the donated material are similar to those of the host. Tissue typing is used to find donors whose MHC proteins are very similar to those of the intended recipient of the tissue.

Organs of the immune system

The immune response is mounted from lymphoid tissue found throughout the body at points vulnerable to invasion (Fig. 4.8). These are connected by a network of small channels called the lymphatic system. There is lymphoid tissue in the liver, spleen, gut (Peyer's patches and appendix), tonsils and adenoids. It is also found in the lymph nodes – small glands distributed throughout the body at junctions between lymph and blood vessels. The cells of the immune system are made in the bone marrow. They differentiate from a single stem cell into several different lines which produce lymphocytes, macrophages and granulocytes (e.g. neutrophils). Once they have matured, the cells migrate to the lymphoid tissue.

Response to invasion by micro-organisms

When a micro-organism reaches a lymph node or other lymphoid tissue, it is trapped and ingested by macrophages. These process the micro-organism and display its antigens on their surface for recognition by T lymphocytes. The T lymphocytes then bind to the antigen and trigger the specific immune response against the invading micro-organism. The lymph nodes closest to the site of infection will mount the immune response and this is apparent when they become swollen and painful; for example, an infection of the leg may cause lymph nodes in the groin to swell, whilst an infection of the upper respiratory tract causes nodes in the neck to swell. Once the micro-

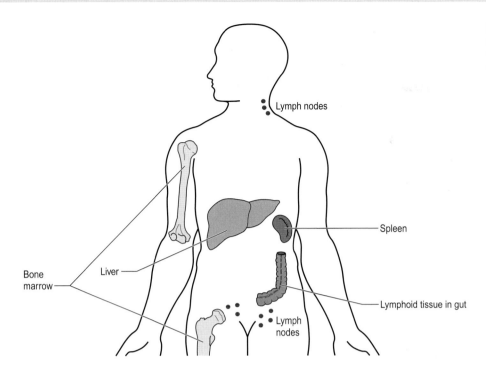

Figure 4.8 The organs of the immune response (reproduced with kind permission from Ackerman & Dunk-Richards 1991).

Lymph nodes

Spleen

Bone marrow

Liver

Lymphoid tissue in gut

Lymph nodes

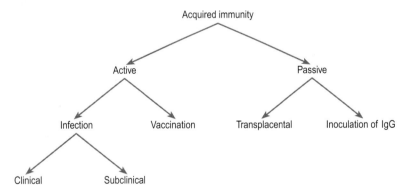

Figure 4.9 Acquired immunity to infection.

Acquired immunity

Active

Passive

Infection

Vaccination

Transplacental

Inoculation of IgG

Clinical

Subclinical

organisms have been destroyed, B and T lymphocyte memory cells remain and are distributed throughout the lymphoid tissue, enabling a rapid response to be made should the pathogen invade again.

IMMUNITY TO INFECTION

The B and T lymphocyte memory cells enable a very rapid response to be mounted against micro-organisms encountered previously. This enables the host to develop immunity to infections. Immunity can be acquired naturally following an infection or artificially by the inoculation of an organism or its products into the body. Immunity can also be conferred by injecting

antibody (IgG) against a specific micro-organism. This is called passive immunity because it does not cause the production of memory cells and the protection lasts only for the lifetime of the IgG. IgG crosses the placenta from mother to fetus so that the baby has some protection against infection for the first few months of life (Fig. 4.9).

Immunization

In the developed world, the ravages of infectious disease have declined dramatically in the last 100 years and immunization is one of several factors that have played a part in this decline (Box 4.2). The

Table 4.4   Types of vaccine in routine use

Type of vaccine	Examples in routine use
Live attenuated organisms	Polio, measles, mumps, rubella, BCG
Killed organisms	Pertussis, cholera, typhoid
Viral proteins	Influenza
Capsule polysaccharide	Meningococcus, pneumococcus
Genetically engineered	Hepatitis B
Inactivated toxin	Diphtheria, tetanus

principles of immunization were developed in the early 1800s. They were pioneered by Edward Jenner, who in 1796 demonstrated that humans could be protected against smallpox by inoculation with a similar virus which caused cowpox in cows; this was the first use of a vaccine (Plate 15).

Vaccines

The aim of vaccination is to induce a specific immune response against a particular micro-organism without causing the actual disease. Most vaccines produce their protective effect by stimulating the production of antibodies, although the bacillus Calmette–Guérin (BCG) vaccine for tuberculosis promotes cell-mediated immunity.

There are a number of different types of vaccine available (Table 4.4). Some are made from dead micro-organisms, others from live micro-organisms that have been altered (attenuated) to prevent them causing infection. A few are made from bacterial products such as altered toxins.

Killed micro-organisms   These can be made from whole cells that have been killed, for example by heat or formaldehyde, or from purified components of the cell such as capsule proteins. Although safe, they are usually less immunogenic and several doses are required to induce immunity.

Live-attenuated   These use live micro-organisms that have been altered to prevent them causing infection. They induce a good immune response because the organism multiplies in the body, resulting in a high level of antigen production. Some live-attenuated vaccines can induce a long-lasting immunity after just a single dose (e.g. measles, mumps, rubella (MMR) vaccine). Attenuated strains occasionally revert to their disease-causing ('wild-type') form and the vaccines can therefore be associated with complications (e.g. encephalitis in association with measles vaccination). The BCG vaccine against tuberculosis is a live-attenuated vaccine of a related organism, *Mycobacterium bovis*. In the future, the deletion of specific genes conferring virulence is likely to be used to produce new live-attenuated vaccines.

Inactivated toxin   Toxins produced by a micro-organism are inactivated by treatment with formaldehyde. Although the resulting toxoid induces an immune response, its toxic activity is destroyed. Adsorption of the toxoid on to aluminium hydroxide reduces the rate at which it diffuses from the site of inoculation and stimulates macrophage activity. *Haemophilus influenzae* type B (HIB) vaccine contains the capsular polysaccharide of *H. influenzae* combined with tetanus and diphtheria toxoids that are used to improve the immunogenicity.

Genetically engineered   Gene manipulation techniques have now been applied to vaccine production. The genes that code for specific microbial antigens (the part of the bacterium or virus recognized by the immune system) are isolated and inserted into a piece of DNA which is transferred into a yeast and cultured in a very large fermenter. The yeast makes the antigen, which is then recovered, purified and made into a vaccine. This method is used to make a vaccine for hepatitis B.

New approaches are based on using live-attenuated micro-organisms as a vector to express the required antigen. For example, antigens for hepatitis B, influenza and herpes simplex virus have been inserted into the vaccinia virus genome and inoculation with vaccinia then used to induce immunity to all the infections. Some organisms present particular problems for vaccine production. The orthomyxoviruses, which cause influenza, undergo minor changes to the proteins on their surface (antigenic drift) and occasionally major changes (antigenic shift). The latter occurs when large sections of chromosome are exchanged with viruses from other animal hosts. Antibody made to the antigens on one strain of influenza may not recognize the antigens on the surface of the next season's strain. When an antigenic shift occurs, the population will have little immunity to the new strain and an epidemic of influenza may result. Influenza vaccine is made from several different viral strains and is prepared each year by identifying the strains most likely to be prevalent. It is recommended mainly for the elderly or those with heart and chest disease who are most vulnerable. The vaccine provides reasonable protection against the selected strains but protection only lasts for about 1 year (DoH 1996).

HIV presents similar problems because when it replicates, the genome is frequently copied inaccurately. Copies of the virus therefore vary slightly which makes it difficult for the immune system to respond effectively.

Administration of vaccines

Injection of a vaccine into an individual who has not previously been exposed to the infection induces a slow production of antibody, mostly IgM. The level rises to a peak within a few weeks and may then fall to undetectable levels. This is called the primary response. Further injections produce a more rapid response to a higher level, for longer; this is called the secondary response. The level of IgM produced is similar to the primary response but a much greater amount of IgG is produced (Fig. 4.10). After a full course of vaccine the level of antibody remains high for months or years. Another single dose of vaccine will increase the level of antibody rapidly because the immune system has been induced to make memory cells. Most immunizations require a course of at least three injections, although some vaccines of live-attenuated micro-organisms (e.g. MMR) produce a high level of antibody after one injection. In many cases, vaccination has been shown to confer protection for at least 15 years (e.g. rubella and BCG). Others may require a booster dose every few years (e.g. cholera).

Passive immunization

The immunity conferred by active immunization with vaccine takes several weeks to establish as it depends on the production of specific antibodies or immuno-globulins. In certain situations, where an individual has been exposed to an infection and is known to have no immunity to it, a more rapid protection against infection is required. The specific antibodies or immunoglobulins made after exposure to particular micro-organisms can be collected from people recently infected or who have high levels of antibody following immunization. If inoculated into another person, these

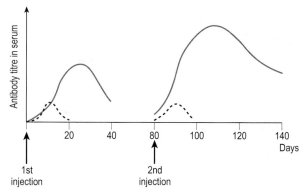

Figure 4.10   Immunization: the primary and secondary response. Small amounts of IgG (–) and IgM (---) are formed after the first injection but disappear fairly rapidly. After the second injection IgG reaches a higher level and persists in the serum for much longer.

specific immunoglobulins will protect against infection, although the protection will be only temporary as they will gradually be lost from the body.

This type of immunization can be used to protect against infection by hepatitis B following a needlestick injury and to protect immunocompromised individuals, who may develop serious illness, from chickenpox following exposure to the virus.

The impact of immunization programmes

Immunization is aimed at protecting individuals against a life-threatening or serious disease, a fetus (for example by the immunization of women against rubella) or the community as a whole through the principle of 'herd immunity'. If sufficient numbers of a population are immune to the disease, the micro-organism is unable to find susceptible hosts in which to cause infection. For herd immunity to be effective, a minimum of 60% of the population must be immune and a higher level if the infection spreads rapidly and is highly contagious.

It is rare for an infection to be completely eradicated through immunization alone. The smallpox eradication programme was started in 1959 by the World Health Organization and not completed until the last case (outside a laboratory) occurred in 1977. Its success depended on an effective vaccine, an easily identifiable disease with no animal or environmental reservoir, and an intensive worldwide surveillance and immunization programme.

It is essential that high rates of immunization are maintained. In instances when diphtheria immu-nization has been relaxed, resurgence of the disease has occurred rapidly. Following fears in the mid-1970s

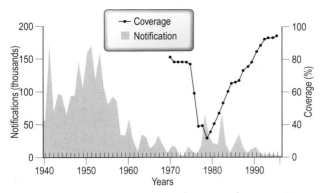

Figure 4.11 Pertussis notifications (1940–1995) and the effect of immunization uptake (DoH 1996) (Crown Copyright; redrawn with permission from the Controller of Her Majesty's Stationery Office).

Table 4.5   Schedule for routine immunization

Vaccine	Age	
Diphtheria, tetanus, pertussis (DTP), polio, *Haemophilus influenzae* (Hib)	2 months 3 months 4 months	1st dose 2nd dose 3rd dose
Measles, mumps, rubella (MMR)	12–15 months	1st dose
Diphtheria, tetanus, polio, measles, mumps, rubella (MMR)	4–5 years	Booster 2nd dose
BCG	10–14 years or infancy	
Tetanus, diphtheria, polio	13–18 years	Booster

about brain damage associated with the pertussis vaccine, the rate of immunization fell from over 80% to 30%. As a result, the number of cases of whooping cough increased from around 2400 in 1973 to over 100 000 in 1977–79 (Fig. 4.11).

As with all medicines, vaccines carry some risk but, even with the pertussis vaccine, the risk is extremely small and less than the risk of serious complications from the disease itself.

In the UK, the Department of Health recommends a schedule of immunization from early childhood and the primary healthcare services are responsible for its implementation (Table 4.5). Detailed information about all aspects of vaccines is available in the Department of Health publication *Immunisation Against Infectious Disease* (DoH 1996). Updates on diphtheria, HIB, pertussis, polio and tetanus were published in 2004.

THE DAMAGED IMMUNE SYSTEM

Individuals vary widely in their ability to resist infection and this depends on many factors, including age, general health, state of nutrition, previous exposure to infection and vaccination. Young children have an immature immune system and are more likely to succumb to infection until they have developed a range of specific memory cells. The elderly also have a diminished immune response, particularly by the T lymphocytes, and are more susceptible to infection.

Physical or emotional stress, for example multiple traumatic injury or major surgery, can affect the immune response through the release of anti-inflammatory hormones such as corticosteroids from the adrenal glands. In major burns, immuno-suppression occurs through the loss of white blood cells and immunoglobulins and reduced phagocytic function. Poor nutrition impairs phagocytosis and reduces the production of white blood cells and antibodies (Conry 1982).

These factors should be taken into account when assessing a patient's risk of acquiring an infection. The immune system of a patient who is malnourished or under stress will be less able to destroy bacteria that invade wounds, intravenous cannulae, etc. Planning the care of patients to improve the activity of their immune system is essential if infection is to be prevented.

Disease associated with immune deficiency

Impairment of the immune response occurs as a result of a variety of genetic disorders, autoimmune disease, chemotherapy and certain viral infections, notably HIV.

The most serious genetic disorder is severe combined immune deficiency disorder in which there is a failure of the bone marrow stem cells to differentiate into B and T cells and as a result, lymphocytes are not produced. It can be treated by bone marrow trans-plantation but the children often die from infection at a few months of age, before the diagnosis has been made.

Autoimmune disorders occur as a result of a malfunction of the body's mechanism for the recognition of cells as 'self', resulting in antibodies being made against host tissue. The damage to the tissue or the deposition of antibody–antigen complexes in joints, blood vessels or kidney causes the symptoms of the disease (Table 4.6).

In rheumatic fever, antibodies formed against *Streptococcus pyogenes* infection in the throat cross-react with tissue on the heart valves that has very similar receptors. The antibodies recognize the heart valves as

Table 4.6   Autoimmune diseases

Autoimmune disease	Self–antigen recognized
Pernicious anaemia	Gastric parietal cells
Juvenile insulin-dependent diabetes	Pancreatic islet cells
Multiple sclerosis	Central nervous system myelin
Lupus erythematosus	DNA, red blood cells, lymphocytes, platelets

an antigen and the resulting damage is called endocarditis.

Chemotherapy can have profound immuno-suppressive effects. Cytotoxic drugs interfere non-specifically in cell division but because bone marrow cells divide very frequently, about once every 12–30 h, the drugs have a major effect on bone marrow and the production of blood cells. Some antibiotics inhibit cellular immunity (e.g. chloramphenicol, tetracycline). Steroids have long-term effects on the production of immunoglobulins by inhibiting the production of cytokines and therefore interfere with the inflammatory response.

Leukaemias are a group of malignant diseases affecting the white cell precursors in the bone marrow. Susceptibility to infection is increased through the overproduction of immature or abnormal white blood cells and the suppression of normal cell production.

Aplastic anaemia is a severe depression of the bone marrow which causes depletion of red blood cells, white blood cells and platelets. There are a variety of causes of aplastic anaemia, including exposure to drugs (e.g. chloramphenicol), chemicals (e.g. benzene) or ionizing radiation.

Human immunodeficiency virus and acquired immune deficiency syndrome

The human immunodeficiency virus (HIV) recognizes and infects cells in the body that carry particular receptor proteins on their surface. The principal cell surface receptor recognized by HIV is a glycoprotein called CD4 that is carried on the surface of T lymphocytes and other immune system cells such as macrophages and dendritic cells of the mucous membranes. Other co-receptors are also necessary to enable the virus to successfully lock onto and infect the cell. These receptors are proteins normally recognized by cytokines (see p. 69). Variants of HIV use different co-receptors: the M trophic variant infects macrophages and monocytes as well as T lymphocytes; T trophic variants only infect T lymphocytes but replicate and

kill cells very rapidly. Individuals infected with HIV will have both variants of the virus.

Once the virus has inserted a DNA copy of its genome into the host cell, hundreds of new copies of the virus are transcribed, packaged into new virus, bud out of the cell membrane and the host cell dies. The transcription process in retroviruses is particularly prone to errors; whilst this means that many copies of the virus are defective, it also enables variants with biological advantages to develop and hampers the ability of both the immune system and drugs to eliminate the infection.

At the time of infection the immune system mounts a response to the virus. Although antibodies and T lymphocyte activity have some success against the virus, the immune system is eventually unable to keep up with the high rate of viral replication. In most people, the gradual damage to the immune system takes many years to become symptomatic. Eventually the decline in T lymphocytes and deterioration in immune response enables a range of organisms and malignancies normally held in check by the immune system to establish infection. Early symptoms include protracted diarrhoea which may be caused by a range of gastrointestinal pathogens, e.g. strongyloides, giardia, candidiasis. Later on, as the immune system becomes progressively impaired, severe, often disseminated infections occur, for example *Pneumocystis jiroveci* (formerly *carinii*), toxoplasmosis, cryptococcus, herpes simplex, tuberculosis and atypical forms of myco-bacteria. At this stage the patient is defined as having acquired immune deficiency syndrome (AIDS).

Antiretroviral therapy aimed at the reverse transcriptase and protease enzymes can be used to slow viral replication. Although these drugs have had a major effect on the survival of people with HIV, they will not cure the infection. Highly active antiretroviral therapy (HAART) involving a combination of at least three drugs is used to treat symptomatic patients, those with very low CD4 counts or very high viral load. However, the side-effects of this treatment are severe and resistance to the drugs can develop, especially where adherence to the drug regimen is incomplete.

Hypersensitivity reactions

Sometimes the immune system responds in an excessive way to an antigen. This is called a hyper-sensitivity reaction. The reaction may be mild, for instance hay fever induced by allergy to pollen, or severe and systemic, as with anaphylactic reactions that are sometimes fatal (e.g. insect stings in a highly sensitized person).

Hypersensitivity reactions are caused by the rapid release of vasoactive amines from mast cells. These are triggered rapidly when exposed to the antigen for a second time and result in local vascular permeability and oedema. If excessive amounts are released into the bloodstream, hypotensive shock, cardiac and respiratory failure may occur.

Delayed hypersensitivity reactions are mediated by T lymphocytes and occur 24–48 h after exposure to an intracellular pathogen. This reaction is the basis of the Heaf test used to determine immunity to *Mycobacterium tuberculosis*.

Organ transplants

It is now possible to treat many illnesses by replacing diseased organs or tissue with healthy tissue from another person, for example kidney, heart, lung and bone marrow. One of the major obstacles to successful organ transplantation is the rejection of the new or 'grafted' material by the recipient's immune system. The surface markers on the foreign tissue cells are recognized as 'non-self' and the foreign material is gradually destroyed, primarily by the T lymphocytes of the cellular immune system. This response is called 'graft versus host disease' or GVHD. Successful transplantation therefore depends on tissue typing, the selection of donor material that is closely related to that of the recipient and less likely to be destroyed, and the use of immunosuppressant drugs that interfere with the activity of T lymphocytes.

One of the most useful of these drugs was originally derived from a fungus and is called cyclosporin A. It blocks the production of lymphokines and therefore affects the immune response to new antigens but not the response by memory cells to previously encountered antigens. Tacrolimus, also derived from a fungus, has a similar but more potent effect. Another commonly used drug, azathioprine, inhibits the synthesis of nucleic acids and therefore prevents cell division. It has a preferential effect on T cells but also affects cells in the bone marrow and intestine.

PREVENTING INFECTION IN THE IMMUNOCOMPROMISED PATIENT

Individuals who have a severely damaged immune system are at particular risk of life-threatening infection acquired either endogenously or exogenously whilst in hospital. They are more likely to be exposed to infection by contact with other patients and staff and through invasive procedures that bypass their defences against micro-organisms.

The immunocompromised host

The expression 'compromised host' is a vague term used to describe an individual who has a severely impaired immune system. Damage to the immune system renders these individuals particularly susceptible to infection, even by 'opportunists', micro-organisms that are not usually able to cause serious infection, such as *Pneumocystis jiroveci* (formerly *carinii*) or *Candida albicans*.

The type of infection associated with immunodeficiency depends on the part of the immune system that is affected. If the cellular or T cell response is reduced, those microbes that cause intracellular infections predominate. Examples are salmonella, listeria, cryptococcus, pneumocystis and viruses that persist in a latent form, such as herpes virus and cytomegalovirus. If the humoral or B lymphocyte response is affected, protection against bacterial pathogens such as *Staphylococcus aureus* and pneumococcus is reduced. The phagocytic cells or granulocytes are important for both the B and T lymphocyte responses; therefore, a reduction in the number of these cells increases susceptibility to a wide range of infections, particularly Gram-negative bacteria, *Staphylococcus epidermidis* and *S. aureus*. Neutrophils account for the largest proportion of granulocytes and in immunocompromised patients, the number of neutrophils circulating in the blood is an important indicator of susceptibility to infection. Granulocytopenic patients are most vulnerable to infection from opportunistic pathogens amongst their own microbial flora. However, they are also more susceptible to infection from inhaled or ingested pathogens, micro-organisms introduced to the tissue via invasive devices such as intravenous cannulae or transferred by equipment or on the hands of staff (Wey 1997).

Bone marrow transplant

Bone marrow transplantation (BMT) has become standard therapy for many blood disorders and some solid tumours. Haematopoietic progenitor cells are infused to re-establish bone marrow function. These cells may be obtained from a compatible donor (allogenic) or taken from the patient prior to high-dose chemotherapy (autologous). Prior to the bone marrow infusion, the patient's own haematopoietic cells must be removed, e.g. by chemotherapy and total body irradiation, so that the grafted cells can become established. The patient is at significant risk of acquiring infection during this time, although the risk varies at different times post transplant, reflecting the predominant deficit in the host defence system (Fig. 4.12).

Patients are most vulnerable to infection in the first month after the transplant when they are severely granulocytopenic with less than 1000 neutrophils per

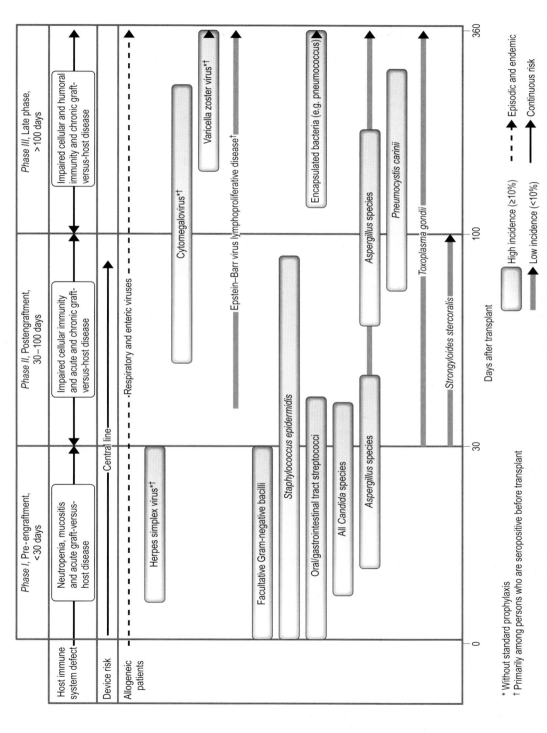

Figure 4.12 Phases of opportunistic infections among allogenic bone marrow recipients (reproduced with permission from US Dept of Health and Human Sciences (2000) *Guidelines for Preventing Opportunistic Infections among Hematopoietic Stem Cell Transplant Recipients*. MMWR, USA).

microlitre of blood (Bodey et al 1966, Tablan et al 1994). Damage to the mucosal progenitor cells which normally protect the mucosa increases susceptibility to pathogens from the gut and oral mucosa, especially candida. Frequent vascular access increases their risk of infection by skin organisms. At this stage both autologous and allogenic recipients are equally vulnerable but once the graft has taken, the immune system of allogenic graft recipients takes much longer to recover, particularly if they develop GVHD and their vulnerability to certain infections is prolonged (Wey 1997).

Severely granulocytopenic patients are vulnerable to infections caused by environmental pathogens such as legionella and the fungus aspergillus. The spores of this fungus are carried in the air and, if inhaled, can cause invasive pulmonary aspergillosis, a serious infection associated with a high mortality rate. The infection may also disseminate to other organs via the bloodstream. Patients most at risk are those who have severe, prolonged granulocytopenia, and outbreaks of aspergillosis have been reported in bone marrow transplant units associated with contamination of hospital ventilation systems and high spore levels as a result of construction work (Tablan et al 1994).

Solid organ transplant

Patients receiving solid organ transplants such as heart or kidney are usually less severely immunosuppressed because more targeted immunosuppression using cyclosporin A or tacrolimus is possible. However, patients may have increased vulnerability to infection because of prolonged chronic illness, such as renal failure, and are at increased risk of acquiring highly antibiotic-resistant strains of bacteria. The risk of infection following transplant depends on the type of organ. For example, renal transplantation is associated with a relatively low risk of serious infection, whilst more than 50% of liver transplant patients are likely to develop infection and many will die as a result (Singh 1997).

Simple protective isolation

Complex methods of preventing infection in immunocompromised patients have been recommended, including the use of sterile equipment, masks, gowns, gloves and overshoes. However, such extensive precautions are expensive and increase the emotional deprivation of the patient and family and there is evidence that they are no more effective in preventing infections than more simple methods (Garner 1996, Mank & Van-der-leilie 2003, Russel et al 2000).

Key to protecting patients who have damaged immune response from infection is reducing their exposure to potential new pathogens. They are most at risk from devices that bypass normal mechanical defences, such as vascular and urinary catheters. The highest standards of infection control should therefore be used routinely for the care of these patients. Box 4.3 summarizes the main infection control procedures required for protective isolation.

Accommodation   Most immunocompromised patients do not require segregation from other patients provided that simple precautions are taken to avoid exposure to other people with infectious diseases (e.g. chickenpox, respiratory tract infection). Common upper respiratory infection such as respiratory syncytial virus can also cause serious illness in patients undergoing bone marrow transplantation. Early identification and isolation of infected patients and restriction of infected visitors and staff are important to prevent transmission (Garcia et al 1997).

If an immunocompromised patient develops an infectious disease, careful adherence to source isolation procedures is essential to prevent spread amongst other vulnerable patients. For infections spread by an airborne route, this may involve restriction to a single room (Hannan et al 2000).

Severely granulocytopenic patients are at risk of aspergillosis which is acquired through inhalation of airborne spores. Single room accommodation, preferably with positive pressure ventilation (i.e. air pressure is higher inside the room to ensure that air flow is directed out of the room), high efficiency particulate air (HEPA) filtered air supply and frequent air changes (at least 12 per hour) are therefore recommended for these patients (Schulster & Chin 2003). Such air handling systems must be regularly monitored to ensure they are operating effectively and the pressure differentials are maintained (Humphries 2004). During periods of construction the levels of airborne aspergillus spores may be extremely high and precautions for bone marrow transplant patients should be reviewed under these circumstances (Schulster & Chin 2003).

There is evidence that patients in protective isolation are able to cope better with the experience than those isolated because of an infectious disease. This may be because the immunocompromised are involved in the decision to isolate and prepared for the experience (Collins et al 1989). However, isolation can cause patients to become demanding and irritable and these behaviours should be recognized as a response to isolation (Denton 1986). Psychosocial care of the patient is important to help them through the period of isolation but is frequently overlooked (Gaskill et al 1997, Knowles 1993) (see Table 14.3). It should form part of the holistic care of all isolated patients.

Box 4.3   Policy for the protective isolation of immunocompromised patients

Indication
Patients with a severely compromised immune system

Aims
- To reduce the risk of an immunologically compromised patient acquiring infection
- To give psychological support and reassurance to the patient whilst in isolation
- To ensure all staff (including domestic staff) are aware of the correct precautions to take

Equipment
- A single room with a washbasin and toilet
- The room must be clean before the patient is isolated

Inside room: soap
paper towels
washbowl
sphygmomanometer
alcohol handrub
disposable clean gloves
disposable plastic aprons
- Display a protective isolation card at the entrance to the room

Practice	Rationale
Patient – explain reason for isolation and give reassurance	To reduce anxiety and gain the patient's co-operation
Apron – put on a disposable plastic apron before contact with the patient and between dirty and clean procedures	To prevent transmission of organisms from clothing to patient
Gloves – not necessary except for aseptic procedures and contact with blood and body fluids. Discard immediately after use	To prevent contamination of vulnerable sites and cross-infection from one site to another
Masks – not necessary	
Hands – always decontaminate hands before entering the room. Repeat after removing gloves, before handling invasive devices or contact with susceptible sites	To remove transient micro-organisms
Staff – exclude staff with infections. Staff who are nursing patients with infections should avoid nursing patients in protective isolation during the same span of duty	To minimize the risk of transferring micro-organisms
Equipment – clean thoroughly with detergent and water before use	To remove micro-organisms
Crockery – use normal utensils and wash in the normal way	The risk of cross-infection is minimal
Visitors – instruct to decontaminate hands on entering room; exclude those with infections	To remove potential pathogens
Other department – should be notified in advance and where possible the patient seen on the ward	To enable appropriate arrangements to be made
Cleaning – ensure that a high standard of cleaning is maintained. Explain the precautions to domestic staff	Dust may harbour micro-organisms. Regular cleaning will remove them
Food – always wash hands and put on a disposable apron before handling food. Food must be served without delay and meals must not be retained for reheating later	These patients are more susceptible to illness from pathogenic bacteria in food. Bacteria multiply in food unless stored at above 65°C or below 5°C
If a microwave is used ensure that the instructions on the packet are followed precisely	To ensure the food reaches an even temperature throughout
Fruit should be washed and peeled	
Fresh tap water and fresh pasteurized milk are permissible	

Handwashing   Handwashing is probably the most important method of protecting the immuno-compromised patient. Hands should be washed thoroughly with soap and water or alcohol handrub before contact with the patient to prevent the transfer of micro-organisms from other patients. Hands should also be decontaminated immediately before direct contact with vulnerable sites on the patient such as intravenous cannulae, urethral catheters and wounds to prevent the transfer of micro-organisms between dirty and clean procedures on the same patient. Handwashing after contact with respiratory secretions or oral mucosa is essential to prevent transmission of respiratory viruses and candida. Patients should also be advised not to share cups, glasses and utensils for this reason.

Protective clothing   Protective clothing should be used to prevent micro-organisms from other patients in the ward and from the patient's own flora gaining access to vulnerable sites. Disposable gloves and aprons should be used for contact with body fluids and changed before contact with wounds, cannulae, catheters or drains. If used appropriately, they can minimize the risk of micro-organisms gaining access to vulnerable sites on the patient. Sterile protective clothing is unnecessary as it is an unlikely source of infection. There is little evidence that masks provide protection against respiratory pathogens (Nauseef & Maki 1981, Taylor 1980). Staff with any symptoms of upper respiratory tract infections should be excluded from direct contact with these patients as this is a safer means of protecting the patient from respiratory pathogens than masks. The use of unnecessary pro-tective clothing should be avoided as this may increase the patient's sense of isolation.

Visitors   Visitors should be asked to decontaminate their hands before seeing the patients but excluded from contact only if they have an infection, in particular symptoms of an upper respiratory tract infection. Visitors do not have contact with invasive devices or other susceptible sites on the patient and therefore do not need to wear protective clothing.

Equipment   In general, there is no reason to treat equipment differently. Low-risk equipment used only on intact skin should be processed in the usual way (e.g. linen, bedpans, crockery). However, some equipment is easily contaminated and often not cleaned thoroughly (e.g. commodes, washbowls). It is therefore preferable to allocate one of these items for use only by the patient and to clean each item thoroughly with detergent and water after each use. There is no need to autoclave items used by immunocompromised patients such as newspapers, toys and books. Toys should be washed with detergent and water regularly. The only equipment that needs to be sterile are items used for invasive procedures.

Cleaning   Dust harbours micro-organisms and should be removed regularly from all horizontal surfaces where it collects. Disinfection of surfaces is probably of no value. Dry floors and surfaces are an unlikely source of infection and contamination is removed only temporarily by disinfectants (Ayliffe et al 1967).

Flowers and pot plants may be contaminated with aspergillus and should not be kept in the rooms of severely granulocytopenic patients (Lass-Florl et al 2000).

Water leaks that result in damp fixtures and fittings can promote the growth of fungus. They should therefore be identified and resolved promptly (Schulster & Chin 2003).

Food   Food normally contains micro-organisms that are not harmful provided they are present in low numbers. Hospital food often contains Gram-negative bacilli (Remington & Schimpff 1981), which can cause serious infection in an immunocompromised host. Whilst it is impractical to sterilize food, particularly as the process may significantly alter the taste, every effort must be made to ensure that food is hygienically prepared and handled (see Ch. 12). Meat should be cooked thoroughly, fruit and vegetables should be washed and peeled before consumption, and hospital-prepared salads should be avoided. Cooked food, opened tins and jars should always be stored in the refrigerator and discarded after 24 h, before micro-organisms have the chance to multiply. Reheating of meals should be avoided because of the risk of increased microbial contamination if stored at ambient temperature for prolonged periods. Ready-to-eat meals should be heated exactly as described by the manufacturer's instructions.

The main foods to avoid are raw or undercooked meat or fish, soft cheeses, patés and freshly cut salads, which may contain listeria (Jones 1990, Lund et al 1989). Eggs should be thoroughly cooked to reduce the risk of salmonella and food containing raw eggs (e.g. mayonnaise) should be avoided (Food Standards Agency 2002).

Tap water from a drinking supply usually contains very few micro-organisms and is probably safe to drink provided it is fresh from the tap and the water supply is free from legionella. Water systems supplying units where highly immunocompromised patients are cared for must be managed to ensure contamination with legionella is avoided (Cooke 2004, Health & Safety Commission 2000, Oran et al 2002).

Ice made in ice-making machines can be more hazardous because the water supplied to the machine may be contaminated, the ice may be present for considerable periods, and ice in the machine may be contaminated by patients or staff using it. Outbreaks of infection caused by Gram-negative bacteria and cryptosporidium have been associated with ice-making machines (King 2001, Medical Devices Directorate 1993). Immunocompromised patients should not use ice from ice-making machines and, where machines are in use, they should be properly connected and maintained (Medical Devices Directorate 1993). Ice should not be removed by hand and vessels used to remove or store the ice should be washed with detergent and water after each use. Bottled water may contain large numbers of bacteria, although probably no more than may be consumed on food. Bottled water should be stored in the refrigerator once opened and drunk within 3 days. It should not be drunk directly from the bottle as this may contaminate the water (Hunter 1993).

Invasive procedures   Probably the most important aspect of the care of the immunocompromised patient is rigorous attention to the care of intravenous cannulae. Nauseef & Maki (1981) suggest that a higher rate of bacteraemia observed when patients were isolated in a single room was related to the reduced attention to intravenous lines afforded to these patients. Total parenteral nutrition, in particular, increases the risk of infection associated with intravenous therapy. The recommended care for intravenous cannulae and urethral catheters is outlined in Chapters 9 and 10.

References

Ackerman V, Dunk-Richards G (1991) *Microbiology – An Introduction for the Health* Sciences. WB Saunders/Baillière Tindall, London.

Ayliffe GAJ, Collins BJ, Lowbury EJL et al (1967) Ward floors and other surfaces as reservoirs of hospital infection. *J. Hyg.*, **65**: 515–36.

Bodey GP, Buckley M, Sathe YS et al (1966) Quantitative relationships between circulating leukocytes and infection in patients with acute leukaemia. *Ann. Intern. Med.*, **64**: 328–40.

Collins C, Upright C, Aleksich J (1989) Reverse isolation: what patients perceive. *Oncol. Nurs. Forum*, **16**(5): 675–9.

Conry K (1982) Anergy: the hidden danger. *Heart Lung*, **11**: 85.

Cooke RDP (2004) Hazards of water. *J. Hosp. Infect.*, **57**: 290–3.

Denton P (1986) Psychological and physiological effects of isolation. *Nursing*, **3**(3): 88–91.

Department of Health (1996) *Immunisation Against Infectious Disease*. Department of Health, London.

Department of Health (2004) *Immunisation Against Infectious Disease. The 'Green Book' Chapters on Diphtheria, Hib, Pertussis, Polio and Tetanus.* Department of Health, London. Available online at: www.immunisation.nhs.uk.

Food Standards Agency (2002) *Eggs: What Caterers Need to Know.* Food Standards Agency, London.

Garcia R, Raad I, Abi-Said D et al (1997) Nosocomial respiratory syncytial virus infections: prevention and control in bone marrow transplant patients. *Infect. Contr. Hosp. Epidemiol.*, **18**: 412–16.

Garner JS (1996) Guideline for isolation precautions in hospital. *Infect. Contr. Hosp. Epidemiol.*, **17**: 53–80.

Gaskill D, Henderson A, Fraser M (1997) Exploring the everyday world of the patient in isolation. *Oncol. Nurs. Forum*, **24**(4): 695–700.

Hannan MM, Azadian BS, Gazzard BG et al (2000) Hospital infection control in an era of HIV infection and multi-drug resistant tuberculosis. *J. Hosp. Infect.*, **44**: 5–11.

Health and Safety Commission (2000) *Legionnaire's Disease: The Control of Legionella Bacteria in Water Systems. Approved Code of Practice and Guidance.* HSE Books, Norwich.

Hunter P (1993) The microbiology of bottled natural mineral waters. *J. Appl. Bacteriol.*, **74**: 345–52.

Humphries H (2004) Positive pressure isolation and the prevention of invasive aspergillosis. What is the evidence? *J. Hosp. Infect.*, **56**: 93–100.

Jones D (1990) Foodborne listeriosis. *Lancet*, **336**: 1171–4.

King D (2001) Ice machines – an audit of their use in clinical practice. *Comm. Dis. Publ. Health*, **4**(1): 49.

Knowles HE (1993) The experience of infectious patients in isolation. *Nursing Times*, **89**(30): 53–6.

Lass-Florl C, Rak P, Niederwieser D et al (2000) *Aspergillus tereus* infection in haematological malignancies: molecular epidemiology suggests an association with in-hospital plants. *J. Hosp. Infect.*, **46**: 31–5.

Lund BM, Knox MR, Cole MB (1989) Destruction of *Listeria monocytogenes* during microwave cooking. *Lancet*, **i**: 218.

Mackowiak PA, Bartlett JG, Borden EC et al (1997) Concepts of fever; recent advances and lingering dogma. *Clin. Infect. Dis.*, **25**: 119.

Mank A, Van-der-leilie H (2003) Is there still an indication for nursing patients with prolonged neutropenia in protective isolation? An evidence-based nursing and medical study of 4 years experience of nursing patients with neutropenia without isolation. *Eur. J. Oncol. Nurs.*, **7**(1): 17–23.

Medical Devices Directorate (1993) Ice cubes: infection caused by *Xanthomonas maltophilia. Hazard*, **93**: 42.

Nauseef WM, Maki DG (1981) A study of the value of simple protective isolation in patients with granulocytopenia. *N. Engl. J. Med.*, **304**(8): 448–52.

Oran I, Zuckerman T, Avivi I et al (2002) Nosocomial outbreak of *Legionella pnuemophila* serogroup 3 pneumonia in a new bone marrow transplant unit: evaluation, treatment and control. *Bone Marrow Transpl.,* **30**(3): 175–9.

Remington JS, Schimpff SC (1981) Please don't eat the salads. *N. Engl. J. Med.,* **304**: 433–5.

Russel JA, Chaudhry A, Booth K et al (2000) Early outcomes after allogenic stem cell transplantation for leukemia and myelodysplasia without protective isolation: a 10-year experience. *Biol. Blood Marrow Transpl.,* **6**(12): 109–14.

Schulster L, Chin RYW (2003) Guidelines for environmental control in healthcare facilities. Recommendations of CDC and the Healthcare Infection Control Practices Advisory Committee. *MMWR,* **52**: RR10.

Singh N (1997) Infections in solid organ transplant recipients. In: Wenzel RP (ed.) *Prevention and Control of Nosocomial Infections,* 3rd edn. Lippincott, Williams and Wilkins, Philadelphia.

Tablan OC, Anderson LJ, Arden NH et al (1994) Guideline for the prevention of nosocomial pneumonia. *Am. J. Infect. Contr.,* **22**: 247–92.

Taylor L (1980) Are face masks necessary in operating theatres and wards? *J. Hosp. Infect.,* **1**: 173–4.

Wey S (1997) Bone marrow transplant patients. In: Wenzel RP (ed.) *Prevention and Control of Nosocomial Infections,* 3rd edn. Lippincott, Williams and Wilkins, Philadelphia

Further Reading

Pratt RJ (2003) *HIV and AIDS. A Foundation for Nursing and Healthcare Practice,* 5th edn. Arnold, London.

Roitt I, Broscroff J, Male D (1998) *Immunology,* 5th edn. Times Mirror Publishers International, London.

Watson R (1998) Controlling body temperature in adults. *Nursing Standard,* **12**(20): 49–53.

Weir DM, Stewart J (1997) *Immunology,* 8th edn. Churchill Livingstone, Edinburgh.

Wigglesworth N (2003) The use of protective isolation. *Nursing Times,* **99**(7): 26–7.

Chapter 5

A guide to antimicrobial chemotherapy

INTRODUCTION

Effective treatment of infection involves the elimination/control of the invading micro-organism whilst, at the same time, not harming the cells of the host. Modern drugs used for antimicrobial chemotherapy affect characteristic features of pro-karyotic cells that are not found (or are different from those) in the eukaryotic cells of humans.

The recognition of bacteria as the cause of fever and infection was soon followed by the search for substances that could destroy them. Chemicals such as carbolic acid and iodine, known to kill bacteria cultured in the laboratory, formed the basis of the antisepsis in surgery used by Lister in the late 19th century. Other chemicals that destroyed bacteria (e.g. mercury) were used to treat infection but invariably caused as much harm to the patient as to the microbe. Ehrlich first perceived that what was required was an agent that was selectively toxic to microbes. In 1904, he succeeded in curing trypanosomiasis (sleeping sickness) with a dye called trypan. He continued his work using a variety of compounds based on arsenic. Then, in 1935, Domagk found that streptococcal infections could be treated with a dye called prontosil. This chemical was actually broken down in the body to form the effective compound sulphonilamide. Other antimicrobial sulphonilamides were developed and widely used in the treatment of infection.

The ability to treat infections was revolutionized by Sir Alexander Fleming's discovery of the first naturally occurring antimicrobial substance. In 1928, Fleming noticed that colonies of *Staphylococcus aureus* were 'dissolved' where they occurred close to a mould, *Penicillium notatum*, which had inadvertently con-taminated the plate. He then grew the same fungus in a broth and found that the broth had a marked inhibitory effect on many types of bacteria. The antibacterial substances were difficult to purify and were unstable but after extensive work by Florey, Chain and co-workers in the 1940s, sufficient penicillin could be made for the treatment of patients. Commercial production of penicillin began during the Second World War and the search then continued for new antimicrobials from a range of micro-organisms living in natural environments. In the 1940s streptomycin, chloramphenicol and tetracycline were isolated from soil organisms and cephalosporin C from a mould found in a sewage outlet in Sardinia. Erythromycin and rifampicin were discovered in the 1950s and gentamicin and fucidin in the 1960s, all from soil organisms.

The term antibiotic was used to describe these naturally occurring substances produced by one microbial species and capable of inhibiting the growth of another species. In the laboratory, small alterations to the chemical structure of naturally occurring antibiotics were found to alter the range of microbes against which the drug was effective (spectrum of activity), the absorption by the body and the duration of action. There are now over 100 antimicrobial drugs available. Many are similar compounds but, with minor modifications, affect different species of bacteria.

An important evolutionary point is worth making here. We have seen that antimicrobial agents are often naturally occurring compounds – produced by micro-organisms themselves, in complex soil ecosystems – no doubt to give the producer organism a means of killing its competitors. It should come as no surprise, therefore, that these competitor organisms should evolve a means (resistance mechanism) to nullify the effects of these substances. So antimicrobial resistance mechanisms existed in bacteria millions of years before humans ever used antimicrobials as therapeutic agents.

Some people use the term 'antibiotic' to refer only to the naturally occurring drugs made by bacteria or fungi. For the purposes of this text, the terms antibacterial or antimicrobial agent will be used for all drugs that are capable of destroying bacteria and other micro-organisms.

CLINICAL APPLICATION OF ANTIMICROBIAL AGENTS

Considerable skill and knowledge are necessary to make the best use of the wide range of antimicrobial agents available. In the UK, advice on antimicrobial therapy is provided by a clinical microbiologist, who is a doctor with a specialist knowledge and training in medical microbiology. Although nurses are not responsible for the prescription of antimicrobial therapy,

they do have an important role to play in administering and monitoring the drugs prescribed and in discussing the treatment with the doctor when therapy seems unnecessary or unsuccessful.

Some of the factors that need to be taken into account when choosing an appropriate antibacterial agent to treat an infection are discussed below.

Indication for treatment

Specific signs and symptoms, such as a fever, rigors, etc., coupled with a rising white blood cell count and C-reactive protein may indicate the presence of infection. These need to be assessed clinically to determine whether treatment with an antimicrobial agent is required. It is important to realize that the isolation of micro-organisms does not always indicate infection. Some sites, in particular the skin and respiratory tract, are normally colonized by bacteria and treatment with an antibacterial is not required if signs of infection are not present. Antibacterial therapy is usually not indicated for the treatment of upper respiratory tract infections, which are mostly caused by viruses, and similarly gastrointestinal infections often do not require specific antibacterial therapy unless the patient is severely ill with evidence of systemic infection.

Micro-organisms causing the infection

In most infections, the help of the microbiology laboratory is required to identify the causative organism and establish the antimicrobial to which it is susceptible. Organisms will be more difficult to detect (or be undetectable) once treatment has commenced and therefore microbiological specimens should be collected (in most cases) prior to starting any antimicrobial therapy. However, there are exceptions to this. For example, it is now recognized that in cases of meningitis it is more important that the GP institutes appropriate antimicrobial therapy immediately, prior to the patient's transfer to hospital, rather than wait until appropriate microbiological specimens (CSF, blood cultures and throat swab) have been taken.

Spectrum of activity

The term 'spectrum' is used to describe the range of organisms against which an antimicrobial is effective. Some antibacterials kill only a few different bacteria (e.g. only Gram-positive bacteria) and are said to have a narrow spectrum of activity. Penicillin is a narrow-spectrum antibacterial because it acts mainly on some Gram-positive bacteria; aztreonam has activity only against Gram-negative bacteria; likewise metronidazole destroys only anaerobic bacteria (and some protozoa).

The modern penicillin derivatives (carbapenems), modern cephalosporins, fluoroquinolones and amino-glycosides are examples of broad-spectrum antibacterials effective against both Gram-negative and Gram-positive bacteria. Broad-spectrum antibacterials are useful when the cause of the infection is unknown and action against a wide variety of organisms may be necessary. This is termed empirical antimicrobial therapy. Unfortunately, broad-spectrum agents kill not only the pathogen but also other bacteria that make up the normal commensal microbial flora of the body. These organisms play an important role in protecting against invasion by more harmful (pathogenic) species and, if destroyed, superinfection by other bacteria or fungi may occur. *Clostridium difficile* is an organism that multiplies in the gut if other normal gut organisms are destroyed by antibacterial therapy. The toxin that it produces causes diarrhoea and can lead to the more serious condition antibiotic-associated colitis (also known as pseudomembranous colitis) which can be life threatening (toxic mega-colon) (see p. 123).

Broad-spectrum antibacterials may also encourage the survival and multiplication (selection) of strains of bacteria that are resistant to these and other anti-microbial agents.

Therefore, once the pathogen and its susceptibility pattern is known, it is important to employ the narrowest spectrum agent available.

Drug combinations

Sometimes it is preferable to treat an infection with a combination of antimicrobials, particularly where the cause of the infection is unknown. Some drug combinations enhance each other's activity – this is known as 'synergy'. An example of this is the use of benzylpenicillin and gentamicin to treat enterococcal endocarditis. Enterococci are resistant to penicillin alone and gentamicin alone, but when used together the combination is bactericidal. Other combinations interfere with one another (e.g. penicillin and tetracycline) or encourage the development of resistant strains (e.g. ampicillin and flucloxacillin). Some antibacterials (e.g. rifampicin or fusidic acid) rapidly select resistant strains and therefore should always be used with another appropriate drug, to ensure that these resistant organisms are destroyed.

So if resistance to a particular antibiotic is likely to develop during treatment, more than one type of drug needs to be given as pathogens are unlikely to develop resistance to both agents at the same time. This is particularly important in antituberculous therapy, where a combination of four drugs is usually prescribed.

Drugs sometimes interact with each other, altering their therapeutic effect or inducing toxicity. Adverse reactions are particularly common where drugs are administered in intravenous fluids and this should be avoided where possible.

Pharmacokinetics

Pharmacokinetics is the term used to describe the absorption, distribution and elimination of a drug by the body. Absorption from the gut occurs mostly by passive diffusion but may be delayed or enhanced by the presence of food in the stomach or by its pH. Some drugs are better absorbed with food because of the accompanying delay in stomach emptying and increase in blood flow (e.g. nitrofurantoin). The absorption of macrolides (such as erythromycin) is reduced by the presence of food because the process is affected by the change in pH. The acid in the stomach alters some drugs and these have to be protected by a capsule that dissolves only in the small intestine.

Intravenous or intramuscular routes of admin-istration are often preferred for antimicrobial agents because of the variability of oral absorption. Some antimicrobials can also be administered topically as creams, ointments and drops or absorbed through the rectal mucosa from suppositories.

The distribution of a drug through the body depends on many factors, including whether it is lipophilic (having an affinity for lipids) or hydrophilic (having an affinity for water). Lipophilic drugs, such as ciprofloxacin, pass readily through plasma membranes and therefore diffuse widely into the tissues. Hydrophilic or highly charged compounds such as the aminoglycosides are restricted to the blood and fluid surrounding cells. Plasma proteins (e.g. albumin) play a part in the distribution of drugs. They bind to compounds, transporting them around the body and affect the rate at which a drug is excreted.

Most antimicrobials do not readily pass through the blood–brain barrier and although they may reach a higher concentration in the brain when the meninges are inflamed, many cannot be used to treat meningitis successfully.

There are two main routes by which drugs are excreted from the body: via the biliary tract into the faeces and via the kidneys into urine. Many drugs are altered, or metabolized, to enable elimination from the body. In particular, lipophilic compounds have to be charged in order to prevent their readsorption in the kidneys.

Antimicrobials are eliminated from the body at different rates. Those that are eliminated fairly rapidly must be given in multiple doses, while others that are excreted slowly can be administered once or twice a day.

Pharmacodynamics

Pharmacodynamics is more complicated but basically concerns the interaction of the antibacterial agent with the bacteria themselves. Pharmacodynamic characteristics of a given antibacterial include: working together with other agents to kill micro-organisms (synergistic killing), concentration-dependent killing and the postantibiotic effect (when there is continued suppression of bacterial growth after the level of the antibacterial has fallen below the minimum inhibitory concentration of that drug). Further discussion on pharmacodynamics is, however, beyond the scope of this book.

Choice of antimicrobial agent

The choice of a suitable agent depends on a number of factors related to both the patient and the known, or most likely, causative organism (British National Formulary 2005).

Patient factors include: history of allergy; renal and liver function; severity of the illness; whether the patient can tolerate oral therapy; whether they are immunocompromised; ethnic origin; age; other drugs they may be taking; and if the patient is a woman, whether she is taking the oral contraceptive, pregnant or breastfeeding.

Organism factors include: the site of infection (urine, chest, intra-abdominal, bone, etc.); where the organism was acquired (community or hospital); and local antimicrobial resistance patterns.

The microbiological, pharmacological and toxicological properties all need to be taken into account before selecting an appropriate antibacterial agent.

Duration of therapy

Antibacterials should be given for long enough to ensure the eradication of the infection but not for too long as this may encourage the development of more resistant strains. Usually treatment should be given for 5–10 days. A single dose of an antimicrobial may cure an uncomplicated urinary tract infection but for serious or systemic infection, prolonged therapy may be necessary. Septicaemia with *Staphylococcus aureus* should receive at least 14 days of appropriate intravenous therapy. There are also specific infections that are more difficult to treat and consequently require even longer therapy. Bacterial endocarditis, an infection of the heart valves, usually is treated for at least 4 weeks. Acute infections that involve the bones or joints are usually treated for 4–6 weeks. Infections that involve prosthetic material require up to 6 weeks of intravenous therapy (coupled with the removal, at that point, of the prosthetic device, e.g. joint or heart valve). In some cases of prosthetic joint infection, it may not be possible to remove the joint and then the patient may be commenced on long-term oral antimicrobial 'suppression'.

Prophylaxis

Antimicrobials can be used to protect patients in situations that markedly increase their vulnerability to infection. These include surgery involving a part of the body heavily colonized with bacteria (e.g. bowel surgery), procedures where subsequent infection could have disastrous consequences (e.g. infection of valve or joint replacement) and during certain treatments (e.g. dental) for people with abnormal heart valves who are at risk of developing endocarditis. Sometimes prophylaxis is indicated to protect intimate contacts of someone who has developed an infectious disease (e.g. meningococcal meningitis). The prophylactic antimicrobial selected should be effective against the bacteria most likely to cause infection. For example, patients undergoing surgery of the large intestine will be most at risk from infection caused by aerobic coliforms and anaerobes of the gut flora. Prophylactic treatment should therefore include metronidazole to kill the anaerobes and gentamicin or a cephalosporin to kill the Gram-negative aerobes. It should be given close to the time of incision to ensure that the level of drug is adequate during the procedure. This may be achieved with a single dose, unless the procedure is prolonged or associated with heavy blood loss. Prophylactic therapy (in these cases) should not be continued for more than 24 h.

On the other hand, antimicrobial prophylaxis taken by patients who have no functioning spleen (who are particularly susceptible to capsulated organisms such as pneumococci) usually continues for life.

HOW ANTIBACTERIAL AGENTS WORK

There are many species of bacteria and it is therefore to be expected that antibacterials may affect each species differently. The effect may be bactericidal, that is, cause the death of the bacterial cell, or bacteriostatic, that is, prevent replication of the bacterium but not kill it. There are a number of different mechanisms of antimicrobial action (Table 5.1).

Table 5.1 Main mechanisms of action of antibacterial agents (Greenwood & Whitely 2003)

Site of action	Antibacterial agent
Cell wall	Penicillins
	Cephalosporins
	Glycopeptides
	Bacitracin
	Isoniazid
	Cycloserine
	Fosfomycin
Ribosomes	Chloramphenicol
	Tetracycline
	Aminoglycosides
	Macrolides
	Lincosamides
	Fusidic acid
	Oxazolidinones
	Mupirocin
Nucleic acid	Quinolones
	Novobiocin
	Rifampicin
	5-Nitroimidazoles (e.g. metronidazole)
	Nitrofurans
Cell membrane	Polymyxins
	Ionophores
Folate synthesis	Sulphonamides
	Diaminopyrimidines (e.g. trimethoprim)

Interference with cell wall synthesis

Bacteria differ from human cells in having a cell wall and this is a useful target for antibacterial agents. A number of different aspects of cell wall synthesis can be affected; for example, the β-lactam agents (penicillins and cephalosporins) bind to enzymes called penicillin binding proteins (PBPs) that are involved in making peptidoglycan, whereas vancomycin prevents the cross-linkage process. The inhibition of cell wall synthesis affects the ability of the cell to withstand osmotic pressures; it therefore swells and eventually breaks open.

Interference with protein synthesis

Several antibacterial agents inhibit protein synthesis by binding to bacterial ribosomes. They are unable to bind on to the much larger eukaryotic cell ribosomes and therefore selectively affect bacteria. Protein synthesis either occurs abnormally or is completely prevented. Some substances do not bind permanently to the ribosome and their action is therefore bacteriostatic (e.g. tetracycline, chloramphenicol).

Aminoglycosides affect both protein synthesis and the permeability of the membrane.

Inhibition of nucleic acid synthesis

Nucleic acid synthesis can be affected in numerous ways. For example, metronidazole inhibits an enzyme involved in nucleic acid production and rifampicin inhibits the transcription of DNA into RNA. The quinolones (e.g. ciprofloxacin) affect an enzyme called gyrase, which controls coiling and uncoiling of DNA strands.

Disruption of the cell membrane

Polymyxins selectively damage the cell membrane of bacteria, causing the cell to swell and burst.

Folate synthesis

The sulphonamides and trimethoprim prevent the synthesis of folic acid, an essential coenzyme in the synthesis of nucleotides. Human cells also use folic acid but because they do not synthesize it and depend on a dietary source, they are not affected by these antibacterials. Bacteria that are able to use pre-formed folic acid are also resistant to these agents.

MAIN GROUPS OF ANTIMICROBIAL AGENTS

The following sections provide an overview of the spectrum of activity and clinical use of common antimicrobial agents. More detailed information can be found in *Antibiotic and Chemotherapy* (Finch et al 2003) and 'Antibacterial therapy and newer agents' (Kaye & Moellering 2004).

Penicillins

The penicillins bind to enzymes, penicillin binding proteins, which are involved in the production of peptidoglycan and, as a result, prevent cell wall synthesis. They are bactericidal. The original, naturally occurring penicillins (e.g. benzylpenicillin) have a quite narrow spectrum of activity and are mainly active against Gram-positive bacteria: including most β-haemolytic streptococci (groups A, B, C and G) and pneumococci. Benzylpenicillin is active against clostridia (the cause of gas gangrene) and anaerobic cocci and is useful in the treatment of anthrax, diphtheria, leptospirosis and Lyme disease. A few Gram-negative organisms are also susceptible, such as meningococci and gonococci, although pneumococci, meningococci and particularly gonococci with reduced sensitivity to penicillin have been isolated.

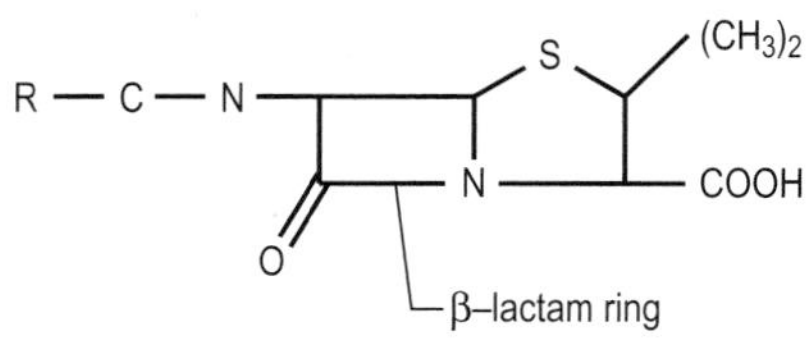

Figure 5.1   The structure of penicillin.

A large number of different penicillin antibiotics have now been synthesized, which have the same basic β-lactam ring structure but, by modification of the side-chain molecules, are able to affect a much wider range of bacterial species (Fig. 5.1). Alterations to the side-chains can also influence the pharmacology of the drugs; for example, benzylpenicillin is destroyed by gastric acid and so must be given intravenously, whereas ampicillin is acid stable and can therefore be given orally.

Penicillins are still very useful antibiotics. They range from the narrower spectrum benzylpenicillin through ampicillin/amoxicillin (which are still useful in the treatment of urinary tract infections and streptococcal/enterococcal infections); co-amoxiclav which is useful for the treatment of skin and soft tissue infections; antistaphylococcal agents such as flucloxacillin and oxacillin; antipseudomonal penicillins such as ticarcillin and piperacillin; to agents such as piperacillin-tazobactam which have a very broad spectrum of activity that includes the more resistant Gram-negative organisms (such as pseudomonas), some extended-spectrum β-lactamase (ESBL) producers (see p. 14), anaerobes, some acinetobacter and many Gram-positive pathogens (except MRSA and glycopeptide-resistant enterococci (Table 5.2).

They reach well into most body tissues and fluids but only poorly into the CSF, unless the meninges are inflamed. Their main adverse effect is a hypersensitivity reaction, which can range from minor rashes to severe anaphylaxis. Allergic reactions occur in up to 10% of those exposed but anaphylaxis occurs in less than 0.05% of cases treated (British National Formulary 2005).

Resistance to penicillin was reported within a few years of its introduction and in certain species is widespread. For example, approximately 90% of *Staphylococcus aureus* isolates in hospitals are resistant to penicillin. Resistant bacteria produce an enzyme, penicillinase (β-lactamase), which breaks open the β-lactam ring and destroys the activity of the antibiotic. Pharmaceutical manufacturers have constantly searched for side-chain modifications that prevent attack by β-lactamases. Flucloxacillin, a β-lactamase-resistant antibiotic, was introduced in the 1960s and is of considerable value for the treatment of *S. aureus*

Table 5.2	Penicillins
Antibacterial	**Principal uses**
Naturally occurring penicillins, e.g. benzylpenicillin	Narrow spectrum. Mainly active against group A, B, C, G β-haemolytic streptococci, pneumococci and clostridia. Also used for penicillin-sensitive meningococci and gonococci
Ampicillin, amoxicillin	Urinary tract infection, sensitive streptococci, enterococci
Co-amoxiclav (Augmentin)	Skin and soft tissue infections
Flucloxacillin	*Staphylococcus aureus* infections (not MRSA)
Ticaracillin, piperacillin	Pseudomonal infections
Piperacillin–tazobactam	Broad-spectrum activity against Gram-positive and -negative bacteria including pseudomonas, some acinetobacter and ESBL producers, anaerobes

infections. Methicillin was a β-lactamase-resistant antibiotic introduced at the same time but, as it was associated with toxicity, was used only in the laboratory to detect flucloxacillin (and therefore β-lactam) resistance in staphylococci. Hence the term **m**ethicillin-**r**esistant *Staphylococcus aureus* – MRSA. Recently, the lack of availability of methicillin has meant that laboratories now use oxacillin as the marker of β-lactam resistance in staphylococci.

Cephalosporins

The cephalosporins have a similar chemical structure to the penicillins. They have a β-lactam ring, an additional side-ring and different side-chains. They also kill bacterial cells by inhibiting cell wall synthesis. The first cephalosporin, cephalothin, was obtained from a fungus in the mid-1960s. These early, or first-generation, cephalosporins had a similar spectrum to ampicillin and some are still used today (e.g. cefalexin) but mainly for urinary tract infections, particularly in pregnancy (Table 5.3). Susceptibility to β-lactamases limited their use until the second generation of β-lactamase-resistant cephalosporins, e.g. cefaclor (oral) and cefuroxime (IV), were introduced in the 1970s. These drugs are more potent and are active against a wider range of bacteria. Cephalosporins generally have no activity against enterococci, listeria, legionella, mycoplasma, coxiella or chlamydia.

Table 5.3   Cephalosporins

Antibacterial	Principal uses
First generation	
Cefalexin	Urinary tract infections
Second generation	
Cefaclor (oral)	Respiratory tract infection, sinusitis, otitis media, skin and soft tissue infections
Cefuroxime (IV)	Prophylaxis in major surgery, penicillin-resistant bacteria, e.g. haemophilus, gonococcus
Third generation	
Ceftriaxone (IV)	Active against Gram-negative bacteria,
Cefotaxime (IV)	less active against *S. aureus*. First-line agents for patients with severe intra-abdominal infections, pneumonia, bacteraemia
Ceftazidime (IV)	Active against many Gram-negative bacteria, including pseudomonas
Fourth generation	
Cefixime (oral)	Active against most enterobacteria, poor activity against staphylococci
Cefpirome (IV)	Active against many Gram-negative bacteria, better antipseudomonal activity than ceftazidime

Cefuroxime is often used for prophylaxis in major surgery and in the treatment of penicillin-resistant strains of bacteria such as the gonococcus, haemophilus and *Staphylococcus aureus* (non-MRSA). Cefaclor has good activity against *H. influenzae* and can therefore be used for respiratory infections, sinusitis and otitis media. It is also used for skin and soft tissue infections.

The third-generation cephalosporins (e.g. ceftriaxone and cefotaxime, both IV), introduced in the early 1980s, are more active against Gram-negative bacteria but less active against *S. aureus*. They have been described as 'workhorse hospital antibiotics' (Livermore & Woodford 2004) 'given as first-line agents to severely ill patients including those with intra-abdominal infections, community-acquired pneumonias and bacteraemias'. As with most other cephalosporins, they have no useful activity against either anaerobic bacteria (especially *Bacteroides* spp.) or pseudomonas. Ceftazidime is a broad-spectrum cephalosporin (IV), which has good activity against many Gram-negative bacteria including *Pseudomonas* spp.

They are expensive agents and many believe that they are subject to widespread misuse in situations where perhaps a cheaper, narrower spectrum antibiotic would be more appropriate. Their use has been linked

to pseudomembranous colitis caused by toxogenic strains of *Clostridium difficile*; to increased resistance in pseudomonas, enterobacter and serratia; and to the 'selection out' of glycopeptide-resistant enterococci (GRE).

Newer cephalosporins (sometimes called fourth generation) include the orally active cefixime and intravenous cefpirome. Cefixime has activity against most enterobacteria but not against *Acinetobacter* spp., *Pseudomonas* spp. or *Bacteroides* spp. and has poor activity against staphylococci. Cefpirome has a similar spectrum of activity as cefotaxime/ceftriaxone but with much more activity against *Pseudomonas aeruginosa*. Consequently it is used in similar situations to ceftazidime.

Resistance to the second and third/fourth generation of cephalosporins is becoming an increasing problem and is often caused by extended spectrum β-lactamases (ESBLs) (see p. 114). If an organism is an ESBL producer, it is resistant to *all* the cephalosporins.

The main side-effect of cephalosporins is hypersensitivity. About 10% of penicillin-allergic patients have some cephalosporin allergy as well.

Other β-lactams

There are a variety of other antibacterial agents that have a β-lactam ring as part of their structure.

The monobactams (e.g. aztreonam)

Aztreonam has activity against a wide range of Gram-negative bacteria (including *Pseudomonas* spp.) but no effect against Gram-positive bacteria or anaerobes. There is little cross-hypersensitivity to other β-lactam agents.

The carbapenems

These intravenous agents (e.g. meropenem/imipenem plus cilastatin/ertapenem) are very potent and effective against a wide range of Gram-positive and Gram-negative bacteria (including anaerobes, acinetobacter and legionella). They are used to treat serious infections caused by resistant bacteria (for instance, those producing extended-spectrum β-lactamases). These drugs have the broadest spectrum available at present but even so, there are organisms that are invariably resistant, e.g. *Stenotrophomonas maltophilia*. Ertapenem is the newest member of the group. It can be given once daily but has little effect against *Pseudomonas aeruginosa* or *Acinetobacter* spp. and is consequently less broad in its spectrum of activity.

β-Lactamase inhibitors and combinations

Since the most important cause of clinically significant resistance to β-lactam antibacterials is the production of the β-lactamase enzyme, it would seem logical to try and negate this by administering a compound which inhibits these enzymes. The β-lactamase inhibitors in current use (clavulanic acid, tazobactam and sulbactam) are all β-lactams themselves but with poor antimicrobial activity. The combined agents available in the UK include amoxicillin-clavulanic acid (co-amoxiclav), piperacillin-tazobactam (Tazocin) and ticarcillin-clavulanic acid (Timentin).

Aminoglycosides

The aminoglycoside antibiotics interfere with protein synthesis by binding to bacterial ribosomes and preventing accurate reading of the messenger RNA. They are bactericidal and active against many Gram-negative aerobic bacteria (including pseudomonas, acinetobacter, ESBL producers) and some Gram-positive bacteria. They are therefore a very important antimicrobial in the treatment of severe Gram-negative sepsis, particularly by the enterobacteria. They are often also used in combination with other antibiotic(s) to provide synergistic activity against a broad range of organisms. This is particularly important in severe infections such as bacteraemia caused by S. aureus (non-MRSA); this would often be treated with the combination of IV gentamicin and flucloxacillin. Similarly, in the treatment of bacterial endocarditis, therapy usually includes an aminoglycoside plus an appropriate penicillin, with the aminoglycoside being stopped after the first 2 weeks of therapy.

Aminoglycosides are not absorbed from the gut and so must be administered parenterally. The concentration of the drug in the blood must be monitored closely (especially in patients with impaired renal function) as aminoglycosides tend to accumulate in the tissues where they can cause damage, particularly to the kidney (nephrotoxicity) and the inner ear (ototoxicity). The aminoglycosides are also synergistically nephrotoxic with other (nephrotoxic) drugs, e.g. vancomycin, amphotericin B and loop diuretics, etc. Resistance to aminoglycosides through the production of enzymes that can modify the molecule is becoming increasingly common.

Glycopeptides

These compounds were originally obtained from actinomyces found in soil. Vancomycin was the only clinically useful glycopeptide until teicoplanin was introduced in the 1980s. Glycopeptides interfere with the synthesis of peptidoglycan, inhibiting the formation of bacterial cell walls.

They are poorly absorbed from the gut and vancomycin given by the intramuscular route is painful, so is usually only administered intravenously. Glycopeptides are active really only against Gram-positive organisms, in particular staphylococci. Their main use is in the treatment of serious staphylococcal infection, including those caused by methicillin-resistant strains. Oral preparations can be used to treat *Clostridium difficile*-associated colitis.

Vancomycin can be nephrotoxic and ototoxic (but much less so than the aminoglycosides) and can cause a reversible neutropenia.

Serum levels must be monitored carefully to avoid these side-effects. Rapid infusion of vancomycin (less than 60 min) can lead to 'red man' syndrome which is caused by the release of histamine from basophils and mast cells.

Teicoplanin is more potent than vancomycin (2–4 times more active) and is associated with fewer (and less severe) side-effects.

Until recently, resistance to glycopeptides was very rare. However, strains of vancomycin (glycopeptide)-resistant enterococci (GRE) have been causing outbreaks of infection since the early 1990s (see p. 112) and vancomycin-resistant strains of *S. aureus*, although at present unusual, have been reported (see p. 108).

Quinolones

These drugs inhibit DNA gyrase, the enzyme responsible for supercoiling microbial DNA molecules, and are rapidly bactericidal. They are synthetic antibiotics, first used in 1962 when nalidixic acid was introduced (Table 5.4). This drug is active against a wide range of Gram-negative bacteria, except pseudomonas, and is used to treat urinary tract infections, although resistance often develops during treatment.

The addition of a fluorine molecule into the compound was found to increase both its potency and spectrum of activity and a new range of compounds, the fluoroquinolones, was subsequently produced (e.g. ciprofloxacin, norfloxacin, ofloxacin). These drugs are effective against most Gram-negative aerobic bacteria, including pseudomonads. They are also active against intracellular pathogens such as mycoplasma, chlamydia, legionella and some mycobacteria. They have poorer activity against staphylococci (they should not be employed as first-line therapy for staphylococcal infections) and streptococci, including pneumococci. Most anaerobic bacteria are not affected.

Quinolones are rapidly absorbed by mouth with similar pharmacokinetics to intravenous administration. They are also distributed widely into tissue and bone, therefore they can be used to treat a wide range of infections in almost any part of the body (O'Donnell & Gelone 2004).

Table 5.4 Quinolones

Antibacterial	Principal uses
Early quinolones	
Nalidixic acid	Urinary tract infections. Active against a wide range of Gram-negative bacteria, not pseudomonas
First fluoroquinolones	
Ciprofloxacin Oxfloxacin Norfloxacin	Active against most Gram-negative aerobic bacteria including pseudomonas, intracellular pathogens (e.g. mycoplasma, chlamydia), some mycobacteria
Newer quinolones	
Levofloxacin Moxifloxacin Gatifloxacin	Use should be restricted to the treatment of respiratory tract infections, including atypical infections, and penicillin-resistant pneumococci

The clinical use of the older fluoroquinolones includes treatment of uncomplicated and complicated urinary tract infections; bacterial prostatitis; sexually transmitted diseases; severe gastrointestinal infections (*Salmonella* spp., typhoid, paratyphoid, *Shigella* spp., *Campylobacter* spp., *Aeromonas* spp.); respiratory infections (although the older agents have poor activity against the pneumococcus); severe Gram-negative sepsis with resistant organisms, e.g. extended-spectrum β-lactamase producers, and pseudomonas (but often in combination with another active agent).

The newer quinolones include levofloxacin, moxifloxacin and gatifloxacin. They have activity against the pneumococcus (including penicillin-resistant strains), *Haemophilus influenzae*, moraxella, group A β-haemolytic streptococci and atypical pathogens.

Resistance to fluoroquinolones is associated with prolonged treatment of chronic infections and excessive prescribing. Many feel that the newer fluoroquinolones should be used judiciously, otherwise overuse will lead to the emergence of resistance. These newer agents can be used for the treatment of upper and lower respiratory infections but their spectrum of activity is much broader than the organisms causing pneumonia. They should therefore perhaps be restricted to treating documented cases of pneumonia.

The quinolones should be used with caution in patients with epilepsy (or conditions that predispose to seizures), pregnant or breastfeeding women, myasthenia gravis, renal impairment and in children or adolescents. This latter caution is because quinolones are known to cause arthropathy in the weight-bearing joints of young animals, although the significance in humans is unclear (British National Formulary 2005).

Macrolides

These drugs inhibit bacterial protein synthesis by binding to the ribosome. They are bacteriostatic as the attachment to the ribosome is reversible. The first of this group of drugs, erythromycin, was isolated from a streptomyces. The naturally occurring macrolides are active against most Gram-positive organisms plus neisseria, haemophilus, moraxella and a range of both Gram-positive and Gram-negative anaerobes. They are also effective against intracellular pathogens such as legionella, chlamydia and rickettsia. They have poor or no activity against enterobacteria and pseudomonas. Erythromycin has been commonly prescribed for patients who are allergic to penicillin, although many *S. aureus* and group A streptococci are now resistant. Their activity against a number of emergent pathogens such as toxoplasma, legionella and helicobacter has recently stimulated interest in this group of antibacterial agents.

Serious side-effects are rare but poor tolerance due to gastrointestinal disturbances (nausea, vomiting, abdominal pain) may occur, especially when erythromycin is given in high doses.

The advanced macrolides are now available, i.e. clarithromycin and azithromycin. These agents are better tolerated, have more favourable pharmacodynamics, once-a-day dosing (azithromycin) and an extended spectrum of activity. Their clinical use includes the treatment of respiratory infections, sexually transmitted diseases and infections caused by *Helicobacter* spp. and *Mycobacterium avium* complex.

Telithromycin

Telithromycin belongs to the new class of macrolides – the ketolides. It shares many of the properties of the advanced macrolides but includes activity against both macrolide/penicillin-resistant pneumococci and macrolide-resistant group A β-haemolytic streptococci. It was specifically developed for the treatment of respiratory infections. The drawbacks of the ketolides are similar to those of the other macrolides which include borderline sensitivity to *Haemophilus influenzae* and the development of resistance (Zuckerman 2004).

Tetracyclines

The name tetracycline is derived from their structure of four rings fused together. They bind to bacterial ribosomes and block protein synthesis by preventing transfer RNA from attaching to messenger RNA. The attachment to the ribosomes is reversible and their effect is therefore bacteriostatic rather than bactericidal.

Available tetracyclines include tetracycline, doxycycline, minocycline and oxytetracycline. A new glycylcycline class compound, tigecycline (IV only), has been developed recently.

Their main side-effect is gastrointestinal disturbance, which is dose dependent. Irritation to the gastric mucosa causes nausea and vomiting and disruption of the normal bowel flora may result in diarrhoea. Tetracyclines are also deposited in developing bones and teeth, causing the teeth to stain yellow. They are therefore contraindicated in pregnant or breast-feeding women and children aged under 12 years. They should be avoided in patients with renal disease. They should not be given intramuscularly as this causes considerable pain.

Tetracyclines are effective against a broad range of Gram-positive and Gram-negative bacteria but increased resistance to them has resulted in a decline in their use. They remain an important treatment for the following infections: those caused by chlamydia (trachoma, psittacosis, salpingitis, urethritis); rickettsial infections (including Q fever); brucellosis; Lyme disease (*Borrelia burgdorferi*); acne vulgaris; and periodontal infection. They are also an alternative agent in the treatment of *Helicobacter pylori*, community-acquired pneumonia, infective exacerbations of chronic pulmonary disease, prostatitis, leptospirosis, plague, tularaemia, Whipple's disease, etc. They are also one of the oral agents that may be used, with a second orally active agent, in the treatment or suppression of infection caused by MRSA (other agents include trimethoprim, fusidic acid and rifampicin).

Resistance to the tetracyclines is mediated by the acquisition of a mechanism that either eliminates the drug from the bacterial cell (efflux mechanism) or that protects the target (the ribosome) from inhibition.

Other antimicrobial agents

Linezolid

Linezolid is the first oxazolidinone (a new synthetic class of antibacterial agents) to become available for clinical use. These agents are unique in acting as inhibitors of protein synthesis by preventing the formation of the 70S ribosomal initiation complex and so far, no cross-resistance with other antibacterial agents has been found.

Linezolid has good activity against most important Gram-positive organisms, including MRSA, vancomycin/glycopeptide intermediate-resistant *Staphylococcus aureus* (VISA/GISA), vancomycin-resistant *S. aureus* (VRSA), vancomycin/glycopeptide-resistant enterococci (VRE/GRE) and penicillin-resistant pneumococci. It also has activity against Gram-negative anaerobes and some activity against *Chlamydia pneumoniae*, *Mycoplasma pneumoniae* and *Legionella* spp. It is bacteriostatic for most organisms but bactericidal for group A β-haemolytic streptococci and *Bacteroides fragilis*.

Linezolid has 100% oral bioavailability with equivalent serum levels when given either orally or intravenously. It penetrates respiratory secretions better than vancomycin with good penetration also of muscle, bone and fat.

The clinical use of linezolid includes the treatment of infections caused by GRE, GISA/VISA or in cases where the patient is intolerant of the glycopeptides, or in treatment failures with the glycopeptides. Linezolid has been used to treat bacteraemias, skin and soft tissue infections and pneumonias caused by these multiresistant organisms. Initial studies suggest that linezolid is more effective than vancomycin in the treatment of MRSA pneumonia (Wunderink et al 2003).

The major side-effect of linezolid is reversible bone marrow suppression and thrombocytopenia (although this is rare in therapy of under 2 weeks). More prolonged therapy is associated with up to a 10% incidence of this side-effect. Therefore weekly full blood counts should be carried out on patients receiving this drug.

Resistance to linezolid is emerging, particularly in enterococci, associated with chronic infection, persistent bacteraemia or peritonitis and the presence of foreign material, such as a catheter.

Linezolid is a costly antibacterial agent; currently a 2-week course would cost over £1200 (British National Formulary 2005). The issue of cost and the worry of overuse/misuse, leading inevitably to increased resistance, have led many to reserve linezolid for glycopeptide-resistant organisms, refractory infections caused by glycopeptide-sensitive organisms and for those patients who are intolerant (have adverse reactions) to the glycopeptides. However, it seems likely that linezolid may well become the treatment of choice for serious MRSA infections even though the organism is glycopeptide sensitive (Lundstrom & Sobel 2004).

Quinupristin–dalfopristin

This agent is a combination of two streptogramins (a new class of antibacterial agents) isolated from *Streptomyces pristinaspiralis*. They inhibit protein synthesis in the bacterial ribosome. It is available for intravenous use only and should be given through a central line to prevent phlebitis. It is usually given every 8 or 12 hours.

Its spectrum of activity includes most important Gram-positive bacterial pathogens except *Enterococcus faecalis*. It also has activity against Gram-negative anaerobes, *Moraxella* spp., *Legionella* spp., mycoplasma and *Chlamydia pneumoniae*. Its main clinical use is in the treatment of vancomycin-resistant *Enterococcus faecium*, though potentially it could be employed for infections caused by VRSA or GISA/VISAs (British National Formulary 2005, Lundstrom & Sobel 2004). Its main side-effects are phlebitis and the development of reversible arthralgias and myalgias.

Chloramphenicol

This drug was originally derived from a streptomyces but is now made synthetically. It is bacteriostatic, preventing protein synthesis by binding reversibly to bacterial ribosomes. It is active against a wide range of bacteria including unusual ones such as rickettsia, spirochaetes, chlamydia and mycoplasma. Its most important side-effect is bone marrow suppression and on rare occasions it may cause aplastic anaemia. It is therefore not used systemically except for life-threatening infections (e.g. bacterial meningitis in patients allergic to mainstream agents) but can be used reasonably safely as a topical preparation for eye infections.

Sulphonamides

These are synthetic chemicals that interfere with para-amino benzoic acid (PABA), an enzyme involved in the production of folic acid, which is an essential ingredient for the production of nucleic acids. Sulphonamides were the first antimicrobials found to be effective against bacteria whilst not harming the patient. Introduced in the 1930s, they are still available today, although resistance and toxicity now significantly restrict their use. Silver sulfadiazine is a topical preparation used to prevent colonization of burns, especially with pseudomonas.

Trimethoprim

Trimethoprim also affects folic acid synthesis and because it enhances the activity of sulphonamides, is often used in the combined form with sulfamethoxazole as co-trimoxazole. As trimethoprim is excreted in the urine, it is a useful treatment for urinary tract infection. It is one of the orally active agents that can be combined with a second orally active agent in the treatment/suppression of MRSA infections (other agents include fusidic acid, rifampicin and tetracycline).

Co-trimoxazole

This is a fixed ratio (1:5) combination of trimethoprim and sulfamethoxazole. Its main clinical indications include the treatment and prophylaxis of *Pneumocystis jiroveci* (formerly *carinii*) pneumonia; urinary tract infections; nocardia infections; shigellosis. It is also used for other infections caused by organisms that are often resistant to most other antimicrobials, including *Acinetobacter* spp., *Burkholderia cepacia*, *Stenotrophomonas maltophilia* and fast-growing mycobacteria such as *M. marinum* and *M. kansasii*. It also has some activity against protozoa, e.g. *Isospora belli*.

Toxicity is almost always due to the sulphonamide component and although serious side-effects are rare, e.g. Stevens–Johnson syndrome, neutropenia, thrombocytopenia and agranulocytosis, they are sufficient to severely restrict the clinical use of co-trimoxazole, especially in the elderly.

Metronidazole

Metronidazole was originally introduced as a treatment for protozoal infections such as trichomonas and giardia. These are anaerobes and their specialized enzymes used for energy production convert metronidazole into toxic substances, which then destroy the cell. Anaerobic bacteria use the same enzymes and metronidazole has now become the main treatment for infections caused by anaerobes (e.g. *Bacteroides* spp.). It is also used as prophylaxis before operation on the bowel or uterus and in combination with other drugs in the treatment of *Helicobacter pylori*.

Metronidazole is distributed throughout the tissues and adverse reactions and resistance are rare, although it should not be taken with alcohol since it causes the 'Antabuse effect'.

Clindamycin

This drug is similar in activity to the macrolides. Its mode of action is probably at the peptidyl transferase stage of protein synthesis. It is active against most Gram positives, particularly staphylococci and streptococci (but not enterococci). It is active against most anaerobes and some protozoa, including toxoplasma and plasmodium. It has no activity against Gram-negative aerobic bacilli.

It is well absorbed by the oral route and is widely distributed, including intracellularly and into bones.

Its major side-effect is an increased risk of antibiotic-associated colitis due to *Clostridium difficile* toxin. This is most common in elderly/middle-aged women. Therapy should therefore be stopped if diarrhoea occurs.

Despite this, clindamycin is an extremely useful antibacterial. It can be used in the treatment of soft tissue, bone and joint infections caused by *Staphylococcus aureus* (non-MRSA) and especially those allergic to the β-lactams. Similarly, it can be used in severe infections caused by group A, C and G β-haemolytic streptococci, again in those allergic to penicillin. It is used for endocarditis prophylaxis in those allergic to penicillin. It can be used for the prophylaxis and treatment of anaerobic infections.

It has an increasing role in the treatment of severe soft tissue infections (including necrotizing fasciitis). Although the mainstay of treatment is surgical debridement, clindamycin should be considered (along with cover for Gram-negative aerobic bacilli) in these situations. This is for two reasons: first, its spectrum of activity includes all the major likely pathogens (group A β-haemolytic streptococci, *Staphylococcus aureus* and anaerobes, including toxigenic clostridia) and second, the theory that its mode of action should quickly shut down the production of the protein exotoxins that are responsible for the high mortality associated with these severe soft tissue infections (Stevens 2000).

Fusidic acid

This is a steroid-like substance which is a product of fermentation by a fungus; it interferes with protein synthesis in bacteria. Fusidic acid is mainly used (as a second active agent) for the treatment of severe staphylococcal infections (including those caused by MRSA), particularly those involving bone, joints and endocarditis. It is well absorbed orally and widely distributed in the tissues. It can also be used topically for treating skin infections. It must be used in combination with another active agent in order to prevent the emergence of resistance.

It causes mild gastrointestinal side-effects (nausea) and in some patients may cause a reversible jaundice. Jaundice is more common with intravenous therapy than oral.

Rifampicin

This is a synthetic derivative of an antibiotic produced by a streptomyces (rifamycin)which inactivates RNA polymerase and is bactericidal. It is used mainly for the treatment of tuberculosis and leprosy (in combination with other active agents); in the elimination of throat carriage of *Neisseria meningitidis* in outbreaks of meningococcal meningitis; as an additional agent in the treatment of Legionnaires' disease (with a macrolide); in severe staphylococcal infections (including MRSA, with a penicillin or glycopeptide); and in severe pneumococcal infections (with a penicillin or glycopeptide). It is also an important component of oral (combination) suppression therapy in cases of prosthetic joint infections not amenable to surgical intervention since it is still active against non-dividing bacterial cells present in the biofilm (unlike agents active on the cell wall, such as the penicillins).

It is virtually entirely absorbed by the oral route and due to its lipid solubility is widely distributed to bones, internal organs and into body fluids such as tears, saliva and ascitic fluid. It penetrates cells and is active against intracellular organisms.

Rifampicin is a potent inducer of the cytochrome P450 enzyme system. This results in the increased metabolism of other drugs. The most important of these are warfarin (oral anticoagulant) and the oral contraceptive pill. In these examples there would be a resultant diminished anticoagulant effect and a possible failure of contraception, respectively. Measures would therefore be required to prevent these problems, i.e an increase in the warfarin dose and an alternative method of contraception.

Rifampicin is relatively non-toxic but patients should be warned that it will turn their body fluids (urine, tears) pink and consequently it will stain soft contact lenses pink too. Its other side-effects include skin reactions (flushing with or without a rash) and transient rises in serum (hepatic) transaminases. In intermittent therapy a flu-like syndrome can occur. Rarer side-effects include a thrombocytopenia (fall in platelets) associated with complement-fixing serum antibodies. The rifampicin must then be discontinued and platelet levels usually return to normal within a few days.

Antituberculous therapy

Tuberculosis is a difficult infection to treat because the mycobacteria grow very slowly and may be protected in cavities within the lungs and within macrophages. A combination of antibiotics must be used to kill both multiplying and intracellular mycobacteria and to prevent resistant bacteria from emerging. The main drugs used are isoniazid, rifampicin, ethambutol and pyrazinamide. The most potent bactericidal agent is isoniazid which kills 90% of sensitive tubercle bacilli in 7 days; the next most potent bactericidal drug is rifampicin. In the UK, for adult respiratory TB, a course of 6 months is given: four drugs together for the first 2 months (rifampicin, isoniazid, pyrazinamide and ethambutol), followed by two drugs (rifampicin and isoniazid) for 4 further months.

The prolonged nature of therapy affects compliance with the treatment regimen but therapy using too few drugs or incomplete courses of treatment encourages resistance to emerge. Although resistance to antituberculous drugs is quite rare in the UK, resistance rates of over 30% to one or more drugs have been reported in some populations in other parts of the world (Mayon-White 2004) (see p. 113).

Patients with AIDS are particularly susceptible to an atypical mycobacterium, *Mycobacterium avium intracellulare*. These bacteria are usually highly resistant to the conventional antituberculous drugs and treatment of the infection can be extremely difficult (Pratt 2003).

ANTIFUNGAL THERAPY

Fungi may cause a variety of infections, ranging from superficial infections of the skin and mucous membranes (often caused by dermatophytes, e.g. *Trichophyton* spp., and yeasts, e.g. *Candida* spp.) to serious invasive/systemic infection (caused by yeasts, e.g. *Candida* spp., and filamentous fungi, e.g. *Aspergillus* spp.) which may be fatal and are usually associated with immune suppression.

The eukaryotic cells of fungi are not susceptible to antibacterial agents and specific antifungal agents are required to treat the infections that they cause. Because they affect eukaryotic cells, these specific antifungal agents are often associated with more toxicity than their antibacterial counterparts.

Not so very long ago, the options for treating severe fungal infection were few, consisting of conventional amphotericin B (with or without flucytosine) or fluconazole. Recently, however, there has been a huge expansion in the available antifungal agents. This is due to the production of new formulations of old agents (lipid-associated amphotericin B, e.g. ambisome, intravenous itraconazole); new drugs within existing classes (triazoles, e.g. voriconazole); and new classes of agents (echinocandins, e.g. caspofungin) (Sinha & Barnes 2003, Warnock 2003).

The effect of the increasing use (and misuse) of broad-spectrum antibacterial agents in increasingly vulnerable patients is not only the selection of increasingly resistant bacteria but also the selection of yeasts and fungi. It should come as no surprise, therefore, to find that there has been an inexorable rise of infections caused by yeasts and fungi in hospitals, both in the USA and Europe, over the last 25 years. *Candida* spp. causes about 75% of these (yeast/fungal) infections. Candidaemia in the UK has an incidence of about three per 100 000 bed days, about 45% of cases occur in the ITU and it has an attributable mortality of some 40% (much higher than other bloodstream infections) (Kibbler et al 2003). If the candidaemia is associated with an intravascular catheter, the treatment should not only be with an appropriate antifungal (for 10–14 days) but the catheter should also be removed. Box 5.1 indicates the patients, in the ITU setting, most at risk of developing systemic candidiasis and in whom antifungal prophylaxis may be necessary. *Candida albicans* remains the commonest cause of hospital-acquired candidaemia in the UK. In ICU patients it is responsible for about 80% of the

Box 5.1   Patients most at risk of developing systemic candidiasis (Singha & Barnes 2003)
• Stem cell transplant patients • Liver transplant patients • Profound neutropenia of >7 days' duration • Necrotizing pancreatitis • Recurrent perforation of the bowel • Breakdown of bowel anastomosis • Oesophageal perforation

bloodstream infections caused by yeasts. Azole resistance is not widespread in ICUs, but occurs more commonly in patients with haematological malignancies or HIV where azoles are used more frequently (Sinha & Barnes 2003).

As the use of azole drugs, such as fluconazole, increases, other *Candida* spp. such as *C. tropicalis, C. parapsilosis, C. glabrata* and *C. krusei* (which are inherently more resistant to fluconazole) are causing an increasing proportion of systemic candida infections.

In severely neutropenic patients (e.g. bone marrow transplant) fungal infections can be difficult to diagnose and careful clinical judgement is required. Patients who are febrile and/or septic may have fungal infection but *with no positive cultures*. Filamentous fungi such as *Aspergillus* spp. do not grow in liquid culture, such as blood cultures. Aspergillus isolated from bronchial specimens may merely indicate colonization while a negative culture does not rule out invasive aspergillosis. Similarly in ITU patients, the risk of a patient having systemic candida infection seems to be related to the number of sites colonized by the same strain of candida (the candida colonization index). Yeasts will grow in blood cultures (but a minimum of 30 ml of blood should be taken) and urine specimens should always be taken. The isolation of yeasts solely from the lower respiratory tract, however, does not predict invasive disease but merely indicates colonization.

The use of newer imaging techniques may be helpful and molecular techniques for the diagnosis of yeast and fungi are becoming available and may prove to be useful.

Polyenes

Amphotericin B and lipid-associated amphotericin B (ambisome, abelcet, amphocil) bind to the sterols of susceptible fungal cells, resulting in the formation of pores in the membrane. Amphotericin B has a wide spectrum that includes most human fungal pathogens. These agents are used to treat aspergillosis, severe candida infections and systemic mycoses such as blastomycosis, histoplasmosis, cryptococcosis and mucormycosis.

Resistance is rare. Common side-effects include fever, chills, headache, backache, nausea, vomiting, anorexia and renal problems. Renal toxicity is the most important side-effect and it should be noted that amphotericin is synergistically nephrotoxic with other nephrotoxic drugs such as the aminoglycosides, cyclosporin and some anticancer agents. Other side-effects include abnormal liver function, rash and anaphylactoid reactions. Renal impairment is significantly less with lipid-associated amphotericin.

Flucytosine

5-Flucytosine is a synthetic fluorinated pyrimidine. It is incorporated into fungal RNA and disrupts protein synthesis. It is available for oral or intravenous use. It has a narrow spectrum, being active against Candida spp. and cryptococcus. It is used for deep and disseminated infections in combination with amphotericin B (or fluconazole). About 10% of Candida albicans are resistant prior to treatment and resistance also occurs during therapy. Gastrointestinal side-effects and rashes are common. Bone marrow toxicity and hepatic dysfunction are important. Levels should be measured if given with amphotericin B as the resultant nephrotoxicity can increase the flucytosine levels. Regular full blood counts should be done if treatment is prolonged.

The azoles

These agents act on the cell wall by inhibiting ergosterol synthesis. Imidazoles (e.g. clotrimazole) are used for the topical treatment of dermatophytoses (caused by *Epidermophyton*, *Microsporum* and *Trichophyton* spp.) and oral, cutaneous and vaginal candida infections.

Triazoles

Fluconazole

Fluconazole is used to treat mucosal, cutaneous and systemic candidiasis; cryptococcal infections; dermatophytic infections; and pityriasis versicolor. It is almost completely absorbed when given orally and it is widely distributed, reaching therapeutic concentrations in most body fluids and tissues. Concentrations in CSF during meningitis are in excess of 60% of serum concentrations. There is also an intravenous preparation. It is active against most strains of *C. albicans* from HIV-negative patients. Resistant strains have been reported but usually in HIV-positive and haematology patients after prolonged treatment. Failure of treatment is normally due to insufficient dose or duration of therapy and

therefore some patients may be on as much as 800 mg per day (Singha & Barnes 2003).

The non-albicans species of candida such as *C. glabrata* are intrinsically resistant to fluconazole, while *C. krusei* can become resistant and *C. tropicalis* has varying degrees of susceptibility. Other fungi are also susceptible to fluconazole, including dimorphic fungi (e.g. histoplasma, blastomycosis, coccidioidomycosis).

Although side-effects include gastrointestinal intolerance, headache, transient liver enzyme abnormalities and rarely serious skin reactions, including Stevens–Johnson syndrome, it has a much better safety profile than amphotericin.

Itraconazole

Itraconazole is used to treat aspergillosis (including prophylaxis and empiric treatment in neutropenic patients); systemic mycoses with dimorphic fungi (e.g. blastomycosis, coccidioidomycosis histoplasmosis); subcutaneous mycoses, e.g. sporotrichosis; mucosal and cutaneous candidiasis; pityriasis versicolor, and dermatophytic infections.

Itraconazole is highly lipophilic and therefore penetrates aqueous fluids poorly. Levels in lung, liver and bone are 2–3 times higher than in serum but low in the CSF. The old oral preparation (capsule) had poor bioavailability; absorption was dependent on a low gastric pH and the presence of food and it took many days for therapeutic levels to be reached in the serum after taking the capsules. A new oral solution combined with cyclodextrin has improved the absorption but has also increased the gastrointestinal side-effects. A new intravenous formulation gives good blood levels but there have been reports of phlebitis and line blockages. Plasma levels of itraconazole should be monitored to ensure that therapeutic levels are being achieved. There is cross-resistance in *Candida albicans* with fluconazole and itraconazole, and itraconazole-resistant *Aspergillus fumigatus* has also been reported.

Side-effects include gastrointestinal intolerance, skin rash, headache and caution is advised in patients with a high risk of developing heart failure. Life-threatening hepatotoxicity is rare but liver function tests should be monitored (British National Formulary 2005).

Voriconazole

This is a newly available synthetic triazole, for either oral or intravenous use. It is well absorbed by the oral route and has wide distribution into body fluids and tissues (including the CSF and brain). It has a very broad spectrum of activity that encompasses most fungi causing infection in humans. It is used for the treatment of life-threatening fungal infections including acute and chronic aspergillosis, candidiasis (including fluconazole-resistant strains) and serious infections caused by *Fusarium* and *Scedosporium* spp. Toxicity and side-effects are few but include mild to moderate visual disturbances, transiently raised liver enzymes and rashes.

Newer triazoles are currently under development including posaconazole and ravuconazole.

Echinocandins

Caspofungin

This is a semisynthetic lipopeptide. It causes cell lysis by interfering with glucan formation. It is available as an intravenous infusion and is widely distributed in the body, the highest concentration being found in the liver where it is metabolized. Dosage reduction is recommended in patients with moderate hepatic dysfunction but no dosage alteration is required in those with renal impairment. It is not removed by dialysis. It can be used for the treatment of invasive aspergillosis in patients who are either refractory or intolerant to other antifungals. It is also licensed for the treatment of invasive candidal infections and for the empiric treatment of systemic fungal infections in patients with neutropenia. It is active against the trophozoite form of *Pneumocystis jiroveci* (formerly *carinii*). Side-effects include fever, rash, itch, nausea, vomiting and transiently raised liver enzymes.

Two other echinocandins, anidulafungin and micafungin, are under development.

Other antifungals

Allylamines, e.g. terbinafine, are the drug of choice for fungal nail infections and also employed for the oral treatment of ringworm infections. Griseofulvin is an oral agent active against dermatophytic infections of the skin, nail and hair (*Epidermophyton*, *Microsporum* and *Trichophyton* spp.).

ANTIVIRAL THERAPY

Viruses are intracellular parasites that use the structures of the host cell to replicate themselves. Antiviral agents must therefore be able to target the virus without damaging the host cell. Some viral infections are self-limiting and cause relatively mild disease; hence active management is rarely necessary. However, the need to find effective treatments for serious viral infections such as HIV and other chronic viral infections (e.g. hepatitis) has stimulated research into antiviral agents. A number of stages in viral replication are now recognized as potential targets for antiviral agents whilst not inter-

Box 5.2 Potential targets for antiviral agents
• Inactivating virus before attachment
• Blocking attachment to cell membrane receptors
• Blocking penetration of the cell
• Preventing virus from uncoating
• Preventing integration into host genome
• Blocking transcription of viral genome
• Blocking translation of viral genome
• Interfering with viral assembly
• Interfering with viral release

fering with the host cell (Box 5.2). The development of rapid diagnostic methods for identifying viruses has also increased the value of antiviral therapy.

The most widely used antiviral agents are analogues of nucleosides, the nitrogen bases linked to sugars that form the building blocks of DNA (see Ch. 1). Nucleoside analogues block the production of nucleic acids by becoming incorporated into the growing viral DNA chain; their structure prevents the phosphate linkage with the next base in the chain so that replication of viral DNA is terminated. They become activated by phosphorylation inside the cell. They also inhibit some mammalian polymerases, especially those found in mitochondria, and this probably explains their toxicity. The more recently developed nucleoside analogues are activated by viral enzymes and because they therefore act specifically on infected cells, are associated with fewer side-effects. Nucleotide analogues mimic the nucleotides found in the DNA chain, they are actively taken up by most cells and are then activated by intracellular phosphorylation. They prevent the formation of viral DNA. However, they also inhibit mitochondrial DNA polymerase. Tenofovir also has activity against HIV reverse transcriptase. Other (non-nucleoside analogue) reverse transcriptase inhibitors work by binding to the enzyme. Oligonucleotides are short nucleotides that mirror sections of mRNA and prevent them being translated into viral proteins.

Protease inhibitors have complex pharmacokinetic properties, cause many side-effects and are associated with drug resistance. They are used in combination with nucleotide analogues to treat HIV and have a synergistic effect. Neuraminidase inhibitors prevent the activity of an enzyme called neuraminidase, which is required for progeny virus to be formed.

Phosphonic acid derivatives, e.g. foscarnet, inhibit the activity of DNA polymerase and are selectively active against viral polymerases such as those of herpes virus.

Interferons are proteins produced by mammalian cells in response to infection by viruses. The drugs are

Table 5.5   Major groups of antiviral agent

Site of action	Antiviral agent	Clinical use
Nucleoside analogues	Aciclovir	Herpes simplex, varicella zoster
	Penciclovir	Herpes zoster, genital herpes
	Idoxuridine (topical)	Herpes simplex
	Ganciclovir	Cytomegalovirus
	Ribavirin	Respiratory syncytial virus, hepatitis C
Reverse transcriptase nucleoside analogue	Dideoxynucleosides • Zalcitabine • Stavudine • Zidovudine • Didanosine • Abacavir • Lamivudine	HIV, hepatitis B
Protease inhibitor	Ritinavir Saquinavir Indinavir Amprenavir Nelfinavir	HIV
Nucleotide analogues	Cidofovir	CMV retinitis
Polymerase inhibitor (RNA and DNA polymerases)	Foscarnet	Cytomegalovirus
Oligonucleotides	Fomivirsen	CMV retinitis
Viral uncoating and assembly	Amantidine Rimantidine	Influenza A
Release of virus from cell	Zanamivir	Influenza A & B
Neuraminidase inhibitors	Oseltamivir Zanamivir	Influenza A & B
Induce cells to resist virus invasion	Interferon Peginterferon	Heptatitis B, hepatitis C

made in *Escherichia coli* using recombinant technology. They activate cytoplasmic enzymes that affect mRNA transcription and protein synthesis but are associated with side-effects such as flu-like symptoms and lymphocytopenia (see Ch. 4).

The main antiviral drugs are listed in Table 5.5.

RESISTANCE TO ANTIMICROBIAL AGENTS

Micro-organisms are not all intrinsically sensitive to all antimicrobials. The terms sensitive and resistant are used to distinguish between those agents that will, or

will not, destroy or prevent the growth of a micro-organism. On a simple level, bacteria can be described as *sensitive* to a particular antibacterial if their growth is inhibited or they are killed by a concentration of the drug that could be achieved by the usual dose regimen. *Resistant* bacteria are not inhibited or killed by this concentration of the drug. However, in practice, it is not always possible to make a clear distinction between sensitive and resistant strains, treatment with a particular antibiotic may still be effective if given at a higher dose. Determining the minimum inhibitory concentration (MIC) of the antibiotic will assess the sensitivity of a particular micro-organism. If the MIC is high, the organism is resistant and unlikely to be affected by treatment with the antibiotic; if it is low, then treatment is likely to be effective provided the antibiotic is able to penetrate the site of infection (Fig. 5.2).

Bacteria may have a *natural resistance* to certain antibiotics because the drug cannot penetrate their cells (e.g. the lipopolysaccharide outer layer of Gram-negative bacteria cannot be penetrated by some antibacterials) or because they do not possess the target to which the drug attaches. Some bacteria are naturally resistant to many antibiotics (e.g. *Pseudomonas aeruginosa, Staphylococcus epidermidis*).

Knowledge of the intrinsic resistance to antimicrobial agents enables appropriate therapy for a specific pathogen to be selected. However, the emergence of strains with acquired resistance to agents that they were previously susceptible to has occurred consistently, since the first antibiotics were introduced in the late 1930s and early 1940s. The prevalence of resistant strains has followed the developments and changes in antimicrobial use. Thus the introduction of flucloxacillin in the 1960s addressed the problem of penicillin-resistant *S. aureus* infections but Gram-negative bacteria then began to emerge as serious pathogens.

Although the propensity to acquire resistance varies between different bacteria, selective pressure is the key to the emergence of resistant strains. When exposed to an antimicrobial agent, sensitive cells will be destroyed but resistant cells survive and continue to multiply until eventually resistant cells replace all the sensitive cells. If an antibacterial agent is administered at a low dose then the resistant bacteria are more likely to outgrow the sensitive ones (Walsh 2000).

Acquired resistance may occur as the result of a mutation in the bacterial chromosome or by the acquisition of new DNA. Mutational resistance occurs when a mistake in DNA replication results in the addition, deletion or substitution of a few base pairs and subsequent alteration of one or more amino acids in a crucial peptide of a target protein. For example, rifampicin resistance in *Mycobacterium tuberculosis* is

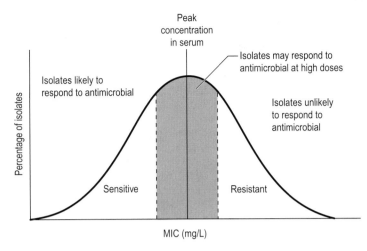

Figure 5.2 Relationship between sensitive, intermediate and resistant bacterial isolates and minimum inhibitory concentration (MIC) of an antimicrobial agent.

due to a mutation in the RNA polymerase. This type of resistance may be induced during therapy. The acquisition of new DNA occurs when genes conferring resistance to one or more antimicrobial agents are transferred from a resistant cell to a previously sensitive one. The transfer of antimicrobial resistance genes frequently occurs on plasmids, small molecules of DNA independent of the chromosome, which can be replicated and transferred between cells by conjugation, transformation or transduction (see p. 10). Plasmids provide a highly effective means of spreading resistance genes, both within a species and to other species.

Resistance genes may also be carried on transposons. These are specific sequences of DNA that can insert into both plasmids and chromosomes and transfer, or jump, between them. They can carry genes encoding for resistance to a wide variety of antibiotics and play a key role in the dissemination of antibiotic resistance, particularly where species develop resistance to more than one drug. Multiple drug resistance is a term used to describe bacteria that have developed resistance to several, unrelated antibiotics, for example Gram-negative bacilli that are resistant to both gentamicin and the β-lactams. These multiresistant bacteria often have one plasmid or transposon that carries several genes conferring resistance to several antibiotics. The antimicrobial resistance genes in MRSA are carried on a transposon (see p. 107).

Integrons are short sequences of DNA located at each end of antimicrobial resistance genes. They act as a framework that enables different resistance genes to be slotted into a plasmid or transposon like a cassette. They carry an enzyme called integrase that facilitates integration of resistance genes.

Inherently sensitive bacteria can *acquire resistance* to antibiotics by means of one or more of the following mechanisms:

- the permeability of the cell membrane changes so that the antimicrobial cannot enter or entry into the cell is slowed (e.g. resistance to imipenem in *Pseudomonas aeruginosa* but this is also in association with the hyperproduction of the chromosomal β-lactamase)
- the drug target may be bypassed through acquiring a new metabolic pathway (e.g. trimethoprim and sulphonamide resistance)
- the target with which the antimicrobial reacts is altered and the drug is unable to affect the cell (e.g. resistance to methicillin, and therefore all β-lactams, in staphylococci and penicillin resistance in pneumococci – both due to alterations in specific penicillin binding proteins)
- the bacterium produces enzymes that inactivate or modify the antimicrobial before or after it enters the cell (e.g. β-lactamases which destroy penicillins and cephalosporins)
- the antimicrobial is actively expelled from the cell – a drug efflux mechanism (e.g. resistance to tetracyclines).

The ability of microbes to acquire resistance to antibiotics was recognized soon after the first drugs were introduced as human therapeutic agents. The development and spread of resistance are the inevitable consequence of widespread use of an antibacterial agent, since the rapid generation time of bacteria gives rise to many mutations with the potential to confer resistance and resistance genes are readily spread within and between species on plasmids. Clinical resistance to an antibacterial agent therefore generally begins to emerge within months or years of its introduction (Walsh 2000).

Initially, the steady supply of new drugs was able to combat the problem. However, although modifications to existing drugs have been made, only a few new classes of antimicrobial agents have been introduced recently. An example includes the oxazolidinones (linezolid), which show much promise. Bacterial genomics holds some hope for the development of other new classes of antimicrobial agents. Many complete genomes of important pathogens such as *S. aureus* and *Strep. pneumoniae* have now been completely sequenced. If genes essential for virulence or for the survival of the cell can be identified, these will provide useful target proteins in the search for effective inhibitors (Chapna et al 1997).

The development of vaccines has also provided some solutions; for example, the vaccination of children against *Haemophilus influenzae* has helped to resolve the problem of emerging resistance in this pathogen. However, vaccines are unlikely to help combat resistance amongst commensal organisms such as enterococci. There is interest in bacteriophages, viruses that destroy specific bacteria, although their use is associated with practical problems such as selecting an appropriate phage and delivery to the site of infection (Barrow & Soothill 1997). Probiotics are harmless commensal micro-organisms which can be used to displace pathogens from certain sites on the body, although their usefulness is limited.

Factors contributing to the emergence of resistance

Although much of the evidence is circumstantial, there are a number of factors considered to play a key role in the development of antimicrobial resistance.

Use of antimicrobial agents

There is considerable evidence to connect heavy use of antimicrobial agents with the emergence of resistance, although at a population level specific links between antibiotic prescribing and resistance can be difficult to prove (DoH 1999, Woodhead et al 2004). The extent of the problem varies considerably between countries. The USA and Japan consume large quantities of antimicrobial agents and have correspondingly higher levels of resistance. In Japan, 70% of *S. aureus* isolates are resistant to methicillin, compared with less than 1% in Scandinavia where antimicrobial usage is much lower. In some countries, particularly South-East Asia and Latin America, problems of overusage are aggravated by poor controls over supplies (Bapna et al 1996). Drugs can be purchased without a prescription and as single, low-dose tablets, which are highly likely to encourage resistance to develop. The use of single-dose therapy for the treatment of gonorrhoea has resulted in the progressive selection of resistant strains, so that around 50% of *Neisseria gonorrhoeae* cases in developing countries are resistant to penicillin and in the UK 9% of isolates are now resistant to either penicillin or ciprofloxacin (DoH 1999, Health Protection Agency 2005a).

Inappropriate prescribing of antimicrobial agents

Many studies have shown that inappropriate use of antimicrobial agents is widespread. In countries where these drugs can be obtained without a prescription, the problem may be endemic. For example, in Mexico people commonly use antibiotics to treat diarrhoea, for which they are both ineffective and unnecessary (Bojalil & Calva 1994). Inappropriate prescribing is also a major problem in the UK. Of the 50 million antibiotic prescriptions dispensed annually in the UK, 80% originate from community practice (general practitioners and dentists). Half of these agents are prescribed for the treatment of minor, upper respiratory tract infections, such as sore throat, otitis media, sinusitis or coughs and wheezes, most of which are caused by viruses and treatment with antibiotics is therefore likely to be unnecessary (Del Mar et al 1997). However, there is evidence that GPs have begun to change their prescribing practice, with a 25% reduction in prescriptions for antibacterial agents between 1997 and 2000 (Wigley & Majeed 2002). Such changes in prescribing practice may have been helped by improving patients' understanding, for example through the use of a 'non-prescription' form which enables the GP to explain why antibiotics are not necessary and provide advice on how the condition the patient has presented with can be managed (House of Lords Select Committee 2001).

In hospitals, antimicrobial agents are frequently given for unnecessarily prolonged periods. For example, when used for prophylaxis in surgery, a single dose of antibiotic is usually adequate, unless evidence of infection is found at the time of operation (see p. 185). However, a recent study in nearly 3000 US hospitals suggested that antibiotic prophylaxis was continued for longer than necessary in 60% of patients (Bratzler et al 2005).

Prolonged antimicrobial therapy favours the growth of resistant strains, which may then become the pathogen, particularly in hospital patients whose defence mechanisms are impaired. Commensal micro-organisms, particularly those in the gut, play an important role in the selection and spread of resistance.

Box 5.3 illustrates some simple principles of good practice in antimicrobial therapy that should be used to help prevent the emergence of resistance.

Transmission of resistance

In many circumstances, the emergence of resistant strains is followed by their spread by cross-infection.

<table>
<tr><td>

Box 5.3   Good practice in antimicrobial therapy

- Do not give for trivial reasons
- Use for prophylaxis only when the risk of infection is high
- Use good infection control to prevent infection rather than use antimicrobials
- Take an appropriate specimen as soon as infection is suspected
- Use antimicrobials only when clinically indicated by signs of infection, not just because of a positive laboratory report
- Use an antimicrobial that has a specific action against the infecting organism rather than one that affects a wide range of organisms
- Administer the correct dose for an adequate period but stop at the end of the course or if there is no obvious clinical response

</td></tr>
</table>

Such transmission is particularly likely to occur in hospitals where invasive devices and underlying illness make patients more vulnerable to infection. Resistant strains are spread to other hospitals when patients are transferred and transmission of strains between countries also occurs frequently. Patients from countries with inadequate controls on antimicrobial consumption are more likely to be infected or colonized by resistant micro-organisms.

Antimicrobial usage in agriculture

Some 50% of antimicrobial agents used in the UK are given to animals, not humans. They are used for three reasons: the treatment of disease, prophylaxis against disease to contain the spread of a particular infection and as growth promoters. The latter practice is highly controversial. In Denmark, pigs treated with a vancomycin derivative growth promoter were found to carry the same strains of vancomycin-resistant enterococcus known to cause infections in humans (Witte 1998). The European Union has banned the use of animal growth promoters that have a human analogue. In some countries their use has been completely banned (e.g. Sweden), whereas in others (e.g. the USA) common human antibiotics such as penicillin and tetracycline are still in use. In the UK there is evidence that the use of antibacterial agents in animals has significantly decreased in recent years (House of Lords Select Committee 2001).

Strategies for preventing antimicrobial resistance

Although reductions in the use of antimicrobial agents have been followed by a decrease in incidence of resistant pathogens, the effect is by no means automatic, may take some time and it is difficult to make clear associations because of other confounding factors such as changes in infection control practice (Davey et al 2003). Selection of resistant strains may continue because several resistance genes may be carried on one plasmid and ongoing use of one antibiotic maintains resistance to the others. Resistance is particularly difficult to eliminate where it is carried by many strains of the same species, rather than by only one epidemic strain, and improvements in prescribing practice may only prevent the situation deteriorating rather than achieve a reduction in the levels of resistance.

However, studies have shown that reducing antibacterial prescribing or changing the antibacterial agent used for empiric treatment has been associated with a decrease in the prevalence of antibiotic resistant bacteria (Bradley et al 1999, Seppala et al 1997).

In the UK the *Antimicrobial Resistance Strategy and Action Plan* (DoH 2000) focuses on three areas: surveillance to monitor the emergence of antimicrobial resistance; encouraging prudent prescribing in both clinical and veterinary practice; and strengthening infection control to prevent spread of resistant pathogens. Key recommendations include measures to change public expectations and attitudes to antibiotics, education of clinicians (especially general practitioners and junior doctors) to improve their awareness of resistance and good prescribing practice; and the development of therapy guidelines. There is some evidence to suggest that these recommendations have begun to have some effect (House of Lords Select Committee 2001).

Antimicrobial policies

More than half the hospitals in the UK have a policy for antimicrobial therapy (BSAC Working Party 1994). These policies are intended to encourage the proper and careful use of antimicrobial agents, to discourage the indiscriminate use especially of broad-spectrum drugs in order to minimize the development of antimicrobial resistance, and to reduce the costs of antimicrobial prescribing (Weinstein 2001). These controls are becoming increasingly important as problems with resistance increase. In addition, they can contribute to minimizing the risk of potentially harmful adverse drug reactions or interactions with other drugs.

Policies should include advice on assessing the need for antimicrobial treatment and prophylaxis, the most appropriate drug to prescribe and the preferred route, dose and duration. The policy may also suggest restricted access to some drugs. The microbiology laboratory plays a key role in encouraging the appropriate use of antimicrobials by reporting only a limited number of sensitivities and may indicate when the organisms are likely to be colonizing rather than causing infection. The consultant clinical microbiologist has an important function in educating and advising doctors and other healthcare professionals in the appropriate use of antimicrobial agents.

Key to the success of any policy is active implementation based on a range of strategies, for example audit and feedback, computerized advice on drug dosage, education and local opinion leaders (Thomson O'Brien et al 2001). Outcome or process measures are required to measure compliance with the policy (Bratzler et al 2005, Scottish Intercollegiate Guidelines Network (SIGN) 1999). Both nurses and clinical pharmacists can play an important part in monitoring the prolonged or inappropriate use of antimicrobials.

CLINICAL PROBLEMS ASSOCIATED WITH ANTIMICROBIAL RESISTANCE

Before the introduction of the first antibiotics, death from sepsis was commonplace, especially amongst hospital patients (Simpson 1869). Until recently, it seemed that new drugs could be found to cope with emerging problems of resistance to antimicrobial agents. However, it is now apparent that this is not the case and widespread resistance amongst major pathogens is seriously threatening our ability to treat some infections.

Hospitals provide a particularly fertile breeding ground for resistant micro-organisms. Antimicrobial usage exerts a selective pressure on commensal micro-organisms, seriously ill patients are particularly vulnerable to infection and resistant strains can spread easily between patients on contaminated hands or equipment.

The key to successful control of antimicrobial-resistant pathogens in hospitals is good isolation techniques, especially rigorous attention to hand hygiene, by *all* members of staff who have contact with patients infected or colonized with resistant pathogens. The aim should be to eliminate infection or colonization as rapidly as possible and ensure the patient's period of isolation is kept to a minimum. The infection control team will co-ordinate the management of outbreaks of resistant pathogens among hospital patients and work closely with the occupational health department to monitor and, where necessary, treat colonized staff. The environment may play a part in the transmission of some pathogens.

Although avoiding exposure to antimicrobial agents is not possible, there is some evidence that

Box 5.4 The development of antibiotic resistance in *Staphylococcus aureus*

1960	Methicillin introduced
1961	Methicillin-resistant *S. aureus* first reported
1970	5% of *S. aureus* isolates methicillin resistant
1976	*S. aureus* resistant to gentamicin and methicillin reported
1980	New penicillins and cephalosporins introduced. Epidemic strain of MRSA reported in London. Incidence of MRSA increases
1990	MRSA affecting most parts of the UK. Many different strains identified
2000	40% of invasive *S. aureus* infections now MRSA; EMRSA types 15 and 16 prevalent

reduction of antimicrobial use and cycling of agents used may provide a potential strategy for reducing the prevalence of antimicrobial-resistant pathogens (John & Rice 2000).

This section reviews the key pathogens for which antimicrobial resistance presents significant problems in healthcare settings both in the UK and many other countries.

Methicillin–resistant *Staphylococcus aureus* (MRSA)

Staphylococci are an important cause of infection. For example, *S. aureus* is responsible for more than one-third of surgical wound infections and approximately 25% of hospital-acquired bloodstream infections (Health Protection Agency 2003a, b). Staphylococci have a remarkable capacity to adapt to the presence of antimicrobials in their environment by developing resistance (Box 5.4). Soon after penicillin became widely available in the late 1940s, strains of *S. aureus* emerged that produced an enzyme (β-lactamase) that destroyed the β-lactam ring. Now resistance to penicillin is almost universal in *S. aureus*.

Modifications to the β-lactam ring were made to prevent attack by β-lactamases and in 1960 methicillin, a penicillin resistant to β-lactamases, was introduced. Methicillin is relatively toxic and was therefore replaced by a similar drug, flucloxacillin, which could also be given orally. Flucloxacillin soon became established as the drug of choice for the treatment of staphylococcal infection, since resistance to other penicillins was widespread.

Soon after the introduction of methicillin, resistant strains of *S. aureus* (MRSA) were reported. The incidence of MRSA increased until the 1970s and caused many serious outbreaks of infection in hospitals. During the early 1970s outbreaks of MRSA diminished but, unfortunately, this was not the end of the problem. In the early 1980s, the third-generation cephalosporins were introduced and used extensively in many countries for treating infections in hospitalized patients. Unfortunately, these broad-spectrum antibiotics had little activity against MRSA strains, their use encouraged the selection of the resistant strain and gradually the *S. aureus* population has become dominated by MRSA strains.

β-lactam antibiotics work by attaching to an enzyme (penicillin binding protein, PBP) that catalyses the formation of cross-bridges in the peptidoglycan of bacterial cell walls. MRSA is resistant to penicillin and other β-lactam antibiotics because it carries a gene (mecA) that encodes an additional PBP that β-lactam antibiotics are unable to attach to and therefore cell wall construction can continue. In MRSA the genes that code for resistance to both β-lactam and non-β-lactam antibiotics are grouped together in a 'cassette' of genes that is incorporated into the cell chromosome. This 'cassette' also contains transposons (see p. 71) that enable it to be readily transferred to other cells. Exposure to antimicrobials triggers the transcription of these genes and confers resistance to many drugs, seriously limiting the treatment options for affected patients. Vancomycin and teicoplanin are the main antimicrobial agents available to treat invasive MRSA infection.

These sophisticated mechanisms for resisting the effects of antibiotics have evolved in *S. aureus* over the last 50 years as it has been presented with new antimicrobial challenges, helped by its ability to readily acquire new genes from other species of staphylococci. The selection of MRSA from a population of *S. aureus* has been promoted by the widespread use of antimicrobials, particularly in the treatment of seriously ill hospital patients whose survival often depends on antimicrobial therapy.

In addition to resistance to many antibiotics, some strains of MRSA carry virulence factors that enhance their capacity to both spread from patient to patient and to cause infection. Recent epidemics of MRSA first occurred in London hospitals in the mid-1980s and subsequently spread throughout the country. Since the 1990s two epidemic strains have emerged in the UK (EMRSA 15 and EMRSA 16); the former is particularly associated with colonization of chronic wounds and urine, the latter with invasive infections such as pneumonia (Cox et al 1995). There has been a marked increase in the number of bloodstream infections caused by MRSA and now more than 40% of *S. aureus* bloodstream infections are caused by MRSA and over 90% of these are EMRSA 15 or 16 (Communicable Disease Report 2004, Johnson et al 2001) (Fig. 5.3). MRSA is also an important problem in many other countries. In Europe, the prevalence of invasive infection caused by MRSA varies considerably, with less than 5% of *S. aureus* isolates resistant to methicillin in northern Europe, compared to over 40% in southern Europe and the UK (Fig. 5.4). However, in many countries, even in northern Europe, prevalence has increased significantly since 1999 (Tiemersma et al 2004).

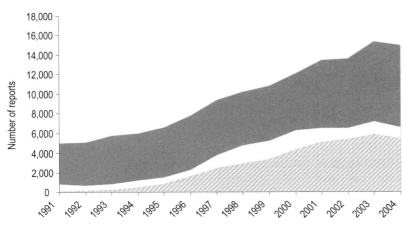

Figure 5.3 *Staphylococcus aureus* bacteraemia reports and methicillin susceptibility (England and Wales 1991–2004) (Source: Health Protection Agency. Available online at: http://www.hpa.org.uk/infections/topics_az/staphylo/lab_data_staphyl.htm).

MRSA (methicillin-resistant *Staphylococcus aureus*)   No sensitivity data   MSSA (methicillin-sensitive *Staphylococcus aureus*)

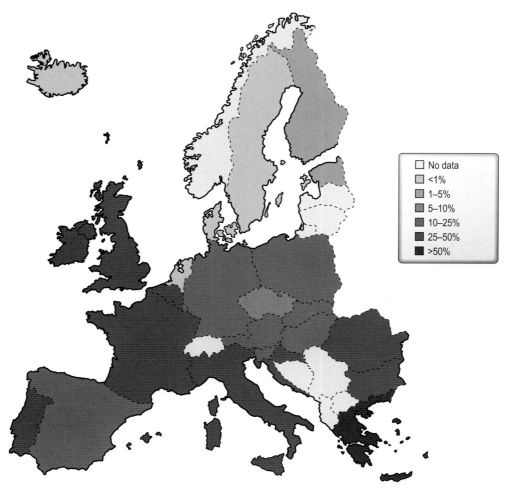

Figure 5.4 Intercountry variation in the proportion of invasive isolates of *Staphylococcus aureus* resistant to methicillin (European Antimicrobial Resistance Surveillance System, EARSS) (reproduced with permission from Tiemersma et al 2004).

Controlling the spread of MRSA presents particular difficulties because *S. aureus* is a normal commensal of skin and many people may become harmlessly colonized with MRSA and act as a reservoir from which the organism can be transferred to other people. MRSA mostly affects patients in hospital, both because of the selective effect of exposure to antibiotics and the many opportunities hospitals provide to transfer *S. aureus* between vulnerable patients and into sites susceptible to infection, such as wounds and invasive devices. Colonization pressure can have a major impact on the ability of a hospital to control the spread of MRSA. A unit that has a high endemic level of MRSA because it admits seriously ill or chronically sick

patients previously colonized with MRSA may find it extremely difficult to prevent transmission and the risk of transmission will be increased during periods of high workload (Grundmann et al 2002).

In the UK the prevalence of MRSA in the community remains low. Maudsley et al (2004) reported a prevalence of less than 1% in elderly patients sampled from the registration list of London GPs and 'previous history of hospitalization' was a key risk factor for MRSA carriage. However, the distinction between hospital and community patients is less clear now than it was in the past. Many more patients are treated in their own home or in community facilities and the chronically sick may move frequently between hospital and residential care. Patients that originally become colonized with MRSA in hospital may return to a nursing home where the organism may be subsequently transferred to other residents.

In the USA there is now evidence of a new type of MRSA in patients with no history of hospital treatment. This strain may have acquired its resistance from *S. epidermidis* (a normal commensal of skin that is intrinsically resistant to many antibiotics) and if disseminated internationally, opens the door to MRSA becoming widespread as a cause of community-acquired as well as hospital-acquired infection (Hiramatsu et al 2001).

There have also been reports of MRSA strains that show intermediate resistance to vancomycin/glycopeptides (VISA/GISA) in the USA, Japan, France and Scotland (Hiramatsu et al 1997, Hood et al 2000, Tenover et al 2001). The first reports of true vancomycin-resistant *S. aureus* (VRSA), i.e. MIC of greater than 256 mg/L, occurred in 2003. Three cases have now been documented, all from the USA and all due to the presence of the Van A gene, presumably acquired from vancomycin/glycopeptide resistant enterococci (Centers for Disease Control 2004, Chang et al 2003). This is potentially very serious as this antibiotic is the main drug used to treat invasive MRSA infection. The increasing use of vancomycin to treat MRSA is likely to drive the inevitable emergence of more VRSA strains.

Epidemiology of Staphylococcus aureus

Staphylococcus aureus is a major cause of both healthcare-associated and community-acquired infections, ranging from mild infection of the skin (boils and abscesses) to serious systemic infection such as bloodstream infection, pneumonia and major wound infection. Methicillin-resistant strains cause a similar range of infections as sensitive strains (see p. 119). Although the virulence of strains may vary, most studies do not suggest that MRSA is more pathogenic than methicillin-sensitive *S. aureus* (MSSA). However, some studies have suggested a higher incidence of septic shock in critically ill patients and an increased case-fatality rate associated with MRSA bloodstream infection (Coello et al 1997, Cosgrove et al 2003).

In addition to causing infection, *S. aureus* is a part of the normal flora of the skin, especially in axillae, groins, perineum and nose. Some people are heavily colonized with *S. aureus* and areas of damaged skin are especially prone to colonization (e.g. wounds, cannula sites). MRSA may replace sensitive strains of *S. aureus* on the skin, which it will colonize to provide a reservoir from which it may spread to other patients or staff. Patients colonized with MRSA have an increased risk of developing serious infection (Coello et al 1997).

Hospitalization is a major risk factor for the acquisition of MRSA; exposure to antibiotics encourages

---

Box 5.5   Types of patient and hospital settings where MRSA colonization/infection is most likely to occur

Hospital settings where patients are at highest risk of becoming colonized/infected with MRSA
- Intensive care units
- Neonatal and special care baby units
- Burns units
- Transplant units
- Cardiothoracic units
- Orthopaedic/trauma wards
- Vascular surgery
- Renal units
- Regional referral/specialist units

Patients with greatest risk of being colonized with MRSA
- Previously known to be MRSA positive
- History of frequent admission to healthcare facilities
- Has been an inpatient in a hospital abroad or UK hospital with known high prevalence
- Admitted from residential care facility with high prevalence of MRSA

Source: BSAC/HIS/ICNA 2005.

---

resistant strains to emerge and the presence of wounds or invasive devices facilitates colonization. Patients in some specialties are more at risk than others (Box 5.5). In long-term care settings, whilst the risk of transmission and serious infection is lower, patients may act as a reservoir of MRSA, bringing the organism into hospital when they are admitted (Fraise et al 1997). Serious staphylococcal infection usually occurs in people made more vulnerable by an underlying illness or medical intervention. Healthy people are unlikely to develop infection, although they may become colonized. Although most patients lose the resistant strain after discharge from hospital, some may remain colonized for prolonged periods, particularly where they are colonized at more than one site (Harbarth et al 2000).

Route of transmission

MRSA is spread in the same way as sensitive strains of *S. aureus*. The most important route of transmission is on the hands of staff who acquire the organism through direct contact with infected or colonized skin and, if carriage is not removed by handwashing, will transfer contamination to the next person or item touched. Pittet et al (2000) reported a reduction in rates of MRSA sustained over 4 years through a major programme aimed at improving compliance with hand hygiene together with a range of other infection control measures such as isolation precautions.

Airborne spread is theoretically possible but there is little direct evidence that it occurs and it is probably not a significant route of transmission unless patients are shedding excessive amounts of skin scales or the standard of cleaning is very low (Barrett et al 1993, Strausbaugh et al 1996).

Heavily contaminated equipment or uniforms could potentially transmit infection. The role of the environment in the spread of infections in hospital is controversial. Although MRSA can be isolated from the environment and inanimate objects such as computer keyboards and door handles, there is little evidence that contamination of the environment plays a significant part in the transmission of infection between patients (Devine et al 2001, Marshall et al 2004). Provided hands are decontaminated before contact with patients, contamination from the environment will not be transferred.

Nonetheless, staphylococci are resistant to desiccation and may survive for many weeks in the environment. Epidemic strains of MRSA may be particularly good at surviving in dust (Wagenvoort et al 2000). If dust is allowed to accumulate in clinical areas it may provide a reservoir of infection. Rampling et al (2001) found that visibly dusty wards contributed to an outbreak of MRSA and implemented a comprehensive cleaning programme targeted at removing dust from surfaces, furniture, floors and equipment. Cleaning should include inaccessible areas that may accumulate dust such as radiators and ventilator grills.

The risk from potentially contaminated equipment or the environment can be eliminated if hands are washed before and after patient contact.

Control of MRSA in hospitals

Attempts to control the spread of MRSA are essential to both retain options for antimicrobial therapy and protect vulnerable patients. The efficacy of different control measures is difficult to evaluate because reports of successful interventions often follow sudden increases in rates of MRSA and subsequent reductions may simply reflect expected fluctuations in numbers of cases (Cooper et al 2003). Usually several interventions are introduced and most are not evaluated against a control group. Many hospitals in the UK now experience high endemic rates of MRSA rather than periodic epidemics and it is not clear how effective control measures directed at controlling outbreaks of MRSA are at reducing rates of endemic infection. However, the literature suggests that there are several key elements that contribute to preventing the transmission and controlling outbreaks of MRSA.

1. *Controlling antimicrobial usage.* Although evidence for the effect of antimicrobial use is conflicting, prudent use of antimicrobials, especially broad-spectrum drugs, may minimize the risk that MRSA will be selected from the population of *S. aureus* (Hiramatsu et al 2001).

2. *Reducing the pool of colonized patients through early detection and decolonization.* Active screening of all patients admitted to high-risk units and high-risk patients admitted to the hospital is recommended (see Box 5.5) (BSAC/HIS/ICNA Working Party 2005). Some units may screen all admissions and then screen all patients in the unit weekly. Swabs from nose and at least one other site, e.g. throat, skin or wound, is a reasonably sensitive method of detecting carriers (Marshall et al 2004). Screening other patients or staff in contact with an MRSA case, or where there is evidence of further spread, may also be necessary to contain spread although the rate of transmission to staff is generally fairly low and frequently transient (Blok et al 2003, Cookson et al 1989).

3. *Preventing transmission from patient to patient.* Single-room isolation for patients found to be colonized or infected with MRSA is generally recommended (Box 5.6). Since the main route of transmission is direct contact, hand hygiene following contact with the patient or their immediate environment is the most important infection control measure. Alcohol handrubs may help to increase compliance with hand hygiene and may be more effective in removing contamination with MRSA (Hoffman et al 2004, Pittet et al 2000). Disposable aprons and gloves should be used for direct contact with the patient and discarded after each use. Although some studies have suggested that masks help to prevent healthcare workers acquiring MRSA, the low rates of acquisition by staff mean that their value is limited (Lacey et al 2001). In some areas of the hospital where the risk of transmission or serious infection is relatively low, e.g. long-stay care of the elderly, psychiatric units, isolation is not necessary provided routine infection control precautions are applied (see Ch. 7) and hands thoroughly washed after direct contact with patients. If the availability of single rooms is limited then patients with MRSA can be cohorted in one ward or part of a ward. The allocation of designated staff to care for them is recommended (BSAC/HIS/ICNA Working Party 1998). Similarly, in intensive care units isolation precautions may have to be applied in the main unit rather than a side room.

Box 5.6   Important principles for controlling MRSA in hospitals

Isolation
- Colonized or infected patients should be nursed in a single room, where available
- Gloves and aprons should be used for contact with the patient and discarded after use. They should also be changed between procedures
- Hands should be washed after contact with patients or their environment
- Alcohol handrub should be available by the bedside and entrance to the room to enable rapid hand decontamination

Cohorting
- A group of several affected patients can be isolated together in a designated part of the ward. This can help to reduce workload for staff and improve adherence to the control measures

Cleaning
- Isolation rooms should be kept clean during use, especially the horizontal surfaces where dust may settle and bacteria accumulate
- Rooms should be cleaned with detergent and water after isolation has been discontinued to remove micro-organisms remaining in the environment

Treatment of affected patients
- Decolonization is recommended prior to surgical procedures and in outbreaks of infection. Recolonization is common
- Apply antistaphylococcal cream to open skin and intranasally (mupirocin, three times per day for 5 days; naseptin, four times a day for 7 days). To prevent resistance to mupirocin emerging, no more than two courses of treatment should be given in any one admission
- Bathe daily for 5 days using antiseptic detergents (e.g. chlorhexidine) to eliminate skin colonization
- Wash hair with antiseptic detergent to eliminate colonization
- Isolation can be discontinued when three sets of negative swabs from all previously positive sites have been obtained
- Clinical infections will require treatment with antibiotics, usually vancomycin or teicoplanin

Readmission
- Previously colonized or infected patients should be rescreened on readmission to hospital as the resistant strain may persist in small numbers
- Notes can be labelled and computer-held records flagged to indicate patients who have had MRSA

Transfer of patients with MRSA
- Avoid moving patients to other wards or departments
- Home care personnel and residential care facilities should be informed of patients with MRSA prior to discharge but this should not affect their transfer

Screening of other patients
- Other patients may need to be sampled for MRSA carriage by taking swabs from the nose, perineum or groin, skin lesions and invasive device insertion sites. This can enable early identification, isolation and treatment of MRSA carriers and help to limit spread
- The extent of screening will depend on the type of clinical area and the number of patients affected
- High-risk units, e.g. ICUs, may screen all patients on admission

Screening of staff contacts
- This is usually necessary only in high-risk areas, such as the intensive care unit, or where the organism continues to spread despite the control measures and a staff carrier may be contributing to transmission
- Swab nose and skin lesions of staff in contact with affected patients
- Staff who are colonized with MRSA should be treated with mupirocin. In high-risk wards, exclusion from work for 48 hours may be necessary

Staffing pressures are acknowledged to affect compliance with infection control measures and increase the risk of MRSA transmission (Grundmann et al 2002). Staff with chronic skin lesions are particularly at risk of becoming colonized with MRSA and should seek advice from the occupational health department if working in direct contact with patients.

Dust should not be allowed to accumulate on horizontal surfaces and particular attention should be paid to areas that are difficult to clean. Keeping the patients' rooms tidy and free from unnecessary equipment helps to facilitate cleaning.

Current guidelines for the control of MRSA in hospitals were originally published in 1998 and updated in 2005. They recommend targeting the approach to infection control according to the level of risk in the clinical area affected (BSAC/HIS/ICNA Working Party 2005).

Decolonization of patients and staff

Staphylococcus aureus can be removed from colonized sites by topical treatment with antistaphylococcal solutions and creams. The most effective of these is mupirocin applied to skin lesions or to the nose for 5 days, three times a day, which is usually sufficient to eliminate MRSA. Unfortunately, resistance to mupirocin has been reported and resistant strains are most likely to emerge when mupirocin is used extensively in settings where MRSA is endemic (Vasquez et al 2000). Mupirocin should therefore not be applied for prolonged periods, particularly to chronic wounds. Recently, tea tree oil has been suggested as a topical treatment for the eradication of MRSA. There is some evidence that it is effective, although this has not yet been demonstrated by clinical trials and little is known about potential toxicity or other side-effects (Chang & London 1998, Dryden et al 2004). Antiseptic skin disinfectant solutions (e.g. chlorhexidine handwash) have been recommended for eliminating *S. aureus* from skin sites but there is limited evidence for their value (Boyce 2001).

Since *S. aureus* commonly colonizes the skin, it is an important cause of surgical wound infection (Health Protection Agency 2003b). Decolonization prior to surgery is therefore recommended for patients known to be colonized with MRSA (BSAC/HIS/ICNA Working Party 2005). Decolonization may also be recommended as part of the measures required to control outbreaks of infection.

Although staff caring for patients with MRSA may acquire the organism, often they are only colonized for a few hours. If there is evidence of more prolonged carriage, they may require treatment with mupirocin. The occupational health department, in conjunction with the infection control team, should arrange this. Staff with infected or colonized lesions should not be in direct contact with patients.

Control of MRSA in community settings

The risk of MRSA transmission in residential care homes, where residents are generally more healthy and have fewer invasive devices than hospital patients, is much lower. Spread of MRSA between residents may occur but is usually associated with colonization rather than infection. Isolation of residents with MRSA is not necessary and they should be able to use communal areas with other residents. They may share a room, provided neither occupant has open lesions, invasive devices or catheters. Routine infection control precautions such as handwashing and the use of disposable gloves and apron for contact with body fluids, dealing with wounds or invasive devices should be sufficient to prevent spread (see Ch. 7). Such precautions are also sufficient for district nurses visiting the homes of patients infected or colonized with MRSA. In community hospitals the risk may be slightly greater as other residents may have open wounds and devices; precautions similar to those used in hospitals are therefore more appropriate (BSAC/HIS/ICNA Working Party 2005).

Colonization with MRSA should not interfere with the admission of a patient into either a hospital or a residential home. However, good communication between staff in hospitals, residential homes and the community is essential to ensure that staff are informed when a patient has MRSA so that appropriate precautions can be taken. The hospital or community infection control nurse (ICN) can help to evaluate the risk to other residents and provide advice on control measures.

Glycopeptide–resistant enterococci (GRE)

Enterococci are normal commensals of the gut and until recently were not a common cause of nosocomial infection. However, their intrinsic resistance to many antibiotics, such as the cephalosporins and quinolones, has enabled them to emerge as major nosocomial pathogens with *Enterococcus faecium* and *Enterococcus faecalis* responsible for most of the infections. Many enterococci have adapted to exposure to antimicrobials in the gut by acquiring resistance. Although *E. faecalis* is generally susceptible to ampicillin and penicillin, most *E. faecium* are not and are also resistant to most other antibiotics, for example tetracyclines, macrolides, trimethoprim and aminoglycosides. The glycopeptides have therefore provided the only effective treatment for infections caused by this organism.

Enterococci take advantage of seriously ill or immunocompromised patients and invasive devices. They can cause septicaemia, endocarditis, urinary tract infection and peritonitis associated with continuous ambulatory peritoneal dialysis (CAPD). Infections caused by GRE are usually associated with specialized units such as intensive care, renal, liver and haematology. Other risk factors for GRE colonization or infection include malignancy, enteral feeding, renal failure and presence of IV lines and mechanical ventilation (Gray & George 2000). GRE infections are associated with high rates of treatment failure and increased mortality (Health Protection Agency 2004).

Acquired resistance to vancomycin was first reported in enterococci in 1988 (Uttley et al 1988) and since then GRE have been reported in many hospitals both in the UK and elsewhere in the world. In England, recent data found 17% of E. faecium and 3% of E. faecalis to be glycopeptide resistant (Health Protection Agency 2004). Resistant strains are selected following exposure to glycopeptides and resistance can then be spread to other strains and species on plasmids. There are virtually no antimicrobial agents currently available to treat infections caused by these highly resistant pathogens and there is also a serious risk that resistance will be transmitted to other important pathogenic bacteria (Chavers et al 2003).

Outbreaks of infection have demonstrated that transmission between patients occurs. The organism is probably readily transmitted on the hands of staff in contact with colonized or infected patients and the environment is also thought to play a role (Weber & Rutala 1997). Enterococci can survive for several days on surfaces and a particularly high level of environmental contamination has been reported where a patient has diarrhoea (Bonilla et al 1995, Noskin et al 1995). A variety of medical equipment has also been implicated in transmission, including fluidized beds, thermometers and defective bedpan washers (Chadwick et al 1996, Weber & Rutala 1997).

Patients whose intestines become colonized with GRE and are otherwise asymptomatic are less likely to contaminate the environment than those who are colonized or infected with GRE at another site or have symptomatic gastrointestinal infection (Gray & George 2000). The latter group of patients should be isolated in a single room to minimize the extent of environmental contamination. Gloves and aprons should be used for contact with the patient or their immediate environment and these should be changed between procedures, particularly after handling material likely to be heavily contaminated with GRE (e.g. stool) and before leaving the room. Hands must also be washed after any contact with these patients or their environment. Equipment such as commodes, stethoscopes and thermometers should be dedicated for use by the isolated patient (Cookson et al 2005, Hospital Infection Control Practices Advisory Committee 1995). Where patients have asymptomatic colonization of the gut, gloves and aprons need be worn only for contact with urine and faeces (Gray & George 2000). Where clusters of GRE cases occur, other patients in the affected unit may need to be screened for GRE carriage by the collection of stool or rectal swabs. As with MRSA, marking medical records of infected or colonized patients and isolation precautions on readmission to hospital are recommended, as the resistant organisms may be carried in the bowel for prolonged periods. High standards of cleanliness are important to minimize environmental contamination and to reduce the risk of transmission between patients.

Multidrug–resistant tuberculosis

Resistance to antituberculous drugs was recognized as a problem when streptomycin was first used in the 1940s. Unlike other bacteria, antimicrobial resistance in mycobacteria is not associated with transmissible plasmids or transposons. Instead, it is due to mutation in single chromosomal genes; for example, resistance to rifampicin is due to a mutation in the gene encoding for RNA polymerase. These mutations occur spontaneously at a low rate within a population of mycobacteria but, if exposed to therapy with a single drug, resistant organisms will eventually predominate. The chances of mycobacteria developing more than one spontaneous mutation that confers resistance to more than one drug are very low. Therapy regimens involving more than one drug were therefore devised to ensure that mutants resistant to one drug would be destroyed by a second drug. However, in populations of mycobacteria already resistant to one drug, mutants to a second drug will be selected by a treatment regimen involving both drugs. Strains resistant to isoniazid and rifampicin, the two most important drugs, are called multidrug-resistant tuberculosis (MDRTB). Once resistant populations of mycobacteria have emerged in one person, they may then be transmitted to others, who will develop a primary drug-resistant infection.

In many parts of the world poor treatment regimens, inadequate supplies of drugs and non-adherence to prescribed therapy have resulted in the widespread emergence of strains resistant to one or more drugs. In a study by the World Health Organization, 10% of cases were found to be resistant to at least one drug. Levels of resistance were particularly high in parts of the former USSR, South America and Africa. In some countries, over 15% of cases were resistant to all four anti-tuberculous drugs and over 50% were resistant to isoniazid and rifampicin (Pablos-mendez et al 1998). Treatment options for MDRTB are extremely limited and the mortality rate is high, especially in patients who are HIV positive (Telzak et al 1995).

In the UK, systems for the diagnosis, treatment and surveillance of *Mycobacterium tuberculosis* have been in place for many years and levels of resistance are relatively low, with approximately 7% of cases resistant to isoniazid and less than 1% MDRTB. However, there has been a gradual increase in the level of drug resistance during the 1990s and problems with non-adherence to therapy have been reported (Interdepartmental Working Group 1998, Morse 1996).

HIV-related drug-resistant tuberculosis

Individuals with HIV are especially vulnerable to *M. tuberculosis*. Although they are probably no more likely to acquire infection if exposed, infection is much more likely to become active and latent infections are also likely to reactivate. Treatment of tuberculosis in HIV-positive patients is complicated by poor absorption of drugs, interaction with other drugs and a high risk of recurrence. HIV is also a major risk factor for MDRTB (Corbett et al 2003). Many outbreaks of tuberculosis amongst patients with HIV nursed together in hospital have been reported. Unfortunately, many of these have involved MDRTB (Hannan et al 2000). In 1998, an outbreak of MDRTB occurred in the UK. The index case did not have HIV but was nursed on the same ward as patients with HIV, seven of whom subsequently acquired MDRTB and two of whom died (Breathnach et al 1998). This outbreak highlighted the importance of adhering to clearly defined infection control policies. Factors that contributed to the spread of infection were an isolation room with airflow directed into the ward and inadequate isolation of suspected cases.

Guidance issued by the Interdepartmental Working Group in 1998 recommends that hospitals have a tuberculosis control plan which includes assessment of the risk of transmission in all patient areas and identifies an appropriate level of isolation facilities to cope with the risk. Systems should be in place to ensure that precautions are taken, with all patients suspected to have tuberculosis until non-infectiousness is proven, and that they are not placed in the same ward as patients with HIV. Patients with suspected or confirmed MDRTB require isolation in a room with negative pressure ventilation (Box 5.7). As they are likely to have mycobacteria in their sputum for months, prolonged isolation is likely to be necessary (Interdepartmental Working Group 1998).

> **Box 5.7   Key infection control measures for patients with multidrug-resistant tuberculosis (Interdepartmental Working Group 1998)**
>
> - Nurse in a negative-pressure isolation room and ensure the efficiency of air handling is monitored regularly
> - Ensure the patient remains in the room with the door closed
> - Restrict the number of staff involved in care of the patient
> - Limit visitors to those who have been in close contact before the diagnosis of MDRTB
> - Only perform aerosol-generating procedures (e.g. sputum induction) in a room with local exhaust ventilation
> - Teach patients to cover their mouth and nose with a tissue when coughing or sneezing
> - Ask patients to wear a mask during transportation to other areas
> - Staff should wear a mask in the isolation room

Extended spectrum β-lactamases (ESBLs)

The term ESBL is used to describe acquired (i.e. from plasmids) class A β-lactamases that hydrolyse, and therefore confer resistance to, the second- and third-generation cephalosporins, e.g. cefuroxime, cefotaxime, ceftriaxone, ceftazidime. These agents are routinely used as first-line agents in patients with, for example, intra-abdominal sepsis, severe community-acquired pneumonias and bacteraemias. Although ESBLs are not the only β-lactamases that confer resistance to the second- and third-generation cephalosporins, they are the most important.

There are essentially three types of ESBLs (Livermore & Woodford 2004):

- those that have arisen from mutations to the cephalosporin-hydrolysing β-lactamases commonly found in enterobacteriaceae, the plasmid-mediated penicillinases known as TEM and SHV. Over 100 variations are known
- those that have evolved separately from the chromosomal β-lactamases from *Kluyvera* spp., known as CTX-M types, of which 30 varieties exist
- obscure types such as VEB, PER and OXA.

In addition to the ESBLs being both clinically important and resistant to common first-line agents, delay in recognizing a pathogen as an ESBL-producer in the laboratory may result in inappropriate therapy and increased mortality (Paterson et al 2001). Because ESBL-mediated resistance is not always obvious (in the laboratory), tighter laboratory methods are required for the screening and confirmation of ESBL-producing organisms so that appropriate therapy is commenced promptly. Many ESBL-producers are now multiresistant, to quinolones, aminoglycosides, etc. Some producer strains have been associated with outbreaks in both hospital and the community.

Recently there has been a worrying change in the epidemiology of ESBL-producing strains in the UK. Until 2001, most ESBL-producers were *Klebsiella* spp. with TEM or SHV mutants and they were generally associated with the most vulnerable patients, i.e. those in intensive care units. However, since 2000 CTX-M ESBLs have emerged in the UK as well as other parts of Europe, Asia and Canada. They are often found in *E. coli* and the predominant CTX-M-15-producing strains are resistant not only to all the cephalosporins but also to the fluoroquinolones, trimethoprim, co-trimoxazole, tetracyclines and amikacin and have variable resistance to gentamicin. The drugs of choice for their treatment are therefore the carbapenems. In addition, infections caused by these CTX-M ESBLs are occurring in patients managed in the hospital/community interface, for example recently hospitalized patients presenting with urinary infections in outpatient clinics. Some cases have had no contact with hospitals (Woodford et al 2004). Others may be admitted with bloodstream infections and have a high mortality if they are put on inappropriate therapy due to a delay in recognizing the isolate as being an ESBL-producer. CTX-M-producing strains of *E. coli* have now been sent to the HPA's antimicrobial reference laboratory from over 60 UK laboratories, with 25% being the type CTX-M-15 enzyme. Guidelines have recently been issued to ensure that ESBL-producing organisms are more widely and effectively identified in laboratory specimens (Livermore & Woodford 2004).

Multidrug–resistant acinetobacter

This small Gram-negative cocco-bacillus is easily isolated from the environment from water, soil, sewage and various foods. About 25% of healthy people have acinetobacter colonizing their skin. *Acinetobacter baumannii* is the species most often associated with true human infection. It is an organism of usually low virulence, it rarely causes death and the prevalence of severe infections is much lower than those caused by MRSA. Acinetobacters are only occasionally invasive, causing nosocomial pneumonia, urinary tract infection, wound infections and bloodstream infections (Health Protection Agency 2005b).

It tends to infect patients who are highly vulnerable with severe immunosuppression and with other serious illnesses often requiring intensive therapy. Acineto-

bacters are selected out in these patients by the use of broad-spectrum antimicrobials that these organisms are already resistant to. In the outbreak situation, acinetobacters can easily be cultured from the hospital environment, other patients and equipment (Health Protection Agency 2005c).

Its intrinsic resistance to many current antimicrobials coupled with its ability to survive easily in the hospital environment means that *Acinetobacter baumannii* is becoming an increasingly important hospital pathogen. Prior to 2000, the incidence of carbapenem resistance in UK strains of *Acinetobacter* spp. was less than 2% but recently there has been an increase in carbapenem-resistant (mostly OXA-23) strains. One particular clone found in over 15 hospitals, mostly in the South-East of England, is highly resistant to β-lactams (including carbapenems and ampicillin-sulbactam), fluoroquinolones and aminoglycosides. Other multiresistant strains (including carbapenem resistant) have been reported from at least 40 hospitals in the London area (Coelho et al 2004). Resistance genes in outbreak strains of acinetobacter have been found to be carried on integrons (see p. 103) (Koeleman et al 2001).

The main treatment for serious infections caused by multiresistant strains of *A. baumannii* is polymyxin, although there are serious concerns related to its toxicity and efficacy. Other agents that may be of limited value are sulbactam (a β-lactamase inhibitor) and the tetracyclines. However, their value in treating severe *A. baumannii* infections is yet to be ascertained. Efforts to prevent infections with these organisms therefore involve the prudent use of broad-spectrum antimicrobials (stopping them removes the selective pressure), careful hand hygiene and the cleaning of the environment.

Other problem species

Streptococcus pneumoniae is an important cause of community-acquired pneumonia, otitis media in children and meningitis. In the past it was highly sensitive to penicillin, which is a useful treatment because of its ability to penetrate the meninges.

Resistance to penicillin began to be reported in the 1970s. In some countries levels of resistance are now extremely high, for example in Spain where 44% of isolates are resistant, probably related to the inappropriate treatment of viral infections in children. In the UK, the rates of resistance are relatively low, at around 7.5%, but increasing (Communicable Disease Report Weekly 2000, DoH 1999).

Resistance amongst enteric pathogens such as salmonella and campylobacter is also emerging and thought to be related to the use of antibiotics as animal growth promoters and in veterinary practice (DoH 1999).

References

Bapna JS, Treipathi CD, Tekur U (1996) Drug utilisation patterns in the third world. *PharmacoEconomics*, **9**: 286–94.

Barrett SP, Teare EL, Sage R (1993) Methicillin-resistant *Staphylococcus aureus* in three adjacent health districts of South-East England 1986–91. *J. Hosp. Infect.*, **24**: 313–25.

Barrow P, Soothill J (1997) Bacteriophage therapy and prophylaxis; rediscovery and reviewed assessment of potential. *Trends Microbiol.*, **5**: 268–71.

Blok HE, Troelstra A, Tita EM et al (2003) Role of healthcare workers in outbreaks of methicillin-resistant *Staphylococcus aureus*: a 10-year evaluation from a Dutch university hospital. *Infect. Contr. Hosp. Epidemiol.*, **24**: 679–85.

Bojalil R, Calva JJ (1994) Antibiotic misuse in diarrhoea. A household survey in a Mexican community. *J. Clin. Epidemiol.*, **47**: 147–56.

Bonilla HF, Zervos MJ, Kauffman CA (1996) Long-term survival of vancomycin-resistant *Enterococcus faecium* on a contaminated surface. *Infect. Contr. Hosp. Epidemiol.*, **17**(12): 770–1.

Boyce JM (2001) MRSA patients: proven methods to treat colonisation and infection. *J. Hosp. Infect.*, **48** (suppl. A): S9–14.

Bradley SJ, Wilson ALT, Allen MC et al (1999) The control of hyperendemic glycopeptide-resistant Enterococcus spp. on a haematology unit by changing antibiotic usage. *J. Antimicrob. Chemother.*, **43**: 261–82.

Bratzler DW, Houck PM, Richards C et al (2005) Use of antimicrobial prophylaxis for major surgery. *Arch. Surg.*, **140**: 174–82.

Breathnach AS, de Ruiter A, Holdsworth GMC et al (1998) An outbreak of multidrug resistant tuberculosis in a London teaching hospital. *J. Hosp. Infect.*, **39**(2): 111–18.

British National Formulary (2005) Royal Pharmaceutical Society, London.

BSAC Working Party (1994) Hospital antibiotic control measures in the UK. *J. Antimicrob. Chemother.*, **34**: 21–42.

BSAC/HIS/ICNA Working Party (1998) Revised guidelines for the control of methicillin-resistant *Staphylococcus aureus* in hospitals. Combined working party of the British Society for Antimicrobial Chemotherapy, Hospital Infection Society and Infection Control Nurses Association. *J. Hosp. Infect.*, **39**(4): 253–90.

BSAC/HIS/ICNA Joint Working Party (2005) Guidelines for the control of methicillin-resistant *Staphylococcus aureus* (MRSA) in hospitals. *J. Hosp. Infect.* (in press). Available online at: www.bsac.org.uk.

Centers for Disease Control and Prevention (2004) Brief report: vancomycin-resistant *Staphylococcus aureus* – New York. *MMWR*, **53**: 322–3.

Chadwick PR, Chadwick CD, Oppenheim BA (1996) Report of a meeting on the epidemiology and control of glycopeptide-resistant enterococci. *J. Hosp. Infect.*, **33**(2): 83–92.

Chang CH, London KW (1998) Activity of tea tree oil on methicillin-resistant *Staphylococcus aureus* (MRSA). *J. Hosp. Infect.*, **39**(3): 244.

Chang S, Sievert DM, Hageman JC et al (2003) Infection with vancomycin-resistant *Staphylococcus aureus* containing the Van A resistance gene. *N. Engl. J. Med.*, **348**: 1342–7.

Chapna L, Hodgson J, Metcalf B et al (1997) The search for antimicrobial agents effective against bacteria resistant to multiple antibiotics. *Antimicrob. Agents Chemother.*, **41**: 497–503.

Chavers LS, Moser SA, Benjamin WH et al (2003) Vancomycin-resistant enterococci: 15 years and counting. *J. Hosp. Infect.*, **53**: 159–71.

Coelho J, Woodford N, Turton J et al (2004) Multiresistant acinetobacter in the UK: how big a threat? *J. Hosp. Infect.*, **58**: 167–9.

Coello R, Glynn JR, Gaspar C et al (1997) Risk factors for developing clinical infection with methicillin-resistant *Staphylococcus aureus* strains among hospital patients initially colonised with MRSA. *J. Hosp. Infect.*, **37**: 39–46.

Communicable Disease Report (2004) *Staphylococcus aureus* bacteraemia: England, Wales and Northern Ireland: October to December 2003. *CDR Weekly*, **14**(12): 1–5.

Communicable Disease Report Weekly (2000) Invasive pneumococcal infection, England and Wales: 2000. *CDR Weekly*, **13**(21).

Cookson B, Peters B, Webster M et al (1989) Staff carriage of epidemic methicillin resistant *Staphylococcus aureus*. *J. Clin. Microbiol.*, **27**(7): 1471–6.

Cookson B, Macrae M, Barrett S et al (2005) Guidelines for the control of glycopeptide-resistant enterococci in hospitals. Available online at: www.his.org.uk/_db/_documents/GRE_WP_distribution.doc.

Cooper BS, Stone SP, Kibbler CC et al (2003) Systematic review of isolation policies in the hospital management of methicillin–resistant *Staphylococcus aureus*: a review of the literature with epidemiological and economic modelling. *Health Tech. Assess.*, **7**(39).

Corbett EL, Watt CJ, Walker N et al (2003) The growing burden of tuberculosis: global trends and interactions with the HIV epidemic. *Arch. Intern.Med.*, **163**: 1009–21.

Cosgrove SE, Sakoulas G, Pereuevich EN et al (2003) Comparison of mortality associated with methicillin-resistant and methicillin-susceptible *Staphylococcus aureus* bacteraemia. A meta-analysis. *Clin. Infect. Dis.*, **36**: 53–9.

Cox RA, Conquest C, Mallghan C et al (1995) A major outbreak of methicillin-resistant *Staphylococcus aureus* caused by a new phage-type (EMRSA 16). *J. Hosp. Infect.*, **29**: 81–106.

Davey P, Nathwani D, Rubinstein J (2003) Antibiotic policies. In: Finch RG, Greenwood D, Ragnar Norrby S, Whitley RJ (eds) *Antibiotic and Chemotherapy. Antiinfective Agents and Their Use in Therapy*, 8th edn. Churchill Livingstone, Edinburgh.

Del Mar C, Glasziou P, Hayem M (1997) Are antibiotics indicated as initial treatment with acute otitis media? A meta-analysis. *BMJ*, **314**: 1526–9.

Department of Health (1999) *The Path of Least Resistance*. Standing Medical Advisory Committee, Subgroup on Antimicrobial Resistance. Department of Health, London.

Department of Health (2000) *Antimicrobial Resistance Strategy and Action Plan*. Department of Health, London.

Devine J, Cooke RPD, Wright EP (2001) Is methicillin-resistant *Staphylococcus aureus* (MRSA) contamination of ward-based computer terminals a surrogate marker for nosocomial MRSA transmission and handwashing compliance? *J. Hosp. Infect.*, **48**: 72–5.

Dryden MS, Dailly S, Crouch M (2004) A randomised controlled trial of tea tree topical preparations versus a standard topical regimen for the clearance of MRSA colonisation. *J. Hosp.Infect.*, **56**(4): 283–6.

Finch RG, Greenwood D, Ragnar Norrby S, Whitley RJ (eds) (2003) *Antibiotic and Chemotherapy. Antiinfective Agents and Their Use in Therapy*, 8th edn. Churchill Livingstone, Edinburgh.

Fraise AP, Mitchell R, O'Brien SJ et al (1997) Methicillin-resistant *Staphylococcus aureus* (MRSA) in nursing homes in a major UK city: an anonymised point prevalence survey. *Epidemiol. Infect.*, **118**: 1–5.

Gray JW, George RH (2000) Experience of vancomycin-resistant enterococci in a children's hospital. *J. Hosp. Infect.*, **45**: 11–18.

Greenwood D, Whitely RJ (2003) Modes of action. In: Finch RG, Greenwood D, Ragnar Norrby S, Whitley RJ (eds) *Antibiotic and Chemotherapy. Antiinfective Agents and Their Use in Therapy*, 8th edn. Churchill Livingstone, Edinburgh.

Grundmann H, Hori S, Winter B et al (2002) Risk factors for the transmission of methicillin-resistant *Staphylococcus aureus* in an adult intensive care unit: fitting a model to the data. *J. Infect. Dis.*, **185**: 481–8.

Hannan MM, Azadian BS, Gazzard BG et al (2000) Hospital infection control in an era of HIV infection and multi-drug resistant tuberculosis. *J. Hosp. Infect.*, **44**: 5–11.

Harbarth S, Liassine N, Dharan S et al (2000) Risk factors for persistent carriage of methicillin-resistant *Staphylococcus aureus*. *Clin. Infect. Dis.*, **31**: 1380–5.

Health Protection Agency (2003a) *Surveillance of Hospital-acquired Bacteraemia in English Hospitals, 1997–2002*. Nosocomial Infection National Surveillance Scheme, London.

Health Protection Agency (2003b) *Surveillance of Surgical Site Infection in English Hospitals, 1997–2002*. Nosocomial Infection National Surveillance Scheme, London.

Health Protection Agency (2004) National Glycopeptide-Resistant Enterococcal Bacteraemia Surveillance Working Group. Report to the Department of Health, August 2004. Available online at: www.hpa.org.uk/infections/publications/pdf/GRE%20bact%20surveillance%20final%20Aug04.pdf.

Health Protection Agency (2005a) The gonococcal resistance to antimicrobials surveillance programme (GRASP) Annual Report. Available online at: www.hpa.org.uk/infection/topics-az/hiv-sti/sti-gonorrhea/publications.

Health Protection Agency (2005b) Available online at: www.hpa.org.uk/infections/topics-az/acinetobacter-b/gen-info.htm.

Health Protection Agency (2005c) Interim working party guidance on the control of multiresistant Acinetobacter outbreaks. Available online at: www.hpa.org.uk/infections/topics_az/acinetobacter_b/guidance.htm.

Hiramatsu K, Hanaki H, Ino T et al (1997) Methicillin-resistant *Staphylococcus aureus* clinical strain with reduced vancomycin susceptibility. *J. Antimicrob. Chemother.*, **40**: 135–6.

Hiramatsu K, Cui L, Kuroda M et al (2001) The emergence and evolution of methicillin-resistant *Staphylococcus aureus*. *Trends Microbiol.*, **9**(10): 486–93.

Hoffman P, Bradley C, Ayliffe G (2004) *Disinfection in Healthcare*, 3rd edn. Blackwell, Oxford.

Hood J, Cosgrove B, Curran E et al (2000) Vancomycin-intermediate resistant *Staphylococcus aureus* in Scotland. Abstracts of the Centers for Disease Control Fourth Decennial Conference on Nosocomial and Healthcare Associated Infections. Centers for Disease Control, Bethesda, Maryland.

Hospital Infection Control Practices Advisory Committee (1995) Recommendations for preventing the spread of vancomycin resistance. *Am. J. Infect. Contr.*, **23**: 87–94.

House of Lords Select Committee on Science and Technology (2001) *Resistance to Antibiotics*. Session 2000–1. Third Report. Stationery Office, London.

Interdepartmental Working Group on Tuberculosis (1998) *The Prevention and Control of Tuberculosis in the United Kingdom. Guidance on the Prevention and Control of Transmission of 1. HIV Related Tuberculosis 2. Drug-resistance, Including Multiple Drug-resistant Tuberculosis.* Department of Health Stores, Wetherby, UK.

John JJ, Rice LB (2000) The microbial genetics of antibiotic cycling. *Infect. Contr. Hosp. Epidemiol.*, **21** (suppl.): S22–S31.

Johnson AP, Auken HM, Cavendish S et al (2001) Dominance of EMRSA-15 and -16 among MRSA causing nosocomial bacteraemia in UK: analysis of isolates from the European Antimicrobial Resistance Surveillance System (EARSS). *J. Antimicrob. Chemother.*, **48**: 143–4.

Kaye D, Moellering RC (eds) (2004) Antibacterial therapy and newer agents. *Infect. Dis. Clin. North Am.*, **18**(3).

Kibbler CC, Soaton S, Barnes RA et al (2003) Management and outcome of bloodstream infections due to candida species in England and Wales. *J. Hosp. Infect.*, **54**: 18–24.

Koeleman JG, Stoof J, Van-Der-Bijl MW et al (2001) Identification of epidemic strains of *Acinetobacter baumannii* by integrase gene PCR. *J. Clin. Microbiol.*, **39**: 8–13.

Lacey S, Flaxman D, Scales J et al (2001) The usefulness of masks in preventing transient carriage of epidemic methicillin-resistant *Staphylococcus aureus* by healthcare workers. *J. Hosp. Infect.*, **48**: 308–11.

Livermore D, Woodford N (2004) Laboratory detection and reporting of bacteria with extended-spectrum ß-lactamases. Available online at: www.hpa.org.uk/srmd/div_nsi_armrl/ESBL_advice_June_2004.pdf

Lundstrom TS, Sobel JD (2004) Antibiotics for gram-positive bacterial infections: vancomycin, quinupristin-dalfopristin, linezolid and daptomycin. *Infect. Dis. Clin. North Am.*, **18**: 651–68.

Marshall C, Wesselingh S, McDonald M et al (2004) Control of endemic MRSA – what is the evidence? A personal view. *J. Hosp. Infect.*, **56**(4): 253–68.

Maudsley J, Stone SP, Kibbler CC et al (2004) The community prevalence of methicillin-resistant *Staphylococcus aureus* in older people living in their own homes: implications for treatment and surveillance in the UK. *J. Hosp. Infect.*, **57**: 258–62.

Mayon-White R (2004) Re-emerging infections. Part 1: Tuberculosis. *Br. J. Infect. Contr.*, **5**(4): 14–16.

Morse DI (1996) Directly observed therapy for tuberculosis. *BMJ*, **312**: 719–20.

Noskin GA, Stosor V, Cooper I et al (1995) Recovery of vancomycin-resistant enterococci on fingertips and environmental surfaces. *Infect. Contr. Hosp. Epidemiol.*, **16**: 577–81.

O'Donnell JA, Gelone S P (2004) The newer fluoroquinolones. *Infect. Dis. Clin. North Am.*, **18**: 691–716.

Pablos-mendez A, Raviglione MC, Laszlo A et al (1998) Global surveillance for antituberculosis drug resistance. *N. Engl. J. Med.*, **338**: 1641–9.

Paterson DL, Ko WC, Von Gottberg A et al (2001) Outcome of cephalosporin treatment for serious infections due to apparently susceptible organisms producing extended-spectrum beta-lactamases: implications for the clinical microbiology laboratory. *J. Clin. Microbiol.*, **39**(6): 2206–12.

Pittet D, Hugonnet S, Harbarth S et al (2000) Effectiveness of a hospital-wide programme to improve compliance with hand hygiene. *Lancet*, **356**: 1307–12.

Pratt RP (2003) *HIV and AIDS. A Foundation for Nursing and Healthcare Practice*, 5th edn. Churchill Livingstone, Edinburgh.

Rampling A, Wiseman S, Davis L et al (2001) Evidence that hospital hygiene is important in the control of methicillin-resistant *Staphylococcus aureus*. *J. Hosp. Infect.*, **49**: 109–16.

Scottish Intercollegiate Guidelines Network (SIGN) (1999) An introduction to SIGN methodology for the development of evidence-based clinical guidelines. SIGN guideline no. 39. SIGN, Edinburgh.

Seppala H, Klaukka T, Vuopio-Varkila J et al (1997) The effect of changes on the consumption of macrolide antibiotics on erythromycin resistance in group A streptococci in Finland. *N. Engl. J. Med.*, **337**: 441–6.

Simpson JY (1869) Some propositions on hospitalisation. *Lancet*, **16 Oct**: 535–8.

Sinha J, Barnes RA (2003) Fungal infections in critical care: the appropriate use of antifungal agents. *Br. J. Intens. Care*, **13**: 89–98.

Stevens DL (2000) Streptococcal toxic shock syndrome associated with necrotising fasciitis. *Annu. Rev. Med.*, **51**: 271–88.

Strausbaugh LJ, Crossley KB, Nurse BA et al (1996) Antimicrobial resistance in long-term care facilities. *Infect. Contr. Hosp. Epidemiol.*, **17**(2): 129–40.

Telzak EE, Sepkowitz K, Alpert P et al (1995) Multidrug resistant tuberculosis in patients without HIV infection. *N. Engl. J. Med.*, **333**: 907–11.

Tenover FC, Biddle JW, Lancaster MV (2001) Increasing resistance to vancomycin and other glycopeptides in *Staphylococcus aureus*. *Emerg. Infect. Dis.*, **7**: 327–32.

Thomson O'Brien MA, Oxman AD, Davies DA et al (2001) Audit and feedback versus alternative strategies: effect on professional practice and healthcare outcomes (Cochrane review). Cochrane Library, Update Software, Oxford.

Tiemersma EW, Bronzwaer S, Lyytikainen O et al (2004) Methicillin-resistant *Staphylococcus aureus* in Europe, 1999–2002. *Emerg. Infect. Dis.*, **10**(9): 1627–34.

Uttley AHC, Collins CH, Naidoo J et al (1988) Vancomycin resistant enterococci. *Lancet*, **i**: 57–8.

Vasquez JE, Walker ES, Franzus BW et al (2000) The epidemiology of mupirocin resistance among methicillin-resistant *Staphylococcus aureus* at a veterans affairs hospital. *Infect. Control Hosp. Epid.* **21**: 459–64

Wagenvoort JHT, Sluijsmans W, Penders RJR (2000) Better environmental survival of outbreak vs. sporadic MRSA isolates. *J. Hosp. Infect.*, **45**: 231–4.

Walsh C (2000) Molecular mechanisms that confer antibacterial drug resistance. *Nature*, **496**: 775–81.

Warnock D (2003) Antifungal agents. In: Finch RG, Greenwood D, Ragnar Norrby S, Whitley RJ (eds) *Antibiotic and Chemotherapy. Antiinfective Agents and Their Use in Therapy*, 8th edn. Churchill Livingstone, Edinburgh.

Weber DJ, Rutala WA (1997) Role of environmental contamination in the transmission of vancomycin-resistant enterococci. *Infect. Contr. Hosp. Epidemiol.*, **18**: 306–9.

Weinstein RA (2001) Controlling antimicrobial resistance in hospitals: infection control and use of antibiotics. *Emerg. Infect. Dis.*, **7**(2): 188–91.

Wigley T, Majeed A (2002) Age and sex-specific antibiotic prescribing patterns in general practice in England and Wales, 1994–1998. *Health Stat. Qual.*, **14**: 14–20.

Witte W (1998) Medical consequences of antibiotic use in agriculture. *Science*, **279**: 996–7.

Woodford N, Ward ME, Kaufmann ME et al (2004) Community and hospital spread of *Escherichia coli* producing CTX-M extended-spectrum beta-lactamases in the UK. *J. Antimicrob. Chemother.*, **54**(4): 735–43.

Woodhead M, Fleming D, Wise R (2004) Antibiotics, resistance and clinical outcomes. *BMJ*, **328**: 1270–1.

Wunderink RG, Rello J, Cammarata SK et al (2003) Linezolid vs vancomycin: analysis of two double-blind studies of patients with methicillin-resistant *Staphylococcus aureus* nosocomial pneumonia. *Chest*, **124**: 1789.

Zuckerman JM (2004) Macrolides and ketolides: azithromycin, clarithromycin, telithromycin. *Infect. Dis. Clin. North Am.*, **18**: 621–49.

Further Reading

Greenwood D (2000) *Antimicrobial Chemotherapy*, 4th edn. Oxford University Press, Oxford.

Finch RG, Greenwood D, Ragnar Norrby S, Whitley RJ (2003) *Antibiotic and Chemotherapy*, 8th edn. Churchill Livingstone, Edinburgh.

Kaye D, Moellering RC (eds) (2004) Antibacterial therapy and newer agents. *Infect. Dis. Clin. North Am.*, **18**(3).

Moellering RC (2002) *New Antibiotics: When to Use and When Not to Use*. American College of Physicians. Available online at: www.acponline.org/ear/vas2002/new_antibiotics.htm.

Walsh C (2000) Molecular mechanisms that confer antibacterial drug resistance. *Nature*, **496**: 775–81.

Chapter **6**

Micro–organisms and their control

INTRODUCTION

There are many different species of bacteria, types of virus and other micro-organisms but only a very small proportion are able to infect a human or animal host and cause disease. This chapter provides a brief outline of some of the pathogenic bacteria, fungi, protozoa and viruses commonly encountered in the healthcare environment. It focuses on the infection control implications of each organism and the precautions that may be required when caring for a patient with the infection.

PATHOGENIC BACTERIA

There are four main groups of bacteria, distinguished by their shape and response to the Gram stain (see p. 20): Gram-positive cocci and bacilli and Gram-negative cocci and bacilli (Plate 2). Other important groups include acid-fast bacilli, spirochaetes and atypical bacteria.

Gram–positive cocci

Staphylococci
The staphylococci are differentiated into coagulase-positive and coagulase-negative species, depending on whether they produce the enzyme coagulase, which clots plasma.

Staphylococcus aureus   This is a coagulase-positive staphylococcus. It is both a commensal of humans and an important pathogen. It causes a range of superficial infections of the skin (Plate 16), such as septic spots, boils, abscesses and impetigo and can also cause more serious infections including osteomyelitis, septicaemia, endocarditis and pneumonia. *S. aureus* is an important cause of healthcare-associated infection. It is responsible for between 40% and 50% of surgical wound infections and approximately 25% of bloodstream infections (Health Protection Agency 2003a, b). *S. aureus* can resist dry conditions and high salt concentrations and is therefore able to colonize skin. It is commonly found on the axillae, groins and perineum. About 20–35% of healthy people persistently carry the organisms in their nose and a further 30–70% carry it intermittently (Williams 1963). Organisms from the nose are then easily transferred to other sites and there is considerable evidence to show that nasal carriers are at increased risk of developing staphylococcal infection, particularly surgical wound infection (Kluytmans et al 1996). Nasal carriage may also increase the risk of infection in patients undergoing haemodialysis (Glowacki et al 1994).

A variety of toxins are produced by different strains of *S. aureus*. Some produce a toxin that attacks cells in the skin, causing it to split and desquamate. These strains sometimes occur in neonates where they cause 'scalded skin syndrome', characterized by large, red, weeping areas where the skin has desquamated. Another toxin is responsible for toxic shock syndrome, associated with retained sanitary tampons. This can cause severe disease, with hypotension, fever, diarrhoea and desquamative skin rash. Other strains produce an enterotoxin which interferes with electrolyte transfer in the gut and causes acute gastroenteritis if eaten with food.

S. aureus is particularly adept at developing resistance to antibiotics (see p. 106). Most isolates are now resistant to penicillin. Methicillin-resistant strains, which are resistant to many other antibiotics used to treat staphylococcal infection, emerged in the 1970s and 1980s and are now a frequent cause of healthcare-associated infection in many countries. Methicillin-resistant *S. aureus* (MRSA) is most likely to emerge in hospital settings because many patients receive antimicrobial therapy and are vulnerable to serious infection due to their underlying illness and presence of susceptible sites such as wounds and invasive devices. Often patients are only colonized with MRSA in their nasal mucosa or on skin sites and can be treated with topical agents but invasive infection may be difficult to treat, as the organism is sensitive to only a few antibiotics. Some strains of MRSA have a particular capacity to spread easily between patients, causing outbreaks of infection. Staff may also become colonized (although usually this is transient) and both staff and patients may act as reservoirs for transmission of the organism to other patients (see Ch. 5, p. 107).

Staphylococcus epidermidis *S. epidermidis* is a coagulase-negative staphylococcus. It colonizes the skin and rarely causes infection. However, although it

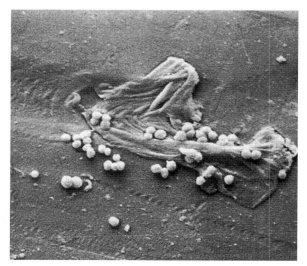

Figure 6.1 *Staphylococcus epidermidis* adhering to a plastic intravenous cannula.

used to be considered as non-pathogenic it is increasingly recognized as an important cause of healthcare-associated infection. It produces an extracellular polysaccharide (slime) which enables it to adhere to and multiply on plastics and metals (Fig. 6.1). It is therefore able to cause infections associated with invasive plastic or metal devices, including peritoneal dialysis catheters, arterial grafts, cardiac prosthetic valves and prosthetic orthopaedic joints. It is also frequently responsible for bloodstream infections associated with intravenous devices (Health Protection Agency 2003b). Immunocompromised patients are particularly vulnerable and the natural resistance of *S. epidermidis* to many antibiotics makes the infections it causes difficult to treat (Koos & Bannerman 1994).

Infection control precautions Staphylococci present on skin and nasal mucosa are able to gain access to, and cause infection in, damaged skin sites such as wounds and cannula insertion sites. The surface of the skin and mucous membranes are the main reservoir of staphylococci and patients who develop an infection may acquire it endogenously from staphylococci colonizing their own body or exogenously from an external source. Staphylococci are most frequently transmitted on the hands and clothing of staff, as the classic experiments of Mortimer et al (1966) eloquently demonstrated. Aseptic technique should always be used to handle invasive devices, which are particularly vulnerable to invasion by both coagulase-negative and coagulase-positive staphylococci.

Occasionally outbreaks of surgical wound infection are caused by a member of staff in the operating theatre who is heavily colonized with *S. aureus* and releases large numbers of organisms into the air on skin scales. Identification and treatment of the member of staff is necessary to prevent further spread.

Although the most common route of transmission is on hands, staphylococci released on skin scales will collect in dust, where they may survive for prolonged periods in the environment (Neely & Maley 2000). The accumulation of dust has been implicated in the spread of MRSA and regular cleaning will reduce the risk of dissemination (Rampling et al 2001).

Handwashing is the most important measure to prevent cross-infection of staphylococci. Elimination of nasal carriage with *S. aureus* has been shown to reduce the risk of postoperative infection and infections associated with continuous ambulatory peritoneal dialysis (CAPD) (Kluytmans et al 1996, Perez-Fontan et al 1993). Mupirocin is usually used to eradicate nasal carriage but its widespread use for prolonged periods should be avoided or resistance is likely to emerge rapidly (Boyce 2001).

Patients with *S. aureus* infection do not usually require isolation unless a large area of open wound is involved. However, special precautions are necessary where a patient is colonized or infected with antibiotic-resistant strains of *S. aureus*. The management of patients with MRSA is discussed in more detail in Chapter 5.

Streptococci

Streptococci are divided into more than 20 different types, called Lancefield groups. Many pathogenic species produce toxins called haemolysins, which lyse red blood cells and, when grown on blood agar, produce a characteristic change in appearance of the agar around the colony (Plate 6). Streptococci that cause complete haemolysis are called β-haemolytic, those that cause incomplete haemolysis are described as α-haemolytic. The most pathogenic species in humans is *Streptococcus pyogenes*, also called group A streptococci. This β-haemolytic streptococcus causes pharyngitis, skin infections and puerperal sepsis and produces a range of toxins which help it to spread through tissue. These include streptokinase, an enzyme that dissolves fibrin, and streptodornase which breaks DNA into small fragments. Streptococci can invade damaged skin, surgical wounds, burns and ulcers and cause invasive infections of the skin (e.g. impetigo), erysipelas (a spreading infection of subcutaneous tissues; Plate 17) and cellulitis (inflammation of connective tissues). Scarlet fever is a pharyngitis caused by a strain of *Strep. pyogenes* that produces an erythrogenic toxin

that results in a characteristic rash affecting skin and mucous membranes.

Puerperal sepsis is a septicaemia that originates from the uterus infected by *Strep. pyogenes* during childbirth. It was a frequent complication of childbirth before the introduction of antibiotics and a more hygienic approach to delivery. Now it is an uncommon, but still serious, infection.

Occasionally, acute rheumatic fever or glomerulo-nephritis occurs after a group A streptococcal infection caused by a hypersensitivity reaction. Antibodies formed against the streptococcus recognize and destroy tissue in the heart muscle, valves or kidneys by mistake. Subsequent streptococcal infection is likely to reactivate rheumatic fever and antibiotic prophylaxis against infection is required to prevent this.

A particular cell surface protein, the M protein, confers resistance to phagocytosis and is an important virulence factor. The antigenic structure of the M protein varies and some types, such as M1 and M3, are associated with a particularly serious form of streptococcal infection called necrotizing fasciitis. This is a serious infection of soft tissue characterized by tissue necrosis. The disease progresses extremely rapidly, probably as a result of the diffusion of toxins through the skin. There is some evidence that strains of *Strep. pyogenes* that cause necrotizing fasciitis have a particular toxin (SpeA) introduced on a bacteriophage (Cartwright et al 1995). Tissue necrosis is accompanied by systemic toxaemia, with hypotension and damage to kidney function and blood coagulation. Necrotizing fasciitis is extremely rare but the fatality rate is high, with 25% of patients dying as a result of the infection. Cases usually occur sporadically, although an outbreak related to a carrier in an operating theatre has been reported (Cartwright et al 1995). Although frequently associated with *Strep. pyogenes*, mixtures of other bacteria, notably bacteroides and coliforms, may also cause necrotizing fasciitis.

Group B streptococci (*Streptococcus agalactiae*) are normal inhabitants of the intestine and sometimes the vagina. They can cause meningitis and septicaemia in the neonate who is exposed to the bacteria in the vagina during delivery. Risk factors for group B streptococcal infection in the newborn include prematurity, prolonged rupture of membranes and evidence of infection in the mother (Heath et al 2004).

Group C and G streptococci are similar to the group A streptococci and, although associated with less serious infection, can cause skin infections, tonsillitis and septicaemia.

The viridans group of streptococci are α-haemolytic and include at least five species that are prevalent amongst the normal flora. *Streptococcus mutans* is responsible for dental caries and can cause endocarditis. This occurs when bacteria lodge on an endocardium previously damaged by rheumatic fever, surgery or congenital defect. The body reacts to their presence by forming a layer of white blood cells and fibrin, which protects the bacteria from the immune system. Endocarditis is therefore a difficult infection to treat. Patients at risk of endocarditis should be given prophylactic antimicrobial therapy before dental treatment. *Streptococcus milleri* forms part of the normal flora of the mouth and gastrointestinal tract but if it gains access to the bloodstream, may cause abscesses, for example in the abdomen or brain.

Streptococcus pneumoniae These bacteria are also known as pneumococci and are characterized by the arrangement of their cells into pairs (diplococci) rather than the chains normally associated with streptococci. Pathogenic strains have capsules made from polysaccharides which protect the cell from phagocytosis. There are many different types of capsule, which are distinguished by antigenic reactions. Non-capsulated strains of pneumococcus are normal inhabitants of the respiratory tract, whilst capsulated strains cause pneumonia, bronchitis, otitis media, sinusitis and meningitis.

Resistance to infection amongst the general population is high but is reduced by underlying heart or lung disease, influenza or immunodeficiency, and epidemics may occur in overcrowded conditions. Pneumococcal pneumonia occurs as a result of aspiration of upper airway secretions. The bacteria can be spread by contact with oral secretions or respiratory droplets. Although illness does not usually occur in contacts, several episodes of cross-infection amongst elderly or immunocompromised patients have been described (Denton et al 1993, Subramanian et al 2003). Vaccination against pneumococcal disease has been recommended for those who are particularly vulnerable, for example people with chronic systemic illness such as cardiac or pulmonary disease (MMWR 1997).

Pneumococcal meningitis mostly affects children under 3 years and adults over 45 years and has a case-fatality rate of 20% or more. Penicillin is the antibiotic of choice for pneumococcal infection but penicillin-resistant *Strep. pneumoniae* now accounts for around 3% of serious pneumococcal infection in the UK (Laurichesse et al 1998).

Infection control precautions Reports of outbreaks of infection in hospital due to streptococci A, B, C and G have been described (Burnett & Norman 1990, Efstratiou 1989, Ramage et al 1996). The bacteria may be acquired on the hands of staff by contact with colonized or infected wounds and skin and transferred to vulnerable sites on other patients. Isolation of patients with these streptococcal infections is therefore recommended until the patient has received appropriate antibiotic therapy for 48 h (see Ch. 14). Longer periods of isolation may be necessary for infections in chronic wounds where the organism is more difficult to eradicate.

Equipment has also been implicated in transmission. Dowsett & Willson (1981) reported an outbreak of infection associated with poor cleaning of baths and damaged enamel surfaces and Takahashi et al (1998) described an outbreak caused by a contaminated bed covering.

Patients with penicillin-resistant strains of *Strep. pneumoniae* should be isolated to reduce the risk of transmission, especially in a ward with a high proportion of elderly or immunocompromised patients (Subramanian et al 2003).

Enterococcus

The main pathogens in the genus are *Enterococcus faecalis* and *E. faecium*. These are normal inhabitants of the bowel but are important causes of urinary tract infection, infective endocarditis, peritonitis and wound infections, especially in seriously ill patients. Occasionally they cause meningitis in neonates and pneumonia.

Enterococci are intrinsically resistant to many antibiotics and glycopeptides are usually used to treat serious infection. Glycopeptide-resistant strains first emerged in the late 1980s and have been reported as causing a number of outbreaks (Johnson 1998) with spread both within and between hospitals (see p. 112).

Infection control precautions Although enterococci that cause infection are usually acquired from the patient's own bowel flora, they can also be spread from patient to patient on the hands of staff. Environmental contamination and other reservoirs of the organism, such as electronic thermometers, may also sometimes be involved in transmission (Gray & George 2000, Weber & Rutala 1997). Outbreaks are particularly likely to occur in intensive care, bone marrow transplant, renal and liver units where patients are particularly vulnerable to infection. Control measures should include the isolation of infected or colonized patients, stringent handwashing, high standards of cleaning and the identification of potential environmental reservoirs (Gray & George 2000, Hospital Infection Control Practices Advisory Committee 1995) (see p. 112).

Gram-positive bacilli

Bacillus

These are aerobic bacteria which form spores. They are widely distributed in soil, water and dust. The main pathogen is *Bacillus anthracis* which causes anthrax, an infection of animals, especially sheep and cattle, and occasionally affects people whose work brings them into contact with animals or animal carcases. It is spread by spores which can survive in soil for many years but decontamination of hides and other animal products has made it an uncommon disease in the UK.

Bacillus cereus causes food poisoning and is usually associated with foods that have been kept for prolonged periods (e.g. rice), although infections associated with dietary supplements prepared in hospital have been reported (Rowan & Anderson 1998). *B. cereus* has occasionally been reported as a cause of surgical wound infections in association with unusual reservoirs of infection (e.g. linen) (Barrie et al 1992, Stansfield & Caudle 1997). It can also cause a severe endophthalmitis following traumatic injury or insertion of contaminated contact lens. Orsi et al (1999) reported an outbreak of endophthalmitis associated with inadequate decontamination of irrigation equipment and Gray et al (1999) described an outbreak of respiratory tract infection in a neonatal unit associated with inadequate decontamination of ventilator circuits.

Clostridia

The clostridia are anaerobic bacteria which form spores. They are mostly found in soil where they play an important role in the decomposition of organic materials and many species are normal commensals of the gut. The pathogenic species cause disease by producing potent toxins that have profound effects on the host.

Clostridium tetani   *Clostridium tetani* is present in the intestinal tract of herbivores and in soil. Tetanus occurs when a wound is contaminated by *C. tetani* spores and the conditions in the tissues are sufficiently anaerobic for them to germinate, multiply and produce toxin. The toxin stimulates motor nerve cells and causes convulsive muscle contractions, beginning near to the site of the wound but spreading progressively throughout the body.

Tetanus is most likely to occur in wounds contaminated with soil or a foreign body, in deep puncture wounds or those with extensive tissue damage. It is associated with a high incidence and mortality rate in countries without immunization programmes or anti-tetanus prophylaxis treatment. In the UK all children should receive immunization and a single booster of toxoid vaccine will protect immune individuals who are at risk of tetanus infection from a potentially contaminated wound. Elderly people are less likely to have been immunized and are at greater risk of acquiring tetanus. Tetanus is not spread from one person to another.

Clostridium perfringens   *Clostridium perfringens* is a normal commensal of the gut but may also cause food poisoning and infection of the soft tissues. Food poisoning occurs when spores of *C. perfringens* contaminating raw meat or poultry survive the cooking process. If ingested, they sporulate and release a toxin that causes abdominal pain and watery diarrhoea. *C. perfringens* is frequently recovered from wounds but rarely causes gas gangrene, a serious infection characterized by muscle destruction, release of gas into the tissues and toxaemia. Gas gangrene occurs only when wounds are contaminated by soil or street dust, or intestinal organisms. It is most likely to develop where there is extensive tissue damage or an impaired blood supply, creating the anaerobic conditions necessary for the organism to multiply. Cases are usually associated with crush injuries, road accidents or underlying vascular disease. More recently, cases have been reported in association with injecting drug users, with both contaminated drugs and injecting equipment as potential sources of the infection (Brett et al 2005).

Gas gangrene is not infectious and does not spread from patient to patient. The organism is acquired endogenously from the gut or the environment and gas gangrene develops only if the conditions in the wound are favourable for its multiplication. Gas gangrene may also be caused by other species of clostridia.

Clostridium difficile   *C. difficile* is commonly found in the intestine of infants where it is carried asymptomatically. Carriage levels then diminish so that only around 3% of healthy adults are colonized. Resistance to colonization is probably influenced by the normal, mostly anaerobic, microbial population of the colon which occupy adhesion sites and compete for nutrients, as the metabolic products they release probably create a hostile environment for *C. difficile*. In addition, there is mounting evidence that the immune system plays a part in defending against colonization by *C. difficile* (Kyne et al 2001). The normal microbial population of the colon declines with age and this together with a diminished immune response may explain why, after the age of 65, rates of *C. difficile* colonization and infection increase. *C. difficile* is now the predominant enteric pathogen amongst the over-65s (Djuretic et al 1999).

It was not recognized as a cause of disease until the late 1970s when it was identified as a cause of hospital-acquired gastrointestinal infections, the symptoms of which range from mild diarrhoea to a severe and sometimes fatal pseudomembraneous colitis, known as *C. difficile*-associated disease (CDAD) (National *Clostridium difficile* Standards Group 2004). The symptoms of CDAD are caused by toxins. Toxin A is both a powerful enterotoxin and a cytotoxin, toxin B is a cytotoxin. Most strains produce both toxins. However, not all strains of *C. difficile* are toxogenic and laboratory tests confirm a diagnosis of CDAD by identifying toxin in the faeces rather than merely the presence of the organism.

The infection usually occurs when the normal gut flora is altered by antibiotic therapy, especially ampicillin, clindamycin and cephalosporins (Kelly & Lamont 1998). Recurrence of symptoms after treatment is common and probably associated with the persistence of spores in the gut. Affected patients may continue to excrete the organism for prolonged periods.

A number of outbreaks of *C. difficile* have been reported, particularly amongst elderly patients, and it is clear that the organism can be transmitted between patients. The main route of transmission is probably on the hands of staff but spores, disseminated in high numbers from infected patients, may survive for several months in the environment. In outbreaks of infection extensive contamination of the environment has been implicated as an important factor in its spread and *C. difficile* has been recovered from floors, toilets, bedpans, bedding and mops (Fekerty et al 1981, Hoffman 1993). Epidemic strains appear to have an enhanced capacity to sporulate and this may contribute to their ability to survive in the environment (Wilcox & Fawley 2000).

Infection control precautions Patients with toxin-producing strains of *C. difficile* in their faeces should be isolated while they have diarrhoea. Protective clothing should be used to handle excreta. Excreta should be discarded promptly into bedpan washer, macerator or toilet and hands washed after any contact with the patient. The spores of *C. difficile* will not be killed by alcohol handrubs so hands should be washed with soap and water after contact with an infected patient or their environment (Hoffman et al 2004).

Regular cleaning with detergent and water should reduce the number of spores present in the environment of affected patients. There is conflicting evidence that disinfectants are more effective for eliminating *C. difficile* from the environment. Some suggest that the disadvantages of using disinfectants (corrosion, inactivation by organic material, adverse effects to staff) outweigh their benefits (Dettenkofer et al 2004). The standard of cleaning should be closely monitored and spillages of excreta promptly removed and the area cleaned thoroughly (Worsley 1993). Equipment such as commodes and mattress covers should also be cleaned thoroughly before use by another patient.

If several patients are affected, cohorting of both patients and staff may be necessary to control the outbreak. Admissions to affected units may also need to be restricted. Measures to control antibiotic usage, such as the use of narrow-spectrum drugs and early discontinuation of antimicrobial therapy, are important to prevent *C. difficile* disease amongst hospital patients. Novel preventive measures for high-risk patients, such as probiotics (organisms that inhibit the effect of *C. difficile* toxins in the gut) and vaccines that produce antibodies against *C. difficile*, are being developed (DoH/PHLS Joint Working Group 1994, National *Clostridium difficile* Standards Group 2004).

Corynebacteria

Many species are commensals that colonize the upper respiratory tract, mucous membranes and skin and are usually referred to as diphtheroids or coryneform bacilli. They occasionally cause serious postoperative infections following cardiac surgery or other infections in immunocompromised patients. The main human pathogen is *Corynebacterium diphtheriae*, the cause of diphtheria. *C. diphtheriae* can be carried asymptomatically in the nose or throat of a healthy person, although not all strains are toxogenic. In susceptible individuals, the organism infects the pharynx and larynx, forming a membrane that may obstruct the airway.

Infection is transmitted by respiratory droplets. Powerful exotoxins cause damage to distant nerves, resulting in paralysis of the soft palate, eye and extremities. The muscles of the heart are also affected. Treatment reverses these effects, although patients remain infectious for several weeks after the symptoms have resolved.

In the UK, routine immunization of children has ensured that cases of diphtheria are now extremely rare. Where a case of diphtheria is suspected, the patient should be isolated.

Listeria

Listeria monocytogenes is the main pathogen of this genus and is commonly found in soil and in the faeces of a variety of animals. It usually causes a mild influenza-like illness. However, infection during pregnancy can cause premature delivery, septicaemia and meningitis in the neonate and is associated with a high mortality. Cross-infection in neonatal units has been reported and extensive environmental contamination may occur following the delivery of an infected baby (Schlech 1991). Serious infections may also occur in immunocompromised patients. The incidence of infection is low with between 100 and 200 cases reported annually. It may be acquired through contact with live animals and raw meat but most infections are acquired by consumption of contaminated food. Soft cheese, coleslaw, fruit, vegetables, ice-cream and salami have all been associated with outbreaks of infection (Jones 1990). Listeria has been found in a variety of chilled foods and can survive and even multiply below normal refrigeration temperatures. However, it is readily destroyed by pasteurization.

Infection control precautions Immunocompromised patients or pregnant women are most at risk of listeriosis. They should eat fresh and well-cooked or thoroughly reheated food and avoid food likely to contain listeria (e.g. soft cheese, paté, uncooked or ready-prepared meals: Food Standards Agency 2002). Isolation of infected patients is necessary only in neonatal units.

Mycobacteria

Mycobacteria, although Gram-positive bacteria, are characterized by their unusual staining properties. They are termed acid-fast bacilli (AFB) because, unlike most bacteria, their waxy cell walls retain the stain after treatment with strong acids. There are many different species; some are found in animals and birds, others in soil and water. The main human pathogens are *Mycobacterium tuberculosis* and *M. leprae*, which cause tuberculosis and leprosy respectively.

Mycobacterium tuberculosis The usual site of infection of this micro-organism is the lungs, where it causes pulmonary tuberculosis (TB). In the past over 90% of children living in cities would develop tuberculosis, although in most the infection would resolve spontaneously with no long-term adverse effects. The incidence of the infection declined during the last century as a result of the improvement in living conditions and the introduction of effective chemotherapy (Fig. 6.2). In the early 1950s, 50 000 cases were reported every year. Now, only about 7000 cases are reported annually, with more than half occurring in people who were born outside the UK. Since the mid-1980s the rate of decline has begun to slow and the incidence is now increasing (Communicable Disease Surveillance Centre 2004a). Most of this rise in TB has occurred in London and is largely focused among new immigrants to the country from sub-Saharan Africa and the Indian subcontinent who have acquired TB before entering the UK (Mayon-White 2004). The HIV epidemic is also an important factor. Worldwide, 9% of TB cases are associated with HIV but in Africa nearly one-third of TB cases occur in people with HIV (Communicable Disease Surveillance Centre 2004b).

Tuberculosis is a chronic, progressive infection which begins as an inflammatory reaction at the point in the lung where inhaled mycobacteria settle. The

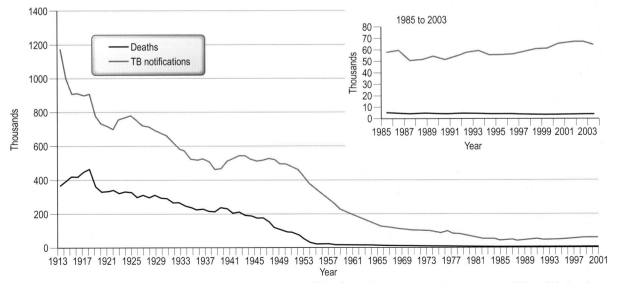

Figure 6.2   Notification of tuberculosis and deaths in England and Wales (reproduced with permission from the Office of National Statistics and Health Protection Agency).

tubercle bacilli are unusual in that they are ingested by phagocytic cells but, instead of being destroyed, multiply within them. The body must therefore respond to the infection by cell-mediated immunity and by the production of specially activated macrophages that are able to kill the phagocytes containing the mycobacteria. The infected phagocytes move to the nearest lymph node, where another inflammatory reaction is initiated. Usually this primary infection resolves without causing disease but leaves a characteristic calcified lesion in the lung visible on a chest radiograph. The tubercle bacilli remain dormant in these lesions but may eventually start to multiply, reactivating the disease. This is most likely to occur later in life as the efficacy of the immune system diminishes.

About 10% of primary infections do not resolve but develop into active tuberculosis. The lesions enlarge to form cavities that fill with pus. When these spread to involve the bronchus, the tubercle bacilli in the cavities are coughed up in sputum. This condition is described as 'open tuberculosis'. The mycobacteria expelled from the respiratory tract may be inhaled by others and can be detected in sputum under the microscope. The expansion and spread of lesions may be brought under control by the immune system but, if not, the patient will eventually die as a result of progressive destruction of lung tissue, haemorrhage from eroded arteries or secondary infection. The disease may also spread to other tissues, including skin, bones, central nervous system, kidney and intestine. Miliary tuberculosis occurs in the immunocompromised when tubercle bacilli are carried in the blood and produce small foci of infection, the size of millet seeds, throughout the body.

The vaccine against tuberculosis, bacille Calmette–Guérin (BCG), is made from a live attenuated strain of *Mycobacterium bovis*. It causes a localized, non-progressive, primary infection that induces cellular immunity. It is considered to be 70–80% effective in protecting against tuberculosis, although transmission to previously immunized individuals may still occur (DoH 1996). In the UK children are vaccinated at 10–14 years of age. Immunization is also offered to immigrants from countries with a high prevalence of the disease and to babies born to them.

The risk of transmission of pulmonary TB is relatively low, occurring in approximately 1% of contacts. Most secondary cases occur in close contacts who have spent at least 8 cumulative hours in the same room as an infected case. Where casual contacts have been screened because a case was considered to be highly infectious or the contacts particularly vulnerable, less than 0.5% have been found to acquire infection (Joint Tuberculosis Committee 2000).

The treatment for tuberculosis is prolonged and complex and requires both specialist knowledge and close supervision. Inadequate or incomplete treatment is the main cause of relapse and facilitates the emergence of multidrug-resistant strains. In the UK, about 7% of cases are resistant to isoniazid and these are often associated with drug use or homelessness where compliance with treatment is poor. Only around 1% of cases are multidrug-resistant tuberculosis (MDRTB) (see p. 113). These are more likely to have been acquired abroad or have a previous history of TB (Communicable Disease Surveillance Centre 2004b).

Outbreaks of infection in hospital have been reported and infection is particularly likely to spread amongst immunocompromised patients (Hannan et al 2000). The very young, elderly or people with HIV infection are at greater risk of developing tuberculosis. The impairment of the immune system caused by HIV infection enables dormant *M. tuberculosis* to reactivate (Watson 1991). Large outbreaks of multidrug-resistant strains have occurred amongst patients with HIV infection in the USA and have also been reported in the UK (Breathnach et al 1998, Hannan et al 1996). The particular problems associated with MDRTB and recommended control measures are discussed in Chapter 5.

Tuberculin skin testing The cellular immunity that develops following a primary infection forms the basis of the tuberculin skin tests (Heaf and Mantoux) used to establish whether an individual has active tuberculosis or is immune to infection. A small amount of protein derived from mycobacteria is inoculated under the skin. If, after a few days, the area is inflamed and blistered, the individual probably has active tuberculosis. A response to the tuberculin indicates immunity to tuberculosis, whilst no response indicates non-immunity (Joint Tuberculosis Committee 2000).

Opportunistic mycobacteria Other species of mycobacteria may infect the lungs of immunocompromised people or those with abnormal respiratory tracts. *Mycobacterium avium intracellulare* (MAI) is a complex of mycobacteria that cause infection in the immunocompromised, especially people with AIDS. It is acquired through the gastrointestinal tract, causes a severe infection affecting both the gastrointestinal tract and lung and is frequently resistant to conventional antimicrobial therapy.

Infection control precautions The control of tuberculosis depends on the early detection of cases, effective treatment and infection control measures whilst the patient is infectious (Joint Tuberculosis Committee 2000). Special planning is required to protect immunocompromised patients as they are particularly vulnerable to acquiring tuberculosis after even brief exposure to an infected person (Hannan et al 2000). The Interdepartmental Working Group on Tuberculosis (1998) has issued specific guidance on the protection of the immunocompromised and the control and prevention of drug-resistant *M. tuberculosis* infection. The working group recommends minimum levels of infection control precautions according to local circumstances (see Table 14.1).

Patients with 'open' tuberculosis (i.e. with sufficient numbers of *M. tuberculosis* in their sputum for bacteria to be seen under the microscope) are infectious. If the bacilli cannot be seen in three separate sputum specimens, the patient may still have tuberculosis but is not exhaling sufficient mycobacteria to be considered infectious. The non-pulmonary forms of tuberculosis are also not infectious.

Transmission occurs by the inhalation of tubercle bacilli in minute airborne droplets (droplet nuclei) expelled from the lungs of an infected person, although close, prolonged contact is usually required for transmission to healthy people to occur. Patients with open tuberculosis are usually treated at home but if nursed in hospital, they should be segregated from other patients, preferably in a single room with a lower air pressure inside the room so that airflow is directed into the room from other patient areas (see Ch. 14, Fig. 14.1). Such negative pressure isolation rooms are essential if MDRTB is suspected or immunocompromised patients are present in the same ward. The door of the room should be kept closed and the patient should not visit communal areas of the ward. Visitors should be restricted to those who had already had close contact before the diagnosis was made.

Masks are not necessary in most situations but should be worn by staff during procedures that involve direct exposure to sputum, for example cough induction, bronchoscopy or where a high-dependency patient requires prolonged periods of intensive care. The masks should be close-fitting, high-efficiency particulate (HEPA) filtering respirator masks able to filter out minute droplet nuclei. The patient should be encouraged to cough into tissues covering the mouth and to wear a mask if required to visit another department. Cough-inducing procedures should never be performed in an open ward area (Interdepartmental Working Group 1998).

Precautions are required for the first 2 weeks of chemotherapy and can then be discontinued provided that the patient's condition is improving and MDRTB is not suspected. The risk of healthcare workers acquiring infection from patients is extremely low and can be minimized by ensuring that all staff who have close contact with potentially infected patients or specimens are tuberculin tested and given vaccination where necessary by the occupational health department (Joint Tuberculosis Committee 2000).

Tracing and screening of close contacts is undertaken to find associated cases or, if the infection is recent, to detect the source case. Rapid diagnosis can be made by using molecular tests (Joint Tuberculosis Committee 2000). This 'contact tracing' is co-ordinated by the local authority proper officer (usually the consultant in communicable disease control) and is initiated following notification of the disease (see p. 44).

All health authorities should have a written policy for tuberculosis prevention and control which describes the measures in place to co-ordinate the surveillance, diagnosis and treatment of cases; the infection control arrangements; contact tracing responsibilities; education of staff; and monitoring procedures. The policy should reflect local epidemiology and ensure the integration of services between hospital and community.

Mycobacterium bovis This organism causes pulmonary tuberculosis in cattle. In humans, infection is usually acquired by drinking unpasteurized milk from cows with tuberculous mastitis. The disease usually involves the gastrointestinal tract, tonsils and related lymph glands, although farmers may acquire pulmonary tuberculosis through contact with infected cattle.

Gram-negative cocci

Neisseria spp.

Neisseria characteristically occur as pairs of cells called diplococci. There are a number of harmless species that form part of the normal flora of the mucous membranes, including the upper respiratory and genital tracts. The two main pathogens are *N. gonorrhoeae* (gonococcus) and *N. meningitidis* (meningococcus).

Neisseria gonorrhoeae This is a sexually transmitted disease which primarily affects the genitourinary tract but may also occur in the anal canal, throat and eyes. *N. gonorrhoeae* is a delicate organism that is susceptible to cold and lack of moisture and therefore unable to survive for long outside the body. Newborn infants may be infected from the mother's birth canal at the time of delivery and subsequently develop conjunctivitis, which damages the sight if not treated promptly. Infections may be asymptomatic, facilitating spread of the infection.

Until recently, the infection could be successfully treated with a single dose of penicillin but penicillin-resistant strains are now becoming increasingly prevalent.

Neisseria meningitidis *N. meningitidis* normally colonizes the nasopharynx and is spread from person to person by nasopharyngeal secretions or respiratory droplets. Close contact, for example kissing within a household, is required for transmission to occur. Carriage is asymptomatic and the proportion of the population who carry the organism varies from around 2% of children under 5 years to about 25% of teenagers. Immunity to *N. meningitidis* develops within 2 weeks of acquiring the organisms in the nasopharynx. Rarely, organisms invade the bloodstream before immunity has developed, causing meningococcal septicaemia, and from the blood, the bacteria may reach the meninges to cause meningococcal meningitis. Both infections may be rapidly fatal if not treated with antibiotics. Risk factors for infection include passive smoking, overcrowding and prior infection with influenza A (PHLS Meningococcus Forum 2002).

Meningococcal disease is most common in infants, declines in children and rises again in teenagers and young adults. The incidence is highest in the winter months. The majority of cases (97%) of meningococcal disease occur in isolation (termed sporadic) and not as part of an outbreak. However, outbreaks, in which two or more related cases occur, sometimes affect schools, universities or other institutions housing large numbers of young people. Those at greatest risk of acquiring infection are people living in the same household as the person with meningitis.

In the UK two strains of *N. meningitidis* are prevalent, serogroups B and C. A vaccine against serogroup C was introduced in 1999 and the incidence of the disease caused by this strain has subsequently fallen (Ramsay et al 2001).

Infection control precautions   In hospital, isolation of infected patients for the first 24 or 48 h of antibiotic therapy is usually recommended, although the risk of transmission is low. Prophylactic antibiotic therapy is recommended for all close contacts, i.e. people living/sleeping in the same household for 7 days prior to onset of illness. Healthcare workers are at risk of infection only if they are intimately exposed to nasopharyngeal secretions (e.g. mouth-to-mouth resuscitation) and prophylactic antibiotics are rarely necessary (Heymann 2004).

Management of outbreaks of meningococcal disease in the community   Cases of meningococcal disease frequently cause immense alarm within a community and a careful and consistent approach to their management is essential. When an isolated case occurs, people living in the same household should be given antibiotic prophylaxis to eliminate meningococcal carriage and reduce the risk of invasive disease. In this situation prophylaxis is not recommended for other nursery or school children as the risk of carriage amongst these contacts is low and chemoprophylaxis may have the adverse effect of eradicating other protective strains of meningococcus from the respiratory tract.

If two or more cases of the same strain of meningococcal infection occur at the same school or other institution within a 4-week period, chemoprophylaxis is likely to be offered to children and staff as well as close household contacts. In schools and universities this is likely to be targeted at subgroups identified as being at increased risk. The consultant in communicable disease control will be responsible for the management of outbreaks and will liaise closely with the Centre for Infections and the regional epidemiologist. It is particularly important to ensure that parents receive adequate information about the disease and how the situation is being managed (PHLS Meningococcus Forum 2002).

Gram–negative bacilli

Enterobacteria

The coliforms   Coliforms is a general term given to a broad group of organisms that are normal inhabitants of the gut, called the Enterobacteriaceae. They can survive in either aerobic or anaerobic environments under a wide range of different temperatures but are commonly associated with warm, moist environments.

The coliform bacteria primarily responsible for infections in hospital are *Escherichia coli* and species of klebsiella, serratia, proteus and enterobacter. They often colonize sites where the normal defence mechanisms are breached, for example intravenous cannulae, urinary catheters and endotracheal or tracheostomy tubes. They can also cause severe infections, including peritonitis, wound infection and urinary tract infection, especially in the seriously ill, immunocompromised or neonates. Many are resistant to a wide range of antibiotics and survive when antibiotic therapy is used to treat other micro-organisms. For example, *Klebsiella pneumoniae* often colonizes the respiratory tract when the normal flora is eradicated by antimicrobial therapy. Outbreaks of infection caused by antibiotic-resistant coliforms are commonly reported (Macrae et al 2001).

E. coli is a normal member of the gut flora but some strains can cause gastroenteritis. Enterotoxogenic *E. coli* is foodborne, common in developing countries and the usual cause of 'traveller's diarrhoea'. Enteropathogenic strains cause severe prolonged diarrhoea in children, especially in developing countries. They can be transmitted via contaminated food, baby milk and water, or on hands through contact with faeces. Verocytotoxin-producing *E. coli* (VTEC) causes a range of symptoms from mild diarrhoea to haemorrhagic colitis, with bloody diarrhoea and severe abdominal pain. Although the illness usually resolves within a few days, about one-third of cases require hospitalization and 2–7% of cases develop haemolytic-uraemic syndrome (HUS), a form of renal failure associated with a high mortality rate. The strain that usually causes disease in humans is called O157. It is a normal inhabitant of animal intestines and outbreaks of infection have been linked to the ingestion of undercooked meat, bathing in contaminated water and handling animals (Coia 1998, PHLS 1995).

Infection control precautions   The hands of staff are often implicated as the route of transmission of Gram-negative coliforms and organisms can remain on hands for prolonged periods (Casewell & Phillips 1977). Colonized or infected patients may have the organism in their faeces and respiratory secretions, as well as in a variety of skin sites and wounds. The opportunity for transmission between patients is therefore high. Hands may also be contaminated by coliforms acquired from the environment, for example by handling towels, washbowls, bed linen and equipment in the sluice (Sanderson & Weissler 1992).

Transmission between patients should be prevented by the use of simple infection control precautions such as handwashing after contact with every patient or potentially contaminated equipment and the wearing of gloves to handle body fluids. However, some antibiotic-resistant strains appear to spread readily and outbreaks are difficult to control even with intensive control measures. Isolation of infected or colonized patients and even temporary ward closure may be required in these circumstances (Macrae et al 2001).

Antibiotic-resistant strains are a particular problem in intensive care or neonatal units where the patients are more susceptible to infection and where frequent staff contact facilitates their spread. Ventilator circuits are prone to contamination from respiratory secretions and hands should be washed after any contact (Gorman et al 1993).

Salmonella   Salmonella are also enterobacteria. There are more than 2000 species, most of which live in the intestines of animals and cause food poisoning in humans. Two species, *Salmonella typhi* and *S. paratyphi*, are strictly human pathogens. They cause enteric fever (typhoid and paratyphoid), a severe illness with symptoms of septicaemia rather than gastroenteritis. The organism multiplies in the reticuloendothelial system, may be excreted in urine and faeces for prolonged periods and sometimes colonizes the gallbladder. Some people become chronic carriers and continue to excrete the organism intermittently for

many years. Typhoid and paratyphoid are usually transmitted by food or water that has been contaminated by untreated sewage or a human carrier. Outbreaks have been associated with shellfish grown in polluted estuaries. In the UK most cases have been acquired abroad.

Other species of salmonella originate in animals but cause food poisoning if ingested. The illness may persist for several days but the organism is usually excreted in the faeces for only 1–2 weeks and long-term carriage is rare.

Infections are associated mainly with foods derived from poultry, which are frequently contaminated with salmonella. Infection occurs if the bacteria are not destroyed by adequate cooking and if contaminated raw food cross-contaminates other food which is then eaten without further cooking. *S. enteritidis*, in particular, has been linked to the consumption of eggs, particularly food containing raw shell eggs, for example mayonnaise, or lightly cooked eggs. Salmonella are a common cause of outbreaks of gastroenteritis in both hospital and community settings (Evans et al 1998).

Infection control precautions   Safe handling of food and strict attention to hygiene in the kitchen are essential to prevent transmission of salmonella on food. People who have a compromised immune system should only eat eggs cooked until the yolk is solid and avoid eating food containing raw eggs. The principles of food hygiene are discussed in greater detail in Chapter 12.

Person-to-person transmission of salmonella may occur but can be prevented by the use of simple infection control measures such as handwashing and the use of protective clothing for direct contact with faeces. Patients with salmonella do not require isolation once they are asymptomatic. Affected individuals should not prepare food for others while they are still likely to be excreting the organism in faeces.

Shigella spp.   These enterobacteria cause bacillary dysentery, a gastrointestinal infection of humans, characterized by bloody mucopurulent stools. Epidemics are associated with low standards of hygiene and are common in developing countries, where *S. dysenteriae* causes a severe disease associated with a high mortality rate. In the UK, most cases are caused by *S. sonnei* and the disease is relatively mild.

As very few organisms are necessary to cause infection, direct physical contact where hands have not been washed after defaecation is frequently responsible for spread of the disease. Transmission also occurs indirectly by the contamination of food. Outbreaks amongst children in nursery schools are sometimes reported (Maguire et al 1998). Shigella is not usually associated with long-term carriage in the faeces after the acute infection.

Infection control precautions Prevention of transmission of infection requires the use of gloves and aprons to handle excreta and thorough handwashing after contact with the patient. Control of outbreaks in schools and nurseries is a particular problem because standards of hygiene amongst young children may be poor and personnel may have frequent, close contact with one another. Staff with shigella infection should not work in these establishments or handle food until they have stopped excreting the organism (up to 4 weeks after illness resolves).

Pseudomonas

Pseudomonas is a strictly aerobic environmental organism commonly found in soil and water. The main pathogenic species is *P. aeruginosa*, which takes advantage of damaged host defences to establish infection in burns, wounds and the urinary tract. It is innately resistant to many antimicrobial agents and has therefore become a major cause of hospital-acquired infection. *P. aeruginosa* is sometimes found in the bowel of healthy people but rapidly colonizes the gut of hospital patients. Pseudomonas is able to multiply in situations where very few nutrients are available such as moist equipment and solutions. Although commonly found in sinks and taps, there is little evidence that organisms from these sources cause infection in patients (Levin et al 1984). Cross-infection has been reported in association with colonized pipework in whirlpool baths (Hollyoaks et al 1995).

The revision of the taxonomy of pseudomonas has resulted in new genera of similar bacteria, notably burkholderia (main pathogen *B. cepacia* which causes respiratory disease in people with cystic fibrosis) and stenotrophomonas (main pathogen *S. maltophilia* which affects the immunocompromised).

Infection control precautions Many infections caused by pseudomonas are acquired from patients' own intestinal colonization, although cross-infection via the hands of staff or contaminated equipment may also occur. Respiratory therapy equipment is prone to contamination and may present a major risk of infection if not decontaminated appropriately and stored dry. Outbreaks of infection have been associated with intensive care equipment such as humidifiers, temperature probes and irrigation tubing (Weems 1993).

Strains of pseudomonas resistant to aminoglycoside antibiotics may cause outbreaks of infection that are difficult to treat, especially in intensive care or burns units. Preventing the spread of these antibiotic-resistant strains may require the isolation of infected or colonized patients.

Acinetobacter

Acinetobacters are aerobic bacteria that are found widely in the environment and are also part of the normal flora of the skin. Like the coliforms, they can cause a range of infections in vulnerable patients, especially those in intensive care units, including pneumonia, meningitis, septicaemia and wound infection. Hospital strains are often resistant to many antibiotics (see p. 115). These are becoming an increasingly important problem because of their capacity to spread between vulnerable patients and the limited options available for treatment (Ayan et al 2003). Acinetobacter have an affinity for warm, moist places and outbreaks of infection related to humidification equipment and damaged mattresses have been reported (Dealler 1998, Loomes 1988). Vegetables are commonly contaminated with acinetobacter and may provide a source of infection in vulnerable hospital patients (Berlau et al 1999). Acinetobacter are also able to survive on dry surfaces for several days. Outbreaks of infection are increasingly reported in intensive care and burns units, where spread between patients on the hands of staff is the most likely route of transmission (Simor et al 2002). The same infection control precautions as those described for coliforms are required to prevent spread of acinetobacter, with a focus on hand hygiene after patient contact and cleaning of room surfaces and equipment (Ayan et al 2003).

Haemophilus

These organisms are commensals of the upper respiratory tract but may also cause infection. Strains with capsules (capsulate) cause serious infection in children (e.g. meningitis, pneumonia, epiglottitis, osteomyelitis, septic arthritis and septicaemia). Non-capsulate strains are particularly associated with chronic bronchitis and otitis media.

Cross-infection in paediatric wards has been reported and outbreaks of *Haemophilus influenzae* pneumonia may also occur on adult wards (Howard 1991). Isolation of infected patients should be considered, particularly if the patient has contact with immunocompromised patients. A vaccine against the capsulate strain (serotype 6) is now given to infants and the incidence of infection has fallen as a result (DoH 2004a).

Legionella

There are several different species of legionella but the main human pathogen is *Legionella pneumophila* which causes a severe respiratory illness called Legionnaires' disease. This usually affects the elderly, mostly men and those with other risk factors such as smoking, chronic bronchitis, emphysema or immunosuppressive treatment. The infection does not respond to conventional antimicrobial therapy and is associated with a high mortality rate. In vulnerable hospital patients, mortality associated with legionella pneumonia is more than 30% (Cooke 2004). A similar but milder disease called Pontiac fever occurs in younger people.

Legionella are ubiquitous environmental organisms with a thermal range for multiplication of 20–45°C. They can also multiply intracellularly in amoeba (Cooke 2004). Infection is acquired through the inhalation of contaminated water aerosols. The build-up of rust, biofilms or algae in water storage tanks, supply pipework or cooling towers can encourage the multiplication of legionella and protect it from chemical biocides. Subsequent aerosolization of the water, for example in showers or air-conditioning vents, exposes people to the risk of legionella infection. Infections are often associated with exposure in large air-conditioned buildings such as hotels, factories and hospitals but water supplies, spa baths and whirlpools have also been implicated as sources of infection (Hutchinson 1990). In the UK, around 200 cases of Legionnaires' disease are reported annually and many of these are acquired in hotels abroad.

Contamination of the water system can be prevented by proper maintenance. This includes regular draining, cleaning and disinfection of tanks and cooling towers, ensuring that stagnant water is not allowed to collect in pipework and maintaining the temperature of the hot water above 50°C to discourage the multiplication of the bacteria (Health & Safety Commission 2000). There is no evidence that the infection can transmit from person to person and therefore isolation of patients with Legionnaires' disease is not necessary.

Curved Gram–negative bacteria

Vibrio
These micro-organisms are commonly found in the environment. The most well-known species, *Vibrio cholerae*, causes cholera. It produces an enterotoxin that causes the severe symptoms of watery diarrhoea and abdominal cramps. Cholera is endemic in South-East Asia and parts of Africa, where it is spread by contaminated water and food. Cases in the UK are usually a result of infections acquired abroad.

Campylobacter
These organisms are found in the intestines of animals. The specialized techniques required to isolate campylobacter were not developed until the 1970s and only since then has *Campylobacter jejuni* been recognized as a major cause of gastroenteritis in humans. Poultry carcases are commonly contaminated with campylobacter and infection is frequently acquired by the ingestion of undercooked poultry (Kessel et al 2001). Only a few organisms are required to cause infection, as they multiply within the gastrointestinal tract. Outbreaks associated with milk or contaminated water have also been reported. Person-to-person spread of campylobacter is unusual (Heymann 2004). Routine infection control precautions are sufficient to prevent transmission in hospitals and affected patients do not require isolation.

Helicobacter
These are spiral-shaped micro-organisms which, since improvement in diagnostic techniques, are now recognized as a cause of gastritis and ulcers. Some 95% of patients with duodenal ulcers are infected with *Helicobacter pylori* and the disease can be cured effectively with antimicrobial therapy (Cottrill 1996). Although the organism is readily destroyed by chemical disinfectants, there is some evidence that it can be transmitted to staff who perform endoscopies. Gloves should be worn during these procedures to minimize the risk of transmission (Williams 1999).

Anaerobic Gram–negative bacilli

These are strictly anaerobic bacteria with two genera of clinical importance.

Fusobacterium and bacteroides
These are normal inhabitants of the intestine, where they are present in considerable numbers, and are also found in the mouth and genital tract. The main pathogenic species are *Fusobacterium necrophorum* and *Bacteroides fragilis* which can cause appendicitis, pelvic inflammatory disease and puerperal sepsis. They may also be responsible for postoperative infection, usually in combination with other organisms, particularly following abdominal or gynaecological surgery. Infection occurs endogenously, rather than as a result of cross-infection.

Mycoplasma

Mycoplasma are very small bacteria that do not have cell walls and therefore do not have a consistent cell shape. They are resistant to a range of antibiotics, including penicillins, which exert their effect on bacterial cell walls. Some species of mycoplasma have been implicated as causes of non-specific urethritis. *Mycoplasma pneumoniae* causes respiratory tract infections which range from mild pharyngitis to pneumonia and bronchitis. Outbreaks of infection have been reported in crowded institutions and within families. Spread of infection occurs through close contact and in hospitals the principal risk is the transmission of infection from staff to patients. Staff suffering from the infection should therefore not work (Kleemola & Jokinen 1992).

Rickettsia

These are very small bacteria that cannot grow outside the cells of their host and, except for Q fever, are transmitted by insects. They cannot be cultured on conventional bacterial culture medium but are grown in the yolk sac of chick embryos. The diagnosis is usually based on serological tests.

Rickettsia prowazeki causes epidemic typhus and is transmitted by the human louse (see p. 308). *R. typhi* is transmitted by rat fleas and lice and causes endemic typhus in urban areas with large rat populations. The microbe multiplies in the intestine of the louse and is excreted in the faeces on to the skin of a new host where it is introduced into the tissues by scratching. Typhus cannot be transmitted directly from person to person and epidemics are usually associated with unusual social conditions where the body louse is able to proliferate in the absence of regular washing of clothes, for example in wars and famines. Patients in hospital suffering with typhus do not require isolation.

Q fever is an atypical pneumonia caused by the inhalation of rickettsia from faeces, milk or the placenta of farm animals.

CHLAMYDIA

These are very small bacteria-like micro-organisms that cannot live outside the cells of their host. There are three main species. *Chlamydia trachomatis* is divided into several groups; one causes a severe blinding conjunctivitis called trachoma, common in South-East Asia, the Middle East and Africa. Other strains cause a sexually transmitted disease which causes non-specific urethritis in males and in females can lead to pelvic inflammatory disease, ectopic pregnancy and infertility. Genital chlamydia is the most commonly reported sexually transmitted disease in the UK (Health Protection Agency 2003c). Infants who acquire the organism from the mother's vagina during delivery may develop pneumonia.

C. psittaci is a parasite of parrots but is also found in other birds (e.g. pigeons, ducks, canaries). In humans it causes respiratory tract infection, which can range from a mild or asymptomatic infection to a severe pneumonia with a high fatality rate. Infection is acquired through the inhalation of infected dust and faeces and usually occurs in people who have close contact with birds (e.g. bird breeders and pluckers). The risk of transmission of psittacosis to patients should be considered when parrots or other caged birds are kept as pets in clinical areas.

C. pneumoniae is associated with community-acquired upper and lower respiratory tract infection, including pneumonia. Outbreaks may occur in schools or other institutions.

FUNGAL INFECTIONS

There are over 70 000 species of fungi, of which only a few are pathogenic. Diseases include superficial infections of the mucosa (e.g. thrush caused by yeasts) or infection by filamentous fungi of the skin, nails and hair (e.g. ringworm). More importantly, fungi can invade the body to cause serious widespread disease, which is often fatal (Bodey 1988). Patients who are immunocompromised and have had multiple courses of antibiotics are particularly vulnerable. The eradication of the normal flora enables fungi to establish infection in these patients (Flanagan & Barnes 1998). In the last few decades infections caused by fungi, particularly candida, have increased significantly (Vincent et al 1995). In most cases, the source of micro-organisms is the gastrointestinal tract, where fungi are normal commensals. Infections are usually acquired endogenously but transmission on the hands of healthcare staff also occurs (Pfaller 1996).

Candida

Most candida infections in humans are caused by *Candida albicans*, found in the normal flora of the mouth, intestinal tract and vagina. Superficial infection of mucous membranes or skin may occur, particularly in neonates and in debilitated adults or those who have received broad-spectrum antibiotic therapy which has destroyed the competing bacteria (Plate 18). In people who are immunocompromised or seriously ill, candida can cause systemic infections such as bloodstream infections, endocarditis and abscesses. Infections may also establish in invasive devices such as intravenous and urinary catheters. These infections can be difficult to treat (Flanagan & Barnes 1998). Candida bacteraemia is most likely to occur in intensive care patients, often in association with intravenous devices, and it has a high mortality (Hobson 2003, Kibbler et al 2003). Although infection is usually endogenous, cross-infection may occur and the use of gloves for oral hygiene and handwashing after the procedure is important to prevent this (Fowler et al 1998).

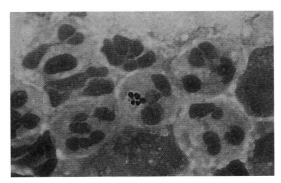

Plate 1   A clump of Gram-positive staphylococci in or on a neutrophil ('pus cell') and surrounded by other neutrophils. (Reproduced with kind permission from Ackerman V, Dunk-Richards G (1991) *Microbiology: An Introduction for the Health Sciences.* W B Saunders, London.)

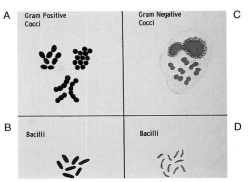

Plate 2   There are four main groups of bacteria: (A) Gram-positive cocci, (B) Gram-positive bacilli (rods), (C) Gram-negative cocci and (D) Gram-negative bacilli (rods). (Reproduced with kind permission of Jennie Wilson.)

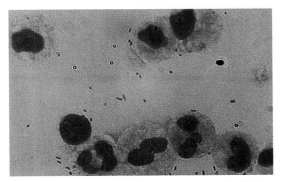

Plate 3   Cerebrospinal fluid from two cases of meningitis. Large mononuclear cells and neutrophils can be seen with a number of small Gram-negative rods. Provisional diagnosis: *Haemophilus influenzae* meningitis. (Reproduced with kind permission from Ackerman V, Dunk-Richards G (1991) *Microbiology: An Introduction for the Health Sciences.* W B Saunders, London.)

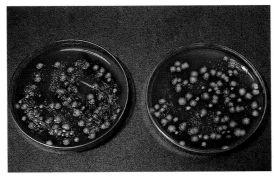

Plate 4   Large colonies of *Bacillus cereus.* (Reproduced with kind permission of Jennie Wilson.)

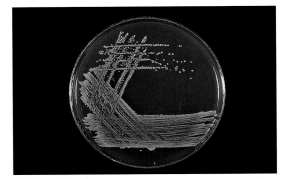

Plate 5   *Staphylococcus aureus.* (Reproduced with kind permission of Dr D Barrie.)

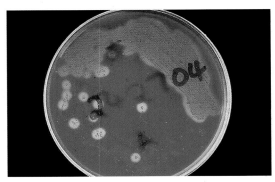

Plate 6   Streptococcus group A. Haemolysins produced by streptococcus lyse the red blood cells in blood agar, producing a clear area around the colonies. (Reproduced with kind permission of Dr D Barrie.)

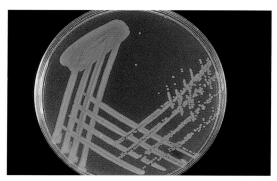

Plate 7 *Pseudomonas aeruginosa*. The colonies of *P. aeruginosa* appear green when grown on nutrient agar. (Reproduced with kind permission of Dr D Barrie.)

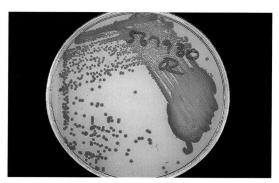

Plate 8 *Serratia marcescens*. The colonies of *S. marcescens* have a characteristic red coloration. (Reproduced with kind permission of Dr D Barrie.)

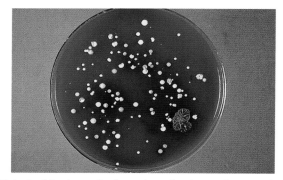

Plate 9 Mixed growth of organisms. Specimens often contain more than one type of bacterium, illustrated by the different forms of colony on this plate. (Reproduced with kind permission of Dr D Barrie.)

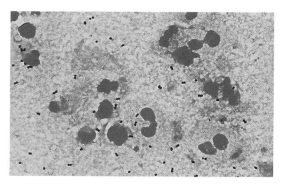

Plate 11 Sputum from a patient with suspected pneumonia. Gram-positive cocci, mostly in pairs, can be seen amongst the numerous, large, pus cells. Provisional diagnosis: pneumococcal pneumonia. (Reproduced with kind permission from Ackerman V, Dunk-Richards G (1991) *Microbiology: An Introduction for the Health Sciences.* W B Saunders, London.)

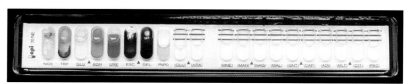

Plate 10 Each chamber contains a different biochemical test. Positive tests are indicated by a colour change and the set of results are used to identify the species of bacteria present. (Reproduced with kind permission of Jennie Wilson.)

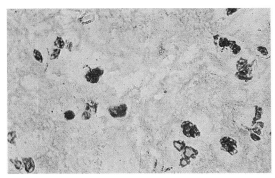

Plate 12 Tubercle bacilli appear as clumps of fine rods. (Reproduced with kind permission from Ackerman V, Dunk-Richards G (1991) *Microbiology: An Introduction for the Health Sciences.* W B Saunders, London.)

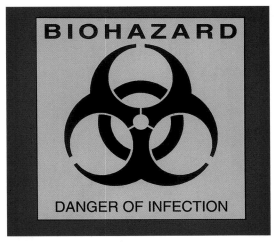

Plate 13 Biohazard label. (Reproduced with kind permission of Jennie Wilson.)

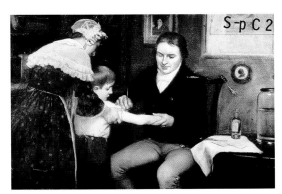

Plate 15 The first vaccination (Edward Jenner). (Reproduced with kind permission of the Wellcome Institute Library, London.)

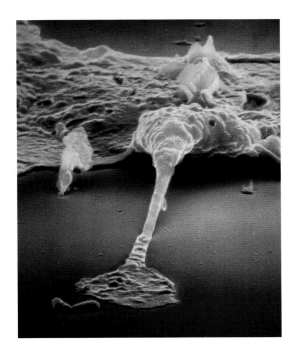

Plate 14 A macrophage extends a pseudopod to ingest a bacterium. (Reproduced with kind permission from Ackerman V, Dunk-Richards G (1991) *Microbiology: An Introduction for the Health Sciences.* W B Saunders, London.)

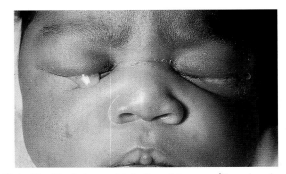

Plate 16 Staphylococcal infection of the eyes. (Reproduced with kind permission of Dr D Barrie.)

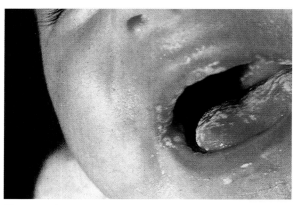

Plate 18   Oral thrush infection caused by the yeast candida. (Reproduced with kind permission of Dr D Barrie.)

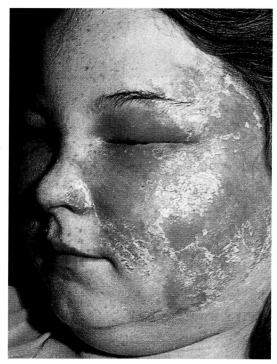

Plate 17   Erysipelas. An acute cellulitis caused by streptococcus. (Reproduced with kind permission of Dr D Barrie.)

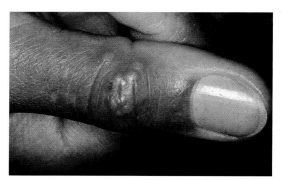

Plate 19   Herpetic whitlow caused by the herpes simplex virus. (Reproduced with kind permission of Dr D Barrie.)

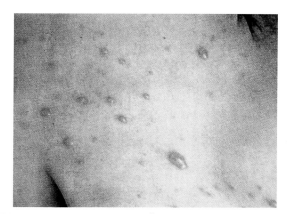

Plate 20   Chickenpox infection. (Reproduced with kind permission of Dr D Barrie.)

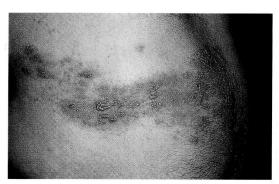

Plate 21   Herpes zoster (shingles). (Reproduced with kind permission from Ackerman V, Dunk-Richards G (1991) *Microbiology: An Introduction for the Health Sciences.* W B Saunders, London.)

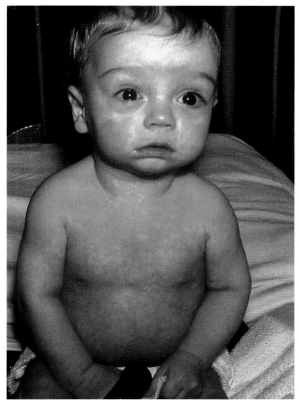

Plate 22 Measles infection. (Reproduced with kind permission of Dr D Barrie.)

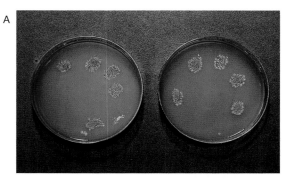

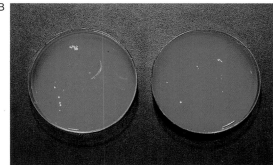

Plate 23 The effect of handwashing. (A) Fingertips pressed on to blood agar before washing. (B) Fingertips pressed on to blood agar after washing with soap and water. (Reproduced with kind permission of Dr D Barrie.)

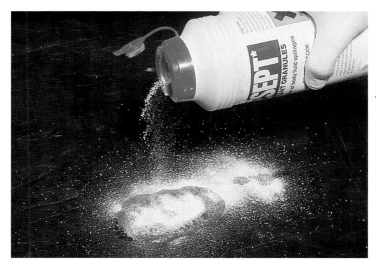

Plate 24 Chlorine-based granules can be used to soak up spills of blood. (Reproduced with kind permission of Jennie Wilson.)

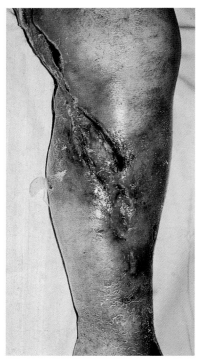

Plate 25 A chronic wound. Slough and superficial pus are present on the surface of the wound but with no signs of infection. (Reproduced with kind permission of Jennie Wilson.)

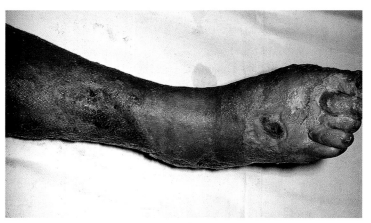

Plate 26 Infection in a surgical wound. (Reproduced with kind permission of Dr D Barrie.)

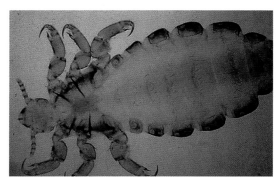

Plate 27 The female head louse (*Pediculus humanus capitis*). (Reproduced with kind permission from Ackerman V, Dunk-Richards G (1991) *Microbiology: An Introduction for the Health Sciences.* W B Saunders, London.)

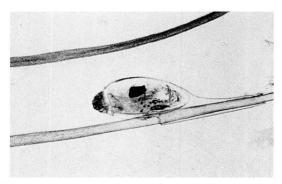

Plate 28 A louse egg (nit) attached to a hair. (Reproduced with kind permission from Ackerman V, Dunk-Richards G (1991) *Microbiology: An Introduction for the Health Sciences.* W B Saunders, London.)

Aspergillus

This saprophytic fungus occurs widely in the environment in dust and soil. It can cause infection in the lungs of people with underlying lung disease, for example cystic fibrosis, and a severe systemic infection in people who are immunocompromised, for example following organ or bone marrow transplant (Manuel & Kibbler 1998). Outbreaks of infection in susceptible patients are often associated with high spore levels in the air derived from environmental sources (e.g. building sites) rather than person-to-person spread (Humphries et al 1991). The regular removal of dust and the use of air filtration have been recommended for the protection of highly immunocompromised patients (Centers for Disease Control 2003) (see Ch. 11, p. 240).

Cryptococcus

Cryptococcus neoformans is a yeast that causes meningitis and brain abscesses but is extremely rare, usually occurring only in patients with severe immuno-deficiency. The main source of the organism is probably soil, although it has been associated with pigeon droppings and infection is acquired through inhalation of dust.

Dermatophytes (ringworm or tinea)

These are fungi that cause superficial infection of the skin, hair and nails and are readily transmitted from person to person. They include species that cause athlete's foot and ringworm of the body or scalp. Outbreaks of ringworm in schools are difficult to eradicate as prolonged treatment of the infection is necessary and infected children are difficult to detect (Communicable Disease Report 1995).

Pneumocystis jiroveci (formerly *carinii*)

This organism used to be considered a protozoon but has recently been reclassified as a fungus. It is found colonizing the lungs of healthy people but in the immunocompromised causes a severe pneumonia.

PROTOZOAL INFECTIONS

Protozoa are an unusual cause of infection in the UK although very common in other parts of the world. Amoeba and giardia cause gastrointestinal infections and are acquired by drinking water contaminated with faeces. Infections are usually associated with poor sanitation and in the UK cases are often acquired abroad. *Trichomonas vaginalis* is a parasite of the vagina which causes a sexually transmitted disease. Some protozoal infections have taken on a new significance because of their ability to cause serious disease in people with AIDS.

Toxoplasma

Toxoplasma gondii is a parasite of the cat family. It lives in the intestine of the cat and cysts are released in faeces. These can remain viable in soil for prolonged periods and may be ingested by humans or other animals. Once ingested, the protozoa reproduce asexually and circulate through the body establishing cysts in other tissue (e.g. brain, muscle and eye). In most cases the infection is mild and immunity develops rapidly.

Primary infection in early pregnancy can cause fetal death or brain damage and in the immuno-compromised, dormant cysts can be reactivated, resulting in large cerebral abscesses or retinitis. In the UK between 30% and 40% of the population has evidence of previous infection (Thomas 1988). Toxoplasma are not directly transmitted from person to person and therefore no special infection control precautions are indicated.

Infection is usually acquired by handling cat faeces or soil contaminated by cat faeces and occasionally by ingesting eggs in raw or undercooked meat.

Cryptosporidium

Cryptosporidium is a waterborne enteric pathogen and a common cause of gastroenteritis, especially in children under 5 years, and is characterized by profuse watery diarrhoea lasting for 1–2 weeks. Infected humans and animals shed large numbers of highly infectious oocysts in their faeces for several weeks and person-to-person spread frequently occurs, especially within households. Oocysts can remain viable in water or damp spoil for many months. They are resistant to water treatment chemicals and filtration must therefore be used to remove them from contaminated water supplies. Large outbreaks of cryptosporidium may occur in association with contaminated swimming pools or public or private water supplies (Communicable Disease Report 1992, 2003). Oocysts from livestock excreta or human sewage can contaminate drinking water supplies. In the immunocompromised, the organism is not easily eradicated from the bowel and prolonged severe disease may result, which has a poor response to antimicrobial therapy.

Plasmodium

Several species of this protozoon are transmitted by mosquitoes and cause malaria. Once inside the human body, the plasmodia replicate in the liver and red blood cells. The red cells rupture as a result, causing bouts of fever, anaemia and tissue hypoxia. Malaria does not occur in the UK but around 2000 cases a year are seen in people returning from abroad. Travellers to areas where malaria is endemic should take antimalarial prophylaxis. However, because resistance to antimalarial drugs is becoming more prevalent, physical protection against mosquitoes is also essential (e.g. hats, insect repellents) (Bradley & Bannister 2003). In endemic areas the local population gradually develops immunity, which reduces the severity of the illness. This immunity diminishes once an individual leaves an endemic area.

VIRAL INFECTIONS

Most viruses cause self-limiting infections, the effects of the disease depending on the particular cells they infect. Table 6.1 lists some important viral pathogens, indicating those of greatest significance for infection prevention and control in clinical settings.

Herpes viruses

These DNA viruses include herpes simplex types 1 and 2, Epstein–Barr virus, varicella zoster virus and cytomegalovirus. An important feature of all herpes viruses is their ability to become latent, causing repeated episodes of infection when reactivated.

Herpes simplex virus (HSV)

There are two types of this virus. Initial infection with HSV-1 usually occurs in infancy or early childhood, often asymptomatically, but it can produce acute gingivostomatitis and ulcers on the gums and oral mucosa. HSV-1 also causes a proportion of genital tract infections, meningoencephalitis, a severe infection that is frequently fatal, and infections of the eye. The virus may remain dormant in local nerve cells, periodically reactivating to cause vesicles on the lip or recurrent eye infections. Herpetic whitlow sometimes affects healthcare workers and occurs when herpes virus contaminates abrasions on the fingers, particularly around the nail bed (Plate 19).

HSV-2 mainly occurs in adults where it causes genital herpes lesions, affecting the penis in the male and vulva, labia and cervix in the female. There is a link between HSV infection of the cervix and cervical cancer. Although the primary infection resolves after a few days, lesions recur when the virus is reactivated by fluctuations in hormone levels, immunity or infection. The risk of transmission is greatest if the mother has a primary herpes infection at delivery. In recurrent herpes infection at the time of delivery, the presence of maternal antibodies helps to protect the neonate. In neonates HSV-2 causes encephalitis and has a high mortality rate so elective caesarean may be considered when the risk of transmission is high.

Both viruses are transmitted by direct contact with lesions, HSV-1 by kissing or touching sores, genital herpes by sexual intercourse although it may also be carried asymptomatically in saliva. Infection with one type of HSV does not provide immunity against the other type.

Infection control precautions   Transmission to healthcare workers or other patients may occur as a result of contact with active lesions. Gloves should be used routinely for contact with mucous membranes (e.g. mouth and vagina) and for contact with active herpes lesions such as cold sores or genital lesions. Care should be taken to prevent transmission from mothers with active genital lesions to their babies. The mother should be advised to wash her hands before handling her baby. Staff with active HSV lesions should not care for immunocompromised patients; those with herpetic whitlow should not undertake any patient's care until the lesion has resolved.

Varicella zoster virus

This virus causes chickenpox as a primary infection, mainly in children (Plate 20). Although usually a mild illness in children, primary chickenpox in adults may be complicated by pneumonia which can cause serious disease. Immunocompromised people may also develop a severe disseminated infection which can be fatal. Virus is secreted in the characteristic vesicles on the skin but it is primarily an infection of the respiratory tract and large amounts of virus are found in respiratory secretions which provide the main route of transmission. It is extremely infectious and in the UK around 90% of people will have had chickenpox by the time they reach adulthood (DoH 1996). The virus travels from the skin along sensory nerves and remains dormant in the ganglion for prolonged periods. If reactivated, it travels back along the sensory nerve and erupts on to the surface of the skin along the nerve pathways, appearing as vesicles. This is called herpes zoster (shingles) (Plate 21). It often causes severe, localized pain. Herpes zoster cannot be caught from people with either shingles or chickenpox; it usually occurs in older adults or the immunosuppressed and represents a reactivation of the primary infection. The fluid from shingles vesicles contains varicella virus and therefore non-immune individuals can acquire chickenpox through contact with people with shingles.

Table 6.1   Some important viral pathogens

Virus group	Disease	Route of entry
Coronaviruses	Common cold, severe acute respiratory syndrome (SARS)	Respiratory tract
Adenoviruses	Respiratory tract infection	Respiratory tract
Rhinoviruses	Common cold	Respiratory tract
Orthomyxoviruses		
Influenza A, B, C	Influenza	Respiratory tract
Paramyxoviruses		
Para-influenza	Para-influenza	Respiratory tract
Respiratory syncytial virus	Bronchiolitis	Respiratory tract
Mumps	Mumps	Respiratory tract
Measles	Measles	Respiratory tract
Caliciviruses		
Norovirus	Gastroenteritis	GIT
Herpes viruses		
Herpes simplex 1	Herpetic skin lesions	Skin, mucosa
Herpes simplex 2	Genital herpes	Sexual intercourse
Varicella zoster	Chickenpox, shingles	Respiratory tract, lesions
Cytomegalovirus	Febrile illness	Mucosa
Epstein–Barr virus	Glandular fever	Mucosa
Enteroviruses (picornaviruses)		
Polio	Polio	GIT
Coxsackie A	Hand, foot & mouth disease	GIT
Coxsackie B	Myo/pericarditis	GIT
Echoviruses	Meningitis	GIT
Calicivirus	Hepatitis A	GIT
Papoviruses		
Human papilloma virus	Warts, genital tract tumours	Skin
Reoviruses		
Rotavirus	Gastroenteritis	GIT
Hepadna viruses	Hepatitis B, D	Blood, sexual intercourse
Hepatoviruses	Hepatitis A	GIT
Flaviviruses	Hepatitis C	Blood
Retroviruses		
HIV-1 and -2	Immune deficiency	Blood, sexual intercourse
HTLV-1	Leukaemia, lymphoma	

GIT, gastrointestinal tract

Chickenpox acquired during the first 3 months of pregnancy may cause fetal abnormalities. A mother who acquires chickenpox a few days before delivery may transmit infection to her non-immune baby, who may subsequently develop severe illness.

Infection control precautions   The main infection control problem presented by patients infected with chickenpox is the risk of transmission to immuno-compromised patients (e.g. patients receiving immunosuppressive therapy, neonates, patients with HIV infection), who may develop serious and life-threatening disease (Stover & Bratcher 1998).

When a patient or member of staff develops chickenpox, the infection control team should be notified so that they can identify other patients who may be at risk of infection and who may need protection with specific immunoglobulin or prophylactic aciclovir if they are found to be non-immune. Immunity to chickenpox can be checked by looking for antibodies to the virus in blood. To minimize the risk of outbreaks of infection in high-risk areas such as maternity units, some occupational health departments routinely check the immunity of healthcare workers without a history of previous infection (Jones et al 1997).

Other herpes viruses

The Epstein–Barr virus (EBV) causes infectious mononucleosis (glandular fever) in teenagers and young adults. The virus invades B lymphocytes and causes fever, sore throat and enlarged lymph nodes. Most cases are mild but the symptoms may be persistent. EBV is transmitted by saliva and may be excreted for a long time after the symptoms have resolved. In parts of Africa EBV is associated with Burkitt's lymphoma and nasopharyngeal cancer.

Cytomegalovirus (CMV) causes a mild disease, similar to glandular fever. It establishes a persistent latent infection which may be periodically reactivated throughout life, resulting in virus being shed in urine and other body fluids. It is a very common infection and 80% of the population have been infected by late middle age (Tookey & Peckham 1991). More serious infection occurs in the immunosuppressed, often as a result of the reactivation of the latent virus. Infection, either primary or reactivation, during pregnancy does not usually cause harm to the fetus but around 1% die or have severe congenital defects.

The virus is excreted in large amounts in saliva and urine and is transmitted by close contact and kissing; most patients excreting the virus will be asymptomatic.

Infection control precautions   Most healthcare workers will be immune to primary CMV infection but may experience reactivation of a latent infection. There is no evidence that healthcare workers are more likely to acquire the virus at work. The routine use of gloves for handling body fluids and handwashing after the removal of gloves minimizes the risk of CMV transmission and additional precautions are not recommended, even for pregnant staff caring for infected patients (Health & Safety Executive 1990, Tookey & Peckham 1991).

Adenoviruses

There are many different types of these DNA viruses. Most cause mild respiratory illness and establish persistent, latent infection in the adenoids and tonsils. Other types cause outbreaks of conjunctivitis and respiratory tract infection, particularly amongst children. The main infection control problem associated with adenovirus is in neonatal intensive care units where they can cause severe viral pneumonia and may spread easily between babies (Piedra et al 1992). The spread of eye infections can be prevented by strict hygiene during eye examinations and the sterilization of equipment (e.g. tonometers).

Severe acute respiratory syndrome (SARS)

This severe form of pneumonia is characterized by high fever and severe cough or shortness of breath. It is caused by a coronavirus (SARS-CoV). The first reported outbreak of SARS started in China in 2002 and probably originated in people who handled wild animals. The primary route of transmission is contact between infectious respiratory secretions and mucous membranes. Although virus is also excreted in other body fluids such as urine and faeces, there is limited evidence that they play a role in transmission (WHO 2003). There is a high risk of transmission in healthcare settings and respiratory isolation precautions are required to prevent and control its spread (see pp. 239, 284).

Other respiratory viruses

There are a number of other viruses commonly encountered in hospitals which, although not related, spread from person to person by respiratory droplets and by respiratory secretions carried on hands (Sattar et al 2002). Respiratory syncytial virus is one of the most important causes of respiratory tract infection in children and can be extremely severe in babies, causing bronchiolitis, croup and pneumonia. Although most people are infected as children, the antibodies formed do not protect against subsequent infection. Adults may therefore acquire the infection and, although the effects are usually mild, it can cause serious, often fatal, infections in the elderly (Crowcroft et al 1999). Outbreaks of infection may occur in paediatric, haematology or bone marrow transplant units. Infected patients should therefore be isolated whilst symptomatic (Jones et al 2000, Madge et al 1992).

Measles (Plate 22), mumps and rubella are also sometimes seen in paediatric units, although the incidence of all of these childhood diseases has declined since the introduction of the combined MMR vaccine in 1988. Measures to reduce the spread of infection should be taken because a proportion of those infected may develop serious complications, especially if they are immunocompromised, for example mumps meningitis and encephalitis, otitis media and pneumonia associated with measles. If possible, infected patients should be discharged home and those that remain should be cared for by staff known to be immune to the infection to avoid secondary spread.

Influenza is caused by orthomyxoviruses. The illness can be serious, especially in the elderly or debilitated, and some people succumb to a secondary bacterial pneumonia. These viruses are easily transmitted by respiratory droplets and outbreaks of infection are common, particularly amongst the elderly (Communicable Disease Report 1998). New strains of the virus emerge almost every year (see p. 76) and severe pandemics occur periodically when a markedly different sub-type emerges that is able to spread readily from person to person. Influenza also causes disease in animals, in particular birds. Exchange of genetic information between avian and human viruses sometimes results in strains of avian influenza that can spread among humans. Since the late 1990s a highly pathogenic strain of avian influenza (H5N1) has been circulating in domestic poultry in Asia. Although this strain has not yet acquired the ability to spread efficiently between humans there is concern that this may occur and be responsible for an influenza pandemic (Health Protection Agency 2005).

Influenza vaccines are prepared annually to protect against the prevalent strain of the virus. Although not completely protective, they reduce the severity of the disease. Vaccination is recommended for residents of nursing homes for the elderly and other vulnerable groups (DoH 1996).

Enteroviruses

Enteroviruses are a large group of picornaviruses that usually infect the gut but then establish infection in lymphoid tissue and spread to other parts of the body in the bloodstream.

Polio viruses

There are three distinct types of polio virus which are transmitted by contact with faeces and pharyngeal secretions. They generally cause a mild febrile illness but in a few cases cause meningitis. In less than 1% of cases the virus invades the spinal cord or brainstem and the resulting damage to motor neurons causes paralysis. Prior to the introduction of mass vaccination in the UK, outbreaks of poliomyelitis were common and several thousand cases of paralytic polio were reported annually. The WHO immunization programme has dramatically reduced the incidence of polio worldwide, from over 30 000 cases in 1988 to less than 700 reported in 2003. Many countries, including the UK, are considered to have completely eliminated the poliomyelitis virus.

Until 2004, a live-attenuated vaccine was used which, because the virus replicates in the gut, had the added benefit of promoting antibody formation in the gut and protecting non-immune contacts through acquisition of the vaccine virus excreted in stool. Rarely, the vaccine virus reverts to a virulent form (or 'wild type') that can cause paralytic disease. Since the early 1990s only one or two cases of paralytic poliomyelitis have been reported each year. These have either been vaccine-associated polio or occurred in vaccine contacts. Since the risk of exposure to wild polio virus through importation of cases or travel abroad is now very low, the recommended vaccine has changed to inactivated polio vaccine and the very small number of vaccine-associated polio cases will be avoided (DoH 2004a).

Coxsackie viruses

Coxsackie A virus causes 'hand, foot and mouth' disease where vesicles erupt on the mouth, hands and feet. Coxsackie B virus causes a myocarditis and pericarditis from which most patients completely recover. Infection is mainly spread through contact with faeces and respiratory secretions. Outbreaks occasionally occur in neonatal units.

Hepatitis A and E

Hepatitis A is a gastrointestinal infection that spreads to the liver. It is characterized by nausea and abdominal pain followed after a few days by jaundice. It is generally a mild illness, often asymptomatic in children, lasting 1–2 weeks and not associated with any long-term adverse effects. The infection is spread by contact with faeces and is sometimes associated with poor sanitation. Recently, there have been major outbreaks of hepatitis A amongst IV drug users and linked to poor social conditions, homelessness and prisons (Perrett et al 2003). The virus is excreted in the faeces for 7–10 days before symptoms develop and for several days afterwards. Hepatitis A can also be transmitted in food and water, particularly sandwiches and salads and molluscs cultivated in contaminated water (Heymann 2004). Hepatitis E is caused by a calicivirus but results in a similar infection to hepatitis A. It is spread by water contaminated with faeces and from person to person via the faecal–oral route. Although rare in developed countries, it is endemic in South-East Asia and Africa.

Infection control precautions   Outbreaks of infection sometimes occur in schools and nurseries. The transmission of infection can be prevented by the use of gloves to handle faeces or change nappies and by strict attention to hand hygiene after using the toilet by both staff and children. During outbreaks of infection in residential institutions or child day-care centres, protection of staff by vaccination or with immuno-globulin may be considered necessary.

Other gastrointestinal viruses

Several other viruses cause gastrointestinal illness in both children and adults and may cause outbreaks of infection in hospital patients. Infections are of greatest concern amongst the very young or the elderly, who easily become severely dehydrated. Rotavirus causes a severe gastroenteritis associated with vomiting, watery diarrhoea and fever usually in children under 5 years, in whom it can cause severe dehydration. Most people acquire the infection during childhood and develop immunity to further infection; however, immunity may diminish with age and outbreaks of rotavirus amongst the elderly also occur (Heymann 2004). Norovirus (previously known as Norwalk-like or small round structured virus) is a calicivirus that causes an acute gastroenteritis characterized by severe vomiting. Cases occur sporadically and in small out-breaks in the community but in healthcare and other institutions, large outbreaks may occur with the virus spreading rapidly from person to person and affecting both patients and staff (Lopman et al 2003). Virus present in vomit may contribute to the spread of infection and virus is also frequently excreted in faeces for several days after the illness has resolved.

Infection control precautions   Outbreaks of infection should be controlled by isolation of patients until at least 48 h after symptoms have resolved. Virus may be particularly easily acquired on the hands through contact with excreta, vomitus, bedding and nappies. Rigorous handwashing and the use of gloves and aprons for contact with affected patients, their body fluids and immediate environment are therefore essential to prevent spread (see Ch. 12). Spills of vomit or faeces from affected patients should be treated with chlorine-based disinfectants to destroy any virus present (Chadwick et al 2000) (see p. 256).

Bloodborne viruses

Viruses transmitted by blood and body fluid are of particular importance to healthcare workers who may be at risk of acquiring infection through contact with body fluid. The most important bloodborne viruses are hepatitis B, hepatitis C and HIV. The hepatitis and HIV viruses are not related but will be considered together because the infection control precautions are similar.

Viral hepatitis

Hepatitis, or inflammation of the liver, has infectious and non-infectious causes. Most primary viral infections of the liver are caused by hepatitis viruses. Hepatitis A and E are transmitted by the faecal–oral route, hepatitis B and C are bloodborne. The hepatitis D virus is not a true virus but can cause a severe, acute hepatitis if it infects an individual already infected with, or carrying, hepatitis B virus. Hepatitis can also be caused by other viruses, including EBV and cytomegalovirus, leptospires and toxoplasma. Hep-atitis causes malaise, nausea and, after a few days, jaundice.

Hepatitis B

Most infections caused by this virus are mild but in a few cases result in extensive liver damage and liver failure that may be fatal. The incubation period is usually between 2 and 3 months, although it may be as long as 6 months. Between 2% and 10% of those infected do not completely eliminate the virus but continue to carry it in their blood. The risk of becoming a chronic carrier is greatest when the infection is acquired as a child. About 90% of those infected perinatally will become chronic carriers (DoH 2002a). In some areas perinatal transmission is common and up to 20% of the population may be chronic carriers of hepatitis B virus (HBV) (e.g. South-East Asia, parts of Africa). Chronic HBV carriers are at increased risk of developing chronic progressive hepatitis, cirrhosis and primary carcinoma of the liver.

The prevalence of HBV varies in different parts of the world. In the UK and most other European countries it is less than 1%. Some groups are at increased risk of acquiring HBV (e.g. residents of institutions for people with learning difficulties whose behaviour may facilitate transmission, haemophiliacs, intravenous drug users who share needles and families of chronic carriers). Patients undergoing haemodialysis are at increased risk of acquiring HBV from blood transfusion or by cross-infection in the dialysis unit (DoH 2002b).

Tests to detect viral components and antibodies formed against them in the blood are used to determine previous infection and the carrier state. The surface antigen HBsAg is found on the outer protein coat of the virus and its presence in blood indicates an active infection or chronic carriage of hepatitis B. Anti-HBs are antibodies formed to the surface antigen and, if present in the blood, indicate that the individual has been infected in the past, the virus has been eliminated by the immune system and the patient is no longer infectious. HBeAg or the 'e' antigen is part of the virus's nuclear material and its presence in blood indicates a high level of viral replication and a highly infectious patient. Usually antibodies (anti-HBe) are formed against this antigen during the first few weeks of infection. The presence of anti-HBe in the blood indicates low infectivity. If anti-HBe is not formed, chronic carriage of the virus develops and the person remains highly infectious. Occasionally a mutation in the virus prevents the production of e antigen. Individuals infected with these mutant viruses appear to be e antigen negative but may in fact be highly infectious chronic carriers (Sundkvist et al 1998).

HBV is transmitted by sexual intercourse and perinatally from mother to baby. It is also transmitted when infected body fluids are inoculated through the skin, on instruments such as needles, via damaged or cut skin, or through contact with mucous membranes.

HBV has been isolated from virtually all body fluids but blood, semen and vaginal fluids are mostly implicated in transmission of the virus. Saliva has been found to contain the virus in much lower concentration than in blood and, although it does not appear to transmit infection through contact with mucous membranes, it has been associated with transmission through biting (Cancio-Bello et al 1982).

Healthcare workers are as much as five times more likely to become infected with HBV than other workers because of their regular and close contact with body fluids. The rate of transmission following needlestick injury with HBeAg-positive blood may be as high as 30% (Royal College of Pathologists 1992). Healthcare workers who are hepatitis B carriers may also transmit the virus to patients during invasive procedures such as surgery and obstetrical procedures and several outbreaks associated with HBV-infected surgeons have been reported (Heptonstall 1991, Sundkvist et al 1998).

Hepatitis B immunization   Vaccination is an effective method of protecting against infection. Healthcare workers who have direct contact with blood, blood-stained body fluids and tissues should be immunized against HBV. Immunization is particularly important for those who perform exposure-prone procedures (Box 6.1). (DoH 2000).

Current guidance recommends universal screening of women in antenatal clinics for HBV to identify carriers and to ensure that their infants are protected against infection by immunization at birth (DoH 2003a). Priority has also been given to HBV vaccination programmes in prisons where the incidence of IV drug use and therefore bloodborne virus infection is high (DoH 2003b).

A course of three injections confers protection in most adults and immunity lasts for at least 15 years (European Consensus Group on Hepatitis B 2000). Specific immunoglobulin (HBIg) can be used to provide immediate, temporary protection against infection with

---

> **Box 6.1   Definition of exposure-prone procedures (EPPs)**
>
> 'Exposure-prone procedures are those where there is a risk that injury to the worker may result in the exposure of the patient's open tissues to the blood of the worker. These include procedures where the worker's gloved hands may be in contact with sharp instruments, needle tips and sharp tissues (spicules of bone or teeth) inside a patient's open body cavity, wound or confined anatomical space where the hands or fingertips may not be completely visible at all times. However, other situations, such as pre-hospital trauma care and care of patients where the risk of biting is predictable (e.g. such as with a disturbed and violent patient or a patient having an epileptic fit), should be avoided by healthcare workers restricted from performing exposure-prone procedures' (DoH 2002e).

---

hepatitis B but it must be administered within 48 h of an exposure.

Hepatitis C

Before the introduction of a serological test for hepatitis C virus (HCV) in 1990, little was known about the epidemiology of a disease previously recognized only as non-A, non-B hepatitis. Although the primary infection with HCV is mild, often asymptomatic and rarely associated with jaundice, about 80% of those infected become chronic carriers of the virus. A significant proportion of those with chronic infection develop liver disease and cirrhosis.

In the UK the prevalence of HCV in the general population is low (0.5%), although in some high-risk groups such as IV drug users, a prevalence of antibody to HCV of 30% has been reported (Hope et al 2001). In 90% of cases of HCV infection where a risk factor is reported, transmission is related to the sharing of contaminated needles and injecting equipment by drug users (DoH 2002c). In the past HCV infection was transmitted by blood transfusions but since the screening of donated blood for HCV was introduced in 1991, the risk from this route is now extremely low. Skin piercing and tattooing have also been associated with transmission. HCV transmits from mother to baby in about 6% of pregnancies where the mother is an HCV carrier. The greatest risk of transmission is at the time of delivery and HCV is not thought to be transmitted by breastfeeding. The virus can also be transmitted by sexual intercourse although the risk of transmission is relatively low, with evidence of infection in approximately 5% of regular sexual partners of individuals with HCV (DoH 2002c).

Healthcare workers are at risk of acquiring HCV from needlestick injuries. The rate of transmission is lower than HBV, with approximately 3% of exposures to infected blood resulting in acquisition of the virus (DoH 2002d). HCV has also been acquired by blood splashing into the eyes (Hosoglu et al 2003). Transmission between patients in renal and haematology units has been reported (Allander et al 1994, 1995).

As with HBV, the virus may also be transmitted to the patient from an infected healthcare worker during exposure-prone procedures (see Box 6.1), although the risk of transmission is lower than that associated with HBV (Duckworth et al 1999). There is currently no vaccine available to protect against HCV, although antiviral treatment successfully clears the virus in at least 50% of carriers (DoH 2002c).

Other hepatitis viruses

Hepatitis D is a defective virus that can only replicate with HBV. It is most prevalent in South America, parts of Russia and the Mediterranean, where co-infection with both viruses often causes serious, chronic illness. More recently, hepatitis G virus has been identified. It is known to be transmitted by blood transfusions and transmission to healthcare workers via needlestick injuries has also been reported (Shibuya et al 1998).

Human immunodeficiency virus (HIV)

HIV is a retrovirus. This means that the genetic information of the virus consists of RNA but it also has an enzyme, reverse transcriptase, that converts the RNA to DNA and then incorporates it into the DNA of the host cell. The virus probably developed from a simian immunodeficiency virus (SIV) in African monkeys that jumped species to humans following exposure to the blood of these animals when they were being killed and butchered. The first documented case of HIV occurred in Africa in 1959 but it is likely that the virus persisted unrecognized in Africa for many decades. Changes in sexual behaviour, population migration to cities and increasing international travel have contributed to the emergence of a worldwide pandemic of HIV (Pratt 2003). Two distinct forms of HIV have been identified: HIV-1 occurs throughout the world while HIV-2 has been found primarily in West Africa. These viruses, although very similar, appear to have evolved from different SIV in monkeys.

HIV infection is diagnosed by detecting antibodies to the virus in the blood. These are not usually detectable until about 3 months after infection when the individual is said to have seroconverted. Tests to detect viral antigens and nucleic acid sequences are also available and play an important role in the management of the infection.

The virus recognizes and infects cells in the body that carry particular receptor proteins on their surface. The principal cell surface receptor recognized by HIV is a glycoprotein called CD4 that is carried on the surface of T lymphocytes and other immune system cells. Although at the time of infection the immune system mounts a response to the virus, it eventually is unable to keep up with the high rate of viral replication and after several years symptoms of immune deficiency become apparent. These include infection caused by opportunistic pathogens, such as *Pneumocystis jiroveci* (formerly *carinii*), and severe disseminated disease of other pathogens such as herpes simplex or tuberculosis. Antiretroviral therapy aimed at the reverse transcriptase and protease enzymes can be used to reduce viral replication but whilst it slows progression of the disease, it does not effect a cure. The reverse transcriptase is associated with a high rate of transcription errors, making it particularly difficult for the immune system to consistently recognize virus agents and hampering efforts to develop an effective vaccine.

Transmission of HIV   Infection with HIV will persist indefinitely. The infected person can transmit HIV to others soon after acquiring the infection but the risk of transmitting infection is greatest from a person with a high level of virus. Viral load is greatest during the primary infection (first 3–4 months after infection) and later once the compromised immune system can no longer control viral replication.

HIV is primarily transmitted by sexual intercourse. However, transmission may also occur by inoculation of infected body fluids through the skin or on to mucous membranes, transplantation of tissues or organs and by transfusion of contaminated blood. In developed countries blood products are now screened and heat-treated to eliminate the risk of HIV infection. The virus is also transmitted from mother to baby through the placenta, during delivery or via breast milk. The greatest risk of transmission is during delivery but this can be significantly reduced by caesarean section prior to the onset of labour (European Mode of Delivery Collaborative 1999). Antiretroviral therapy and avoiding breastfeeding also reduce the risk of mother-to-child transmission. Rates of transmission of 2% or less are now reported in Western Europe where these precautions are widely used (European Collaborative Study 2001).

The greatest concentration of virus is found in blood or body fluid containing visible blood. The virus has also been found in semen, vaginal secretions, tissues, cerebrospinal fluid, amniotic fluid and

Table 6.2   Proportion of adults living with HIV/AIDS by region (reproduced with permission from United Nations Programme on AIDS 2004)

Region	Prevalence of HIV/AIDS (%)
Sub-Saharan Africa	7.4
North Africa/Middle East	0.3
Asia	0.4
Latin America	0.6
Caribbean	2.3
Eastern Europe/Central Asia	0.8
Western Europe/North America	0.4
Oceania	0.2

In 2004 there were an estimated 39 million people in the world infected with HIV.

Table 6.3   Prevalence of HIV infection in different population groups within the United Kingdom (reproduced with permission from Health Protection Agency 2003c)

Group	Prevalence of HIV (%)
Pregnant women	0.14
– Sub-Saharan women	2.5
Homosexual men attending GUM clinic	
– London	5.4
– Outside London	2.4
– Under 24 years old	4.0
Heterosexuals attending GUM clinic	
– All heterosexuals	0.8
– Sub-Saharan African	4.9
Injecting drug users in contact with services	
– London	3.6
– Outside London	0.18

synovial fluid. HIV is also found in breast milk and in developed countries where safe alternatives to breast milk are available, HIV mothers are advised not to breastfeed. HIV has also been found in saliva and tears, although in much lower concentrations, and these fluids have not been associated with transmission of the infection unless they contain visible blood (Centers for Disease Control 1991, UK Health Departments 1998).

The HIV pandemic   HIV began to spread worldwide in the late 1970s. Initially cases of AIDS were recognized in Western industrialized countries in North America, Western Europe and Australasia, mostly affecting homosexual men. In sub-Saharan Africa, heterosexual contact was the main route of transmission and with growing numbers of women affected, prenatal transmission is also common. By the 1990s the pandemic had spread to Asia, Eastern Europe and the Middle East. In many Westernized countries, health education, condom use and the availability of treatment have minimized the impact of HIV. However, 90% of people with HIV live in developing countries that lack the resources required to control the spread of the virus and have much greater prevalence of HIV (Table 6.2).

HIV in the UK   Approximately 50 000 people in the UK have HIV with about 5000 new diagnoses made each year. Over half of these people live in London. The prevalence of diagnosed HIV infection varies among different risk groups (see Table 6.3). Homosexual contact is the most common route of transmission (see Fig. 6.3). Estimates made from unlinked anonymous testing suggest that 30% of people with HIV do not realize that they have the infection. The prevalence of HIV infection has been increasing since the late 1990s. Much of this increase is due to transmission among homosexual men and the migration of HIV-infected heterosexual people from sub-Saharan Africa. However, the number of people acquiring HIV heterosexually in the UK, although low, is also increasing (Health Protection Agency 2003c).

The unlinked anonymous HIV Survey provides data on the prevalence of HIV in England and Wales by testing specimens obtained from genitourinary medicine clinics, injecting drug users, hospital patients and pregnant women. The tests are taken from leftover blood that has been taken for other, routine clinical tests and all patient-identifying information is removed before testing; the results cannot therefore be linked to the source patient. The data obtained from this testing programme are used to monitor the spread of the disease, to target health promotion programmes and to monitor their efficacy (DoH 1998b).

Transmission of HIV to healthcare workers   The first documented case of a healthcare worker who acquired HIV occupationally was reported in 1984 (Anonymous 1984). Many other reports have subsequently been published (PHLS HIV & STD Centre 1999). In the UK there have been very few documented cases of a healthcare worker acquiring HIV following an occupational exposure. A surveillance system for monitoring occupational exposure to bloodborne viruses was started in 1997 (Health Protection Agency 2004).

Most occupational transmissions of HIV have followed inoculation of infected body fluid into the

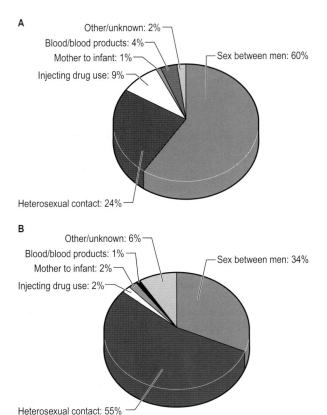

A

Other/unknown: 2%
Blood/blood products: 4%
Mother to infant: 1%
Injecting drug use: 9%
Sex between men: 60%
Heterosexual contact: 24%

B

Other/unknown: 6%
Blood/blood products: 1%
Mother to infant: 2%
Injecting drug use: 2%
Sex between men: 34%
Heterosexual contact: 55%

Figure 6.3 Recent changes in epidemiology of HIV in the United Kingdom. (A) Exposure category of HIV infections diagnosed, 1992–1999 (*n* = 41 387). (B) Exposure category of HIV infections diagnosed, 2000–2002 (*n* = 14 336) (reproduced with permission from Health Protection Agency 2003).

skin by a needle or other sharp instrument, although some have occurred after contamination of damaged skin or mucous membranes by infected body fluids. Follow-up of healthcare workers exposed to HIV-infected body fluids indicates that the rate of HIV transmission is much lower than that of hepatitis B. The risk of acquiring HIV from a needlestick injury with HIV-infected blood is estimated as 0.32%, although the volume of blood inoculated and the infectivity of the blood will influence whether transmission occurs. The risk of transmission associated with mucocutaneous exposure is lower, at around 0.03% (PHLS AIDS & STD Centre 1999). Although there is no vaccine available to protect against HIV infection, postexposure prophylaxis with antiretroviral drugs is recommended should a healthcare worker have an injury involving HIV-infected material (see p. 168) (DoH 2004b).

As with other bloodborne viruses, there is a risk of healthcare workers infected with HIV transmitting infection to others, although it is extremely low (DoH 2002e). Transmission of HIV from an infected dentist to five of his patients has been reported, although the exact route of transmission remains unclear (Centers for Disease Control 1991). Transmission of HIV from an infected orthopaedic surgeon to a patient has been reported in France (Dorozynski 1997).

Infection control precautions for bloodborne viruses
The screening of blood donors for hepatitis B, treatment of blood products and the targeting of high-risk groups for immunization against hepatitis B, particularly infants born to infected mothers, have reduced the incidence of the infection in the UK (DoH 1996). The risk of acquiring HIV from blood products has been virtually eliminated by screening. However, the absence of a vaccine against HIV means that controlling the spread of infection depends on education to discourage behaviour that may transmit infection, such as unprotected sexual contact and the sharing of used needles to inject drugs.

Frequent contact with body fluids places many healthcare workers at particular risk of acquiring bloodborne viruses (BBV). Workers may be infected in the following ways:

- inoculation of infected blood or body fluid through the skin on contaminated sharp instruments
- contamination of mucous membranes such as the eyes or mouth with infected blood or body fluid
- contamination of broken skin with infected blood or body fluid.

In line with the Control of Substances Hazardous to Health Regulations, the risk of exposure to hazardous biological agents such as BBV should be assessed and methods of minimizing the risk identified. Infection cannot be transmitted by social contact with patients. Protective clothing is therefore only necessary for direct contact with blood or body fluids and not for the routine care of the patient. Healthcare workers can avoid exposure by using safety equipment, employing safe procedures and using protective clothing when exposure to body fluid is anticipated. The main risk is from contaminated sharp instruments. Healthcare workers are often unaware of patients who are infected with BBV and any blood and most body fluids must therefore be considered potentially infectious and precautions used routinely in all situations (UK Health Departments 1998). The main principles are listed in Box 6.2 and discussed in more detail in Chapter 7.

Patients known to be infected with BBVs do not generally require isolation unless contamination of the environment is likely (e.g. profuse bleeding). However, they may require isolation if they have another

Box 6.2   Preventing the transmission of bloodborne viruses

Routine infection control precautions to be used in the care of all patients to prevent the transmission of bloodborne viruses from patient to healthcare worker and between patients. First recommended by the Centers for Disease Control in 1987, they have now been widely adopted and are also recognized as a means of minimizing the risk of transmission of other pathogens (Garner 1996, Wilson & Breedon 1990).

Sharps safety
- Safety equipment
- Safe handling disposal procedures
- Provide hepatitis B vaccination
- Manage and report injuries/exposures

Protective clothing
- Use to protect against direct contact with body fluid
- Assess risk of procedure and select appropriate protection

Maintain integrity of skin
- Cover cuts with waterproof dressing
- Seek advice from occupational health if extensive damaged skin

Handwashing
- After gloves removed
- After contact with body fluid

Decontamination
- Equipment contaminated with body fluid
- Spills of body fluid
- Launder soiled linen
- Render safe/incinerate hazardous waste

infection that presents a risk to other patients, for example tuberculosis, and there is also evidence for the spread of opportunistic infections such as *Pneumocystis jiroveci* (formerly *carinii*) and cryptosporidium amongst patients with AIDS in hospital (Laing 1999).

The use of long-term intravenous access to provide nutrition or therapy also places patients with AIDS at increased risk of bloodstream infection and a high standard of care must be used to minimize the risk. Isolation may be indicated for such patients for the duration of their illness with these secondary pathogens.

Equipment that enters a sterile area of the body or has close contact with mucous membranes (e.g. fibreoptic endoscope) has the potential to transmit BBVs between patients. Chant et al (1993) reported an outbreak of HIV infection related to minor surgical procedures in private surgical consulting rooms and

Bronowicki et al (1997) reported HCV transmission on endoscopes used to perform colonoscopies. Such equipment must be decontaminated appropriately after each use to prevent cross-infection. Chapter 13 discusses methods of disinfection and sterilization in more detail.

Injury with a contaminated sharp instrument is the most likely route of transmission to healthcare workers and every hospital should have a policy outlining the procedures to be followed in the event of a needlestick injury (see Fig. 7.5). Staff with extensive areas of damaged skin, e.g. active eczema, should seek advice from the occupational health department.

Exposure–prone procedures (EPPs) Transmission of BBVs from an infected healthcare worker to a patient may occur during procedures in which injury to the healthcare worker could result in blood contaminating the patient's open tissue, for example when hands are in contact with sharp instruments, bone or teeth (see Box 6.1). Since 1993, healthcare workers who perform EPPs have been required to be immunized against HBV and have their antibody response tested. Those who are HBeAg positive (or eAg negative but have evidence of active infection) are not able to perform EPPs. Healthcare workers who are HCV carriers (i.e. have had a positive test for HCV RNA) should not perform EPPs unless they respond successfully to treatment. Healthcare workers who are infected with HIV are not able to perform EPPs (DoH 2000, 2002d, e, 2004b). Healthcare workers who think that they may be infected with a BBV should seek advice from the occupational health department and may need to modify their practice or avoid performing invasive procedures. Postexposure prophylaxis may need to be offered to patients exposed to the blood of a hepatitis B or HIV-infected healthcare worker (DoH 2000, 2004b).

Preventing transmission of BBVs in dialysis units Transmission of hepatitis B amongst patients undergoing renal dialysis was recognized as a major problem in the 1970s. Improved infection control, particularly the management of sharps and equipment, has reduced the incidence of infection. However, outbreaks of HBV and HCV in haemodialysis and haematology units are still reported (Allander et al 1994, 1995, Roll et al 1995).

Recent guidance suggests that patients undergoing renal dialysis are protected from HBV by immunization and should be tested for HBV and HCV at least 3 monthly. HIV testing should be undertaken if indicated by a risk assessment. Where possible, patients with BBVs should be dialysed in a separate area from other patients, using designated staff for each shift. A dialysis machine should be designated for patients with HBV but this is not necessary for HCV or HIV where the risk of transmission is much lower. Dialysis machines should undergo routine decontamination procedures between patients but in addition, the surface of the machines used to dialyse patients with BBVs should also be decontaminated after use (DoH 2002b).

Virus–like agents: prions

Prions are abnormal proteins. They are not conventional infectious agents and have no nucleic acid. They appear to cause disease by replacing normal proteins on the surface of host cells, gradually compromising their function. They are associated with some rare diseases in humans and animals that cause progressive degeneration of the nervous system. Scrapie is a prion disease of sheep that has been recognized in the UK for many years, although with no evidence of transmission to humans. An epidemic of a prion disease in cattle, bovine spongiform encephalopathy (BSE), was first recognized in the UK in the mid-1980s and is thought to have affected a million cattle (Patterson & Painter 1999). The epidemic was probably related to changes in the methods used to render animal carcases, which reduced heat and chemical decontamination and enabled the prion proteins to enter the meat and bone meal used as cattle feed supplements (Haywood 1997).

The main prion disease in humans is Creutzfeldt–Jakob disease (CJD). This is a spongiform encephalopathy associated with destruction of brain tissue and presenile dementia. This is mostly a sporadic disease affecting 30–50 people a year in the UK. Although the cause is unknown, genetic factors appear to play a part. A familial form of CJD accounts for 10–15% of cases and is genetic in origin, caused by a mutation of the prion protein gene. Iatrogenic cases of CJD have occurred in association with grafting of human-derived tissues, e.g. cornea, pituitary hormones and dura mater grafts, and, more rarely, neurosurgical instruments.

In 1996 a new form of CJD was identified and termed variant CJD (vCJD). This generally affects young people under 30 years of age and causes a range of different neurological changes and symptoms (DoH 1998a). By 2003 over 140 cases of vCJD had been reported. It is likely that these cases of vCJD are linked to exposure to BSE. It is difficult to estimate how the epidemic may progress, as little is known about the risk of transmission, incubation period or susceptibility to the disease, although a slight decline in the number of cases has been reported since 2002 (Advisory Committee on Dangerous Pathogens 2003, Patterson & Painter 1999).

Unlike conventional CJD where the presence of abnormal protein in patients with clinical disease is confined to the central nervous system, there is evidence that vCJD affects the lymphoreticular systems. It can therefore be detected in lymph nodes, tonsils and spleen and has been detected in the appendix of an affected patient 24 months before the disease became clinically apparent (Hilton et al 2002). Infectivity of tonsils and spleen has been demonstrated experimentally (Bruce et al 2001). Prion proteins are highly resistant to conventional methods of decontamination, including cooking, irradiation, most chemical disinfectants and formaldehyde. In addition, the standard autoclave cycle of 134°C for 3 min does not reliably destroy the prion protein even if put through the cycle several times.

Infection control precautions   Currently there is no evidence that CJD is transmitted from person to person by close contact and the routine precautions taken with blood and body fluids from all patients are sufficient for the care of patients known or suspected to have CJD (see Box 6.2). There is no evidence that body secretions, excreta or saliva are infectious. Clinical waste (e.g. sharps, dressings) generated during the care of known or suspected patients, whether in hospital or the community, should be treated as normal clinical waste. Nervous tissue (e.g. cerebrospinal fluid) does present a risk and although conventional CJD is not transmitted by blood, there is some experimental evidence to suggest that vCJD could be transmitted by blood transfusion. People at risk from CJD (e.g. symptomatic, blood relative with CJD, recipients of human-derived tissue) are no longer able to donate blood; white cells are removed from donated blood and plasma for blood products is sourced from outside the UK (Advisory Committee on Dangerous Pathogens 2003).

The main risk in healthcare settings is presented by invasive procedures, particularly those that involve the nervous system (e.g. lumbar puncture, neurosurgery) and the potential risk of transmission to other patients on contaminated instruments. Because the CJD agent is unusually resistant to conventional sterilization and disinfection processes, instruments used on patients known or suspected to have CJD should be destroyed after use (and where possible single-use instruments should be used), together with any protective clothing worn by those involved in the procedure. Instruments used on patients with symptoms of CJD but no definite diagnosis should be quarantined until a diagnosis is made (see p. 277, Ch. 13) (Advisory Committee on Dangerous Pathogens 2003).

Haemorrhagic fevers

Although viral haemorrhagic fevers such as Lassa fever, Marburg and Ebola viruses do not occur in the

UK, they are occasionally seen in patients recently returned from abroad. They are associated with a high rate of mortality. The viruses are transmitted to humans from animals such as rats and monkeys but transmission to healthcare workers through handling of infected blood and body fluids has also been reported. Acute hospitals should have a policy outlining the management of any patient admitted with unexplained

fever. If viral haemorrhagic fever is strongly suspected, the patient should be transferred to a high-security isolation unit. Otherwise, routine blood and body fluid precautions should be used until a diagnosis has been confirmed (see Box 6.2). Most patients returning from abroad with unexplained fever have malaria and it is important to exclude this diagnosis (Advisory Committee on Dangerous Pathogens 1997).

References

Advisory Committee on Dangerous Pathogens (1997) *Management and Control of Viral Haemorrhagic Fevers.* PL(97)1. Stationery Office, London.

Advisory Committee on Dangerous Pathogens (2003) *Transmissible Spongiform Encephalopathy Agents: Safe Working and the Prevention of Infection.* Spongiform Encephalopathy Advisory Committee. Department of Health, London.

Allander T, Medin C, Jacobson SH et al (1994) Hepatitis C transmission in a haemodialysis unit: molecular evidence for spread of virus among patients not sharing equipment. *J. Med. Virol.*, **43**: 415–19.

Allander T, Gruber A, Naghavi M et al (1995) Frequent patient-to-patient transmission of hepatitis C in a haematology ward. *Lancet*, **345**: 603–7.

Anonymous (1984) Needlestick transmission of HTLV-III from a patient infected in Africa. *Lancet*, **ii**: 1376–7.

Ayan M, Durmaz R, Aklas E et al (2003) Bacteriological, clinical and epidemiological characteristics of hospital-acquired *Acinetobacter baumanii* in a teaching hospital. *J. Hosp. Infect.*, **54**: 39–45.

Barrie DB, Wilson JA, Hoffman PN et al (1992) *Bacillus cereus* meningitis in two neurosurgical patients: an investigation into the source of the organism. *J. Infect.*, **25**: 291–7.

Berlau J, Auken HM, Houang E et al (1999) Isolation of *Acinetobacter* spp including *A. baumannii* from vegetables: implications for hospital-acquired infections. *J. Hosp. Infect.*, **42**: 201–4.

Bodey GP (1988) The emergence of fungi as major pathogens. *J. Hosp. Infect.*, **11** (suppl. A): 411–26.

Boyce JM (2001) MRSA patients: proven methods to treat colonisation and infection. *J. Hosp. Infect.*, **48** (suppl. A): S9–14.

Bradley DJ, Bannister B, on behalf of the Health Protection Agency Committee on Malaria Prevention for UK Travellers (2003) Guidelines for malaria prevention in travellers from the United Kingdom for 2003. *Comm. Dis. Public Health*, **6**(3): 180–99.

Breathnach AS, de Ruiter A, Holdsworth GMC et al (1998) An outbreak of multidrug resistant tuberculosis in a London teaching hospital. *J. Hosp. Infect.*, **39**(2): 111–18.

Brett M, Hood J, Brazier JS et al (2005) Soft tissue infections caused by spore-forming bacteria in injecting drug users in the United Kingdom. *Epidemiol. Infect.*, **133**: 575–82.

Bronowicki JP, Vernard V, Botte C et al (1997) Patient-to-patient transmission of hepatitis C during colonoscopy. *N. Engl. J. Med.*, **337**(4): 237–40.

Bruce ME, McConnell I, Will RG et al (2001) Detection of Creutzfeldt–Jakob disease infectivity in extraneural tissues. *Lancet*, **358**: 208–9.

Burnett IA, Norman P (1990) *Streptococcus pyogenes*: an outbreak on a burns unit. *J. Hosp. Infect.*, **15**(2): 173–6.

Cancio-Bello TP, de Medina M, Shorey J et al (1982) An institutional outbreak of hepatitis B related to a human biting carrier. *J. Infect. Dis.*, **146**(5): 652–6.

Cartwright K, Logan M, McNulty C et al (1995) A cluster of cases of streptococcal necrotising fasciitis in Gloucestershire. *Epidemiol. Infect.*, **115**: 387–97.

Casewell MW, Phillips I (1977) Hands as a route of transmission for Klebsiella species. *BMJ*, **2**: 1315–17.

Centers for Disease Control (1991) Update: transmission of HIV infection during invasive dental procedures – Florida. *MMWR*, **40**: 378–81.

Centers for Disease Control (2003) Guidelines for environmental control in healthcare facilities. *MMWR*, **52**: RR10.

Chadwick PR, Beards C, Brown D et al (2000) Management of hospital outbreaks of gastro-enteritis due to small round structured viruses. *J. Hosp. Infect.*, **45**: 1–10.

Chant K, Lowe D, Rubin G et al (1993) Patient to patient transmission of HIV in private surgical consulting rooms. *Lancet*, **342**: 1548–9.

Coia JE (1998) Nosocomial and laboratory acquired infections with *Escherichia coli* O157. *J. Hosp. Infect.*, **40**(2): 107–14.

Communicable Disease Report (1995) Scalp ringworm in London. *CDR*, **5**(38): 179.

Communicable Disease Report (1998) An outbreak of influenza in four nursing homes in Sheffield. *CDR*, **8**(16): 139.

Communicable Disease Report (1999) Cryptosporidiosis associated with swimming pools. *CDR Weekly*, **9**(48): 423.

Communicable Disease Report (2003) Large summer and autumn peak of cryptosporidiosis in England and Wales 2003. *CDR Weekly*, **13**(41). Available online at: www.hpa.org.uk/CDR/archives/2003/cdr4103.pdf

Communicable Disease Surveillance Centre (2004a) Preliminary report on tuberculosis cases reported in 2002 in England, Wales and Northern Ireland. March 2004. Available online at: www.hpa.org.uk.

Communicable Disease Surveillance Centre (2004b) Tuberculosis update. Available online at: www.hpa.org.uk.

Cooke RDP (2004) Hazards of water. *J. Hosp. Infect.*, **57**: 290–3.

Cottrill MRB (1996) *Helicobacter pylori. Prof. Nurse*, **12**(1): 46–8.

Crowcroft NS, Cutts F, Zambon MC (1999) Respiratory syncytial virus: an underestimated cause of respiratory tract infections, with prospects of a vaccine. *Commun. Dis. Public Health*, **2**(4): 234–41.

Dealler S (1998) Nosocomial outbreak of multi-resistant *Acinetobacter* spp. on an intensive care unit: possible association with ventilator equipment. *J. Hosp. Infect.*, **38**: 147.

Denton M, Hawkey PM, Hoy CM et al (1993) Co-existent cross-infection with *Streptococcus pneumoniae* and group B streptococci on an adult oncology unit. *J. Hosp. Infect.*, **23**: 271–8.

Department of Health (1996) *Immunisation Against Infectious Disease*. HMSO, London.

Department of Health (1998a) *New Variant CJD – Patients Who have Received Implicated Blood Products*. PL(CO)(98) 1. Department of Health, London.

Department of Health (1998b) *Prevalence of HIV in England and Wales 1997*. Summary Report from the Unlinked Anonymous Surveys Screening Group. Department of Health, London.

Department of Health (2000) *Hepatitis B Infected Healthcare Workers*. HSC 2000/020. Department of Health, London.

Department of Health (2002a) *Children in Need and Blood-Borne Viruses: HIV and Hepatitis*. Department of Health, London.

Department of Health (2002b) *Good Practice Guidelines for Renal Dialysis/Transplant Units. Prevention and Control of Blood-Borne Virus Infection*. Department of Health, London.

Department of Health (2002c) *Hepatitis C Strategy for England*. Department of Health, London.

Department of Health (2002d) *Hepatitis C Infected Healthcare Workers*. HSC 2002/010. Department of Health, London.

Department of Health (2002e) *AIDS/HIV Infected Health Care Workers: Guidance on the Management of Infected Health Care Workers and Patient Notification*. Department of Health, London.

Department of Health (2003a) *Screening for Infectious Diseases in Pregnancy. Standards to Support the UK Antenatal Screening Programme*. Department of Health, London.

Department of Health (2003b) *DH & HM Prison Service. Guidance on Developing Local Prison Health Delivery Plans*. Department of Health, London.

Department of Health (2004a) *Immunisation Against Infectious Disease (update)*. Chapters on diphtheria, Hib, pertussis, polio and tetanus. Department of Health, London. Available online at: www.immunisation.nhs.uk.

Department of Health (2004b) *HIV Post-Exposure Prophylaxis: Guidance from the UK Chief Medical Officers' Expert Advisory Group on AIDS*. Department of Health, London.

Department of Health/Public Health Laboratory Service Joint Working Group (1994) *Clostridium difficile Infection. Prevention and Management*. Health Publications Unit, Heywood, UK.

Dettenkofer M, Hauer T, Daschner FD (2004) Detergent versus hypochlorite cleaning and *Clostridium difficile* infection. *J. Hosp. Infect.*, **56**: 78–9.

Djuretic T, Wall PG, Brazier JS (1999) *Clostridium difficile*: an update on its epidemiology and role in hospital outbreaks in England and Wales. *J. Hosp. Infect.*, **41**: 213–18.

Dorozynski A (1997) French patient contracts AIDS from surgeon. *BMJ*, **314**: 250.

Dowsett EG, Willson PA (1981) An outbreak of *Streptococcus pyogenes* infection in a maternity unit. *CDR*, **81**(17): 3.

Duckworth GJ, Heptonstall J, Aitkin C et al (1999) Transmission of hepatitis C virus from a surgeon to a patient. *CDR*, **2**: 188–92.

Efstratiou A (1989) Outbreaks of human infections caused by the pyogenic streptococci of Lancefield group C and group G. *J. Med. Microbiol.*, **29**: 207–19.

European Collaborative Study (2001) HIV-infected women and vertical transmission in Europe since 1986. *AIDS*, **15**: 761–70.

European Consensus Group on Hepatitis B (2000) Are booster immunisations needed for lifelong hepatitis B immunity? *Lancet*, **355**(9203): 561–5.

European Mode of Delivery Collaborative (1999) Elective caesarean section versus vaginal delivery in prevention of vertical HIV transmission: a randomised clinical trial. *Lancet*, **353**: 1035–9.

Evans BG, Gill ON, Gleave SR et al (1991) HIV-2 in the United Kingdom – a review. *CDR*, **1**(2): R19–23.

Evans HS, Madden P, Douglas C et al (1998) General outbreaks of infectious intestinal disease in England and Wales: 1995 and 1996. *Commun. Dis. Public Health*, **1**(3): 165–71.

Fekerty R, Kim KH, Brown D et al (1981) Epidemiology of antibiotic associated colitis. *Am. J. Med.*, **70**: 906–8.

Flanagan PG, Barnes RA (1998) Fungal infection in the intensive care unit. *J. Hosp. Infect.*, **38**(3): 163–77.

Food Standards Agency (2002) *Eating While You Are Pregnant*. Food Standards Agency, London.

Fowler SL, Rhoton B, Springer SC et al (1998) Evidence for person-to-person transmission of *Candida lusitaniae* in a neonatal intensive care unit. *Infect. Contr. Hosp. Epidemiol.*, **19**(5): 343–5.

Garner JS (1996) Hospital Infection Control Practices Advisory Committee Guideline for isolation precautions in hospitals. *Infect. Contr. Hosp. Epidemiol.*, **17**(1): 54–80.

Glowacki LS, Hodsman AB, Hammerberg O et al (1994) Surveillance and prophylactic intervention of *Staphylococcus aureus* nasal colonisation in a haemodialysis unit. *Am. J. Nephrol.*, **14**: 9–13.

Gorman LJ, Sanai L, Notman W et al (1993) Cross-infection in an intensive care unit by *Klebsiella pneumoniae* from ventilator condensate. *J. Hosp. Infect.*, **23**(1): 27–34.

Gray JW, George RH (2000) Experience of vancomycin-resistant enterococci in a children's hospital. *J. Hosp. Infect.*, **45**: 11–18.

Gray J, George RH, Durbin GM et al (1999) An outbreak of *Bacillus cereus* respiratory tract infections on a neonatal unit due to contaminated ventilator circuits. *J. Hosp. Infect.*, **41**: 19–22.

Hannan MM, Bell A, Easterbrook P et al (1996) An outbreak of multi-drug resistant tuberculosis in a London teaching hospital HIV/GUM unit: outbreak investigations, infection control issues and molecular epidemiology. *Genitourin. Med.*, **72**: 307–8.

Hannan MM, Azadian BS, Gazzard BG et al (2000) Hospital infection control in an era of HIV infection and multi-drug resistant tuberculosis. *J. Hosp. Infect.*, **44**: 5–11.

Haywood AM (1997) Transmissible spongiform encephalopathies. *N. Engl. J. Med.*, **337**: 1821–8.

Heymann D (ed.) (2004) *Control of Communicable Disease in Man*, 18th edn. American Public Health Association, Washington, DC.

Health and Safety Commission (2000) *Legionnaire's Disease: The Control of Legionella Bacteria in Water Systems. Approved Code of Practice and Guidance.* HSE Books, Norwich, UK.

Health and Safety Executive, Advisory Committee on Dangerous Pathogens (1990) *Statement on Cytomegalovirus and the Pregnant Woman.* HMSO, London.

Health Protection Agency (2003a) *Surgical Site Infection. Analysis of Surveillance in English Hospitals, 1997–2002.* Health Protection Agency, London.

Health Protection Agency (2003b) *Hospital-acquired Bacteraemia. Analysis of Surveillance in English Hospitals 1997–2002.* Health Protection Agency, London.

Health Protection Agency (2003c) *Renewing the Focus. HIV and Other Sexually Transmitted Infections in the United Kingdom in 2002. An update: November 2003.* Health Protection Agency, London. Available online at: www.hpa.org.uk/infections/topics_az/bbv/bbmenu.htm.

Health Protection Agency (2004) *Surveillance of Significant Occupational Exposure to Bloodborne Viruses in Health Care Workers. England, Wales and Northern Ireland: Six-Year Report: March 2004.* Health Protection Agency, London. Available online at: www.hpa.org.uk/infections/topics_az/bbv/bbmenu.htm.

Health Protection Agency (2005) Influenza pandemic contingency plan. Version 8.0. October 2005. Available online at: www. hpa.org.uk/infections/topics_az/influenza/pdfs/.

Heath PT, Balfour G, Weisner AM et al (2004) Group B streptococcal disease in UK and Irish infants younger than 90 days. *Lancet*, **363**: 292–3.

Heptonstall J (1991) Outbreaks of hepatitis B virus infection associated with infected surgical staff. *CDR*, **1**: R81–5.

Hilton DA, Ghani AC, Conyers L et al (2002) Accumulation of prion protein in tonsil and appendix: review of tissue samples. *BMJ*, **325**: 633–4.

Hobson RP (2003) The global epidemiology of invasive candida infections. Is the tide turning? *J. Hosp. Infect.*, **55**(3): 159–68.

Hoffman P (1993) *Clostridium difficile* and the hospital environment. *PHLS Microbiol. Digest*, **10**(2): 91–2.

Hoffman P, Bradley C, Ayliffe G (2004) *Disinfection in Healthcare*, 3rd edn. Blackwell Publishing, Oxford.

Hollyoaks V, Allison D, Summers J (1995) *Pseudomonas aeruginosa* wound infection associated with a nursing home's whirlpool bath. *CDR*, **5**(7): R100–2.

Hope VD, Judd A, Hickman M et al (2001) Prevalence of hepatitis C among injecting drug users in England and Wales. Is harm reduction working? *Am. J. Public Health*, **91**(1): 38–42.

Hosoglu S, Celen MK, Akalin S et al (2003) Transmission of hepatitis C by blood splash into conjunctiva in a nurse. *Am .J. Infect. Contr.*, **31**: 502–4.

Hospital Infection Control Practices Advisory Committee (1995) Recommendations for preventing the spread of vancomycin-resistance. *Am. J. Infect. Contr.*, **23**:87–94.

Howard AJ (1991) Nosocomial spread of *H. influenzae. J. Hosp. Infect.*, **19**(1): 1–4.

Humphries H, Johnson EM, Warnock DW et al (1991) An outbreak of aspergillosis in a general ITU. *J. Hosp. Infect.*, **18**(3): 167–78.

Hutchinson DN (1990) Nosocomial legionellosis. *Rev. Med. Microbiol.*, **1**: 108–15.

Interdepartmental Working Group on Tuberculosis (1998) *The Prevention and Control of Tuberculosis in the United Kingdom: UK Guidance on the Prevention and Control of Transmission of 1. HIV Related Tuberculosis and 2. Drug-resistant, Including Multiple Drug-resistant, Tuberculosis.* Department of Health, London.

Johnson AP (1998) Antibiotic resistance among clinically important Gram positive bacteria in the UK. *J. Hosp. Infect.*, **40**: 17–26.

Joint Tuberculosis Committee of the British Thoracic Society (2000) Control and prevention of tuberculosis in the United Kingdom, Code of Practice. *Thorax*, **55**: 887–901.

Jones BL, Clark S, Curran ET et al (2000) Control of an outbreak of respiratory syncytial virus infection in immunocompromised adults. *J. Hosp. Infect.*, **44**: 53–7.

Jones D (1990) Foodborne listeriosis. *Lancet*, **336**: 1171–4.

Jones EM, Barnett J, Perry C et al (1997) Control of varicella-zoster infection on renal and other specialist units. *J. Hosp. Infect.*, **36**: 133–40.

Kelly CP, Lamont JP (1998) *Clostridium difficile* infection. *Ann. Rev. Med.*, **49**: 375–90.

Kessel AS, Gillespie IA, O'Brien SJ et al (2001) General outbreaks of infectious intestinal disease linked with poultry, England and Wales 1992–1999. *Comm. Dis. Public Health*, **3**: 171–7.

Kibbler LC, Seaton S, Barnes RA et al (2003) Management and outcome of bloodstream infection due to Candida species in England and Wales. *J. Hosp. Infect.*, **54**: 18–24.

Kleemola M, Jokinen C (1992) Outbreak of *Mycoplasma pneumoniae* infection amongst hospital personnel studied by a nucleic acid hybridisation test. *J. Hosp. Infect.*, **21**(3): 213–22.

Kluytmans JAJW, Mouton JW, Van den Bergh MFQ et al (1996) Reduction of surgical site infections in cardiothoracic surgery by elimination of nasal carriage of *Staphylococcus aureus. Inf. Contr. Hosp. Epidemiol.*, **17**: 780–5.

Koos WE, Bannerman TL (1994) Update on clinical significance of coagulase-negative staphylococci. *Clin. Micro. Rev.*, **7**: 117–40.

Kyne L, Warny M, Qamar A et al (2001) Association between antibody response to toxin A and protection against recurrent *Clostridium difficile* infection. *Lancet*, **357**: 189–93.

Laing RBS (1999) Nosocomial infections in patients with HIV disease. *J. Hosp. Infect.*, **43**: 179–85.

Laurichesse H, Grimand O, Wraight P et al (1998) Pneumococcal bacteraemia and meningitis in England

and Wales: 1993 to 1995. *Commun. Dis. Public Health*, **1**(1): 22–7.

Levin MH, Olsen B, Nathan C et al (1984) Pseudomonas in the sinks of an intensive care unit: relation to patients. *J. Clin. Pathol.*, **37**: 424–7.

Loomes S (1988) Is it safe to lie down in hospital? *Nursing Times*, **84**(49): 63–5.

Lopman BA, Adak GK, Reacher MH et al (2003) Two epidemiologic patterns of norovirus outbreaks: surveillance in England and Wales, 1992–2000. *Emerg. Infect. Dis.*, **9**(1): 71–7.

Macrae MB, Shannon KP, Rayner DM et al (2001) A simultaneous outbreak on a neonatal unit of two strains of multiply antibiotic resistant *Klebsiella pneumoniae* controllable only by ward closure. *J. Hosp. Infect.*, **49**: 183–92.

Madge P, Payton JY, McColl JH et al (1992) Prospective controlled study of four infection control procedures to prevent nosocomial infection with respiratory syncytial virus. *Lancet*, **340**: 1079–83.

Maguire HC, Seng C, Onauters S et al (1998) Shigella outbreak in a school associated with eating canteen food and person to person spread. *Commun. Dis. Public Health*, **1**(4): 279–80.

Manuel RJ, Kibbler CC (1998) The epidemiology and prevention of invasive aspergillosis. *J. Hosp. Infect.*, **39**: 95–109.

Mayon-White D (2004) Re-emerging infections Part 1: Tuberculosis. *Br. J. Infect. Contr.*, **5**(4): 14–16.

Morbidity & Mortality Weekly Report (1997) Prevention of pnuemococcal disease: recommendations from the Advisory Committee on Immunisation Practices (ACIP). *MMWR*, **46**: 1–24.

Mortimer EA, Wolinsky E, Gonzaga AJ et al (1966) Role of airborne transmission in staphylococcal infections. *BMJ*, **1**: 319–22.

National *Clostridium difficile* Standards Group (2004) Report to the Department of Health. *J. Hosp. Infect.*, **56** (suppl. 1): 1–138.

Neely AN, Maley MP (2000) Survival of enterococci and staphylococci on hospital fabrics and plastic. *J. Clin. Microbiol.*, **38**(2): 724–6.

Orsi GB, Aureli P, Cassonet J et al (1999) Post surgical *Bacillus cereus* endophthalmitis outbreak. *J. Hosp. Infect.*, **42**(3): 250–1.

Patterson WJ, Painter MJ (1999) Bovine spongiform encephalopathy and new variant Creutzfeldt–Jakob disease: an overview. *Commun. Dis. Public Health*, **2**: 5–13.

Perez-Fontan M, Garcia-Falcon T, Rosales M et al (1993) Treatment of *Staphylococcus aureus* nasal carriers in continuous ambulatory peritoneal dialysis with mupirocin: long term results. *Am. J. Kidney Dis.*, **22**: 708–12.

Perrett K, Granerod J, Crowcroft N et al (2003) Changing epidemiology of hepatitis A: should we be doing more to vaccinate injecting drug users? *Comm. Dis. Public Health*, **6**(12): 97–100.

Pfaller MA (1996) Nosocomial candidiasis: emerging species, reservoirs and modes of transmission. *Clin. Infect. Dis.*, **22** (suppl.): S89–94.

Piedra PA, Kasel JA, Norton JH et al (1992) Description of an adenovirus type 8 outbreak in hospitalised neonates born prematurely. *Pediatr. Infect. Dis. J.*, **11**(8): 460–5.

Pratt RJ (2003) *HIV and AIDS. A Foundation for Nursing and Healthcare Practice*, 5th edn. Arnold, London.

Public Health Laboratory Service (1995) Interim guidelines for the control of infections with verocytotoxin producing *Escherichia coli* (VTEC). *CDR Rev.*, **5**(6): R77–80.

Public Health Laboratory Service AIDS & STD Centre at the Communicable Disease Surveillance Centre (1999) *Occupational Transmission of HIV. Summary of Published Reports*. Available online at: www.hpa.org.uk/infections/topics_az/hiv_and_sti/publications.

Public Health Laboratory Service Meningococcus Forum (2002) Guidelines for public health management of meningococcal disease in the UK. *Comm. Dis. Public Health*, **5**(3): 187–202.

Ramage L, Green K, Pyskir D et al (1996) An outbreak of fatal nosocomial infections due to group A streptococcus on a medical ward. *Infect. Contr. Hosp. Epidemiol.*, **17**: 429–31.

Rampling A, Wiseman S, Lacey L et al (2001) Evidence that hospital hygiene is important in the control of methicillin-resistant *Staphylococcus aureus*. *J. Hosp. Infect.*, **49**: 109–16.

Ramsay ME, Andrews N, Kaczmarski EB et al (2001) Efficacy of meningococcal serogroup C conjugate vaccine in teenagers and toddlers in England. *Lancet*, **357**: 195–6.

Roll M, Norder H, Magnius LO et al (1995) Nosocomial spread of hepatitis B virus (HBV) in a haemodialysis unit confirmed by HBV DNA sequencing. *J. Hosp. Infect.*, **30**: 57–63.

Rosen HR (1997) Acquisition of hepatitis C by a conjunctival splash. *Am. J. Infect. Contr.*, **25**: 242–7.

Rowan NJ, Anderson JG (1998) Growth and enterotoxin production by diarrhoegenic *Bacillus cereus* in dietary supplements prepared for hospitalized HIV patients. *J. Hosp. Infect.*, **38**: 139–46.

Royal College of Pathologists (1992) *HIV Infection: Hazards of Transmission to Patients and Health Care Workers During Invasive Procedures*. Royal College of Pathologists, London.

Sanderson PJ, Weissler S (1992) Recovery of coliforms from the hands of nurses and patients: activities leading to contamination. *J. Hosp. Infect.*, **21**: 85–94.

Sattar SA, Springthorpe VS, Tetro J et al (2002) Hygienic hand antiseptics: should they not have activity and label claims against viruses? *Am. J. Infect. Contr.*, **30**: 355–72.

Schlech WF (1991) Listeriosis: epidemiology, virulence and the significance of contaminated foodstuffs. *J. Hosp. Infect.*, **19**(4): 211–24.

Shibuya A, Takeuchi A, Sakurai K, Saigenji K (1998) Hepatitis G virus infection from needle-stick injuries in hospital employees. *J. Hosp. Infect.*, **40**: 287–90.

Simor AE, Lee M, Vearnacombe M et al (2002) An outbreak due to multiresistant *Acinetobacter baumanii* in a burn unit: risk factors for acquisition and management. *Infect. Contr. Hosp. Epidemiol.*, **23**: 261–7.

Stansfield R, Caudle S (1997) *Bacillus cereus* and orthopaedic surgical wound infection associated with incontinence pads manufactured from virgin wood pulp. *J. Hosp. Infect.*, **37**(4): 336–7.

Stover BH, Bratcher DF (1998) Varicella-zoster virus: infection control and prevention. *Am. J. Infect. Contr.,* **26**: 369–84.

Subramanian D, Sandoe JAT, Keer V et al (2003) Rapid spread of penicillin-resistant streptococcus pneumoniae among high-risk hospital inpatients and the role of molecular typing in outbreak confirmation. *J. Hosp. Infect.,* **54**(2): 99–103.

Sundkvist T, Hamilton GR, Rimmer D et al (1998) Fatal outcome of transmission of hepatitis B from an e antigen negative surgeon. *Commun. Dis. Public Health,* **1**(1): 48–50.

Takahashi A, Yomoda S, Tarimoto K et al (1998) *Streptococcus pyogenes* hospital acquired infection within a dermatological ward. *J. Hosp. Infect.,* **40**(2): 135–40.

Thomas CGA (1988) *Medical Microbiology,* 6th edn. Baillière Tindall, London.

Tookey P, Peckham CS (1991) Does cytomegalovirus present an occupational risk? *Arch. Dis. Child.,* **66**: 1009–10.

UK Health Departments (1998) *Guidance for Clinical Health Care Workers: Protection Against Infection with Blood-borne Viruses. Recommendations of the Expert Advisory Group on AIDS and the Advisory Group on Hepatitis.* Department of Health, Wetherby, UK.

United Nations Programme on AIDS and World Health Organization (2004) *AIDS epidemic Update 2004.* UNAIDS, Geneva. Available online at: www.unaids.org.

Vincent JL, Bihari DJ, Suter PM et al (1995) The prevalence of nosocomial infection in intensive care units in Europe. Results of the European prevalence of infection in intensive care units in Europe study. *JAMA,* **274**: 639–44.

Watson JM (1991) Tuberculosis in perspective. *CDR Rev.,* **1**(12): R129–31.

Weber DJ, Rutala WA (1997) Role of environmental contamination in the transmission of vancomycin-resistant enterococci. *Infect. Contr. Hosp. Epidemiol.,* **18**: 306–9.

Weems JJ (1993) Nosocomial outbreak of *Pseudomonas cepacia* associated with contamination of reusable electronic ventilator temperature probes. *Infect. Contr. Hosp. Epidemiol.,* **14**(10): 583–6.

Wilcox MH, Fawley WN (2000) Hospital disinfectants and spore formation by *Clostridium difficile. Lancet,* **356**: 1324.

Williams CL (1999) *Helicobacter pylori* and endoscopy. *J. Hosp. Infect.,* **41**: 263–8.

Williams REO (1963) Healthy carriage of *Staphylococcus aureus*: its prevalence and importance. *Bacteriol. Rev.,* **27**: 56–71.

Wilson J, Breedon P (1990) Universal precautions. *Nursing Times,* **86**(37): 67–70.

World Health Organization (2003) *Consensus Document on the Epidemiology of Severe Acute Respiratory Syndrome (SARS).* World Health Organization, Geneva.

Worsley MA (1993) A major outbreak of antibiotic-associated diarrhoea. *PHLS Microbiol. Digest,* **10**(2): 97–9.

Further Reading

Greenwood D, Slack RCB, Peutherer JF (eds) (2002) *Medical Microbiology. A Guide to Microbial Infections: Pathogenesis, Immunity, Laboratory Diagnosis and Control,* 16th edn. Churchill Livingstone, Edinburgh.

Health Protection Agency website: www.hpa.org.uk.

Mims C, Playfair J, Roitt I, Wakelin D, Williams R (1998) *Medical Microbiology,* 2nd edn. Mosby, London.

Pratt R (2003) *HIV and AIDS: A Foundation for Nursing and Healthcare Practice,* 5th edn. Arnold, London.

SECTION 2

Practice

Chapter **7**

Standard infection control precautions

INTRODUCTION

Infection is a common but often avoidable complication of healthcare which has a major impact on the patient and the health service. It has been estimated that up to one-third of hospital-acquired infections could be prevented by improved infection control practice (Haley et al 1985, Harbarth et al 2003, National Audit Office 2000).

As discussed in Chapter 3, patients receiving healthcare are at increased risk of acquiring infection due to invasive procedures, devices or conditions that impair normal defences against infection. In addition, the healthcare environment provides plenty of opportunities for micro-organisms to transfer between patients and for antimicrobial resistant strains to emerge and spread.

Some patients may be recognized as having a communicable infection and special precautions implemented to prevent transmission. However, often these patients will be infectious before the illness becomes apparent. For example, patients with chicken-pox are infectious for two or three days before the rash appears and bloodborne viruses such as human immunodeficiency virus (HIV), hepatitis B and C are associated with prolonged asymptomatic carriage of which even the patient may be unaware. Similarly, patients may be colonized with antibiotic-resistant pathogens such as methicillin-resistant *Staphylococcus aureus* but remain undetected for prolonged periods.

Many infections occur because micro-organisms colonizing the patient are inadvertently transferred to a vulnerable site on the same or another patient. The implementation of special precautions only on diagnosis of infection may therefore not prevent cross-infection. Practices to prevent patients acquiring infection and to minimize the risk of transmission should therefore be incorporated into routine practice, not just implemented for those patients known to have an infection.

Infection control procedures are also important to protect staff from infection. Healthcare workers are healthy and are generally less susceptible to infection than their patients. However, they may acquire skin infections caused by streptococci, staphylococci, herpes simplex, fungi and scabies (Greaves et al 1980, Ross et al 1998), respiratory infections such as chickenpox, respiratory syncytial virus and *Mycobacterium tuberculosis* and enteric infections, particularly viral gastroenteritis. Healthcare workers are also at risk from the bloodborne viruses such as hepatitis B and C and HIV (Health Protection Agency 2005).

Healthcare workers infected with bloodborne viruses may transmit infection to their patients, although the main risk of transmission is associated with invasive procedures in which injury to the healthcare worker could result in blood entering the patient's open tissues (DoH 2000, 2002a, b).

Background to routine precautions

In the past, infection control precautions tended to be focused on special measures intended to prevent the transmission of infection from patients known to have infectious disease. The concept of using a range of infection control precautions routinely in the care of all patients, regardless of whether they are known to have an infection, was first recommended in the late 1980s (Centers for Disease Control 1987). This approach, called universal precautions, was developed in response to the emerging HIV epidemic which highlighted the problem of identifying patients with infection (see Box 7.1). Universal precautions were originally applied to all body fluids but when it became clear that bloodborne viruses were not transmitted by all fluids (e.g. faeces, urine, sputum), a recommendation to exclude those fluids from universal precautions, unless they contained visible blood, was made (Centers for Disease Control 1988).

As body fluids are involved in the transmission of a wide range of other pathogens, the introduction of universal precautions stimulated interest in the use of routine precautions to prevent the transmission of other hospital-acquired infections (Wilson & Breedon 1990). However, if universal precautions were to be effective in preventing cross-infection between patients, as well as protecting staff from bloodborne viruses, then it was important that protective clothing was both used and changed appropriately. Thus, by changing protective clothing after each procedure, micro-organisms acquired during contact with body fluid would not be

Box 7.1   Universal precautions

Universal precautions were first recommended by the Centers for Disease Control in Atlanta, USA, in 1985 in response to growing concerns about the risk to healthcare workers from the human immunodeficiency virus (HIV) (Centers for Disease Control 1987). Until then, special precautions had been taken only with body fluids from patients known or suspected to be infected with bloodborne viruses. HIV had highlighted the difficulty of identifying people who were incubating a disease and were infectious but who had no outward signs of the infection. Universal precautions recognized that there were a few simple practices that could be used in the care of all patients that would minimize the risk of bloodborne viruses being transmitted to healthcare workers. These included the safe management of sharps, the use of protective clothing in situations where open skin lesions or mucous membrane may have contact with blood or body fluid, the use of waterproof dressings to cover cuts and handwashing after any contact with body fluids.

Since universal precautions were first proposed, other workers have recognized their benefit as a means of protecting staff and patients from other pathogens that have a propensity to spread in clinical settings (Lynch et al 1990, Wilson & Breedon 1990).

introduced to a susceptible site on the same or another patient. A number of studies have subsequently demonstrated a reduction in infection rates associated with the routine use of gloves and other protective clothing (Johnson et al 1990, Klein et al 1989).

In 1987, Lynch et al proposed a simplified approach to isolation procedures for patients known to have an infection on the basis that a system of universal precautions with all moist body substances should be in place. Healthcare workers were required to use clean gloves where contact with moist body substances was anticipated, for contact with mucous membranes and non-intact skin and to change them after each procedure. By ensuring that these basic precautions were taken to prevent transmission from patients who are unknowingly incubating infection or colonized with pathogens, isolation procedures for patients known to have infectious disease could be simplified and focused on a smaller number of pathogens (Jackson & Lynch 1985).

The value of applying standard infection control precautions both to protect healthcare workers from bloodborne viruses and to minimize the risk of transmission of other pathogens is now generally accepted. In the recent guideline on isolation precautions (Garner 1996), the principles of universal precautions and body substance isolation have been synthesized with a level of 'standard precautions' recommended for use with the care of all patients. UK guidelines contain similar advice (Pellowe et al 2003, Pratt et al 2001).

PRINCIPLES OF INFECTION CONTROL

The core principles of infection control are:

- effective and timely hand hygiene
- the appropriate use of protective clothing
- maintenance of a clean environment.

These represent the standard of care that should be used routinely in the care of all patients to minimize the transmission of pathogens between patients and to staff. They are applicable in all healthcare settings, in hospitals, clinics, surgeries or the patient's own home (Pellowe et al 2003, Pratt et al 2001). These standard precautions are summarized in Box 7.2. More specific measures required to prevent infections associated with invasive devices, equipment and infectious diseases are covered in subsequent chapters.

Isolation precautions were originally developed to prevent the spread of infectious disease amongst vulnerable hospital patients and are used to prevent or control outbreaks or epidemics of infection in hospital, for example micro-organisms transmitted by an airborne route. They are initiated when an infectious disease meriting additional control measures is diagnosed in a particular patient and are discussed in more detail in Chapter 14.

Risk assessment

Risk assessment should underpin the principles of standard infection control precautions. Assessment of the risk of transmitting infection should form part of every clinical activity. It should consider the risk to both patients and healthcare workers and result in an appropriate level of infection control precautions being taken (Box 7.3).

As highlighted in Chapter 3, systems to analyse and manage risks to both patients and staff are recognized as essential to providing safe, high-quality care and systems must be in place to ensure that potential risks in relation to the transmission of infection are identified and managed (see p. 53, Ch. 3).

Health and safety regulations require employers to identify hazards in the workplace and assess them for

---

Box 7.2   Standard principles for preventing healthcare–associated infections (adapted from Pellowe et al 2003 and Pratt et al 2001)

Hand hygiene
- Decontaminate hands before and after contact with patients
- Decontaminate hands after gloves are removed
- Decontaminate hands after contact with body fluid

Maintain integrity of skin
- Cover cuts to skin with waterproof dressing
- Dry skin properly and use handcream
- Staff with active skin conditions seek advice from occupational health

Protective clothing
- Use to protect against direct contact with body fluid
- Assess risk of procedure and select appropriate protection
- Change after each procedure

Sharps safety
- Use equipment with safety devices
- Use safe handling and disposal procedures
- Provide hepatitis B vaccination for staff at risk
- Report exposures to blood or body fluid

Safe handling of clinical waste
- Use safe handling and disposal procedures
- Discard excreta directly into drainage system
- Incinerate/render safe hazardous waste

Decontamination of equipment
- Clean and decontaminate equipment after use
- Disinfect used linen by laundering
- Use protective clothing whilst handling and cleaning

Decontamination of environment
- Keep environment clean and free from dust
- Disinfect spills of body fluid

---

their potential to cause harm. The Control of Substances Hazardous to Health (COSHH) Regulations (Health & Safety Executive 2002) apply to hazardous micro-organisms present in body fluids or tissues as well as chemicals and carcinogens. They apply to situations where micro-organisms are being used or worked on, for example in laboratories, as well as activities that may result in incidental exposure such as refuse disposal, food production and healthcare. Assessments should take into account the type of biological agent that may be present (Box 7.4).

Box 7.3   Example of risk assessment in practice

Activity
- Emptying a urine drainage bag

Infection hazard
- Urine and bag likely to be heavily contaminated with micro-organisms. These will be acquired on the hands and may be transferred to other patients
- Pathogens that may be on the hands must not be introduced to the drainage bag as these may gain access to the bladder and cause infection

Risk management
- Wash hands to remove transient organisms
- Put on clean gloves and empty urine into clean container
- Discard urine into sluice, disinfect container, remove and discard gloves
- Wash hands to remove transient micro-organisms

Box 7.4   Biological agents: hazard groups (Health & Safety Executive 2002)

Group 1	Unlikely to cause human disease
Group 2	Can cause human disease and may be a hazard; is unlikely to spread to the community; there is usually effective prophylaxis or treatment available
Group 3	Can cause severe human disease and may be a serious hazard; may spread to the community but there is usually effective prophylaxis or treatment available
Group 4	Causes severe human disease and is a serious hazard; likely to spread to the community and there is usually no effective prophylaxis or treatment available

---

Where a hazard is identified, a hierarchy of controls to prevent or minimize the risk associated with it should be devised. These should begin by considering whether the hazard can be eliminated completely, for example whether a hazardous chemical can be replaced by a safer one. If this is not possible, other controls such as those illustrated in Table 7.1 should be implemented.

Risk assessments should be made in all areas of work to identify those procedures likely to involve a risk of infection to either patients or healthcare workers and the options available to minimize the risk. The identification of hazards and the development of associated control measures should involve a multidisciplinary group of staff familiar with the clinical area under consideration. This will help to ensure that control measures are practical and relevant.

It may sometimes be possible to avoid or minimize risks by changing work practices, for example using disposable instruments or sending reusable ones to a central sterile supply department for automatic decontamination, rather than cleaning them by hand. There may also be equipment available with safety features that can prevent injury to staff, such as blunt

Table 7.1   Hierarchy of controls to prevent or minimize risks in the workplace (Gerberding 1993, Health & Safety Executive 2002)

Control	Description	Example
1. Eliminate or substitute hazard	Avoid activity or substance or replace with a safer one	Use peracetic acid in place of glutaraldehyde to disinfect endoscopes
2. Engineering controls	Use equipment that may prevent injury	Shielding devices, blunt-tipped needles
3. Work practice controls	Adopt systems of work that prevent or minimize risk	Discard used sharps directly into sharps container
4. Protective clothing	Select appropriate clothing for activities likely to result in exposure to a hazard	Use gloves to clean instruments, wear eye protection during surgical procedures
5. Administrative controls	Ensure relevant personnel know about hazards and recommended controls	Policy, training programme
6. Monitoring and prevention	Record and analyse accident data, provide health surveillance where indicated	Monitor sharps injuries

suture needles or needles with automatic resheathing devices.

First aid equipment should be available to enable prompt treatment if inadvertent exposure to a hazardous substance occurs (e.g. eye wash solutions). In addition, administrative controls should be in place. These should include systems for ensuring that staff know about the risks, are trained to comply with controls and are aware of the actions to take should exposure to the hazard occur, for example following a needlestick injury. Mechanisms for monitoring adherence to health and safety policies and for recording accidents should be in place and the information used to evaluate and review practice (Gerberding 1993).

STANDARD INFECTION CONTROL PRECAUTIONS

The infection control precautions outlined below represent the standard of care that should be used routinely with all patients to minimize the spread of pathogens between patients and staff and between staff and patients.

Handwashing

The hands of staff are the most common vehicle by which micro-organisms are transmitted between patients and hands are frequently implicated as the route of transmission in outbreaks of infection (Box 7.5).

Box 7.5   Hands and the spread of infection

Over a period of 1 month the same type of *Klebsiella pneumoniae* was isolated from the respiratory secretions of six patients in an intensive care unit. Four patients developed infections caused by the organism. During the investigation to identify the source of the organism, it was noticed that the water traps collecting condensate from ventilator tubing were emptied into foil dishes. These remained by the bedside until full when they were emptied into the sink. Although hands were washed after contact with tracheal secretions, hands were not washed after handling the condensate.

Klebsiella was found in samples of the condensate and in the foil bowls and was also recovered from the hands of staff. No further cases of infection occurred once staff had been alerted to the hazard of the condensate and handwashing after contact with ventilator tubing and traps had been instituted (Gorman et al 1993).

It is difficult to find direct evidence that hands are involved in passing micro-organisms from one person to another. However, it is generally accepted that pathogens are frequently acquired on the hands in clinical settings and that handwashing is essential to remove them if their transfer between patients is to be avoided (Boyce & Pittet 2002, Pratt et al 2001).

There are two categories of micro-organisms present on the skin: the transient and the resident flora.

Transient skin flora

Microbes acquired on the surface of the skin through contact with other people, objects or the environment are known as transient skin flora. They are particularly easily acquired on the hands when the object touched is moist (Marples & Towers 1979). The composition of this transient flora varies but reflects the extent of contact with patients or their environment and the prevalent micro-organisms. For example, methicillin-resistant *Staphylococcus aureus* (MRSA) is frequently found on the skin of nurses caring for patients infected with the organism. The antibacterial properties of skin generally prevent these transient micro-organisms surviving for more than a few hours (Reybrouck 1983) but within this time the organisms can be readily transferred to other people or objects (Mackintosh & Hoffman 1984).

The potential for transmission has been demonstrated by experiments using a fluorescent powder, visible only under ultraviolet light, to represent micro-organisms. This study demonstrated that 2 h after the powder was applied to a baby, traces of it were found on the hands of all the nurses responsible for the care of the baby, the hands of at least one other nurse and in the environment (Scanlon & Leikkanen 1973).

Pathogens are likely to be acquired on the hands in greatest number when handling moist, heavily contaminated substances such as body fluids (Pittet et al 1999). However, Casewell & Phillips (1977) showed that, even during routine procedures such as touching, lifting or washing a patient, transient bacteria are easily acquired on the hands. They are also acquired simply by touching the buttocks of a baby, even if the nappy is not soiled (Sprunt et al 1973) and have been recovered from hands after bedmaking, handling curtains or using the sluice (Sanderson & Weissler 1992). Pathogens present on the skin surrounding an infected wound are readily transferred to the hands even if forceps are used to dress the wound (Tomlinson 1987). Viruses are also easily acquired, for example during nappy changing (Samadi et al 1983), and hands are commonly contaminated by respiratory viruses (Sattar et al 2002).

Resident skin flora

The skin is an inhospitable environment for most micro-organisms as it is dry, acidic and poor in nutrients (Hoffman & Wilson 1994). However, some micro-organisms have adapted to these conditions and exist in stable populations known as the resident or normal flora. These organisms live in deep crevices in the skin, in hair follicles and sebaceous glands. The type and distribution of organisms vary according to humidity, temperature, body site and the person's general health. The micro-organisms present in largest numbers are Gram-positive bacteria, mainly coagulase-negative staphylococci, micrococci and coryneforms. Although not conventionally considered part of the resident flora, some Gram-negative bacilli appear able to survive in some areas, notably moist areas beneath rings (Hoffman et al 1985).

Removing micro-organisms from the hands

Washing with soap   The majority of transient micro-organisms can be easily removed mechanically by washing with soap and water, even by a brief, 10 s wash (Lucet et al 2002) (Plate 23).

The removal of resident skin flora during routine clinical care is not necessary in many situations as these micro-organisms are not readily transferred to other people or surfaces and most are of low pathogenicity. However, some resident bacteria could cause infection if introduced during invasive procedures into normally sterile body sites or on to particularly vulnerable individuals (e.g. neonates).

The resident microbial flora are not easily removed by the mechanical action of washing with soap but their numbers can be reduced by the combination of a detergent and a microbiocide, such as chlorhexidine, povidone-iodine or triclosan. Microbiocides, in particular chlorhexidine, can have a persistent effect on the resident flora, suppressing their regrowth for several hours (Lowbury & Lilley 1973). This can be particularly useful in situations where maintaining low levels of resident flora for prolonged periods is desirable, such as during surgery. Microbiocides vary in their activity against different types of micro-organisms. For example, chlorhexidine and triclosan have better activity against Gram-positive than Gram-negative organisms. Povidone-iodine has good activity against Gram-negatives, Gram-positives, viruses and fungi but less persistent activity than other agents (Boyce & Pittet 2002).

Antiseptic soap solutions are only slightly more effective at removing transient skin flora than soap and water (Ayliffe et al 1988). Many studies promulgating their efficacy as handwashing agents are misleading because count reductions do not distinguish between transient and resident flora (Lucet et al 2002). Antiseptic solutions were originally designed for use by surgeons only a few times a day; when used frequently for handwashing in ward situations, they have been associated with damage to skin and increased levels of bacteria on the hands (Ojajärvi et al 1977). Their use is therefore best restricted to situations where the removal of resident flora is indicated, such as in operating theatres and before invasive procedures, although they may also be of value for controlling outbreaks of infections, especially those caused by antimicrobial resistant pathogens (Pellowe et al 2003, Webster et al 1994, Zafar et al 1995). Box 7.6 provides a simple guide to selecting hand decontamination agents.

Gram-negative micro-organisms may grow on soap bars and in solutions, even in the presence of disinfectants (Archibald et al 1997a). Soap should therefore be supplied in liquid form in a dispenser fitted with disposable cartridges. Recently Sartor et al (2000) reported an outbreak of *Serratia marcescens* associated with contaminated soap pumps. The micro-organisms were transferred from one soap bottle to another on the contaminated pump and then multiplied in the soap. Disposable sealed pumps and

---

Box 7.6   Guide to selecting hand–cleaning preparations

	Soap	Alcohol rub or gel	Antiseptic soap
		Handwashing preparation	
Removes transient micro-organisms	✓	✓	✓
Removes resident micro-organisms		✓	✓
Effective on physically soiled hands	✓		✓
Routine use in clinical areas	✓	✓	
Preoperative hand preparation		✓	✓
Hand preparation before invasive procedures		✓	✓

General principles

- Use liquid soap for routine use to wash physically soiled hands
- Use alcohol handrub or gel for routine use to decontaminate physically clean hands and as a preoperative hand preparation
- Use antiseptic soap solution to remove transient and resident flora before surgical or invasive procedures

small-volume soap cartridges are recommended to avoid this problem.

Alcohol handrubs or gels   There is increasing interest in the value of alcohol-based handrubs for routine hand decontamination (National Patient Safety Agency 2005); 60–95% alcohol solutions are rapidly microbiocidal and active against Gram-negative and -positive bacteria, fungi and some viruses. Although there is doubt about their efficacy against non-enveloped viruses, both 70% ethanol and 70% propanol appear to be effective in eliminating norovirus from hands (Gehrke et al 2004). However, alcohol handrubs are not effective against spores and should therefore not be relied on for routine hand-washing after contact with patients with *Clostridium difficile* (Hoffman et al 2004). Although not considered to have a residual effect, alcohol does appear to suppress bacterial growth on the skin for a few hours after application and is effective against both resident and transient skin flora (Boyce & Pittet 2002).

Since alcohol handrubs do not mechanically remove organic material, they are not suitable for cleansing visibly soiled hands. However, there is evidence that they are more effective than soap at removing transient micro-organisms (Ojajärvi 1980). Their main advantage is that they are quicker and easier to use and when made widely available, have been associated with an increased frequency of hand decontamination among healthcare workers (Boyce 2001, Pittet et al 2000). They also achieve higher reductions in bacterial counts on hands than either soap or antiseptic soap solutions and cause less skin irritation and dryness provided they contain adequate emollients (Boyce et al 2000). They are available as rinses, gels and foams but there is currently little evidence on the comparative efficacy of different formulations.

Handwashing technique

Hands should be washed properly to ensure micro-organisms are removed. Taylor (1978) observed that nurses washed their hands for an average time of 20 s and that large areas of the skin were frequently left unwashed (Fig. 7.1). Micro-organisms may remain on parts of the hands not exposed to soap and water or alcohol and would still be available for transfer to other patients. The greatest concentration of micro-organisms is found beneath fingernails (McGinley et al 1988). There is evidence that nurses with long fingernails are more likely to become colonized with Gram-negative pathogens and to transmit infection to vulnerable patients (Moolenaar et al 2000). Long fingernails may also interfere with the handwashing process.

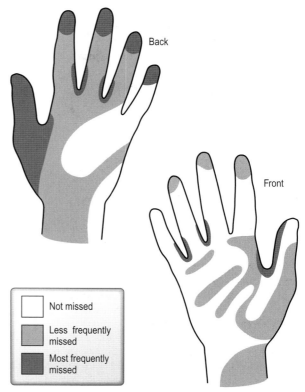

Figure 7.1   Parts of the hands most frequently missed during handwashing (redrawn with permission from Taylor 1978).

Hands should be washed by systematically rubbing all parts of the hands and wrists with soap and water, being particularly careful to include the areas that are most frequently missed (see Fig. 7.1). Similarly, the efficacy of alcohol handrubs or antiseptic soap solutions depends on the adequacy of the handwash; micro-organisms will be removed by these solutions only if all parts of the hands are reached. Some infection control teams recommend a six-stage technique for ensuring that all parts of the hands are covered (Ayliffe et al 1978). However, because even a brief handwash appears to remove transient micro-organisms effectively (Lucet et al 2002), the relevance of such a detailed technique is debatable, particularly if it acts to discourage handwashing taking place.

Thorough drying afterwards is also an important part of the procedure. More bacteria are probably removed by the towel or hot-air drier (Ansari et al 1991) and moisture remaining on the skin may cause it to become dry and cracked.

Hand cleansing prior to surgery has traditionally involved several minutes of scrubbing of the hands using an antiseptic soap solution. However, a short (1–2 min) scrub with 4% chlorhexidine followed by an alcohol handrub is just as effective, as is the application of chlorhexidine and alcohol without scrubbing (Mulberry et al 2001).

Alcohol handrubs should only be applied to hands that are free of organic material and the hands rubbed together vigorously, covering all surfaces, until all the alcohol has evaporated.

Care of the skin

Frequent handwashing, especially with antiseptic soap solutions, depletes skin lipids and damages the skin barrier. Even repeated exposure to water can irritate the skin. Contact dermatitis of the hands has been reported to affect up to 30% of healthcare workers (Kampf & Loffler 2003) and damaged skin is twice as likely to be colonized with potential pathogens (Larson 2001, Norton-Hughes & Pyrak 1998). Although alcohol handrubs are associated with less skin irritation than soaps, if applied to already damaged skin they can cause a burning sensation. Therefore, one of the prime considerations in ensuring that handwashing takes place is selecting a handwash preparation that is acceptable to the users and contains adequate emollients and moisturizers to minimize skin damage (Hoffman & Wilson 1994, Larson 2001).

Soap should always be applied to wet hands to minimize irritation to the skin and hands should be properly dried. Regular use of handcreams may help to prevent skin damage and enable hands to be washed more frequently (McCormack et al 2000). Communally used creams should be avoided as they may become a potential source of infection (Morse & Schonbek 1968).

Intact skin protects tissue from invasion by micro-organisms. Damaged skin may become infected superficially by bacteria or fungi and bloodborne viruses may enter the body through damaged skin. Whilst at work, healthcare workers should therefore always protect any damaged skin, particularly on the hands and forearms, with a waterproof dressing. Staff with any form of active dermatitis/eczema are at particular risk of acquiring infection and may become colonized by hospital pathogens such as MRSA, increasing the risk that they will transmit infection to patients. They should therefore seek advice from the occupational health department.

Long or artificial nails may increase the number of bacteria present on the hands and interfere with glove use and handwashing. They should therefore be discouraged where staff are working in clinical areas (Jeanes & Green 2001).

When should hands be decontaminated?

In clinical situations, transient micro-organisms acquired on the hands through contact with patients, their body fluids or environment need to be removed if cross-infection is to be avoided. Ideally, hands should be washed to remove these organisms before and after each episode of patient care that involves any direct contact with their skin, dressings or devices (Pratt et al 2001). However, as a minimum, they should always be washed *before* an activity that could introduce infection to a susceptible site on the patient (e.g. handling an invasive device or wound) and *after* an activity that could result in the hands becoming contaminated by micro-organisms (e.g. contact with urine or faeces) (Box 7.7).

A single episode of care may involve both clean and dirty procedures on the same patient. Micro-organisms may be transferred from a contaminated site, e.g. bowel or respiratory tract, to a susceptible site, e.g. wound, intravenous device on the same patient, if hands are not decontaminated between procedures. Hands must also be washed after gloves are removed because, although gloves reduce microbial contamination, hands may still be contaminated through punctures in the glove or as the gloves are removed (Olsen et al 1993).

In many situations contact with a patient does not result in hands becoming visibly soiled. Alcohol handrubs provide a quick and effective means of removing transient micro-organisms acquired through contact. They can also be applied readily to ensure micro-organisms are removed from hands prior to contact with a susceptible site such as wound or invasive device. Handrubs should be placed by every patient's bed to ensure access to hand decontamination is readily available.

Box 7.7   Indications for handwashing

Hands should be decontaminated before any direct contact with patients and especially:
- before and after handling invasive devices
- before and after dressing wounds
- before and after contact with immunocompromised patients
- before and after handling food/drink
- after handling equipment contaminated with body fluid
- after contact with blood or body fluid
- after handling clinical waste and used laundry
- after removing gloves
- after using the toilet
- before leaving the clinical area

Factors that influence hand hygiene

Unfortunately, research has shown that healthcare staff frequently do not wash their hands at all after contact with patients, even after dirty procedures. Medical staff have been found to be especially unlikely to wash their hands (Glynn et al 1997, Pittet et al 1999, 2000). Handwashing activity may not reflect the risk of contamination or cross-infection. Pittet et al (1999) found that staff were more likely to decontaminate their hands after an activity associated with a low risk of acquiring micro-organisms than before an activity associated with a high risk of introducing infection. Hands were washed between a dirty and clean body site on only 11% of occasions. This suggests that the risk to the patient of transferring micro-organisms into a susceptible site was not appreciated or was being overlooked.

Commonly, healthcare workers believe they wash their hands far more frequently than they are actually found to (Harris et al 2000). A number of factors influence handwashing frequency, notably staff workload, shortage of sinks, lack of soap, hand towels or water temperature controls (Archibald et al 1997b, Kaplan & McGuckin 1986, Pittet et al 1999). Williams & Buckles (1988) demonstrated that, even though handwashing frequency increased significantly after an extensive promotional campaign, 6 months later the rate of handwashing had decreased to the previous level. This finding has been confirmed by Larson et al (1997), who found that focus groups, automated sinks and feedback on handwashing frequency had a minimal long-term effect on handwashing practice.

The time required for handwashing is a key inhibitory factor in clinical areas where levels of direct patient contact, and hence expected handwashing frequency, are high. A single handwash with soap and water takes about 1 min to perform properly, more if there is some distance between the patient and the nearest sink. Voss & Widmer (1997) estimated that if handwashing was performed on all recommended occasions, this would consume 16 h of nursing time in an ICU with 12 staff per shift.

This study also estimated that the time taken to decontaminate hands could be reduced by three-quarters if alcoholic handrubs are available at every patient's bed. Other studies have confirmed that compliance with hand hygiene is improved by making alcohol handrubs widely available. Pittet et al (2000) achieved both a sustained increased compliance with hand hygiene and a decrease in transmission of MRSA through a combination of posters promoting hand hygiene, the use of bedside alcohol handrubs and strong management support for the hospital-wide programme. This study highlighted the value of providing alcohol handrubs as a means of making hand decontamination quicker and easier. However, the study also showed that for sustained improvement in hand hygiene, a multimodal approach is required that takes account of a range of influences on the behaviour of individuals, the climate of the institution and the constraints of the environment (Kretser & Larson 1998, Pittet et al 2000). Other studies confirm the importance of a multifaceted approach to improving handwashing compliance (Naikoba & Hayward 2001).

Prieto (2003) found that deficiencies in understanding of basic microbiology and principles of infection control affected the ability of healthcare workers to appropriately assess the risk of hand contamination and recognize situations where handwashing or other infection control measures are required. Raising the profile of handwashing as a key infection control measure and finding novel ways of encouraging staff to wash their hands remains an important challenge. Education programmes need to address the importance of hand hygiene in preventing healthcare-associated infection and provide clear guidance on situations when hands should be washed.

Protective clothing

Many excretions and secretions of the body are a major source of pathogenic micro-organisms associated with hospital-acquired infection (Box 7.8). Protective clothing should therefore be worn for any direct contact with these body fluids, to protect the skin of staff from contamination with body fluid and micro-organisms and to reduce the risk of transmission of micro-organisms between patients and staff.

Box 7.8   Potentially infectious body fluids

Body fluids that may contain bloodborne viruses
Blood
Blood-stained body fluids
Semen
Vaginal secretions
Tissues
Cerebrospinal fluid
Amniotic fluid, synovial fluid, pleural fluid, etc.

Body fluids that may contain other pathogens
Faeces
Urine
Vomit
Sputum
Saliva

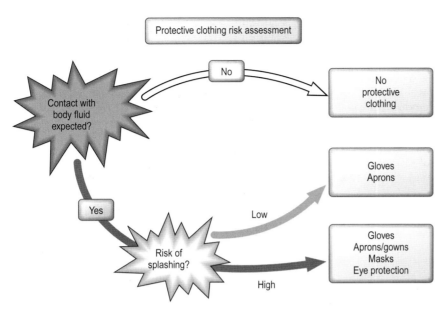

Figure 7.2 The selection of protective clothing.

The protective clothing selected depends on the anticipated risk of exposure to body fluid during the particular activity. This assessment should consider the risk both to the patient and to the healthcare worker. Many clinical activities involve no direct contact with body fluid and do not require the use of protective clothing, for example washing a patient or taking a pulse, blood pressure or temperature. Other procedures may result in contamination of the hands or clothing and require the use of gloves and a plastic apron, for example assisting a patient with a commode or handling specimens. Procedures in which there is a risk of splashing of blood or body fluid require the use of a mask and eye protection to protect these mucous membranes and a water-resistant gown will be necessary. In the operating theatre, waterproof boots or shoes may also be required in some situations. Figure 7.2 illustrates the principles of risk assessment in the selection of protective clothing. They should be applied in all situations, with all patients and in all areas of clinical practice.

To prevent the transmission of infection to other patients, protective clothing should be changed between caring for different patients. In addition, it should be changed between contact with body secretions and a susceptible site, such as a wound or intravenous device, on the same patient.

Gloves

The contribution that the hands of staff make to the transmission of infection in healthcare settings has already been demonstrated (see p. 157). The use of disposable gloves for direct contact with body fluids and moist body sites provides a reliable method of reducing the acquisition on hands of micro-organisms from these sources (Pittet et al 1999, Tenorio et al 2001). Some studies have demonstrated a reduction in the incidence of infection where gloves are used routinely for handling body fluids (Johnson et al 1990, Lynch et al 1990). Gloves will also help to protect the healthcare worker from infection if cuts and abrasions are present on the hands. Gloves should be worn for procedures involving direct contact with mucous membranes, for example mouth care and vaginal examination. Micro-organisms colonizing or infecting mucous membranes may easily be transmitted on hands and infect another person, for example papilloma virus or candida in the vagina, herpes simplex virus or candida in the mouth (Burnie et al 1985).

Gloves should be worn for any activity where body fluid may contaminate the hands but to prevent transmission of infection, gloves must be discarded after each procedure. This principle even applies for procedures on the same patient. For example, gloves worn for tracheal suction must be changed before dressing a wound otherwise micro-organisms colonizing the respiratory tract may be transferred into the wound and establish infection.

Gloves must always be changed between patients, even if being used for routine procedures such as emptying urine drainage bags. Failure to change gloves appropriately has been associated with cross-infection (Patterson et al 1991). Washing gloves between patients is not recommended; the gloves may be damaged by the soap solution and, if punctured unknowingly, may cause body fluid to remain in direct contact with skin for prolonged periods (Adams et al 1992, Centers for Disease Control 1993).

Although gloves significantly reduce the risk of hand contamination, they do not eliminate it completely; they may be punctured and hands are easily contaminated as the gloves are taken off (Olsen et al 1993, Pittet et al 1999). Hands should therefore always be decontaminated after gloves have been removed.

Type of glove material   Disposable gloves must be readily available in all clinical areas. Medical gloves are made from rubber latex, synthetic latex (copolymer, nitrile) or vinyl. Each type has slightly different properties and may be suited to a different range of activities.

Latex gloves conform to the hands and are most suitable for procedures requiring a degree of dexterity, although sensitization to latex is increasingly recognized as a problem amongst healthcare workers (Booth 1996) (Box 7.9). They should also be changed regularly during prolonged procedures as hydration of the latex may cause the gloves to become porous (UK Health Departments 1998). Synthetic formulations of latex (e.g. copolymer), with similar conforming properties, are becoming more widely available.

Vinyl gloves are looser fitting but not associated with adverse skin reactions. Korniewicz et al (2002) have suggested that vinyl and copolymer gloves are more likely to develop holes during use than latex gloves, although their study used prolonged simulated tests and identified significant differences in quality between manufacturers. Latex does have some resistance to puncture and resealing properties, so these gloves are probably more appropriate for procedures involving the handling of sharp instruments. De Groot-Kosolcharoen & Jones (1989) demonstrated that a proportion of both latex and vinyl medical gloves have small holes in them before use. This points to the importance of ensuring that good-quality gloves are purchased. Medical gloves should comply with British Standard EN455 (British Standards Institution 2000), should be free from pinholes and not split or tear easily. Nonetheless, they should be regarded as a means of minimizing the risk of acquiring pathogens on the hands rather than as an impermeable barrier. Gloves do not need to be sterile unless used in a sterile body site (e.g. surgical or other invasive procedures).

Gloves with very long cuffs are available for procedures where blood contamination of the arms is likely (e.g. obstetrics).

Box 7.9   Latex allergy

Latex gloves are made from natural rubber latex. The latex is treated with chemicals called accelerators to increase its strength and flexibility and to enable it to retain its moulded shape. When dry, the gloves are washed to remove residual traces of chemicals and latex proteins. Cornstarch powder is commonly added to latex gloves to improve the ease with which they can be put on and removed. Since the introduction of universal precautions in the 1980s, the use of gloves has increased considerably and there has been a corresponding increase in reports of allergy to latex (Yessin et al 1994). Users may react to latex proteins, chemical accelerators or the cornstarch powder. Allergy to the latex proteins is mediated by immunoglobulin (Ig) E and causes an itchy rash on exposed skin, itching eyes and nose, wheezing or asthma (Johnson 1998, Medical Devices Agency 1996). Allergy to accelerators causes contact dermatitis with red, cracked and thickened skin developing a few hours after contact with the gloves. Cornstarch powder can absorb latex proteins and enable them to become airborne when gloves are put on or removed; this can expose other sensitized people to the allergens in areas where gloves are being used. Cornstarch powder in gloves has also been linked with adhesions in surgical wounds and poor healing (Medical Devices Agency 1998). People who are 'atopic', that is, they are predisposed to producing IgE on exposure to an allergen (e.g. hayfever, asthma, eczema), may be more easily sensitized to latex. There is also a link between latex sensitization and some foods (Medical Devices Agency 1996).

In recognition of these problems, reputable glove manufacturers produce powder-free latex gloves, coated with hydrogel polymer for donning and removal. They will also use thorough washing processes to ensure that the levels of accelerators and extractable latex proteins in the gloves are low.

Local supplies departments should convene a multidisciplinary group to consider these issues in relation to the purchase of gloves for clinical use and ensure that gloves comply with the relevant British Standard (British Standards Institution 2000, Medical Devices Agency 1996). The Medical Devices Agency recommends that only powder-free gloves should be purchased (Medical Devices Agency 1998).

Gloves and the prevention of percutaneous injury
Whilst disposable gloves cannot prevent percutaneous injury, there is evidence that they can help to reduce the risk of injury (Palmer & Rickett 1992, UK Health Departments 1998). A number of studies in operating

theatres have demonstrated that wearing two pairs of latex gloves (double-gloving) significantly reduces the risk of exposure to blood. Gerberding et al (1990) found that where two pairs of gloves were worn, 17% of outer gloves were punctured during the procedure but only 5% of the inner gloves, and Tokars et al (1992) recorded a 70% reduction in exposure to blood in surgeons who double-gloved. Wearing two pairs of gloves does not appear to have a significant effect on comfort but the recommended combination is an outer glove of the usual size and inner glove half a size larger (Telford & Quebberman 1993). Double-gloving is recommended for procedures associated with a high risk of glove tear or percutaneous injury (e.g. gynaecology and orthopaedic surgery, obstetric procedures) (Tanner & Parkinson 2004, UK Health Departments 1998). Indicator glove systems are available that use a coloured inner glove to alert the user to punctures of the outer glove (Zimmerman & Junghans 1996).

Gloves should also be worn for venepuncture, especially by inexperienced personnel. Several healthcare workers have acquired bloodborne viruses as a result of blood exposure during venepuncture (Health Protection Agency 2005, UK Health Departments 1998).

Masks and eye protection

Masks were introduced at the turn of the 20th century to protect patients from micro-organisms expelled from the respiratory tract of staff during surgical procedures and to provide protection for staff caring for patients with infectious disease. Evidence of their ineffectiveness followed much later. It is now recognized that, unless the mask fits closely around the mouth and nose, air is inhaled and exhaled around its edge and is therefore not filtered. If masks are worn for prolonged periods, moisture, which collects in the fabric, interrupts the passage of air through the mask and increases the flow around the outside (Belkin 1997).

Masks are also of limited value in protecting sites on the patient that are susceptible to infection as healthy staff expel few micro-organisms from the respiratory tract (Ayliffe 1991). Although still used in operating theatres for this purpose, there is little evidence that they reduce the risk of surgical wound infection (Hubble et al 1996). However, staff are vulnerable to infection by bloodborne viruses and other pathogens if infected body fluid is splashed on to the mucous membranes of the eyes and mouth (PHLS AIDS & STD Centre 1999).

Eye protection and a mask should be worn for any activity where there is a risk of body fluid splashing into the face (Fig. 7.3). Such activities are not commonly

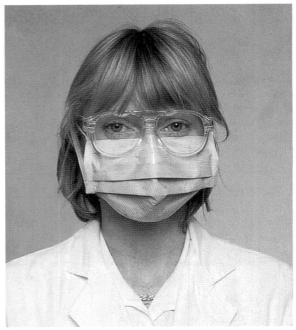

Figure 7.3 Eye protection. Mask and eye protection should be worn for procedures where there is risk of splashing of blood or body fluids.

encountered in ward settings, where the main risks are associated with respiratory suction, if excessive secretions are present, or cleaning of instruments and equipment. Staff at greatest risk from splashing of blood or other body fluids are those involved in surgical or obstetrical procedures. Tokars et al (1995) found that contact between blood or other infective fluids and the eyes or mouth of surgical staff occurred in 2% of surgical procedures, particularly orthopaedic and gynaecological. Short & Bell (1993) reported a high risk of splashing into the face associated with obstetrical procedures.

In common with people in other occupations whose work involves a risk of damage to the eyes, healthcare workers are often reluctant to protect their eyes properly. Masks and eye protection must be readily available in any clinical area where such procedures are performed. In the past, eye protection has been cumbersome to wear but now a variety of types is available and some look similar to conventional spectacles. Information on different types of eyewear can be found in British Standard BS7028 (British Standards Institution 1999).

High-efficiency respirator masks are occasionally recommended for some aspects of care of patients with infections transmitted in droplet nuclei by the airborne route, e.g. multidrug-resistant tuberculosis and severe acute respiratory syndrome (SARS), but are not generally necessary for patients with other infectious diseases (see p. 296).

Water-repellent aprons or gowns

There is evidence to suggest that the clothing of healthcare workers is vulnerable to contamination by pathogenic micro-organisms. Contamination is especially likely when healthcare workers have contact with body secretions/excretions (Callaghan 1998, Perry et al 2001). Because the front of the body is the part most frequently contaminated by body fluid, plastic disposable aprons provide adequate protection in most circumstances (e.g. dealing with body fluid spills, handling bedpans, dressing wounds). Plastic aprons should be readily available in all clinical areas and must be replaced after each procedure to prevent the transfer of micro-organisms to susceptible sites or to other patients. Cotton gowns are not water repellent and, when wet, micro-organisms pass through them easily (Callaghan 1998, Holborn 1990).

Exposure to body fluid during surgical procedures varies; minor surgery such as biopsy, lump removal or laparoscopy involves little exposure to body fluid. Some orthopaedic, abdominal and cardiac procedures may result in considerable contamination with blood or body fluid and then a water-repellent gown should be worn (Tokars et al 1995, UK Health Departments 1998). Gowns with water-repellent sleeves, together with a plastic apron underneath, may also provide adequate protection.

Water-repellent gowns may be disposable or reusable and made from specially woven or treated cotton. The most impervious have a plastic layer but are expensive. For procedures where the legs and feet may be contaminated (e.g. obstetrics), the gown must be long enough to cover the legs and calf-length over-boots should be worn rather than clogs.

All contaminated clothing must be removed before leaving the area and any blood that has inadvertently contaminated the skin washed off immediately.

Safe handling of sharp instruments

'Sharps' include needles, scalpels, broken glass or other items that may cause a laceration or puncture. Sharp instruments frequently cause injury to healthcare workers and are a major cause of transmission of bloodborne viruses (Health Protection Agency 2005). They are reported to account for 16% of occupational injuries in hospitals but since many go unreported, this figure is likely to be a considerable underestimate (National Audit Office 1999).

The risk of transmission following a single sharps (percutaneous) injury depends on the type of blood-borne virus involved. The risk is one in three when the instrument is contaminated with hepatitis B virus from a patient who is e antigen positive (see p. 138), approximately one in 30 when the instrument is contaminated by hepatitis C, and one in 300 when contaminated by HIV. The risk of acquiring HIV depends on the infectivity of the source patient; this is highest at the time of seroconversion and during the later stages of HIV disease when the level of virus is high (DoH 1997). Hollow 'sharps', such as hypodermic needles or cannulae, are more likely to transmit infection than solid items such as suture needles and scalpels (PHLS AIDS & STD Centre 1999, Royal College of Pathologists 1992).

Causes of sharps injuries

A number of studies have investigated the causes of percutaneous injuries in healthcare workers. Injuries are commonly associated with venepuncture; the disassembly of devices such as vacuum blood-taking systems or intravenous cannulae; recapping of needles; transfer of used sharps to point of disposal; sharps not discarded after use; or overfilled sharps containers (Castella et al 2003, Weltman et al 1995). Resheathing of needles is particularly dangerous because if the needle misses the sheath, it will puncture the hand holding it.

Preventing needlestick injuries

Used sharps must be handled as little as possible to avoid injury. Needles should not be disconnected from syringes but discarded as one unit. In situations where resheathing is essential, a device should be used (Fig. 7.4). If such a device is unavailable, the sheath should be placed on a flat surface and the needles inserted without holding the sheath by hand.

Immediate disposal of used sharps diminishes the risk that they will cause injuries. Disposal of used sharps in inappropriate places may present a considerable risk to other people, for example used needles left on trolleys or blood glucose lancets left on lockertops. Every healthcare worker has a responsibility to ensure proper disposal of the sharps that they have used. Sharps should always be discarded immediately into appropriate containers and these should be readily accessible at the point where sharps are used. Small, portable sharps bins are available that can be carried to the bedside or used in the patient's home. Containers used for sharps should conform to the British Standard for sharps containers (British Standards Institution 1990), which is summarized in

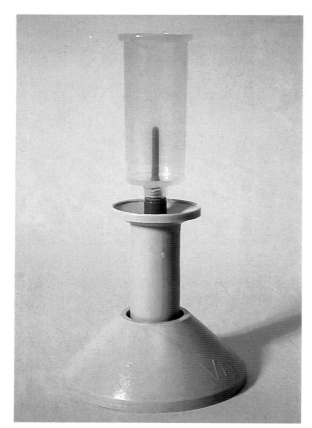

Figure 7.4 A resheathing device. If it is essential to resheathe a needle, a resheathing device should be used.

Box 7.10. Containers must be assembled properly and sealed securely for disposal before discarded sharps protrude from the aperture. In areas where children may be present, containers must be kept out of their reach. Box 7.11 outlines the principles of good practice for the safe management of sharp instruments.

Many devices for preventing needlestick injuries are available but not all are effective; some have limited application or are more difficult to use. Some devices have been shown to reduce the risk of needlestick injury but injuries may still occur, especially if the device is used incorrectly (Pratt et al 2001, Trim & Elliot 2003).

Each clinical area should take a systematic approach to minimizing percutaneous injuries by undertaking a risk assessment of local practices and instituting appropriate controls (see Table 7.1). Data collected from injury reports can help to pinpoint the important hazards in a particular area. If sharp instruments cannot be replaced, for instance by blunt needles, then engineering controls such as safety devices or retractable needles and changes to work practices, such as arrangements for sealing and closing bins when three-quarters full, should be considered. A clear, written policy outlining recommended practices and control measures should be available to all staff, together with information on the management of injuries (Fig. 7.5).

Handling sharps in operating departments

The risk of percutaneous injury is particularly high during surgical procedures. A comprehensive study undertaken by Tokars et al in 1992 found that a percutaneous injury occurred during 7% of surgical procedures. In vaginal hysterectomies the rate was as

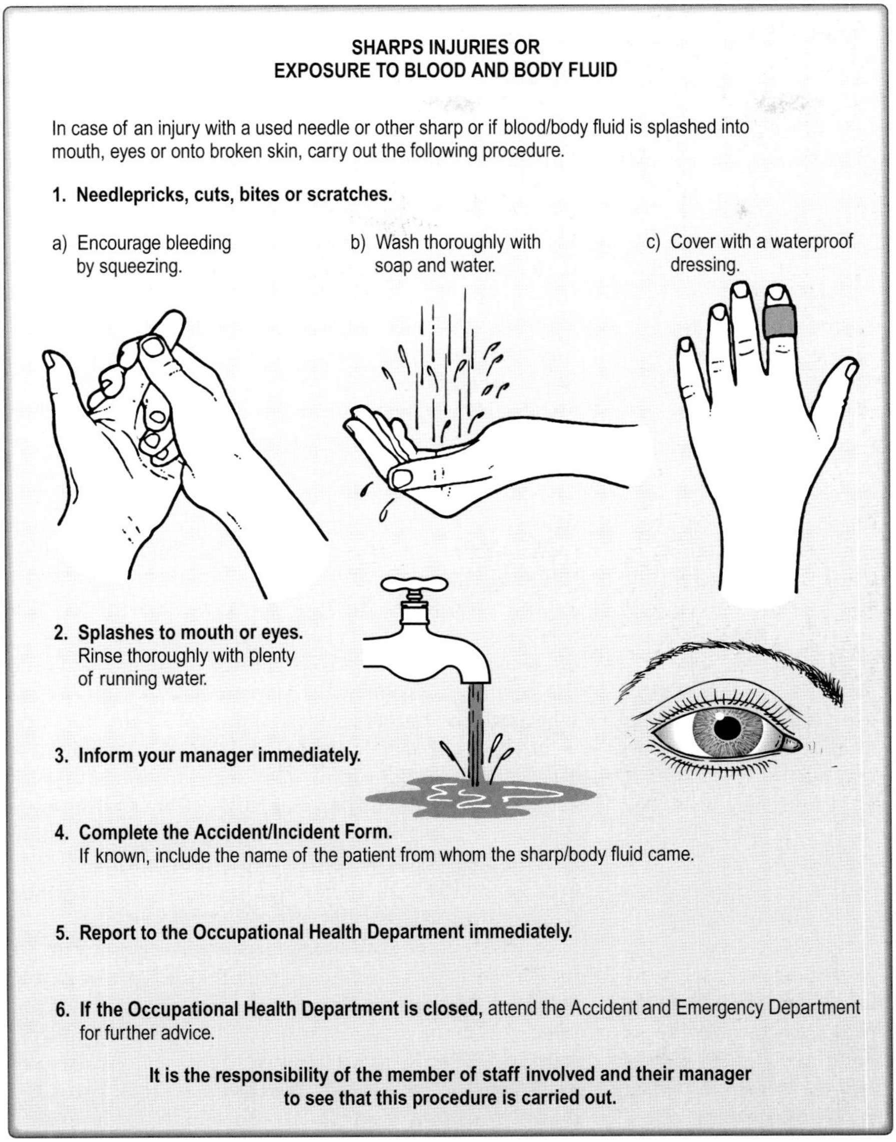

Figure 7.5 Management of sharps injuries or exposure to blood or body fluid (reproduced with permission from Riverside Health Authority; original artwork by Linda Foreman).

**SHARPS INJURIES OR
EXPOSURE TO BLOOD AND BODY FLUID**

In case of an injury with a used needle or other sharp or if blood/body fluid is splashed into mouth, eyes or onto broken skin, carry out the following procedure.

1. Needlepricks, cuts, bites or scratches.

a) Encourage bleeding by squeezing.

b) Wash thoroughly with soap and water.

c) Cover with a waterproof dressing.

2. Splashes to mouth or eyes.
Rinse thoroughly with plenty of running water.

3. Inform your manager immediately.

4. Complete the Accident/Incident Form.
If known, include the name of the patient from whom the sharp/body fluid came.

5. Report to the Occupational Health Department immediately.

6. If the Occupational Health Department is closed, attend the Accident and Emergency Department for further advice.

**It is the responsibility of the member of staff involved and their manager
to see that this procedure is carried out.**

---

high as 21%, probably because of the poor visibility associated with this procedure. Suture needles caused 77% of injuries; commonly these were inflicted on the index finger of the non-dominant hand as it was used to guide the needle. One-quarter of injuries were inflicted on a co-worker. This type of study provides an important insight into factors associated with injury and where preventive measures should be directed. Blunt suture needles are now available and can be used to suture most tissues, apart from skin.

Needle-holders with needle-tip guards, blade removal devices and safety containers for storage of used sharps should be used routinely (Davies 1994, Stafford et al 1995). Double-gloving can also be employed to reduce the risk of sharps penetrating the skin (see p. 164). Systems of work should be established to ensure that sharp instruments are not handed directly to co-workers but passed on a tray or via a neutral zone. Magnets should be used to pick up blades or needles that have fallen on to the floor (Box 7.12).

Box 7.12   Prevention of percutaneous injuries in operating departments

- Use blunt suture needles where possible and remove sharp needles before tying the suture
- Use a device to handle needles and remove blades
- Store used needles and blades in a safety container
- Do not pass sharps from hand to hand
- Use instruments, not fingers, to retract tissue
- Use double gloves for procedures where there is a risk of sharps injury
- Ensure sharps containers of an appropriate size are available

---

Vacuum blood collection systems   These systems are now widely used for venepuncture and are generally considered safer than taking blood with a needle and syringe, as blood is drawn directly into the specimen bottle and not injected in after collection.

Some vacuum collection systems incorporate a reusable barrel from which the needle has to be unscrewed. This can be done safely only if the needle is resheathed in a resheathing device and it is better if the barrel and needle are discarded together.

Hepatitis B vaccination

A safe and effective vaccine against hepatitis B is available and recommended for immunization of healthcare workers who have direct contact with blood, blood-stained body fluids or tissues; for staff and clients in residential homes; for people with learning difficulties, where there is known to be a high prevalence of hepatitis B carriage and where behavioural problems increase the risk to staff. Immunization should also be considered for other staff who may not directly handle blood but who are at risk from injury by blood-contaminated sharps (DoH 1993).

Exposure-prone procedures

Healthcare workers who perform exposure-prone procedures (EPPs) (see Box 6.1) are not only at increased risk of acquiring bloodborne viruses from patients but if infected themselves, may transmit the virus to the patient during the procedure. Healthcare workers who perform EPPs should be immunized against hepatitis B virus (HBV) and their response to the vaccine checked (DoH 1993 – addendum 1996). A small proportion of people do not respond to HBV vaccine and can only perform EPPs provided they have been investigated to exclude HBV infection. Healthcare workers infected with HIV or who are HBV e antigen positive may not perform EPPs. Healthcare workers who are infected with HBV and e antigen negative must have further tests to ensure that the viral infection is not active. Healthcare workers infected with HCV cannot carry out EPPs unless the infection responds adequately to antiviral treatment (DoH 2000, 2002b, 2004).

Management of blood exposure incidents (percutaneous or mucocutaneous)

Exposure to blood or body fluid, from a sharps injury, bite or from splashing into the eyes, mouth or broken skin, must always be followed up properly because of the risk of infection from bloodborne viruses (BBV) (see Fig. 7.5). There should be local policies in place that specify the arrangements for risk assessment, management and advice to healthcare workers following blood exposures (DoH 2004).

The risk assessment and expert advice on the management of blood exposures should be provided by a designated, expert practitioner (usually within the occupational health department) who will assess whether any action is necessary to prevent infection with BBV. If occupational health is closed, risk assessment to determine the appropriate course of action should be undertaken by another competent person, for example ward manager or consultant microbiologist. If the source of the blood or body fluid is known, the patient should tested, with informed consent, for BBV.

If the risk of BBV transmission is assessed to be high the affected member of staff should go straight to A&E for immediate treatment and follow-up. If the injured person is not immune to hepatitis B, specific immunoglobulin can be given. This will prevent or moderate the infection by hepatitis B virus, provided that it is administered quickly, preferably within 48 h of the injury. A full course of hepatitis B vaccination should also be given. Although there is currently no vaccine or specific immunoglobulin against hepatitis C, active management is recommended as early antiviral therapy can effectively clear the virus and prevent chronic infection (Health Protection Agency 2005).

A baseline sample of blood should be stored and follow-up samples taken to establish whether a BBV has been acquired as a result of the incident. There is a legal requirement for employers to keep records of accidents to staff and the records provide an important method of identifying hazardous procedures or inadequate equipment. Healthcare workers who acquire a BBV at work are considered eligible for industrial injury compensation. Accurate records of the time of the injury are essential if compensation is to be awarded. Unfortunately, a significant proportion of needlestick injuries are not reported. One reason commonly cited for non-reporting is lack of knowledge about the risk or standard procedures (Leliopoulou et al 1999). This illustrates the importance of clear, accessible policies and regular training for all groups of staff on sharps injuries, their significance, prevention and management.

An incident where a patient is exposed percutaneously or mucocutaneously to the blood of a healthcare worker should be assessed and managed in the same way as described for healthcare workers (DoH 2004).

Management of percutaneous or mucocutaneous exposure to material known, or strongly suspected, to be infected with HIV

The risk of acquiring HIV following a needlestick injury with infected blood is small and even smaller for mucocutaneous exposures. The risk of transmission is increased where the injury is deep, involves a large volume of blood (e.g. hollow bore needle) or if visible blood is present on the device that caused the injury, and it also depends on the viral load of the source patient (DoH 2004).

There is evidence that the risk can be reduced by up to 80% by rapidly commencing prophylactic antiretroviral therapy. Postexposure prophylaxis (PEP) should be considered when a healthcare worker has a percutaneous or mucocutaneous exposure to blood or other high-risk body fluid (see Box 7.8). If the source patient is known, they should be asked for consent for HIV testing. If the source is unknown, a risk assessment of the likelihood of it being an HIV-positive source should be made. If PEP is recommended, it is important that the first dose is taken within 1 h of the exposure. If the source patient is subsequently found to be HIV negative, the PEP can be discontinued. PEP comprises a combination of antiviral drugs and should be administered for 4 weeks. However, the side-effects can be severe and the healthcare worker will require close monitoring and support during this time.

The risk assessment requires expert advice, which is usually provided by the occupational health department. However, because PEP should be commenced within 1 h of the injury, starter packs containing the relevant drugs should be available in a designated place (e.g. A&E) and specific staff given appropriate training to administer the drugs. The decision about whether treatment should be continued can then be made once expert advice is available.

Every healthcare organization should have a policy describing how to obtain immediate advice and treatment and who is responsible for long-term follow-up. Healthcare workers exposed to HIV should have follow-up counselling, medical evaluation and postoperative testing regardless of whether they have received PEP (DoH 2004).

The safe disposal of waste

Waste from hospitals, clinics, surgeries, veterinary practices or pharmacies which may be toxic, hazardous or infectious is described as clinical waste (Box 7.13). Clinical waste needs to be properly segregated, handled, transported and disposed of to ensure it does not harm staff, patients, the public or the environment. The responsibilities of those who produce waste are described in the Environmental Protection Act 1990 (DoE 1991) and the Environmental Protection (Duty of Care) Regulations 1991. These Regulations require the producers of waste to manage it safely and to transfer it only to an authorized person. They also include duties to control polluting emissions and discharges to sewers and producers must be satisfied that arrangements for treatment and disposal are appropriate.

Most clinical waste is classified as controlled waste, requiring those who keep, treat or dispose of it to be licensed by the Environment Agency. Since the new regulations on hazardous waste came into force in July 2005 there is a requirement to segregate hazardous and non-hazardous waste. Hazardous waste is material that is potentially toxic or dangerous to people or the environment, and includes infectious substances that are known (or reliably believed) to cause disease. Waste that is hazardous must be segregated and is subject to stringent controls over its transportation and disposal. It will be disposed of by incineration or by treatment to

---

Box 7.13 Definition of clinical waste (Controlled Waste Regulations 1992)

- Human or animal tissue
- Blood, other body fluids and excretions
- Drugs, other pharmaceutical products
- Soiled surgical dressings, swabs and instruments
- Discarded syringes, needles, cartridges, broken glass and other sharp surgical instruments in contact with the above
- Other waste arising from medical, nursing, dental, veterinary, pharmaceutical or other similar practice that may cause infection to persons coming into contact with it

render it safe prior to landfill. Much of the waste generated in healthcare facilities is acknowledged to carry a low risk of infection and can be treated as 'offensive waste' which does not require incineration but must be disposed of in deep landfill sites (Collins & Kennedy 1992, DEFRA 2005, Hazardous Waste 2005).

Segregation of waste

Disposing of waste safely and cost-effectively depends on the proper segregation of different types of waste. This can be achieved by ensuring that waste is discarded into an appropriate colour-coded bag which must conform to NHS performance specifications (Table 7.2). Information about where different waste items should be discarded should be clearly displayed and all staff should receive training. A considerable proportion of waste generated in clinical areas is not hazardous and can be safely disposed of as household waste. It is important to ensure that this waste is not sent for incineration to minimize both disposal costs and damage to the environment (Audit Commission 1997).

Handling and storage

Waste containers should be closed and sealed when three-quarters full to prevent spillage of the contents. Clinical waste should be labelled with the point of origin so that any problems that arise during disposal can be investigated. Sharps bins should be clearly

Table 7.2 Colour coding for the disposal of clinical waste (Health Services Advisory Committee 1999)

Colour of bag	Type of waste
Black	Household waste, treated clinical waste (e.g. paper, food, flowers, etc.)
Yellow*	Clinical waste (e.g. material contaminated with blood or body fluid, human or animal tissue)
Yellow sharps containers	Needles, syringes, broken glass and any other contaminated sharp item
Blue or transparent with blue inscription	Waste for autoclaving (e.g. pathology specimens)
Yellow, black stripes	Non-infectious human waste (e.g. sanitary towels, incontinence pads)

*Colour may change to reflect new hazardous waste regulations.

visible and not enclosed inside plastic bags. If leakage of body fluids is likely, a second bag or a special impervious container should be used. This particularly applies to the disposal of human tissue, which should not be mixed with other waste. The safest method of waste handling uses containers to transport waste bags and automatically discharges them into collection containers at the disposal point.

Training

Training is of key importance in ensuring safe and effective waste management and should include all grades of staff involved in the process. It should cover the procedures specific to their work and the actions to take in an emergency, such as how to deal with and report accidents or spills. First aid kits and protective clothing must be readily available.

Waste policy

A local policy, accessible to all staff and taking account of different levels of knowledge, must be available. This should form part of the overall risk management strategy for the organization and should clearly define the responsibilities of line managers (e.g. for staff training). A waste manager should be designated to monitor, evaluate and review the policy regularly (Health Service Advisory Committee 1999, NHS Executive 1999).

Efforts to minimize the volume of clinical waste produced are essential, as incineration is both costly and damaging to the environment. Alternatives to incineration are being developed, such as sterilization and gasification, and increasing the use of reusable and recyclable materials has been proposed (Daschner & Dettenkofer 1997, Phillips 1999). There is little evidence to suggest that most clinical waste is any more hazardous than household waste (Collins & Kennedy 1992).

Disposal of clinical waste in the home

The situation in the home is different as the amounts of clinical waste generated are much smaller and householders are exempt from the 'duty of care' for their own household waste. Waste produced and handled only by the patient or his or her family can usually be discarded with the normal household waste where, because it is mixed with large amounts of ordinary waste, it does not present a hazard. Used needles, such as those used by insulin-dependent diabetics, must not be discarded into household waste even if a device is used to destroy them. Arrangements for disposal should be made with local hospitals, clinics, pharmacies or local authorities (Health Services Advisory Committee 1999).

Healthcare workers who produce clinical waste in the home, for example community nurses or dialysis technicians, are obliged under the Health and Safety at Work Act to transport and dispose of the clinical waste safely but are exempted from being registered carriers. Small amounts of waste can be discarded into sharps bins and discarded via the employer's clinical waste disposal system. Employers may need to make arrangements for the collection and disposal of larger amounts (Environmental Protection Act 1990; DoE 1991). In Scotland, the importance of risk assessment in choosing a safe method of disposal for clinical waste has been emphasized (NHS in Scotland 1998). This approach is particularly helpful for staff working in the community where a large proportion of clinical waste generated in the patient's home is of low risk and small volume.

Local authorities have a legal obligation to provide a collection service for infectious waste if requested but this usually applies only to waste from dialysis patients or those known to be infected with bloodborne viruses. This in itself presents difficulties to the client who may fear possible loss of anonymity if an infected waste collection service is arranged for them. They may prefer to make their own arrangements to take waste to a health centre or GP surgery.

Linen

Used hospital linen may become contaminated with micro-organisms from patients with infection or when soiled by blood, excreta or other body fluids. It is decontaminated in the laundry process by a combination of detergent, dilution and mechanical action to remove particles at temperatures that destroy micro-organisms. The process must include sufficient time for all parts of the load to reach an adequate temperature, for example 71°C for 3 min or 65°C for 10 min. Failure in the process has been associated with outbreaks of infection, notably with spore-forming bacteria such as *Bacillus cereus* (Barrie et al 1992).

Laundries that process hospital linen have to comply with Department of Health guidance on disinfection, staff protection and effluent control (NHS Executive 1995). Most linen will be washed in large tunnel washers that carry several batches at one time in a continuous process (Barrie 1994). Laundry staff sort linen by hand into batches of sheets, pillow cases, towels, etc. before washing and may be exposed to potential pathogens on soiled linen, particularly where instruments or 'sharps' are carelessly discarded with linen (Fig. 7.6). The risks may be minimized by the use of protective clothing and the segregation of particularly hazardous linen for disinfection by washing prior to sorting, for example linen from patients infected with enteric pathogens or heavily blood-stained linen (Table 7.3). This infected linen should be sealed in a water-soluble or soluble stitched bag and distinguished from other linen by placing it in a red outer bag. The water-soluble bag can then be removed from the outer bag and placed directly into a designated washing machine without opening (NHS Executive 1995).

Micro-organisms that remain after washing may also be destroyed by tumble drying and ironing. Some fabrics are damaged by high wash temperatures and must be decontaminated by the addition of a chemical disinfectant to the rinse cycle instead. Bedlinen made from these types of fabrics should be avoided because these chemicals damage the fire retardancy of the fabric.

Contaminated linen may release pathogens on lint and should be handled carefully on the ward prior to disposal (Overton 1988). See Guidelines for practice above.

Guidelines for practice: safe handling of linen

- Wear a plastic apron during bedmaking and discard afterwards
- Wash hands after contact with soiled linen
- Place linen carefully into an appropriate linen bag
- Use linen bags that comply with Health Service guidance (HSG(95)18; NHS Executive 1995)
- Place linen that is heavily soaked in body fluid in a plastic bag to prevent leakage
- Securely fasten the linen bag when full

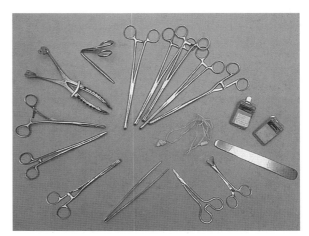

Figure 7.6 Sharps found in laundry bags. These sharps present a considerable hazard to laundry staff.

Table 7.3 Categories of hospital linen (NHS Executive 1995)

Category	Bag colour	Description	Recommended process
Used	White linen or clear plastic	Used, soiled and foul linen	Thermal disinfection by washing at 65°C for 10 min or 71°C for 3 min
Infected	Water-soluble bag, with red outer bag	Linen used by patients with certain infectious diseases or as advised by Infection Control Team	Not sorted prior to washing, thermal disinfection as used linen
Heat-labile	Orange stripe	Fabrics likely to be damaged by thermal disinfection (e.g. wool)	Wash at 40°C and add hypochlorite to penultimate rinse

Some wards use domestic washing machines to wash patients' clothing. Whilst satisfactory for this purpose, they should not be used to wash bedlinen or other items that will be used by different patients. The normal wash temperatures of 40°C or 60°C may not achieve satisfactory heat disinfection and the items can be difficult to dry quickly and thoroughly.

Duvets are sometimes used in clinical areas. Fabric duvets must withstand a wash temperature of 71°C and comply with Department of Health standards of fire retardancy. The duvet cover should be washed between patients and when soiled. The duvet should be washed when soiled and at least once every 3 months (Croton 1990). PVC-coated duvets should be cleaned with detergent and water between patients in the same way as mattresses.

In the home, contaminated linen can be decontaminated in a hot wash of a domestic washing machine (UK Health Departments 1998).

Uniforms

Uniforms worn by staff in clinical areas may become contaminated by a range of pathogens, especially after contact with body fluids, infected wounds or burns (Hambreaus 1973, Perry et al 2001). The front of the uniform is the most likely part to become contaminated and the risk can be reduced by appropriate use of disposable plastic aprons (Babb et al 1983). Healthcare workers who have direct contact with patients should wear a clean uniform every day. These can be decontaminated by washing in hot water, preferably at least 50°C, either in hospital or domestic washing machines (Callaghan 1998).

Excreta

Excreta and other body fluids may contain considerable numbers of pathogens and must be discarded safely to minimize the risk of transmission of infection to others. Excreta should be discarded directly into the bedpan washer, macerator or toilet. There is no advantage in adding disinfectant to excreta prior to disposal as it is unlikely to penetrate the organic material. Pathogens are constantly introduced to the drainage system from infected people in the community and there is therefore no value in attempting to remove them from the relatively small amounts entering the system from hospitals.

To prevent the transmission of micro-organisms between patients on bedpans, these should be decontaminated in a bedpan washer with a heat-disinfection cycle. The bedpan is disinfected during the cycle by flushing with water at a temperature of 80°C for a few minutes after washing. Faults in these machines must be reported promptly.

Disposable bedpans should be discarded into bedpan macerators. These should have an effective seal around the door to prevent the escape of aerosols that may contain pathogenic micro-organisms.

Decontamination of equipment

There are numerous examples of infection transmitted between patients on inadequately decontaminated equipment and concerns about the transmission of bloodborne viruses have highlighted the need to ensure that equipment used for invasive procedures is properly decontaminated after every patient, not only those known to be infected.

The method selected should be sufficient to prevent transmission of any pathogens and usually it should not be necessary to use a higher level of decontamination after equipment has been used on patients known to have an infection.

In some instances it is possible to reduce exposure to equipment contaminated by body fluid by changing practice. For example, swabs used during operations present a considerable hazard to staff who handle and count them on to a swab rack. This risk can be reduced if such swabs are counted directly into clear plastic bags so that contamination of the swab rack can be avoided.

Departments such as intensive care and theatres, which use suction frequently, may choose a disposable suction system to avoid the need to decontaminate suction jars.

Any equipment contaminated by body fluid that requires servicing or repair must be decontaminated before it is given to the engineer or returned to the manufacturer (NHS Management Executive 1993). The principles of decontamination of both equipment and the environment are discussed in more detail in Chapter 13.

Treatment of spills of blood or body fluid

Dealing with spills of blood or body fluid may expose the healthcare worker to bloodborne viruses or other pathogens. The task can be carried out more safely if any pathogens in the spillage are first destroyed by a disinfectant (Coates & Wilson 1989).

High-concentration chlorine-releasing compounds provide the most economical and effective method of treating many spills, especially large spills of blood (Box 7.14). Chlorine-releasing granules have the advantage of containing the spill rather than adding to it; they have a longer shelf-life than hypochlorite solutions and are more portable (Plate 24). In the home, good-quality thick bleaches, such as Domestos

or Parazone, contain a high concentration of available chlorine (see p. 272) and can be diluted and used to treat spills. However, chlorine compounds are corrosive to many materials and will bleach the colour from fabrics. They should not be used on carpets or furnishings and residual disinfectant should be removed from surfaces with detergent and water. If chlorine disinfectants cannot be used, spills should be removed using detergent and hot water.

Unfortunately, acidic solutions such as urine may react with the hypochlorite and cause the release of chlorine vapour. Hypochlorite solutions should therefore not be used on large urine spills (DoH 1990).

It may be impractical to treat large spills of blood or body fluid, such as may occur in labour wards or operating theatres, with hypochlorite. The spill should be soaked up with disposable paper towels or wipes and discarded into a yellow waste bag. The area should then be cleaned with detergent and water.

EDUCATION AND TRAINING

The adoption of a routine standard of infection control is essential for the safety of both patients and staff. Employers have an obligation to protect workers from hazards encountered during their work, including microbiological hazards (COSHH Regulations: Health & Safety Executive 2002).

The health and safety legislation acknowledges the importance of training and the provision of suitable equipment in establishing safe working practices. The adoption of a routine standard of infection control depends on regular and appropriate education and training to ensure that all healthcare workers understand the procedures and know what standards are expected (Fahey et al 1991). Gershon et al (1995), in their assessment of compliance with universal precautions amongst hospital staff, identified organizational commitment to safety as a key factor in increasing compliance.

Written policies or standards should be developed to clarify the local arrangements for minimizing the risks from hazards identified by the risk assessment process, for example situations where the use of protective clothing is indicated, local arrangements for the disposal of sharps and recommended methods of passing used instruments in theatre. Gerberding (1993) emphasizes the importance of involving all groups of staff in the process of identifying hazards and risk management solutions. These policies can form the basis for informing and training all staff who work in the area and then need to be the subject of regular monitoring and review.

Box 7.14   Methods of treating body fluid spills

Chlorine–releasing granules*
- Put on disposable gloves and apron
- Cover fluid completely with chlorine granules
- Leave for 2 min
- Remove granules and discard into yellow waste bag
- Wash the area with detergent and water

Hypochlorite solution*
- Put on disposable gloves and apron
- Cover spill with disposable paper towels
- Pour hypochlorite (10000 ppm available chlorine) over the towels
- Leave for 2 min
- Remove towels and discard into a yellow waste bag
- Wash area with detergent and water

Detergent and water
- Put on disposable gloves and apron
- Soak up spill with disposable paper towels
- Discard into a yellow waste bag
- Wash area with detergent and water

*Do not use for large spillages of urine

References

Adams D, Bagg J, Limaye M et al (1992) A clinical evaluation of glove washing and re-use in dental practice. *J. Hosp. Infect.*, **20**: 153–62.

Ansari SA, Springthorpe VS, Sattar SA et al (1991) Comparison of cloth, paper and warm air drying in eliminating viruses and bacteria from washed hands. *Am. J. Infect. Contr.*, **9**: 243–9.

Archibald L, Corl A, Shah B et al (1997a) *Serratia marcescens* outbreak associated with extrinsic contamination of 1% chloroxylenol soap. *Infect. Contr. Hosp. Epidemiol.*, **18**: 704–9.

Archibald LK, Manning ML, Bell LM et al (1997b) Patient density, nurse-to-patient ratio and nosocomial infection risk in a pediatric cardiac intensive care unit. *Pediatr. Infect. Dis. J.*, **16**: 1045–8.

Audit Commission (1997) *Getting Sorted – The Safe and Economic Management of Hospital Waste*. Bookpoint, Oxon.

Ayliffe GAJ (1991) Masks in surgery? *J. Hosp. Infect.*, **18**: 165–6.

Ayliffe GAJ, Babb JR, Quoraishi AH et al (1978) A test for hygienic hand disinfection. *J. Clin. Pathol.*, **31**: 923.

Ayliffe GAJ, Babb JR, Davies JG et al (1988) Hand disinfection: a comparison of various agents in laboratory and ward studies. *J. Hosp. Infect.*, **11**: 226–43.

Babb JR, Davies JG, Ayliffe GAJ (1983) Contamination of protective clothing and nurses' uniforms in an isolation ward. *J. Hosp. Infect.*, **4**: 49–57.

Barrie D (1994) How hospital linen and laundry services are provided. *J. Hosp. Infect.*, **27**(3): 219–36.

Barrie D, Wilson J, Hoffman PN, Kramer J (1992) *Bacillus cereus* meningitis in two neurosurgical patients: an investigation into the source of the organism. *J. Infect.*, **25**: 291–7.

Belkin NL (1997) The evolution of the surgical mask: filtering efficiency versus effectiveness. *Infect. Contr. Hosp. Epidemiol.*, **18**(1): 49–56.

Booth B (1996) Latex allergy: a growing problem in healthcare. *Prof. Nurse*, **11**: 316–19.

Boyce JM (2001) Antiseptic technology: access, affordability and acceptance. *Emerg. Infect. Dis.*, **7**(2): 231–3.

Boyce JM, Pittet D (2002) Guideline for hand hygiene in health-care settings: recommendations of the Healthcare Infection Control Practices Advisory Committee and the HICPAC/SHEA/APIC/IDSA Hand Hygiene Task Force. *Infect. Contr. Hosp. Epidemiol.*, **23**(12): S1–S40.

Boyce JM, Kelliher S, Vallande N (2000) Skin irritation and dryness associated with two hand-hygiene regimens: soap and water handwashing versus hand antisepsis with an alcoholic hand gel. *Infect. Contr. Hosp. Epidemiol.*, **211**: 442–8.

British Standards Institution (1990) *Specification for Sharps Containers*. BS 7320. British Standards Institution, London.

British Standards Institution (1999) *Eye Protection for Industrial and Other Uses. Guidance on Selection, Use and Maintenance*. BS 7028. British Standards Institution, London.

British Standards Institution (2000) *Medical Gloves for Single Use*. BS EN455. BSI, London.

Burnie JP, Odd FC, Lee W et al (1985) Outbreak of systemic *Candida albicans* in intensive care unit caused by cross-infection. *BMJ*, **290**: 746–8.

Callaghan I (1998) Bacterial contamination of nurses' uniforms: a study. *Nursing Standard*, **13**(1): 37–42.

Casewell M, Phillips I (1977) Hands as a route of transmission for *Klebsiella* species. *BMJ*, **ii**: 1315–17.

Castella A, Vallino A, Argentero PA et al (2003) Preventability of percutaneous injuries in healthcare workers: a year-long survey in Italy. *J. Hosp. Infect.*, **55**(4): 290–4.

Centers for Disease Control (1987) Recommendations for the prevention of HIV transmission in healthcare settings. *MMWR*, **36**: 2S.

Centers for Disease Control (1988) Update: universal precautions for prevention of transmission of human immunodeficiency virus, hepatitis B virus and other bloodborne pathogens in healthcare settings. *MMWR*, **37**: 24.

Centers for Disease Control (1993) Recommended infection control practices in dentistry. *MMWR*, **42**: RR1–8.

Coates D, Wilson M (1989) Use of dichloroisocyanurate granules for spills of body fluids. *J. Hosp. Infect.*, **13**: 241–52.

Collins CH, Kennedy DA (1992) The microbiological hazards of municipal and clinical wastes. *J. Appl. Bacteriol.*, **73**: 1–6.

Croton CM (1990) Duvets on trial. *Nursing Times*, **86**(26): 63–7.

Daschner FD, Dettenkofer M (1997) Protecting the patient and the environment – new aspects and challenges in hospital infection control. *J. Hosp. Infect.*, **36**: 7–16.

Davies MS (1994) Blunt-tipped suture needles. *Inf. Contr. Hosp. Epidemiol.*, **15**(4): 191.

DEFRA (2005) Hazardous waste regulations – guidance on mixing hazardous waste. Available online at: www.defra.gov.uk/environment/waste/special.

De Groot-Kosolcharoen J, Jones JM (1989) Permeability of latex and vinyl gloves to water and blood. *Am. J. Infect. Contr.*, **17**: 196–201.

Department of Health (1990) Spills of urine: potential risk of misuse of chlorine-releasing disinfecting agents. *Safety Advice Bull.*, **59**(90): 41.

Department of Health (1993) *Protecting Health Care Workers and Patients from Hepatitis B: Recommendations of the Advisory Group on Hepatitis*. HSG(93)40. Addendum (1996) EL(96)77. Department of Health, London.

Department of Health (1997) *Guidance on Post-exposure Prophylaxis for Health Care Workers Occupationally Exposed to HIV*. PL/CO(97)1. Department of Health, London.

Department of Health (2000) *Hepatitis B Infected Healthcare Workers*. HSC 2000/020. Department of Health, London.

Department of Health (2002a) *AIDS/HIV Infected Health Care Workers: Guidance on the Management of Infected Health Care*

Workers and Patient Notification. Department of Health, London.

Department of Health (2002b) *Hepatitis C Infected Healthcare Workers.* HSC 2002/010. Department of Health, London.

Department of Health (2004) *HIV Post-Exposure Prophylaxis: Guidance from the UK Chief Medical Officers' Expert Advisory Group on AIDS.* Department of Health, London.

Department of the Environment (1991) *Environmental Protection Act 1990. Waste Management: The Duty of Care. A Code of Practice.* HMSO, London.

Fahey BJ, Koziol DE, Banks SM et al (1991) Frequency of nonparenteral occupational exposures to blood and body fluids before and after universal precautions training. *Am. J. Med.*, **90**: 145–53.

Garner JS (1996) Hospital Infection Control Practices Advisory Committee. Guideline for isolation precautions in hospitals. *Infect. Contr. Hosp. Epidemiol.*, **17**(1): 54–80.

Gehrke C, Steinmann J, Goroncy-Bermes P (2004) Inactivation of feline calcivirus, a surrogate of norovirus (formerly Norwalk-like viruses), by different types of alcohol in vitro and in vivi. *J. Hosp. Infect.*, **56**: 49–55.

Gerberding JL (1993) Procedure-specific infection control for preventing intra-operative blood exposures. *Am. J. Infect. Contr.*, **21**: 364–7.

Gerberding JL, Littell C, Tarkington A et al (1990) Risk exposure of surgical personnel to patients' blood during surgery at San Francisco general hospital. *N. Engl. J. Med.*, **322**: 1788–93.

Gershon RM, Vlahor D, Felknor SA et al (1995) Compliance with universal precautions among healthcare workers at three regional hospitals. *Am. J. Infect. Contr.*, **23**: 225–36.

Glynn A, Ward V, Wilson J (1997) *Hospital Acquired Infection: Surveillance, Policies and Practice.* PHLS, London.

Gorman LJ, Sanai L, Notman W et al (1993) Cross-infection in an intensive care unit by *Klebsiella pneumoniae* from ventilator condensate. *J. Hosp. Infect.*, **23**(1): 27–34.

Greaves WL, Kraiser AB, Alford RH et al (1980) The problem of herpatic whitlow among hospital personnel. *Infect. Contr.*, **1**: 181–5.

Haley RW, Culver DH, White JW et al (1985) The efficacy of surveillance and control programs in preventing nosocomial infections in US hospitals. *Am. J. Epidemiol.*, **121**: 182–205.

Hambreaus A (1973) Transfer of *Staphylococcus aureus* via nurses' uniforms. *J. Hyg. Camb.*, **71**: 799–814.

Harbarth S, Sax H, Gastmeier P (2003) The preventable proportion of nosocomial infections: an overview of published reports. *J. Hosp. Infect.*, **54**: 258–66.

Harris AD, Sanmore MH, Natziger D et al (2000) A survey on handwashing practice and opinions of healthcare workers. *J. Hosp. Infect.*, **45**: 318–21.

Hazardous Waste (England & Wales) (2005) Statutory Instrument 894. Available online at: http://www.opsi.gov.uk/legislation/.

Health and Safety Executive (1992) *Personal Protective Equipment at Work Regulations* (EEC Directive). HMSO, London.

Health and Safety Executive (2002) *The Control of Substances Hazardous to Health. Approved Code of Practice and Guidance*, 4th edn. Health and Safety Executive, London.

Health Protection Agency (2005) *Eye of the Needle. Surveillance of Significant Occupational Exposure to Bloodborne Viruses in Healthcare Workers. Seven-Year Report.* Health Protection Agency, London.

Health Services Advisory Committee (1999) *Safe Disposal of Clinical Waste.* HSE Books, Sudbury.

Hoffman PN, Wilson JA (1994) Hands, hygiene and hospitals. *PHLS Micro. Dig.*, **11**(4): 211–16.

Hoffman PN, Cooke EM, McCarville MR et al (1985) Micro-organisms isolated from skin under wedding rings worn by hospital staff. *BMJ*, **290**: 206–7.

Hoffman PN, Bradley C, Ayliffe G (2004) *Disinfection in Healthcare*, 3rd edn. Blackwell Publishing, Oxford.

Holborn J (1990) Wet strike through and the transfer of bacteria through operating barrier fabrics. *Hygiene Med.*, **15**: 15–20.

Hubble MJ, Weale AE, Perez JV et al (1996) Clothing in laminar flow operating theatres. *J. Hosp. Infect.*, **32**: 1–7.

Jackson MJ, Lynch P (1985) Isolation practices: a historical perspective. *Am. J. Infect. Contr.*, **13**: 21–31.

Jeanes A, Green J (2001) Nail art: a review of current infection control issues. *J. Hosp. Infect.*, **49**: 139–42.

Johnson G (1998) Latex allergy: reducing the risks. *Nursing Times*, **94**(44): 69–73.

Johnson S, Gerding DN, Olsen MM et al (1990) Prospective controlled study of vinyl glove use to interrupt *Clostridium difficile* nosocomial transmission. *Am. J. Med.*, **88**: 137–40.

Kampf G, Loffler H (2003) Dermatological aspects of a successful introduction and continuation of alcohol-based hand rubs for hygienic hand disinfection. *J. Hosp. Infect.*, **55**(1):1–7.

Kaplan LM, McGuckin M (1986) Increasing handwashing compliance with more accessible sinks. *Infect. Contr.*, **7**: 408–9.

Klein BS, Perloff WH, Maki DG (1989) Reduction of nosocomial infection during pediatric intensive care by protective isolation. *N. Engl. J. Med.*, **320**: 1714–21.

Korniewicz DM, El-Masri M, Broyles JM et al (2002) Performance of latex and non-latex medical examination gloves during simulated use. *Am. J. Inf. Contr.*, **30**(2): 133–8.

Kretzer EK, Larson EL (1998) Behavioural interventions to improve infection control practices. *Am J. Infect. Contr.*, **26**: 245–53.

Larson EL (2001) Hygiene of skin: when is clean too clean? *Emerg. Infect. Dis.*, **7**(2): 225–9.

Larson EL, Bryan JL, Adler LM et al (1997) A multifaceted approach to changing handwashing behaviour. *Infect. Contr. Hosp. Epidemiol.*, **25**: 3–10.

Leliopoulou C, Waterman H, Chakrabarty S (1999) Nurses failure to appreciate the risk of infection due to needle stick accidents: a hospital based survey. *J. Hosp. Infect.*, **42**: 53–9.

Lowbury EJL, Lilley HA (1973) Use of 4% chlorhexidine detergent solution (Hibiscrub) and other methods of skin disinfection in wards. *J. Hyg. (Camb.)*, **76**: 75.

Lucet JC, Rigaud MP, Mentre F et al (2002) Hand contamination before and after different hand hygiene techniques: a randomized clinical trial. *J.Hosp. Infect.*, **50**(4): 276–80.

Lynch P, Jackson MM, Cummings MJ et al (1987) Rethinking the role of isolation practices in the prevention of nosocomial infections. *Ann. Intern. Med.*, **107**: 243–6.

Lynch P, Cummings MJ, Roberts PL et al (1990) Implementing and evaluating a system of generic infection control precautions: body substance isolation. *Am. J. Infect. Contr.*, **18**: 1–13.

Mackintosh CA, Hoffman PN (1984) An extended model for the transfer of micro-organisms and the effect of alcohol disinfection. *J. Hyg.*, **92**: 345–55.

Marples RR, Towers AG (1979) A laboratory model for the investigation of contact transfer of micro-organisms. *J. Hyg.*, **82**: 237–48.

McCormack RD, Buchman TL, Maki DG (2000) Double-blind randomised trial of scheduled use of a novel barrier cream and a oil-containing lotion for protecting the hands of healthcare workers. *Am. J. Infect. Contr.*, **28**: 302–10.

McGinley KL, Larson EL, Leyden JJ (1988) Composition and density of microflora in the subungual space of the hand. *J. Clin. Microbiol.*, **26**: 950–3.

Medical Devices Agency (1996) *Latex Sensitisation in the Healthcare Setting (Use of Latex Gloves)*. DB9601. Department of Health, Wetherby, UK.

Medical Devices Agency (1998) *Powdered Latex Medical Gloves (Surgeons and Examination)*. Safety Notice SN9825. HMSO, London.

Moolenaar RL, Crutcher JM, San Joaquin VN et al (2000) A prolonged outbreak of *Pseudomonas aeruginosa* in a neonatal intensive care unit: did staff fingernails play a role in disease transmission? *Infect. Contr. Hosp. Epidemiol.*, **21**: 80–5.

Morse LJ, Schonbek LE (1968) Hand lotions and potential nosocomial hazard. *N. Engl. J. Med.*, **278**: 376–8.

Mulberry G, Snyder AT, Heilman J et al (2001) Evaluation of a waterless scrubless chlorhexidine gluconate/ethanol surgical scrub for antimicrobial efficacy. *Am. J. Infect. Contr.*, **29**: 377–82.

Naikoba S, Hayward A (2001) The effectiveness of interventions aimed at increasing handwashing in healthcare workers – a systematic review. *J. Hosp. Infect.*, **47**: 173–80.

National Audit Office (1999) *The Management of Medical Equipment in Acute NHS Trusts in England*. Stationery Office, London.

National Audit Office (2000) *The Management and Control of Hospital Acquired Infection in Acute NHS Trusts in England. Report by the Comptroller and Auditor General*. Stationery Office, London.

National Patient Safety Agency (2005) Clean Your Hands Campaign. Available online at: www.npsa.nhs.uk/cleanyourhands/campaign/about

NHS Executive (1995) *Hospital Laundry Arrangements for Used and Infected Linen*. HSG(95)18. HMSO, London.

NHS in Scotland (1998) *Management and Disposal of Clinical Waste*. Scottish Hospital Technical Note No. 3. Estates Environment Forum, April 1998.

NHS Management Executive (1993) *Decontamination of Equipment Prior to Inspection, Service or Repair*. HSG(93)26. HMSO, London.

Norton Hughes CA, Pyrak JD (1998) Changes in bacterial flora associated with skin damage on hands of healthcare personnel. *Am J. Infect. Contr.*, **26**: 513–21.

Ojajärvi J (1980) Effectiveness of hand washing and disinfection methods in removing transient bacteria after patients nursing. *J. Hyg. (Lond.)*, **85**: 193–203.

Ojajärvi J, Mäkelä P, Rautasalo I (1977) Failure of hand disinfection with frequent handwashing: a need for prolonged field studies. *J. Hyg. (Camb.)*, **79**: 107–12.

Olsen RJ, Lynch P, Coyle MB et al (1993) Examination gloves as barriers to hand contamination in clinical practice. *JAMA*, **270**(3): 350–3.

Overton E (1988) Bed-making and bacteria. *Nursing Times*, **85**(9): 69–71.

Palmer JD, Rickett JWS (1992) The mechanisms and risks of surgical glove perforation. *J. Hosp. Infect.*, **22**: 279–86.

Patterson JE, Vecchio J, Pantelick EL (1991) Association of contaminated gloves with transmission of *Acinetobacter calcoaceticus* var. *anitratus* in an intensive care unit. *Am. J. Med.*, **91**: 479–83.

Pellowe CM, Pratt RJ, Harper P et al (2003) Evidence-based guidelines for preventing healthcare-associated infections in primary and community care in England. *J. Hosp. Infect.*, **55** (suppl. 2): S1–S27.

Perry C, Marshall IR, Jones IE (2001) Bacterial contamination of uniforms. *J. Hosp. Infect.*, **48**: 238–41.

Phillips G (1999) Microbiological aspects of clinical waste. *J. Hosp. Infect.*, **41**: 1–6.

Pittet D, Dharan S, Touveneau S et al (1999) Bacterial contamination of the hands of hospital staff during routine patient care. *Arch. Intern. Med.*, **159**: 821–6.

Pittet D, Hugonnet S, Harbarth S et al (2000) Effectiveness of a hospital-wide programme to improve compliance with hand hygiene. *Lancet*, **356**: 1307–12.

Pratt RA, Pellowe CM, Loveday HP et al (2001) The Epic project: developing national evidence-based guidelines for preventing healthcare associated infections. *J. Hosp. Infect.*, **47** (suppl.: S1–82).

Prieto JA (2003) Influencing infection control practice: assessing the impact of supportive intervention for nurses. PhD thesis, University of Southampton.

Public Health Laboratory Service AIDS & STD Centre at the Communicable Disease Surveillance Centre (1999) *Occupational Transmission of HIV. Summary of Published Reports*. Available online at: www.hpa.org.uk/infections/topics_az/hiv_and_sti/publications

Reybrouck G (1983) Role of the hands in the spread of nosocomial infections. *J. Hosp. Infect.*, **4**: 103–10.

Ross DJ, Cherry NM, McDonald JC (1998) Occupationally acquired infectious disease in the United Kingdom: 1996 to 1997. *Commun. Dis. Public Health*, **1**(2): 98–102.

Royal College of Pathologists (1992) *HIV Infection: Hazards of Transmission to Patients and Health Care Workers During Invasive Procedures*. Royal College of Pathologists, London.

Samadi AR, Huq MI, Ahmed QS (1983) Detection of rotavirus in handwashings of attendants of children with diarrhoea. *BMJ*, **286**: 188.

Sanderson PJ, Weissler S (1992) Recovery of coliforms from the hands of nurses and patients: activities leading to contamination. *J. Hosp. Infect.*, **21**: 85–93.

Sartor C, Jacomo V, Duvivier C et al (2000) Nosocomial *Serratia marcescens* infections associated with extrinsic contamination of liquid non-medicated soap. *Infect. Contr. Hosp. Epidemiol.*, **21**: 196–9.

Sattar SA, Springthorpe VS, Tetro J et al (2002) Hygienic hand antiseptics: should they not have activity and label claims against viruses? *Am. J. Infect. Contr.*, **30**: 355–72.

Scanlon JW, Leikkanen M (1973) The use of fluorescein powder for evaluating contamination in a newborn nursery. *J. Pediatr.*, **82**: 966–71.

Short LJ, Bell DM (1993) Risk of occupational infection with bloodborne pathogens in operating and delivery room settings. *Am J. Infect. Contr.*, **21**: 343–50.

Sprunt K, Redman W, Leidy G (1973) Antibacterial effectiveness of routine handwashing. *Pediatrics*, **52**: 264–71.

Stafford K, Kitchen VS, Smith JR et al (1995) Reducing the risk of bloodborne infection in surgical practice. *Br. J. Obstet. Gynaecol.*, **102**(6): 439–41.

Tanner J, Parkinson H (2004) Double gloving to reduce cross infection (Cochrane Review). The Cochrane Library. Issue 2. John Wiley, Chichester.

Taylor L (1978) An evaluation of handwashing techniques. *Nursing Times*, **74**: 108–10.

Telford GL, Quebberman EJ (1993) Assessing the risk of blood exposure in the operating theatre. *Am. J. Infect. Contr.*, **21**: 351–6.

Tenorio AR, Badri SM, Sahgal NB et al (2001) Effectiveness of gloves in the prevention of hand carriage of vancomycin-resistant enterococcus species by healthcare workers after patients care. *Clin. Infect. Dis.*, **32**: 826–9.

Tokars JI, Bell DM, Culver DH et al (1992) Percutaneous injuries during surgical procedures. *JAMA*, **267**: 2899–904.

Tokars JI, Culver DH, Mendelson MH et al (1995) Skin and mucous membrane contacts with blood during surgical procedures: risk and prevention. *Infect. Contr. Hosp. Epidemiol.*, **16**: 703–11.

Tomlinson D (1987) To clean or not to clean? *Nursing Times*, **83**: 71–5.

Trim JC, Elliot TSJ (2003) A review of sharps injuries and preventative strategies. *J. Hosp. Infect.*, **53**(4): 237–42.

UK Health Departments (1998) *Guidance for Clinical Health Care Workers: Protection Against Infection with Blood Borne Viruses. Recommendation of the Expert Advisory Group on AIDS and Advisory Group on Hepatitis*. Department of Health, Wetherby, UK.

Voss A, Widmer AF (1997) No time for handwashing! Handwashing versus alcohol rub: can we afford 100% compliance? *Infect. Contr. Hosp. Epidemiol.*, **18**(3): 205–8.

Webster J, Faagali JL, Cartwright D (1994) Elimination of methicillin-resistant *Staphylococcus aureus* from a neonatal unit after handwashing with triclosan. *J. Paed. Child Health*, **30**: 59–64.

Weltman AC, Short LJ, Mendelson MH et al (1995) Disposal-related sharps injuries at a New York City teaching hospital. *Infect. Contr. Hosp. Epidemiol.*, **16**: 268–74.

Williams E, Buckles A (1988) A lack of motivation. *Nursing Times*, **84**: 60–4.

Wilson J, Breedon P (1990) Universal precautions. *Nursing Times*, **86**: 67–70.

Yessin MS, Lieri MB, Fischer TJ et al (1994) Latex allergy in hospital employees. *Ann. Allergy*, **72**(3): 245–9.

Zafar AB, Butler RC, Reese DJ et al (1995) Use of 0.3% triclosan (Bact-Stat) to eradicate an outbreak of methicllin-resistant *Staphylococcus aureus* in a neonatal nursery. *Am. J. Infect. Contr.*, **23**: 200–8.

Zimmermann C, Junghans K (1996) Use of a new peroration indicator system. *Hyg. Med.*, **21**: 9.

Further Reading

Infection Control Nurses Association (1999) *Glove Usage Guidelines*, ICNA, Bathgate, West Lothian.

Infection Control Nurses Association (2002) *Guidelines for Hand Hygiene*. ICNA, Bathgate, West Lothian.

Larson E (1988) A causal link between handwashing and risk of infection? Examination of the evidence. *Infect. Contr. Hosp. Epidemiol.*, **9**(1): 28–36.

Truscott W, Stoessel KB (2003) Factors that impact on the infections control capability of gloves. *Prof. Nurse*, **18**(9): 507–11.

Chapter **8**

Preventing wound infection

CHAPTER CONTENTS

INTRODUCTION

A wound has been defined as a loss of continuity of skin or tissue (Ayton 1985) and may result from accidental trauma, an underlying disease process (e.g. venous ulceration) or a surgical procedure. When considering the prevention of infection in wounds, it is important to distinguish between wounds healing by secondary intention, in which there is loss of tissue and the remaining tissues are exposed for many days or weeks, and the surgical wound where exposure of the underlying tissue occurs for only a few minutes or hours and healing is by primary intention (Fig. 8.1). In healing by secondary intention, the gap must be gradually filled from the base by new tissue. This process is accelerated by contraction; contractile cells in the wound gradually move the edges of the wound into the centre and decrease its size.

Epithelial cells are constantly shed and replaced from the surface of the skin. When skin is damaged, these cells migrate across the living tissue, towards areas where cells are lost or depleted. This process is called epithelialization and is particularly important for healing by secondary intention. Epithelial cells can only migrate over healthy viable tissue. If the surface of the wound is dry they migrate to moist layers beneath the surface.

The processes that take place in a wound as it heals are summarized in Box 8.1.

THE SURGICAL WOUND

Surgical wound infections account for between 10% and 20% of infections acquired by patients in hospital (Emmerson et al 1996, Haley et al 1985a). Infections may affect the superficial cutaneous layer, the deep fascial layers or nearby organs and other sites such as

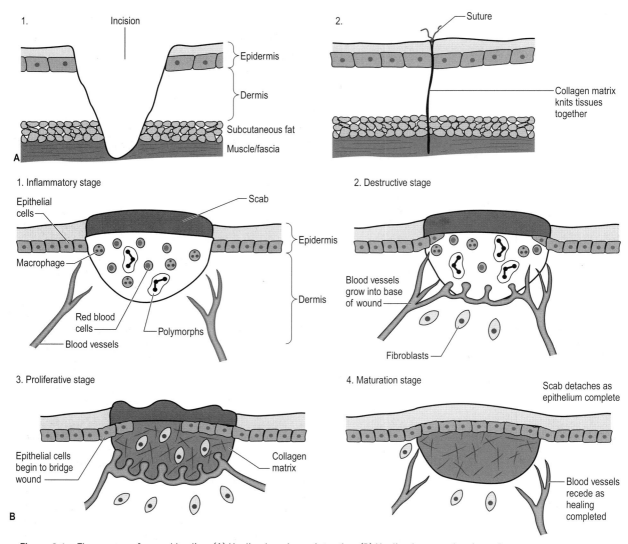

Figure 8.1   The process of wound healing. (A) Healing by primary intention. (B) Healing by secondary intention.

joints or abdomen manipulated during the procedure. Most infections are acquired at the time of operation (Kluytmans 1997). The bacteria may be introduced from a variety of sources but the most common source is the patient's own microbial flora (Box 8.2). Intra-abdominal wound infection caused by Gram-negative bacteria can be particularly serious because the endotoxins released may trigger a systemic inflammatory response and subsequent multiorgan failure (Henderson et al 1996). The risk of infection developing in a surgical wound depends on a delicate balance between the host immune defences and the number of bacteria present in the wound at the end of the operation. This balance is influenced by the condition of the wound and the susceptibility of the patient to infection (Box 8.3).

Factors that affect the risk of wound infection

Bacterial contamination of the wound

Wounds are able to heal despite the presence of quite large numbers of bacteria. Kriezek & Robson (1975) found that wound infection occurred only if more than 100 000 bacteria per gram of tissue were present when the wound was closed.

As the bacteria that cause surgical wound infections are frequently derived from the patient's own normal flora, the number of bacteria in the wound at the end of

Box 8.1   Stages in wound healing

These stages overlap and the wound may move backwards and forwards through several phases before it finally heals.

Stage 1 (0–3 days) Inflammation phase	Injured blood vessels thrombose; clot forms. Damaged tissue releases histamine, causing vasodilation. Increased blood supply brings macrophages and polymorphonucleocytes. Epithelialization begins with the formation of fibrinogen
Stage 2 (2–5 days) Destructive phase	Polymorphs and macrophages remove dead tissue and stimulate multiplication of fibroblasts. Cytokines released by macrophages play an important role in orchestrating wound healing
Stage 3 (3–24 days) Proliferation phase	Fibroblasts and epithelial cells proliferate. Fibroblasts begin to produce fibrin filaments. These are coated with fibronectin (a plasma protein) to build a framework (collagen matrix) for the epithelial cells and fibroblasts. New capillary loops grow into the collagen to form granulation tissue, which has a red uneven appearance
Stage 4 (24 days to 1 year) Maturation phase	Epithelial cells migrate over the wound surface. Contractile fibroblasts pull the edges of the wound together and more collagen fibres are made and reorganized to increase the strength of the scar

Box 8.2   Surgical wound infections: potential sources of bacteria

Patient	Theatre	Ward
Skin	Staff	Staff
Colonized hollow organs	Instruments	Wound dressings
Other infection	Airborne particles	Airborne particles

Box 8.3   Factors that increase the risk of surgical wound infection

In the wound	In the patient
Number of bacteria	Malnourishment
Dead tissue	Obesity
Haematoma	Underlying illness (e.g. diabetes, vascular insufficiency)
Tissue damage during procedure	
Foreign material	Immune deficiency
	Infection at a remote site

the procedure depends on the site of the body involved. Procedures involving sterile tissues, for example orthopaedic surgery, are likely to encounter few colonizing bacteria and the risk of surgical wound infection developing is relatively small (Fig. 8.2; Table 8.1).

Some parts of the body, for example the intestines, are colonized by large numbers of bacteria which readily enter the wound when surgery is performed on the bowel. Before operating on the colon, various methods are used to reduce the number of bacteria in the bowel (e.g. elemental diets, purgatives, antibiotics).

Surgery involving a site with pre-existing infection, or where necrosed tissue is present, is significantly more likely to result in wound infection. For example, Figure 8.2 demonstrates the high rate of infection following limb amputation. Many of these procedures will be undertaken on patients with extremely poor perfusion of their lower limbs and consequently they will have an increased vulnerability to infection.

However, it is often difficult to separate the risks associated with the procedure from those related to the patient. The risk of wound infection in partial hip replacements is higher than in total hip replacements. However, when all the main risk factors are taken into account, this increased risk is found to be related to the greater age and number of co-morbidities in the group undergoing partial replacements rather than differences in the procedure itself (Ridgeway et al 2005).

Foreign bodies

The presence in tissue of even a small amount of foreign material has a dramatic effect on the immune

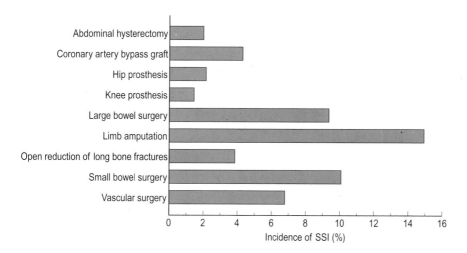

Figure 8.2 Incidence of surgical site infection (SSI) by category of surgical procedure (reproduced by permission from CDR Weekly 2004).

Table 8.1 Classification of wound contamination

Category	Description	Type of surgery	Approximate rate of surgical wound infection (%)
Clean	GI, GU or respiratory tract not entered; no evidence of inflammation or infection; no break in technique	Orthopaedic; neurosurgery; cardiac surgery	2–5
Clean-contaminated	GI, GU or respiratory tract entered but no spillage of contents	Abdominal hysterectomy; resection of prostate	4–8
Contaminated	Open traumatic wounds; major break in technique; spillage from GI tract; inflamed tissue encountered	Reduction of open fracture; some large bowel surgery	15
Dirty	Delayed treatment of traumatic wounds; pre-existing clinical infection, perforated viscera at site of operation	Drainage of abscess	40

GI, gastrointestinal; GU, genitourinary.

defences. This was first demonstrated by Elek & Conen (1957), who inoculated the forearms of medical students with *Staphylococcus aureus*. They found that only 100 bacteria were necessary to produce infection in the presence of a silk suture, compared with the 6.5 million bacteria required without a suture. This effect is demonstrated by the occurrence of small areas of inflammation around skin sutures on surgical wounds.

Some bacteria, e.g. *S. epidermis*, are able to adhere to implanted material such as joint replacements and prosthetic heart valves where they can multiply to produce infection and sometimes devastating consequences for the patient (Schierholz & Beuth 2001).

Susceptibility of the patient to infection
The risk of patients acquiring a wound infection is influenced by their susceptibility to infection and the ability of the wound to heal.

Underlying disease may depress the response of the immune system and patients with serious underlying illness are more susceptible to infection.

Diabetes mellitus interferes with phagocytosis by white blood cells and causes a general increase in susceptibility to infection, as well as an increased risk of surgical wound infection (Slaughter et al 1993). The risk of surgical wound infection appears to be highest in insulin-dependent diabetics. Since the risk appears to be related to perioperative blood glucose levels, controlling hyperglycaemia may be an important measure for reducing the risk of wound infection in diabetic patients undergoing surgery (Kluytmans et al 1995, Lathan et al 2001).

Immunosuppressive therapy or steroid treatment also depresses the immune response and enables bacteria to multiply more easily in the wound. There is a significant correlation between increasing age and the risk of developing wound infection, probably related to slower immune responses and other underlying diseases. Impairment in tissue oxygenation such as may occur with vascular insufficiency or diabetes will delay healing and increase the risk of infection (Bowler et al 2001, Desia 1997, Ridgeway et al 2005). Poor nutrition and nicotine use have been associated with delayed wound healing. Obesity has been shown to be an important risk factor for surgical wound infection (Cruse & Foord 1973, Nicholson et al 1994). Deep layers of adipose tissue can increase the complexity of the procedure and reduce the blood flow to the wound during healing (Mangram et al 1999, Wilson & Clark 2003). In breast surgery, larger breast size also increases the risk of surgical wound infection (Rotstein et al 1992).

Patients who already have an infection, for example pneumonia or urinary tract infection, at the time of operation are more prone to develop a wound infection and existing infections should be treated before surgery is performed, if possible (Valentine et al 1986).

An awareness of the underlying factors that predispose patients to infection can help to identify patients at greatest risk, enhance their resistance to infection as much as possible before operation and observe them closely after operation for early signs of infection.

Nasal colonization with Staphylococcus aureus

Although *S. aureus* is an important pathogen, it is also commonly present as part of the normal flora of the skin and nose. About 20% of people carry *S. aureus* in their nose all the time and a further 60% some of the time (Williams 1963). *S. aureus* is an important cause of surgical wound infection, accounting for approximately 50% of infections (Health Protection Agency 2003a). An association between nasal carriage of *S. aureus* and the development of surgical wound infection has been recognized for many years but a number of more recent studies have emphasized its importance as a major risk factor (Kluytmans et al 1995).

Reducing the risk of surgical wound infection

In seminal work on monitoring the rate of surgical wound infections, Cruse & Foord (1980) suggested 10 key elements for minimizing the risk of surgical wound infection (see Box 8.4). These recommendations still represent the cornerstone of good practice for preventing surgical wound infection (Mangram et al 1999). More recently, new evidence has emerged about other potentially valuable practices such as preoperative warming and nasal decolonization. These are discussed below, together with the principles of good operating theatre practice.

Preoperative hospitalization

From the time of admission to hospital, the normal harmless flora of the patient's skin is gradually replaced by hospital pathogens, which may then be introduced into the surgical wound (Noone et al 1983). Cruse & Foord (1980) demonstrated that the longer a patient stayed in hospital before operation, the greater the probability that the wound would become infected. When the preoperative stay was 1 day, 1.2% of wounds became infected, whilst 3.4% of wounds became infected if the patient had been in hospital for more than 2 weeks. However, some of this increase in risk is probably linked to the patient's underlying illness. More seriously ill patients are more likely to require preparation and treatment in hospital before surgery (Mangram et al 1999).

Box 8.4   Key elements for minimizing the risk of surgical wound infection (Cruse & Foord 1980)

- Short preoperative stay
- Disinfectant shower before operation
- Shaving kept to a minimum
- Contamination of the wound avoided
- Punctilious surgical technique
- An operation performed as quickly as is safe
- Scrupulous care in operations on the elderly, obese, malnourished or diabetic
- No drains brought out through the operative wound
- Meticulous coagulation technique
- Information to each surgeon on his/her wound infection rate compared to the average of his/her peers

For most patients, hospital stay can be reduced to a minimum by performing essential preoperative investigations in assessment clinics and admitting them on the day before or the day of surgery.

Preoperative bathing

Bacteria present on the patient's skin can be introduced into the wound during operation. Reducing bacterial colonization of the skin before incision has therefore been advocated as a means of minimizing the risk of infection. A bath or shower using an antiseptic such as chlorhexidine or povidone-iodine before operation reduces the number of bacteria on the skin but a clear association with reduction in wound infection rate has not been demonstrated (Ayliffe et al 1983, Lynch et al 1992).

Alcoholic solutions of iodine or chlorhexidine should be used to cleanse around the site of the incision to reduce the number of skin bacteria present when the incision is made and to minimize the risk of introducing them into the wound (Mangram et al 1999). Single-use containers of antiseptic are preferred as multiuse bottles may become contaminated (Woodhead et al 2002). The solution should be allowed to dry completely on the skin before using diathermy to avoid the risk of igniting the alcoholic vapour.

Shaving the skin

A number of studies have shown that shaving the skin before operation increases the risk of wound infection (Alexander et al 1983, Cruse 1986). Bacteria multiply in microabrasions caused by the razor on the surface of the skin, particularly if the skin is shaved some hours before surgery. Removal of hair with an electric shaver is associated with a lower infection rate but shavers present their own cross-infection problems if used between patients (Millward 1992). Where hair removal is essential (for example, to visualize the operative site) hair clippers may provide a suitable alternative since they significantly reduce the risk of wound infection (Ko et al 1992), especially if the hair is clipped on the same day as surgery (Alexander et al 1983). The use of depilatory creams instead of razors reduces the risk of wound infection but they can cause an allergic reaction and may not remove hair of male patients (Seropian & Reynolds 1971). Some studies have suggested that any form of hair removal increases the risk of infection (Winston 1992).

Hair is no more heavily colonized with microbial flora than the skin and the criteria for hair removal should be based on the need to view or access the operative site rather than to remove bacteria. If hair removal is essential, the best approach is to remove the minimum amount of hair as near to the time of operation as possible (Mangram et al 1999).

Preoperative warming

Hypothermia has been suggested to affect platelet function and have an immunosuppressive effect on neutrophils that results in delayed wound healing and predisposes to wound infection (McNally et al 2001). A randomized controlled trial of preoperative warming using either a warm air blanket or radiant heat dressing in the planned wound area in clean surgery was found to both significantly increase the body temperature and reduce the rate of surgical wound infection (Melling et al 2001). Kurz et al (1996), also in a controlled trial, achieved a three times lower rate of infection in colorectal surgery when patients were warmed to maintain a core body temperature of 36°C before, during and after the operation and warmed IV fluids were administered.

Surgical technique

A considerable proportion of surgical wound infection has been attributed to the technique of the surgeon (Cruse 1986, Holzheimer et al 1997, Kluytmans 1997). Minimizing the amount of trauma to the tissue improves wound healing and reduces the risk of infection (Holzheimer et al 1997). Important factors include maintaining a good blood supply, removing devitalized tissue, minimizing bleeding and preventing tissues from drying out by using saline irrigation. Control of haemorrhage is also important because of the increased surgical wound infection rate associated with blood transfusion. This is thought to be due to an adverse effect on cell-mediated immunity: the risk increases for each unit administered but is significantly lower when autologous blood is used (Heiss et al 1993). In a study on major vascular surgery, the rate of surgical site infection increased to over 50% if five or more units of blood were given (Verwaal et al 1992). The presence of haematomas and dead tissue in the wound encourages the multiplication of bacteria which may then be able to establish infection. Inadvertent breaks in surgical technique, for example spillage of bowel contents, are also likely to increase the risk of subsequent wound infection.

Duration of operation

The longer that tissues are exposed, the greater the chance that bacteria carried by airborne particles will settle on to the tissues or be carried into the wound on hands or instruments (Whyte et al 1982). Longer procedures also provide more opportunity for tissue damage or a break in surgical technique to occur. The time taken to perform an operation may be affected by both the skill of the surgeon and the complexity of the procedure. However, a rapidly performed procedure may be associated with poor technique and increased risk of infection (Haley et al 1985a). The duration of operation is therefore an important risk factor for wound infection (Culver et al 1991).

Wound drains

A wound is more likely to become infected if a drain is inserted leading from the tissues out through the skin, as it will provide a route through which bacteria can enter the wound (Cruse 1986). However, drains can facilitate wound healing by preventing the formation of haematomas. When required, a closed drainage system, for example emptying directly into a bag or bottle, is recommended because this reduces the risk of bacteria entering the wound. Making a separate incision for the drain has also been advocated so that the main incision is not affected when the drain is shortened or if it becomes infected (Mangram et al 1999). Drains should not be left in place for too long as this may enable bacteria to colonize the site (Drinkwater & Neil 1995).

Postoperative care

Although the first signs of infection in a surgical wound become apparent during postoperative care, usually 4–10 days after operation, most of these infections will probably have been introduced during surgery. As soon as the wound has been sutured, a loose mesh of fibrin is formed and is gradually infiltrated by fibroblasts and collagen. In most cases this structure will become impervious to the entry of bacteria within a few hours and, provided the dressing applied in theatre remains undisturbed for the first 48 hours, pathogens are unlikely to gain access to the wound. However, the wound may not seal completely if it continues to exude serous fluids and in obese patients poor oxygen perfusion may delay the healing process (Wilson & Clark 2003). Particular care must be taken to avoid contamination of the surgical wound postoperatively until the wound surface has sealed completely. Ensuring the wound is as well perfused as possible postoperatively minimizes the risk of infection (Hunt & Hopf 1997).

Antibiotic prophylaxis

The efficacy of antimicrobial prophylaxis depends on the timing of administration (Holzheimer et al 1997). In general, the use of antibiotics to prevent infection is recommended for surgery associated with a high risk of infection such as clean-contaminated procedures, or for clean procedures involving the insertion of a prosthesis where the consequences of infection could be serious. The aim is to inhibit bacterial growth in the wound and other areas prone to postoperative infection. For example, an appendectomy for an inflamed appendix may be complicated by an infected wound and peritonitis, and antibiotic prophylaxis is intended to prevent both. Prophylactic antibiotics have undoubtedly had a major effect in reducing the risk of surgical wound infection but their efficacy depends on selecting an appropriate agent and time of administration. The choice of antibiotic should be based on the species of bacteria most likely to contaminate the wound. In some circumstances more than one agent may be required to prevent infection by bacteria resistant to common antibiotics, such as enterococci (Korten & Murray 1993). The administration of the antibiotics should be timed to achieve the right levels in blood and tissue before bacterial contamination occurs and to maintain them during operation. The first dose should therefore be given before the incision is made. Further doses should not be continued for more than a few hours after operation as this will encourage the selection of resistant bacteria (Holzheimer et al 1997).

Topical mupirocin to remove nasal carriage before operation has been used successfully to reduce surgical site infections following major surgery (Kluytmans 1998). However, evidence from randomized controlled trials is required to demonstrate its efficacy and assess the long-term impact on resistance to mupirocin (Kalmeijer et al 2002, Kluytmans & Voss 2002).

Procedures in the operating department

Ventilation and air filtration   Air contains microorganisms on airborne particles such as skin squames, dust, lint or respiratory droplets. In theatre, the main source of airborne bacteria is the staff, although power tools can also create aerosols from tissues (Hoffman et al 2002).

The number of airborne microbial particles in an operating room is proportional to the number of humans present and their level of activity. Each person has been estimated to emit approximately 10 000 organisms per minute at rest, increasing to 50 000 per minute during activity as friction of clothing against the skin releases more squames (Howarth 1985). These particles may settle on to instruments or gloved hands or into the wound itself and subsequently result in wound infection (Hambreaus 1988, Whyte et al 1982). Barrie et al (1992) reported an unusual outbreak of surgical wound infection caused by linen contaminated with *Bacillus cereus*. Lint from the contaminated linen was thought to have entered the wound directly or after settling on instruments but infection occurred during two neurosurgical operations which lasted for many hours and provided ample opportunity for bacteria to enter the wound and establish infection.

Special ventilation systems are used to filter out airborne micro-organisms, to prevent micro-organisms from entering the theatre in the air supply from corridors or other parts of the hospital, and to dilute contaminated air in the room by replenishing with fresh filtered air (Hoffman et al 2002). Air is forced into the theatre through filters in the ceiling which remove particles and bacteria; the volume of air in the room will be changed approximately 20 times an hour (less frequently in scrub-up and anaesthetic rooms). Theatres are plenum ventilated; that is, a higher pressure is maintained in the room to prevent unfiltered air from outside flowing in through the doors (Fig. 8.3).

The air handling and filtration system should be checked by the infection control team after any substantial modification to an operating theatre and before new theatres are used (Hoffman et al 2002).

The number of airborne particles can be reduced by keeping the number and activity of people present during operation to a minimum and ensuring that the ventilation system is not disrupted by opening operating room doors during the procedure. Dust should not be allowed to collect on surfaces where it may be disturbed and become airborne. Ultra-clean air systems have been recommended to reduce the incidence of infection in orthopaedic surgery,

particularly prosthetic hip and knee replacements. Such procedures are susceptible to infection even if only small numbers of bacteria are introduced into the wound (Gosden et al 1998). These systems direct a laminar flow of filtered air over the operating table and use over 600 air changes per hour (Lidwell et al 1982). Early studies demonstrated a significant reduction in wound infection rates, although some suggest that similar results may be achieved by using only prophylactic antibiotics (Mangram et al 1999).

Handwashing The transfer of micro-organisms from the surgeon's hands to the wound may be reduced by handwashing. Whilst soap removes the transient flora of the skin, microbicidal detergents (surgical scrubs) are used to reduce the resident microbial flora of the skin (see Ch. 7). To achieve maximum reduction, the hands and arms should be washed thoroughly, ensuring that all parts are covered with the detergent.

There is little conclusive evidence to define the optimal duration of washing but a scrubbing brush should not be used as this may cause skin abrasion (Woodhead et al 2002).

Chlorhexidine and povidone-iodine have a persistent effect on skin micro-organisms; therefore repeated washes through the day gradually reduce the number of bacteria on the skin (Ojajärvi 1976, O'Shaughnessy et al 1991). Alcohol handrub solutions

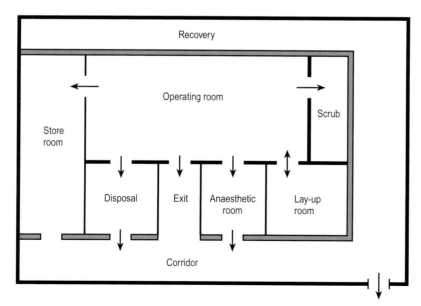

Figure 8.3 Ventilation of an operating theatre. Air moves from the cleanest areas to the least clean areas. Arrows indicate direction of air flow.

are equally effective on clean hands and could be used in place of surgical scrubs for repeated washing (Woodhead et al 2002). Artificial nails can increase bacterial colonization of the hands and outbreaks of wound infections associated with artificial nails have been reported (Passaro et al 1997).

Operating room clothing   Micro-organisms are constantly shed from skin; therefore, personnel directly involved in the operation wear sterile gowns to limit the transmission of their microbial skin flora into the open wound. Although gowns provide some protection against contamination by body fluid, they do not completely prevent bacteria shed from the skin escaping from the openings at the neck, ankles and wrists as well as through pores in the fabric (Whyte et al 1976). The passage of bacteria is enhanced if the material becomes wet (Hoborn 1990). Gowns made of non-woven materials or close-woven polyester fabrics can reduce the dispersal of bacteria (Matthews et al 1985, Whyte et al 1990) and are often recommended for orthopaedic surgery.

Sterile occlusive drapes can be used to reduce the transfer of bacteria from the patient's skin into the wound. The permeability of drapes used to cover the patient varies according to the type of material. Impermeability is lost if the material becomes wet (Blom et al 2002). Johnson et al (1987) showed that iodophor-impregnated adhesive plastic sheets applied to the operative field may reduce recolonization of the skin; however, there is no evidence for their effect on rates of wound infection.

Waterproof disposable gowns and drapes have been shown to reduce bacterial contamination of the wound (Woodhead et al 2002). A European Standard (EN13795) details performance standards expected of surgical gowns and drapes (Wigglesworth 2003).

Masks are conventionally worn to prevent bacteria from the upper respiratory tract entering the wound. There is little evidence to suggest a significant risk of transmission by this route (Ayliffe 1991a). The mask rubbing against the skin may actually increase the shedding of skin squames and, unless it fits very well, exhaled air will escape from the sides. Air flow around the sides will increase as the material becomes wet with moist exhaled air (Belkin 1997, Schweizer 1976). Masks are, of course, necessary to protect those close to the operating site from blood or body fluid splashing on to mucous membranes but the value of masks to other personnel in the theatre is questionable (Hubble et al 1996, Mitchell & Hunt 1991). Splash shields that protect at-risk staff from splashing of blood or tissues may provide a more practical alternative (Belkin 2002).

Whilst head covers may prevent bacteria on hairs from entering the operative sites, they probably have limited impact on counts of bacteria in the air (Humphries et al 1991a). They are therefore probably of little value for non-scrubbed staff assisting most types of surgery. Overshoes also appear to have no effect on bacterial counts on the floor (Humphries et al 1991b) and, because the open wound has no contact with the floor, there seems to be no logical reason for their use.

Sterile gloves are worn to prevent the transmission of the operator's skin flora into the wound. Evidence from operations performed with punctured gloves suggests that there is no increase in the rate of wound infection as a result of bacteria leaking out of the glove from the skin (Cruse 1986, Whyte et al 1991). Gloves are essential to protect the operator from exposure to blood and may provide some protection against needlestick injury (see Ch. 7). The use of two pairs of gloves (double-gloving) can significantly reduce the risk of puncturing the inner glove and is recommended for procedures associated with a high risk of injury (e.g. gynaecology) (Tanner & Parkinson 2004, UK Health Departments 1998).

Instruments and equipment   Items used for invasive procedures should be sterile when used (see Ch. 13). The sterility of packs can be maintained indefinitely, provided they remain intact and are not exposed to moisture, direct sunlight or heat. Those who are working close to the operation field must adhere to the principles of asepsis to minimize the risk of surgical wound infection.

Cleaning   In a modern well-managed theatre, the risk of infection from the environment is low (Ayliffe 1991b). Smears of blood and body fluid on surfaces should be removed with detergent and water after each operation and large spills removed using chlorine-releasing granules (see Ch. 7). Horizontal surfaces, which readily collect dust, should be cleaned daily and the minimum amount of equipment should be kept in the operating room to prevent the collection of dust and avoid unnecessary cleaning. Tacky mats outside the entrance to the theatre do not reduce the risk of wound infection (Ayliffe 1991b).

There is usually no need to allocate infected patients to the end of an operating list provided that spills of blood or body fluid are removed at the end of the operation, dust is removed from surfaces and ventilator tubing is changed. There is no evidence to support special cleaning procedures or for the theatre to be left empty for any more than 10–15 min (Mangram et al 1999, Woodhead et al 2002). Suspended particles will be rapidly removed by the air filtration system and the next patient can be brought into the room as soon as it has been cleaned.

Surveillance of wound infection

Surgical wound infections are an important problem: they delay the recovery of the patient, increase the length of hospital stay and may result in readmission to hospital for further treatment. These factors have obvious economic consequences. A study by Plowman et al (1999) found that patients with a surgical wound infection had an additional hospital stay of 6.5 days and their hospital costs were doubled.

Surveillance of the incidence of surgical site infections in England has demonstrated marked differences in infection rates between hospitals even when the rates are adjusted by the most important risk factors for infection (Health Protection Agency 2003a). Although some of these differences may reflect variations in patient mix or case finding, the standard of clinical practice in the operating theatre and ward and skills of the operating surgeon have a major effect.

A major study of the efficacy of infection control measures in the USA in the 1980s demonstrated the value of surveillance of surgical wound infection and reporting the rates of infection to individual surgeons (Haley et al 1985b). In hospitals with organized infection control programmes, intensive surveillance and rates of surgical wound infection reported to surgeons, surgical wound infection rates were 20% lower. If a doctor with specialist knowledge of infection control was involved in feeding back data then rates of surgical wound infection were 38% lower. The feedback of these data to surgeons focuses attention on the importance of good surgical technique in preventing wound infection and can be used to motivate change in practice where high rates are identified (Cruse & Foord 1980, Gaynes et al 2001, Haley 1986). Major reductions in wound infection rates have been reported when such surveillance and feedback programmes are used (Cruse 1986, Olsen & Lee 1990).

A scheme enabling hospitals to participate in a surveillance programme for surgical site infections was started in England in 1997 (Cooke et al 2000). This was based on a similar system, the National Nosocomial Infection Surveillance System, which had been established in the United States for several decades (Gaynes 1997). Similar surveillance systems have been developed in other parts of the United Kingdom and Europe (Wilson et al 2005). Making valid comparisons between rates of surgical wound infection requires the use of standard definitions such as those described in Box 8.5 and reliable methods of

finding cases of infection. Hospitals participating in the Surgical Site Infection Surveillance Service in England are able to compare their results by category of surgical procedure with the results aggregated from all participating hospitals. The ability of hospitals to measure their own performance against others is key to ensuring that poor performance is identified and action taken to review and improve practice (National Audit Office 2000). Data quality is of paramount importance if the results of surveillance are to truly inform clinical practice. Active methods of surveillance that use designated, trained staff to identify cases of infection are more reliable than passive methods that rely on other staff to report infections (Gaynes et al 2001, Wilson et al 2002) (see p. 56, Ch. 3).

Data required to identify surgical wound infections are not routinely available and are therefore resource intensive to collect. Surveillance may therefore need to be targeted and part of a programme of activity planned over several years.

One of the problems associated with surgical wound infection surveillance is the difficulty of detecting infections that develop after the patient has been discharged from hospital. The 60% reduction in length of hospital stay that has occurred in the UK and other developed countries over the past two decades and the increasing use of day-case surgery exacerbate this problem (Appleby 1997). As many as 50% of wound infections may develop post discharge and this can result in a significant underreporting of infection rates unless some form of postdischarge surveillance is included, although the proportion of infections that develop after discharge depends on the average length of postoperative stay and this varies for different types of surgery (Plowman et al 1999, Stockley et al 2001).

Management of surgical wounds

The dressing placed on the surgical wound in the operating theatre should not be disturbed for at least the first 48 h as bacteria may enter the wound from adjacent skin until the wound surface has sealed. If the dressing is dislodged or cannot contain the wound exudate, it should be changed using an aseptic technique (see Box 8.7).

After 48 h the dressing can be removed and wounds that are not leaking exudate and are not drained can be left exposed or protected with a transparent film dressing; the patient is able to shower or bathe (Chrintz et al 1989). Leaving the wound exposed enables the early signs of wound infection to be detected and saves dressing materials and nursing time. However, patients may experience less pain from the wound where a transparent film dressing is used (Briggs 1996). Some

Box 8.5   Definitions of surgical site infections (Health Protection Agency 2004)

Superficial incisional infection
This is defined as a surgical site infection that occurs within 30 days of operation, involves only the skin or subcutaneous tissue of the incision and meets at least one of the following criteria.

Criterion 1   Purulent drainage from the superficial incision
Criterion 2   The superficial incision yields organisms from the culture of aseptically aspirated fluid or tissue or from a swab and pus cells are present
Criterion 3   At least two of the following symptoms and signs: pain, tenderness, localized swelling, redness or heat

and

- the superficial incision is deliberately opened by a surgeon to manage the infection, unless the incision is culture negative *or*
- the clinician diagnoses a superficial incisional infection

Deep incisional infection
This is defined as a surgical site infection involving the deep tissues (i.e. muscle and fascial layers) that occurs within 30 days of operation if no implant is in place or within 1 year if an implant is in place, appears to be related to the surgical procedure and meets at least one of the following criteria.

Criterion 1   Purulent drainage from the deep incision
Criterion 2   The deep incision yields organisms from the culture of aseptically aspirated fluid or tissue or from a swab and pus cells are present
Criterion 3   A deep incision that spontaneously dehisces or is deliberately opened by a surgeon when the patient has *at least one* of the following symptoms or signs: fever (>38°C), localized pain or tenderness, unless the incision is culture negative
Criterion 4   An abscess or other evidence of infection involving the deep incision that is found by direct examination during reoperation or by histopathological or radiological examination
Criterion 5   Clinician's diagnosis of deep incisional wound infection

Organ or space infection
This is defined as a surgical site infection involving any part of the anatomy other than the incision opened or manipulated during the procedure, that occurs within 30 days of operation if no implant is in place or within 1 year if an implant is in place, appears to be related to the surgical procedure and meets at least one of the following criteria.

Criterion 1   Purulent drainage from a drain that is placed through a stab wound into the organ or space
Criterion 2   The organ or space yields organisms from the culture of aseptically aspirated fluid or tissue or from a swab and pus cells are present
Criterion 3   An abscess or other evidence of infection involving the organ or space that is found by direct examination, during reoperation or by histopathological or radiological examination
Criterion 4   Clinician's diagnosis of organ/space wound infection

wounds continue to seep serous fluid for several days. These wounds should be covered with a sterile dressing and managed using an aseptic technique, as the superficial layer of the skin will not seal until leakage of fluid has stopped. A dressing will be required to absorb excess exudate from the surface of the skin (which is not contributing to the healing process occurring under the skin). The frequency of dressing change should be dictated by the amount of exudate. The site should be cleaned, if necessary with sterile, normal saline.

Wound drains should be attached to a sterile drainage bottle which should be changed when necessary, without touching the connections and washing hands thoroughly before and after the procedure.

WOUNDS HEALING BY SECONDARY INTENTION

The term healing by secondary intention is used to describe the process of healing in wounds when there is tissue loss and the gap must be gradually filled from the base by new tissue (see Fig. 8.1). This type of wound is often referred to as a chronic wound and includes ulcers, pressure sores, burns and some surgical wounds in which closure by suture is delayed (e.g. blast injuries, dehisced wounds).

Underlying disease processes such as impaired blood supply or drainage predispose to chronic wounds that then often heal slowly and unpredictably. The exposed tissue provides a favourable environment for colonization by micro-organisms from the surrounding skin, mucosa or environment. Effective management of these wounds depends on creating an optimum environment for wound healing to take place and minimizing the adverse impact of the underlying pathophysiology, e.g. by compression bandaging of limbs to improve the blood supply (Cullum et al 2004).

Epithelialization, the formation of new granulation tissue and microcirculation are all encouraged by maintaining a moist environment at the wound bed since epithelial cells can only migrate across moist, healthy tissue (Collier 2002, Winter 1962). However, it is also important to absorb excess moisture that may otherwise cause surrounding skin to become excoriated or macerated. Modern dressing materials, such as alginates, hydrocolloids and hydrogels, are designed to absorb excess exudate whilst at the same time providing the warm, moist environment that is most likely to promote wound healing (Box 8.6). Attempting to discourage bacterial growth in a wound by removing exudate and keeping the wound surface dry is inappropriate for wounds healing by secondary intention. Wound exudates contain macrophages. These not only play a role in destroying bacteria and preventing infection of the tissues but also, through the release of cytokines, they co-ordinate the wound healing process. Their activity requires oxygen and warmth and is enhanced if the wound is occluded (Buchan et al 1980, Clarke 1985). Research has shown that modern occlusive dressings can be safely used on wounds without increasing the risk of infection or encouraging the growth of anaerobic bacteria (Gilchrist & Reed 1989).

The volume of wound exudate generally decreases as healing takes place so it is important to regularly review the dressing to ensure optimum exudate control (Thomas 1997).

Removing the dressing reduces the temperature of the wound and may disrupt the delicate new tissue; dressing changes should therefore be kept to a minimum. Because bacteria are not removed from the surface of the wound by cleaning but are simply redistributed (Tomlinson 1987), dressings should not be changed simply to 'clean' the wound. Dressings on

---

Box 8.6   Properties of an ideal wound dressing for wounds healing by secondary intention

- Maintains a high humidity. Epithelial cells require moist conditions to migrate
- Provides thermal insulation. Tissue repair occurs best at a constant temperature of 37°C
- Is impermeable to bacteria. Helps to prevent cross-infection
- Allows gaseous exchange. Promotes healing
- Removes excess exudate. There is a balance between removal of exudate to prevent tissue maceration whilst maintaining a moist environment. Exudate contains white blood cells, which protect the wound from invasion by bacteria
- Is non-adherent, preventing the removal of newly formed tissue and capillaries when dressings are changed
- Is non-toxic and non-allergenic. Avoids interference with healing
- Comfortable and acceptable to the patient

---

large wounds healing by secondary intention can be removed more easily and with less damage to the underlying tissue, by irrigation with a syringe of normal saline or by soaking off with water in a bath or shower (Fernandez et al 2004).

The presence of ischaemic or necrotic tissue delays wound healing and because host defences are impaired in poorly perfused or hypoxic tissue, microorganisms can readily grow and multiply (Bowler et al 2001). Devitalized tissue should therefore be removed to minimize the risk of infection and accelerate healing (NICE 2001). There are a number of approaches to debridement including surgical removal, chemicals or enzymes and dressings that encourage the normal wound debriding processes such as hydrocolloids, hydrogels and alginates. These also have the advantage of reducing pain from the wound without impairing healing (Benbow 2002).

The use of chemicals (e.g. hypochlorite, hydrogen peroxide) to debride wounds should be avoided as there is little evidence to support their ability to remove dead tissue and some evidence to suggest that they delay wound healing (Brennan et al 1986, Gruber et al 1975, Leaper 1986). Recently, interest in the old remedies of using maggots and leeches to clean wounds of dead and necrotic material has increased. Maggots are bred in sterile conditions and then put into a wound at a ratio of 10 maggots per square centimetre. They use powerful proteolytic enzymes to liquefy dead tissue, which they then digest (Cork 1997).

The care of the wound should not be directed solely at the dressing procedure. Adequate nutrition is essential to encourage rapid wound healing and thereby reduce the possibility of wound infection. Collagen, the principal building material for the repair of wounds, is a protein; vitamin C is essential for collagen synthesis and other trace elements, such as zinc and copper, are also important for the healing process. Nutrition is particularly important to aid wound healing in patients with a poor nutritional state caused by malignancy, malabsorption syndromes or temporary starvation (Shepherd 2003).

Promoting a good blood supply to the wound will also aid healing. The relief of pressure from pressure sores is essential if an adequate blood supply is to reach the wound.

Burns

Burns are always colonized by a variety of micro-organisms. Although most do not usually interfere with healing, some may invade the tissues and cause septicaemia, a frequent and serious complication of patients with severe burns. *Streptococcus pyogenes* and *Pseudomonas aeruginosa* may interfere with skin grafting and cause invasive infections that are sometimes fatal (Lowbury & Cason 1985).

Patients with 60% or more of their body surface affected by burns are most vulnerable to infection. Two-thirds will develop infection on the burnt area and most will also develop secondary bloodstream infection (Weber et al 1997). Bacterial multiplication is enhanced because of impaired neutrophil and lymphocyte activity (Dong et al 1993). Pathogens encountered in burn wounds change over time. Initially Gram-negative bacteria predominate but these are replaced after the first few days by Gram-negative species. Occasionally burns may be infected by fungi such as candida and aspergillus, or viruses (e.g. herpes simplex).

The modern approach to the treatment of burns is prompt excision of the burn wound and covering with a skin graft or skin substitute. This reduces the time during which the wound is exposed and has had a marked effect on the incidence of infection associated with burns (Mozingo et al 1998).

Cross-infection is a major problem in burns units, particularly with *S. aureus*, pseudomonas and other Gram-negative bacilli such as acinetobacter. The main risk of transmission is on the hands of staff. Contaminated equipment has also been implicated in outbreaks of infection in burns units. Kolmos et al (1993) reported an outbreak of infection associated with tubes used to irrigate wounds.

All staff should wear appropriate protective clothing for contact with patients, discard it after each use and wash hands thoroughly between patients.

The large surface area of damaged skin increases the probability of micro-organisms being introduced from an airborne route, particularly those bacteria that are more resistant to desiccation such as staphylococci and acinetobacter. The use of single-bed rooms may help to minimize the risk of cross-infection but special ventilation is probably not necessary for most types of infection (Mozingo et al 1998). Large numbers of bacteria may be released during dressing changes and the use of a dressing room supplied with filtered air at around 10 changes per hour has been recommended (Ayliffe & Lilly 1985).

For patients who are not critically ill, cleansing is most easily achieved in a shower. Topical antimicrobial solutions are used to control colonization and reduce the mortality rate associated with burns. Commonly used agents are based on silver compounds, usually bonding silver with an antimicrobial agent called sulphonamide (silver sulfadiazine). Silver impairs the electron transport system of bacteria and is generally considered as a safe, broad-spectrum antimicrobial agent (Lansdown 2002). It is often used in a slow-release oil-based cream which should be cleansed from the wound and reapplied every 12 hours. A range of other dressing formulations containing silver have now also been developed although their efficacy as antimicrobial agents depends on the amount of silver they release (Demling & DeSanti 2001).

THE 'ASEPTIC TECHNIQUE'

When the normal defences of the body are breached, the tissues are vulnerable to invasion by micro-organisms. The aseptic technique (Box 8.7) aims to prevent micro-organisms on hands, surfaces or equipment from being introduced to such a susceptible site. It should also prevent micro-organisms from the patient being transferred to staff or other patients. The aseptic technique has become incorporated into nursing ritual and is often based more on tradition than on rational reason or research evidence. It is frequently performed without reference to the underlying principles of infection prevention or to the requirements of the situation to which it is being applied (Walsh & Ford 1989).

A good example of this is the preparation of the trolley. There is no evidence that bacteria on the trolley are transferred into the wound, or vice versa, and routine cleaning of trolleys with alcohol between patients probably serves no useful purpose provided the surface of the trolley is regularly

Box 8.7   Aseptic technique

Aim

To minimize the risk of introducing pathogenic organisms into a wound or other susceptible site and to prevent the transfer of pathogens from the wound to other patients or staff.

Indications

- Wounds healing by primary intention (before surface skin has sealed)
- Intravenous cannulation
- Urinary catheterization
- Suturing
- Vaginal examination during labour
- Medical invasive procedures

Principles

1. Ensure that all equipment required is readily available and there is a clear field in which to carry out the procedure
2. Explain the procedure to the patient, obtain oral consent and position the patient so that the procedure can be performed easily
3. Wash hands or decontaminate clean hands with an alcohol handrub
4. Open the sterile pack carefully to prevent contamination of the contents
5. Wear sterile gloves for the procedure to prevent the introduction of pathogenic bacteria to the site or direct contact with body fluids
6. Use aseptic principles to ensure that:
   - only sterile items come into contact with the susceptible site
   - sterile items do not come into contact with non-sterile objects
7. After completion, discard waste contaminated with body fluid into an appropriate plastic bag and sharps into a sharps container
8. Discard protective clothing and wash hands to prevent cross-infection to others

However, forceps are cumbersome to use and do not prevent the transfer of bacteria from the wound to the hands (Tomlinson 1987). The procedure can be performed more easily holding sterile swabs in the hands (Briggs 1994), using gloves to prevent direct contact between hands and a vulnerable site.

The purpose of cleaning a wound is to remove excess exudate and necrotic tissue in order to minimize the amount of material present that could support the growth of micro-organisms. Antiseptics are of little value since they are only in contact with the wound for a short time (White et al 2001).

Assessment of the circumstances of individual patients is vital (Briggs et al 1996). In many situations a modified aseptic or 'clean' technique is more appropriate (Box 8.8), for example during the removal of sutures from a sealed surgical wound or the application of dressings to wounds healing by secondary intention. In the latter situation, the wound probably already contains large numbers of different bacterial species and will frequently be exposed to new bacteria from the environment. The greatest concern is to ensure that potential pathogens are not transferred to another patient. Clean, rather than sterile, gloves are usually acceptable as when removed from the dispensing box they are likely to be contaminated only by very small numbers of bacteria of low pathogenicity (Rossof et al 1993). In chronic wounds healing by secondary intention dressings are probably best removed by bathing or irrigation with saline or tap water and the use of a rigorous aseptic technique is unnecessary (Fernandez et al 2004, Hollinworth & Kingston 1998).

Preventing cross-infection

Preventing the transmission of micro-organisms from one patient to another is a particular problem with heavily colonized or infected wounds. An organism colonizing the wound of one patient may be transmitted to cause infection in another patient and, as illustrated by Tomlinson (1987), bacteria are easily acquired on the hands whilst cleaning a wound, even if forceps are used.

The use of disposable gloves minimizes the risk of acquiring bacteria on the hands but hands should still be washed before and after dressing wounds.

Bacteria acquired on the clothing during the procedure may be transferred into the wound of another patient; therefore a clean disposable apron should be used for each dressing procedure.

If dressings are removed by soaking in bathwater or bowls, the bath or bowl should be thoroughly cleaned with detergent and then dried to ensure that

cleaned with detergent and water (Thompson & Bullock 1992).

The important principles are that the susceptible site should not come into contact with any item that is not sterile and that any items that have been in contact with the wound may be contaminated and should be discarded safely or decontaminated. Because hands are not sterile, forceps have traditionally been used for the procedure, probably because disposable gloves are a relatively recent introduction to medical care.

Box 8.8   Clean technique

Aim

To avoid the introduction of pathogens to a susceptible site and to prevent the transfer of pathogens to other patients or staff.

Indications

- Dressing of wounds healing by secondary intention
- Removal of sutures
- Dressing intravenous lines
- Removal of drains
- Endotracheal suction
- Dressing tracheostomy site

Principles

1. Ensure that all equipment required is ready and that a clean area on which to place it is available
2. Explain the procedure to the patient, obtain verbal consent and position the patient so that the procedure can be performed easily
3. Wash hands and disinfect with alcohol handrub
4. If direct contact with blood or body fluid is anticipated, wear clean gloves and a plastic apron
5. Use sterile swabs to clean the site or irrigate with saline or water and apply a sterile dressing
6. Avoid touching any unclean area while performing the procedure
7. On completion of the procedure, dispose of all waste contaminated with body fluid into an appropriate plastic bag
8. Discard gloves and apron and wash hands to prevent cross-infection to others

pathogens are removed before use by the next patient.

In the past it has been recommended that wounds should not be redressed when cleaning or bedmaking is in progress because of the risk of airborne contamination. However, it has been shown that although such activities increase the number of bacteria in the air, the increase is not sufficient to present a risk of infection by organisms settling on to a dressing trolley (Ayliffe et al 1999).

Dressing clinics Particular care must be taken to prevent cross-infection between patients attending ulcer treatment or dressing clinics where there are plenty of opportunities for transmission to occur and the rapid turnover of patients may encourage inadequate cleaning of equipment between patients. Bacteria in the wound will have contaminated the

dressings and the surrounding skin and hands must always be washed after touching dressings or skin. Gloves and a plastic apron should be worn for the removal and application of dressings and must be changed after each patient. Creams and dressing materials must be used for one patient only. Equipment such as buckets for soaking off dressings and scissors must be thoroughly cleaned with detergent and water and dried after each patient.

DETECTION AND TREATMENT OF WOUND INFECTION

The diagnosis of wound infection is based on the presence of clinical signs rather than the isolation of micro-organisms from a wound swab, since micro-organisms may only be colonizing the wound and not invading the tissues (Box 8.9). Surgical wounds should be inspected regularly for signs of infection so that prompt treatment with systemic antimicrobial therapy can be initiated (Plate 25).

Detection of infection in wounds healing by secondary intention is more difficult. Slough is easily mistaken for pus and in some situations pus collects on the surface of the wound but without evidence of tissue invasion (Plate 26). The most significant indicator of infection is inflammation spreading from the margins of the wound, local oedema, the patient reporting a marked increase in pain in the wound or a pyrexia where no other focus of infection can be identified (Hutchinson & Lawrence 1991). Other

Box 8.9   Signs of wound infection

- Pain
- Inflammation at wound margins
- Oedema
- Pyrexia
- Purulent exudate

Additional criteria to be considered in wounds healing by secondary intention*

- Delayed healing
- Discoloration
- Friable granulation tissue that bleeds easily
- Unexpected pain/tenderness
- Pocketing at base of wound
- New epithelium fragile, blue-coloured
- Abnormal smell
- Wound breakdown

* Source: Cutting & Harding 1994.

criteria may also need to be considered such as delayed healing, friable granulation tissue or discoloration. However, the relationship between these and infection has not been tested in some types of chronic wounds such as leg ulcers and burns (Cutting & Harding 1994) (see Box 8.9). Wound culture may be indicated for chronic wounds that are persistently failing to respond to appropriate wound care (Kingsley 2003).

Purulent fluid or tissue samples provide the best guide to organisms responsible for wound infection. However, swabbing the surface of a wound that has been pre-cleaned to remove traces of occlusive dressing or antimicrobials can still provide a useful assessment of potential causative micro-organisms (Health Protection Agency 2003b). Although anaerobic bacteria do not appear to usually impair healing of chronic wounds, they should not be overlooked as a cause of infection or failure to heal (Bowler et al 2001).

Clear clinical information is essential to help the microbiologist decide which tests should be undertaken. For example, a sacral sore is more likely to be infected by faecal organisms; a malodorous wound may indicate infection by anaerobes and special tests are required to detect these (Health Protection Agency 2003a) (see Ch. 2).

Whilst antimicrobial agents should not be prescribed routinely for chronic wounds, their use is indicated for overt infection since topical antiseptic solutions are unlikely to reach organisms that are invading the tissue and their antibacterial activity is probably lost rapidly in the presence of blood and tissue.

However, whilst not recommended for the treatment of overt infection, antiseptics may have a place in the management of non-healing wounds where high levels of bacteria colonizing the wound are suspected to be contributing to delayed healing. Slow-release, low-concentration formulations of iodine (cadexomer iodine) or silver in combination with occlusive dressings have been recommended for short-term use on non-healing wounds until the wound begins to show signs of healing (Sunberg & Meller 1997, White et al 2001).

Antiseptic solutions should be used with caution as many have not been well researched and their effects on wound healing and on bacteria in the wound are unknown (O'Meara et al 2001). Hypochlorites may be toxic to granulation tissue and delay healing (Brennan et al 1986) and there are also concerns about chlorhexidine and povidone-iodine which have been shown to destroy fibroblasts in tissue culture (Gruber et al 1975, Leaper 1986, Neidner & Schopf 1986).

References

Alexander JW, Fischer JE, Boyajian M et al (1983) The influence of hair-removal methods on wound infections. *Arch. Surg.*, **118**: 347–52.

Appleby J (1997) The English patient. *Health Service J.*, **10 April**: 36–7.

Ayliffe GAJ (1991a) Masks in surgery? *J. Hosp. Infect.*, **18**: 165–6.

Ayliffe GAJ (1991b) Role of the environment of the operating suite in surgical wound infection. *Rev. Infect. Dis.*, **13**(10): 5800–4.

Ayliffe GAJ, Lilly HA (1985) Cross-infection and its prevention. *J. Hosp. Infect.*, **6** (suppl. B): 47–57.

Ayliffe GAJ, Noy ME, Davies JG et al (1983) A comparison of pre-operative bathing with chlorhexidine-detergent and a non-medicated soap in the prevention of wound infection. *J. Hosp. Infect.*, **4**: 237–44.

Ayliffe GAJ, Babb JR, Taylor LJ (1999) *Hospital Acquired Infection – Principles and Prevention*, 3rd edn. Butterworth, London.

Ayton M (1985) Wounds that won't heal. *Nursing Times*, **81**(46) (suppl.): 16–19.

Barrie D, Wilson JA, Hoffman PN et al (1992) *Bacillus cereus* meningitis in two neurosurgical patients: an investigation into the source of the organism. *J. Infect.*, **25**: 291–7.

Belkin NL (1997) The evolution of the surgical mask: filtering efficiency versus effectiveness. *Infect. Contr. Hosp. Epidemiol.*, **18**(1): 49–57.

Belkin NL (2002) Surgical masks in the operating theatre: are they still necessary? *J. Hosp. Infect.*, **50**: 233.

Benbow M (2002) Necrotic wounds. *Nurse2Nurse*, **12**(11): 54–6.

Blom AW, Gozzardi C, Heal J et al (2002) Bacterial strike-through of re-usable surgical drapes: the effect of different wetting agents. *J. Hosp. Infect.*, **52**: 52–5.

Bowler PG, Duerdin BI, Armstrong DG (2001) Wound microbiology and associated approaches to wound management. *Clin. Microbiol. Rev.*, **14**(2): 244–69.

Brennan SS, Foster ME, Leaper DJ (1986) Antiseptic toxicity in wounds healing by secondary intention. *J. Hosp. Infect.*, **8**: 263–7.

Briggs M (1994) Examining equipment for wound care: the use of forceps and cotton wool in dressing packs. *Accid. Emerg. Nurs.*, **2**(4): 237–9.

Briggs M (1996) Surgical wound pain: a trial of two treatments. *J. Wound Care*, **5**(10): 156–60.

Briggs M, Wilson S, Fuller A (1996) The principles of aseptic technique in wound care. *Prof. Nurse*, **11**(12): 805–8.

Buchan IA, Andrews JK, Lang SM et al (1980) Clinical and laboratory investigation of the composition and properties of human skin wound exudate under semi-permeable dressings. *Burns*, **7**: 326–34.

Chrintz H, Vibits H, Cordtz TO et al (1989) Need for surgical wound dressing. *Br. J. Surg.*, **76**: 204–5.

Clarke RAF (1985) Cutaneous tissue repair: basic biological considerations I. *J. Am. Acad. Dermatol.*, **13**: 701–25.

Collier M (2002) Wound-bed management: key principles for practice. *Prof. Nurse*, **18**(4): 221–5.

Communicable Disease Report Weekly (2004) Surgical site infection surveillance in England. *CDR Weekly*, **14**(21): 1–5.

Cooke EMC, Coello RC, Sedgwick J et al (2000) A national surveillance scheme for hospital-associated infections in England. *J. Hosp. Infect.*, **46**: 1–3.

Cork A (1997) Maggots that munch. *Hosp. Equip. Supplies Suppl.*, **August**: 28.

Cruse PJE (1986) Surgical infection: incisional wounds. In: Bennett JV, Brachman PS (eds) *Hospital Infections*, 2nd edn. Little, Brown, Boston, MA.

Cruse PJE, Foord R (1973) A five-year prospective study of 23649 surgical wounds. *Arch. Surg.*, **107**: 206.

Cruse PJE, Foord R (1980) The epidemiology of wound infection – a 10 year prospective study of 62939 wounds. *Surg. Clin. North Am.*, **60**(1): 27–40.

Cullum N, Nelson EA, Fletcher AW et al (2004) Compression for venous leg ulcers (Cochrane Review). The Cochrane Library. Issue 2. John Wiley, Chichester.

Culver DH, Horan TC, Gaynes RP et al (1991) Surgical wound infection rates by wound class, operative procedure and patient risk index. *Am. J. Med.*, **91** (suppl. 3B): 152S–157S.

Cutting KF, Harding KG (1994) Criteria for identifying wound infection. *J. Wound Care*, **3**(4): 198–201.

Demling RH, DeSanti L (2001) The role of silver in wound healing. Part 1: effects of silver on wound management. *Wounds*, **13** (suppl. 1): A3–A15.

Desia H (1997) Aging and wounds. Part 2. *J. Wound Care*, **6**(5): 237–9.

Dong YL, Abdullah K, Yan TZ et al (1993) Effect of thermal injury and sepsis on neutrophil function. *J. Trauma*, **34**: 417–21.

Drinkwater LJ, Neil MJ (1995) Optimal timing of wound drain removal following joint arthroplasty. *J. Arthroplasty*, **10**(2): 185–9.

Elek SD, Conen PE (1957) The virulence of *Staphylococcus pyogenes* for men: a study of the problems of wound infection. *Br. J. Exper. Pathol.*, **38**: 573–86.

Emmerson AM, Enstone JE, Griffin M et al (1996) The second national prevalence survey of infection in hospitals – overview of the results. *J. Hosp. Infect.*, **32**: 175–90.

Fernandez R, Griffiths R, Ussia C (2004) Water for wound cleansing (Cochrane Review). The Cochrane Library. Issue 2. John Wiley, Chichester.

Gaynes R (1997) Surveillance of nosocomial infections: a fundamental ingredient for quality. *Infect. Contr. Hosp. Epidemiol.*, **18**(7): 175–8.

Gaynes R, Richards C, Edwards J et al (2001) Feeding back surveillance data to prevent hospital-acquired infections. *Emerg. Infect. Dis.*, **7**(2): 295–301.

Gilchrist B, Reed C (1989) The bacteriology of leg ulcers under hydrocolloid dressings. *Br. J. Dermatol.*, **121**: 337–44.

Gosden PE, MacGowen AP, Bannister GC (1998) Importance of air quality and related factors in the prevention of infection in orthopaedic implant surgery. *J. Hosp. Infect.*, **39**: 173–80.

Gruber RB, Vistnes L, Pardoe R (1975) The effect of commonly used antiseptics on wound healing. *Plast. Reconstr. Surg.*, **55**: 472–6.

Haley RW (1986) *Managing Hospital Infection Control for Cost-effectiveness*. American Hospital Publishing, Chicago.

Haley RW, Culver DH, Morgan WM et al (1985a) Identifying patients at risk of surgical wound infection: a simple multivariate index of patient susceptibility and wound contamination. *Am. J. Epidemiol.*, **121**(2): 206–15.

Haley RW, Culver DH, White JW et al (1985b) The efficacy of infection surveillance and control programs in preventing nosocomial infection in US hospitals (SENIC Study). *Am. J. Epidemiol.*, **121**(2): 182–205.

Hambreaus A (1988) Aerobiology in operating rooms. *J. Hosp. Infect.*, **11** (suppl. A): 68–76.

Health Protection Agency (2003a) *Surveillance of Surgical Site Infection in English Hospitals 1997–2002*. Nosocomial Infection National Surveillance Scheme, London. Available online at: www.hpa.org.uk.

Health Protection Agency (2003b) *Investigation of Skin and Superficial Wound Swabs*. BSOP 11. Issue 3.1. Standards Unit, Evaluations and Standards Laboratory. Health Protection Agency, London. Available online at: www.hpa.org.uk/srmd/div_esl_su/sops_docs/bsops/bsop11i3.1.pdf.

Health Protection Agency (2004) *Protocol for Surveillance of Surgical Site Infection. Version 3.4*. Health Protection Agency, London. Available online at: www.hpa.org.uk.

Heiss MM, Mempel W, Jauch KW et al (1993) Beneficial effect of autologous blood transfusion on infectious complications after colorectal cancer surgery. *Lancet*, **342**: 1328–33.

Henderson B, Poole S, Wilson M (1996) Microbial/host interactions in health and disease: who controls the cytokine network? *Immunopharmacology*, **35**: 1–21.

Hoborn J (1990) Wet strike-through and transfer of bacteria through operating barrier fabrics. *Hyg. Med.*, **15**: 15–20.

Hoffman PN, Williams J, Stacey A et al (2002) Microbiological commissioning and monitoring of operating theatre suites. A report of a working party of the Hospital Infection Society. *J. Hosp. Infect.*, **52**: 1–28.

Hollinworth H, Kingston JE (1998) Using a non-sterile technique in wound care. *Prof. Nurse*, **13**(4): 226–9.

Holzheimer RG, Haupt W, Thriede A et al (1997) The challenge of post-operative infections. Does the surgeon make a difference? *Infect. Contr. Hosp. Epidemiol.*, **18**: 449–56.

Howarth FH (1985) Prevention of airborne infection during surgery. *Lancet*, **i**: 386–8.

Hubble MJ, Welae AE, Perez JV et al (1996) Clothing in laminar flow operating theatres. *J. Hosp. Infect.*, **32**: 1–7.

Humphries H, Russell AJ, Marshall RJ et al (1991a) The effect of surgical theatre head-gear on air bacterial counts. *J. Hosp. Infect.*, **19**: 175–80.

Humphries H, Marshall RJ, Ricketts VE (1991b) Theatre overshoes do not reduce operating floor bacterial counts. *J. Hosp. Infect.*, **17**: 117–24.

Hunt TR, Hopf HW (1997) Wound healing and wound infection. What surgeons and anaesthetists can do. *Surg. Clin. North Am.*, **77**(3): 587–606.

Hutchinson JJ, Lawrence JC (1991) Wound infection under occlusive dressings. *J. Hosp. Infect.*, **17**: 83–94.

Johnson DH, Fairclough JA, Brown EM et al (1987) Rate of bacterial decolonization of the skin after preparation: four methods compared. *Br. J. Surg.*, **74**: 64.

Kalmeijer MD, Coertjens H, van Nieuwland-Bollen PM et al (2002) Surgical site infections in orthopaedic surgery: the effect of mupirocin nasal ointment in a double-blind, randomised placebo-controlled study. *Clin. Infect. Dis.*, **35**: 353–8.

Kingsley A (2003) Audit of wound swab sampling: why protocols should improve practice. *Prof. Nurse*, **18**(6): 338–43.

Kluytmans J (1997) Surgical infections including burns. In: Wenzel RP (ed.) *Prevention and Control of Nosocomial Infection*, 3rd edn. Williams and Wilkins, Baltimore, MD.

Kluytmans J (1998) Reduction of surgical site infections in major surgery by elimination of nasal carriage of *Staphylococcus aureus*. *J. Hosp. Infect.*, **40** (suppl. B): S25–S30.

Kluytmans J, Voss A (2002) Prevalence of post surgical infection: some like it hot. *Curr. Opin. Infect. Dis.*, **15**: 427–32.

Kluytmans J, Moulon JW, Ijzerman EPF et al (1995) Nasal carriage of *Staphylococcus aureus* as a major risk factor for wound infections after cardiac surgery. *J. Infect. Dis.*, **171**: 216–19.

Ko W, Lazenby WD, Zelano JA et al (1992) Effects of shaving methods and intraoperative irrigation on suppurative mediastinitis after bypass operations. *Ann. Thorac. Surg.*, **53**: 301–5.

Kolmos HJ, Thuesen B, Nielsen SV et al (1993) Outbreak of infection in a burns unit due to *Pseudomonas aeruginosa* originating from contaminated tubing used for irrigation of patients. *J. Hosp. Infect.*, **24**: 11–21.

Korten V, Murray BE (1993) The nosocomial transmission of enterococci. *Curr. Opin. Infect. Dis.*, **6**: 498–505.

Kriezek TJ, Robson MC (1975) Biology of surgical infection. *Surg. Clin. North Am.*, **55**: 1262–7.

Kurz A, Sessler DI, Lenhardt R et al (1996) Pre-operative normothermia to reduce the incidence of surgical wound infections and shorten hospitalisation. *N. Engl. J. Med.*, **334**(19): 1209.

Lansdown A (2002) Silver: its antibacterial properties and mechanisms of action. *J. Wound Care*, **11**(4): 125–3.

Lathan R, Lancaster AD, Covington JF et al (2001) The association between diabetes and glucose control with surgical site infection among cardiothoracic surgery patients. *Infect. Contr. Hosp. Epidemiol.*, **22**: 607–12.

Leaper DJ (1986) Antiseptics and their effect on healing tissue. *Nursing Times*, **82**(22): 45–7.

Lidwell OM, Lowbury EJL, Whyte W et al (1982) Effect of ultraclean air in operating rooms on deep sepsis in the joint after total hip or knee replacement; a randomised study. *BMJ*, **285**: 10–14.

Lowbury EJL, Cason JS (1985) Aspects of infection control and skin grafting in burned patients. In: Westerby S (ed.) *Wound Care*. Heinemann Medical, London.

Lynch W, Davey PG, Malek M et al (1992) Cost-effectiveness analysis of the use of chlorhexidine detergent in preoperative whole-body disinfection in wound infection prophylaxis. *J. Hosp. Infect.*, **21**: 179–91.

Mangram AJ, Horan TC, Pearson ML et al (1999) Guideline for the prevention of surgical site infections, 1999. *Am. J. Infect. Contr.*, **27**: 97–134.

Matthews J, Slater K, Newsom SWB (1985) The effect of surgical gowns made with barrier cloth on bacterial dispersal. *J. Hyg.*, **95**: 123–30.

McNally HB, Cutter GR, Ruttenber A et al (2001) Hypothermia as a risk factor for pediatric cardiothoracic surgical site infection. *Paed. Infect. Dis. J.*, **20**: 459–62.

Melling AC, Ali B, Scott EM, Leaper DJ (2001) Effects of pre-operative warming on the incidence of wound infection after clean surgery: a randomised controlled trial. *Lancet*, **358**: 876–8.

Millward S (1992) The hazards of communal razors. *Nursing Times*, **88**(6): 58–62.

Mitchell NJ, Hunt S (1991) Surgical face masks in modern operating rooms – a costly and unnecessary ritual? *J. Hosp. Infect.*, **18**: 239–42.

Mozingo DW, Mcmanus AT, Pruitt BA Jr (1998) Infections of burn wounds. In: Bennett JV, Brachman PS (eds) *Hospital Infections*, 4th edn. Lippincott-Raven, Philadelphia.

National Audit Office (2000) *The Management and Control of Hospital Acquired Infection in Acute NHS Trusts in England. Report of the Comptroller Auditor General*. Stationery Office, London.

National Institute for Clinical Excellence (2001) *Guidance on the Use of Debriding Agents and Specialist Wound Clinics for Difficult to Heal Surgical Wounds*. Technology Appraisal Guidance No. 24. National Institute for Clinical Excellence, London.

Neidner R, Schopf E (1986) Inhibition of wound healing by antiseptics. *Br. J. Dermatol.*, **115**(S31): 41–4.

Nicholson ML, Dennis MJ, Makin GB et al (1994) Obesity as a risk factor in major reconstructive vascular surgery. *Eur. J. Vasc. Surg.*, **8**: 209–13.

Noone MR, Pitt TL, Bedder M et al (1983) *Pseudomonas aeruginosa* colonization in an intensive therapy unit: role of cross infection and host factors. *BMJ*, **286**: 341–4.

Ojarjärvi J (1976) An evaluation of antiseptics used for hand disinfection in wards. *J. Hyg. (Camb.)*, **76**: 75–82.

Olsen MM, Lee JT Jr (1990) Continuous 10-year wound infection surveillance. Results, advantages and unanswered questions. *Arch. Surg.*, **125**: 794–803.

O'Meara SM, Cullum NA, Majid M et al (2001) Systematic review of antimicrobial agents used for chronic wounds. *Br. J. Surg.*, **88**: 4–21.

O'Shaughnessy M, O'Malley VP, Corbett G et al (1991) Optimum duration of surgical scrub-time. *Br. J. Surg.*, **78**: 685–6.

Passaro DJ, Waring L, Armstrong R et al (1997) Postoperative *Serratia marcescens* wound infection traced to an out-of-hospital source. *J. Infect. Dis.*, **175**(4): 992–5.

Plowman R, Graves N, Griffin M et al (1999) *The Socio-economic Burden of Hospital-acquired Infection*. Public Health Laboratory Service, London.

Ridgeway S, Wilson J, Charlet A et al (2005) Surgical site infection after hip arthroplasty. *J. Bone and Joint Surgery*, **87-B**: 844–50.

Rossof LJ, Lam S, Hilton E et al (1993) Is the use of boxed gloves in an intensive care unit safe? *Am. J. Med.*, **94**(6): 602–7.

Rotstein C, Ferguson R, Cummings KM et al (1992) Determinants of clean surgical wound infection for breast procedures at an oncology center. *Infect. Contr. Hosp. Epidemiol.*, **13**: 207–14.

Schierholz JM, Beuth J (2001) Implant infections: a haven for opportunistic bacteria. *J. Hosp. Infect.*, **49**: 87–93.

Schweizer RT (1976) Mask wiggling as a potential source of wound contamination. *Lancet*, **ii**: 1129–30.

Seropian R, Reynolds BM (1971) Wound infections after preoperative depilatory versus razor preparation. *Am. J. Surg.*, **121**: 251–6.

Shepherd A (2003) Nutrition for optimum wound healing. *Nursing Standard*, **18**(6): 55–8.

Slaughter MS, Olsen MM, Lee JT et al (1993) A 15-year wound surveillance study after coronary artery by-pass. *Ann. Thorac. Surg.*, **56**: 1063–8.

Stockley JM, Allen RM, Thomlinson DF et al (2001) A district general hospital's method of post-operative infection surveillance including post-discharge follow-up, developed over a 5-year period. *J. Hosp. Infect.*, **49**: 48–54.

Sunberg J, Meller R (1997) A retrospective review of the use of cadexomer iodine in the treatment of chronic wounds. *Wounds*, **9**(3): 68–86.

Tanner J, Parkinson H (2004) Double gloving to reduce cross infection (Cochrane Review). The Cochrane Library. Issue 2. John Wiley, Chichester.

Thomas S (1997) Assessment and management of wound exudate. *J. Wound Care*, **6**(7): 327–30.

Thompson G, Bullock D (1992) To clean or not to clean? *Nursing Times*, **88**(34): 66–8.

Tomlinson D (1987) To clean or not to clean? *Nursing Times*, **83**(9): 71–5.

UK Health Departments (1998) *Guidance for Clinical Health Care Workers: Protection Against Infection with Blood Borne Viruses. Recommendations of the Expert Advisory Group on Hepatitis.* HMSO, London.

Valentine RJ, Weigelt JA, Dryer D et al (1986) Effect of remote infection on clean wound infection rates. *Am. J. Infect. Contr.*, **14**: 64–7.

Verwaal VJ, Wobbes T, Koopman van Gemert AW et al (1992) Effect of perioperative blood transfusion and cell saver on the incidence of postoperative infective complications in patients with an aneurysm of the abdominal aorta. *Eur. J. Surg.*, **158**: 477–80.

Walsh M, Ford P (1989) *Nursing Rituals, Research and Rational Actions*. Butterworth-Heinemann, Oxford.

Weber JM, Sheridan RL, Pasternack MS et al (1997) Nosocomial infections in pediatric patients with burns. *Am. J. Infect. Contr.*, **25**: 145–201.

White RJ, Cooper R, Kingsley A (2001) Wound colonization and infection: the role of topical antimicrobials. *Br. J. Nurs.*, **10**(9): 563–78.

Whyte W, Vesley D, Hodgson R (1976) Bacterial dispersion in relation to operating room clothing. *J. Hyg.*, **76**: 367–78.

Whyte W, Hodgson R, Tinkler J (1982) The importance of airborne bacterial contamination of wounds. *J. Hosp. Infect.*, **2**: 349–54.

Whyte W, Hamblen DL, Kelly IG et al (1990) An investigation of occlusive polyester surgical clothing. *J. Hosp. Infect.*, **15**: 363–74.

Whyte W, Hambreaus A, Laurell G et al (1991) The relative importance of routes and sources of wound contamination during general surgery. 1. Non-airborne. *J. Hosp. Infect.*, **18**: 93–107.

Wigglesworth N (2003) The new European Standard for surgical drapes and gowns: issues and implications. *Br. J. Inf. Contr.*, **4**(5): 35–6.

Williams REO (1963) Healthy carriage of *Staphylococcus aureus*: its prevalence and importance. *Bacteriol. Rev.*, **27**: 56–71.

Wilson JA, Clark JJ (2003) Obesity: impediment to wound healing. *Crit. Care Nurs. Qterly*, **26**(2): 119–32.

Wilson J, Ward V, Coello R et al (2002) A user evaluation of the National Nosocomial Infection Surveillance System: surgical site infection module. *J. Hosp. Infect.*, **52**: 114–21.

Wilson J , Suetens C, De Laet C et al (2005) Hospitals in Europe Link for Infection Control Through Surveillance (HELICS). Intercountry comparison of rates of surgical site infection: opportunities and limitations. Society of Hospital Epidemiologists of America, 15th Annual Conference. Abstract 05-A-523.

Winston KR (1992) Hair and neurosurgery. *Neurosurgery*, **31**(2): 320–9.

Winter GD (1962) Formation of the scab and the rate of epithelialisation of superficial wounds in the skin of the young domestic pig. *Nature*, **193**: 293–4.

Woodhead K, Taylor EW, Bannister G et al (2002) Behaviours and rituals in the operating theatre. *J. Hosp. Infect.*, **51**: 241–55.

Further Reading

Briggs M (1997) Principles of closed surgical wound care. *J. Wound Care*, **6**(6): 288–92.

Hampton S, Collins F (2004) *Tissue Viability*. Whurr, London.

Health Protection Agency (2003) *Standard Operating Procedure. Investigation of Abscesses and of Post-operative Wound and Deep-seated Infections*. BSOP 14, Issue 3.1.

Standards Unit, Evaluations and Standards Laboratory. Health Protection Agency, London. Available online at: www.hpa.org.uk.

Little K, Rutherford M, Jenkins M (1999) Ritual or reason? *Nursing Times*, **95**(20): 57–9.

Rainey J (2002) *Wound Care. A Handbook for Community Nurses*. Whurr, London.

Chapter 9

Preventing infection associated with intravascular therapy

INTRODUCTION

Intravascular (IV) catheters are now an indispensable part of medical care used to administer fluids, blood products and nutritional support and for haemo-dynamic monitoring. Over 60% of patients admitted to hospital are likely to receive therapy via an IV catheter and in the UK almost all patients in intensive therapy units have at least one catheter inserted into a central vein or artery (Glynn et al 1997).

The most important infections associated with IV catheters are bloodstream infections (BSI) which, although they affect less than 5% of patients admitted to hospital, are associated with considerable mortality and morbidity, especially amongst the critically ill (Emmerson et al 1996, Plowman et al 2001).

The management of IV catheters has an important effect on the incidence of catheter-associated infection and there is considerable potential to prevent infections through the application of the best principles of practice (Coello et al 2003, MMWR 2000). Eggiman et al (2000) were able to demonstrate significant reductions in rates of IV catheter-related infections in critically ill patients by an education and surveillance programme targeted at the insertion and maintenance of vascular access catheters.

INFECTIONS ASSOCIATED WITH INTRAVASCULAR CATHETERS

Infection associated with IV catheters may affect the skin surrounding the insertion site or the bloodstream.

Bloodstream infections (BSI) or bacteraemia

Bacteraemia affects at least three patients in every 1000 admitted to acute hospitals and accounts for 6% of hospital-acquired infections (Emmerson et al 1996,

Health Protection Agency 2003). Some BSI occur as a secondary infection from another primary focus such as a respiratory tract, urinary tract or surgical wound infection. IV catheters cause BSI when bacteria colonizing the surface of the catheter are released into the bloodstream. IV catheters are reported as the source of around 48% of BSI, although the risk depends on the patient, the type of catheter, duration of use and how frequently it is manipulated (Coello et al 2003, O'Grady et al 2002). The critically ill are particularly vulnerable to BSI, with around 10 infections per 1000 patient-days reported in intensive care units and 6 per 1000 patient-days in haematology departments. More than half of BSI in these patients are likely to be IV catheter related. The source of most (approximately 90%) of IV catheter-associated BSI is central vascular catheters (Coello et al 2003). However, although the risk of BSI is much lower for peripheral catheters, the frequency with which they are used means that they can still be responsible for considerable morbidity (O'Grady et al 2002).

Bloodstream infections are associated with a case fatality rate of at least 20%; in the critically ill this rises to about 35% although frequently it is difficult to determine the extent to which BSI contributes to the death of these patients as they have many other underlying conditions that may contribute to mortality (Pittet & Wenzel 1995, Pittet et al 1994).

The presence of bacteria in the bloodstream may be accompanied by systemic symptoms such as fever, hypertension, chills or rigors and this is termed septicaemia. In children aged less than 1 year, symptoms may include hypothermia, apnoea or bradycardia (PHLS 1998). Once introduced into the bloodstream from the IV catheter, bacteria may lodge on other tissues to cause secondary endocarditis or osteomyelitis (Fang et al 1993).

Infection at the insertion site

Superficial infection may develop at the point where the catheter enters the skin, indicated by erythema or the presence of pus. There is considerable evidence to suggest a link between the presence of bacteria at the insertion site and subsequent catheter-related BSI (Cercenardo et al 1990, Mermel et al 1991). Bacteria colonizing the skin site gain access to the blood vessel by migrating along the outside of the catheter.

Phlebitis, inflammation of the vein where the catheter is sited, develops in approximately one-third of patients who have a peripheral catheter but rarely in association with central vascular catheters (Maki et al 1991a). The signs include tenderness, erythema, swelling or palpable cord. Usually, phlebitis is caused by the mechanical irritation of the tissues by the catheter or chemical irritation by the infusate. The risk of phlebitis is influenced by the catheter material and size, quality of insertion and time for which the catheter remains in place. The presence of phlebitis increases the risk of infection and, if infection develops, the catheter should be removed. Occasionally a purulent suppurative phlebitis occurs in a peripheral vein. This is an extremely serious infection that requires surgical treatment and is associated with a high mortality rate (Hammond et al 1988).

SOURCES OF INTRAVASCULAR CATHETER–ASSOCIATED INFECTION

The two main routes by which micro-organisms gain access to the bloodstream via an IV catheter are by migrating along the outside of the catheter from the insertion site and by travelling through the catheter lumen (Fig. 9.1). The importance of the external route is demonstrated by the strong association between catheter-related BSI, the culture of micro-organisms from the skin at the site of insertion and micro-organisms cultured from the outside of the catheter tip if the catheter is removed (Maki et al 1977).

Contamination of the internal surface of the catheter usually begins at the hub and colonized hubs are responsible for a significant proportion of catheter-related BSI (Linares et al 1985). Bacteria are protected from the immune defences of the host as they migrate through the lumen to the catheter tip. Colonization of the internal surface of the catheter increases with the duration of catheterization. Thus, in patients with short-term catheters the skin at the insertion site is the most likely source of catheter-related BSI, whereas in the long-term catheterized the hub is a more likely source (Raad et al 1993b).

More rarely, the source of BSI may be contaminated infusate. Good quality control in manufacturing has reduced the risk from commercially prepared fluids but in-use contamination may still occur, especially where fluids are accessed frequently (Maki et al 1987). In some cases, the external surface of the catheter tip becomes colonized by bacteria circulating in the blood from another focus of infection (e.g. the respiratory or urinary tract). This is called haematogenous seeding. The bacteria may then multiply on the catheter tip and subsequently cause BSI.

The role of biofilms

Micro-organisms are able to attach to surfaces, including medical devices, forming a biofilm. Micro-organisms adhering to the surface produce extracellular polysaccharide and other polymeric substances. These

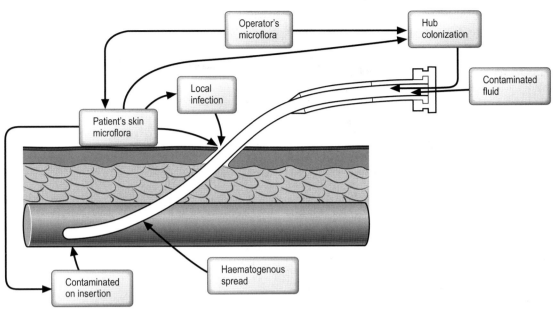

Figure 9.1   Sources of infection in IV catheters. Schematic cross-section of the skin and underlying tissue at the site of catheterization (reproduced with permission from Elliott 1988).

form a matrix that surrounds the bacterial cells and facilitates their adhesion to the catheter surface. Biofilms can form rapidly (within 24 hours) on virtually all IV catheters, although the extent and location of the biofilm depend on how long it is in place. The most common colonizing organisms are *S. epidermidis*, *S. aureus*, candida, pseudomonas, klebsiella and enterococcus which originate from the microflora of the patient or from healthcare workers. Micro-organisms within a biofilm are protected from the effect of antimicrobial agents and neutrophils. Bacteria are therefore able to multiply freely in the biofilm on the catheter surface from where they are released into the bloodstream (Donlan 2001).

Microbiology

Most IV catheter-associated infections are acquired endogenously from micro-organisms colonizing the patient's skin, although micro-organisms may also be introduced into the hub or administration set during manipulation by healthcare staff (Table 9.1). Coagulase-negative staphylococci, predominantly *S. epidermidis*, are the organisms that most commonly colonize IV catheters and when they cause infection, are associated with a high mortality rate (Daschner & Frank 1989). The proportion of catheter-related BSI caused by *S. epidermidis* has increased since the 1980s as a result of

Table 9.1   Micro-organisms most commonly responsible for IV device-related infection

Micro-organism	Source
Staphylococcus epidermidis	Common skin commensal
Staphylococcus aureus	Skin commensal
Enterococcus spp.	Gut flora, colonizes skin sites in the critically ill
Klebsiella Pseudomonas Escherichia coli Serratia	Gram-negative organisms, colonize the skin of hospitalized patients; colonize upper respiratory tract of ventilated patients; carried transiently on the hands of staff, may contaminate pumps, transducers, etc.
Candida	May colonize skin when normal flora altered by antibiotic therapy; associated with haemodialysis or parenteral nutrition

more IV device use and the improved survival rate of the critically ill, especially neonates (O'Grady et al 2002).

S. epidermidis, although part of the normal flora of the skin, is not usually pathogenic in healthy people. Its ability to cause infection in IV catheters is related to the production of a glycocalyx called 'slime', which enables the bacteria to adhere to the catheter surface (see biofilms, Fig. 6.1).

Staphylococcus aureus is also a common cause of BSI, accounting for about a quarter of these infections (Health Protection Agency 2003). *S. aureus* is able to colonize IV devices by forming biofilms. Although a skin commensal, *S. aureus* is also able to cause serious infection and bacteraemia may subsequently result in osteomyelitis and endocarditis (Richet et al 1990). In the UK, approximately 50% of *S. aureus* causing catheter-related BSI are methicillin resistant (Coello et al 2003).

Gram-negative micro-organisms are less common causes of IV catheter-associated infection but may affect the critically ill whose skin flora is altered by antibiotic therapy. Catheters such as transducers or heparin pumps may also be a source of these bacteria (Cheeseborough & Catlow 1999). Other pathogens emerging as important causes of catheter-related BSI are fungi and enterococci (Beck-Sague & Jarvis 1993, Health Protection Agency 2003).

DIAGNOSIS OF CATHETER-RELATED INFECTION

One of the difficulties of quantifying the risks of IV catheters is defining what constitutes a catheter-related infection. Some studies use the incidence of septicaemia or bacteraemia as a measure; others use the occurrence of phlebitis or colonization of the catheter. However, the immunocompromised or critcally ill can have a BSI but no fever, or a fever that is not related to infection. Frequently, the source of micro-organisms in the blood cannot be established. It is therefore difficult to make a precise diagnosis of catheter-associated bloodstream infection and often the main indication is a pyrexia that has no other apparent cause and is unresponsive to antibiotic therapy (Elliot 1993) (see Box 9.1).

A standard method of diagnosing catheter-related infection is by culture of the catheter tip. The method used is semiquantitative: it involves an estimation of the number of bacteria present and takes account of inadvertent contamination when the catheter is removed (Maki et al 1977). Growth is considered significant when more than 15 bacteria are found, confirming the catheter as the source of clinical symptoms of infection. However, this is not a practical method in many circumstances because it is often not possible to remove the catheter to confirm it as the

---

Box 9.1   Example of a case definition of catheter–related, bloodstream–associated infection (Hospitals in Europe Links for Infection Control through Surveillance 2004)

1. **Local CVC–related infection (no positive blood culture)**
   Quantitative CVC culture $\geq 10^3$ CFU/ml or semiquantitative CVC culture >5 CFU
   and pus/inflammation at the insertion site or tunnel

2. **General CVC–related infection (no positive blood culture)**
   Quantitative CVC culture $\geq 10^3$ CFU/ml or semiquantitative CVC culture >5 CFU
   and clinical signs improve 48 h after catheter removal

3. **CVC–related bloodstream infection* (positive blood culture)**
   Bloodstream infection occurring when catheter in place (or 48 h before or after removal)
   and positive culture with the same organisms of either:
   - Quantitative CVC culture $\geq 10^3$ CFU/ml or semiquantitative CVC culture >5 CFU
   - Quantitative blood culture ratio CVC blood sample/peripheral blood sample >5
   - Differential delay in positivity of blood culture: CVC blood sample positive at least 2 h before peripheral blood culture (blood samples drawn at same time)
   - Positive culture of the same micro-organism from blood and from pus at the insertion site

---

* Bloodstream infection Patient has at least one of the following signs or symptoms: fever (>38°C), chills or hypotension *and* a recognized pathogen isolated from one or more blood cultures *or* a common skin contaminant (e.g. coagulase-negative staphylococcus, *Micrococcus* spp., *Bacillus* spp., *Corynebacterium* spp., *Proprionibacterium acnes*) isolated from two blood cultures from two separate blood samples drawn within 48 h.

---

source of fever. Skin culture of the insertion site may be a useful alternative as there is a high correlation between skin colonization and catheter-related infection (Raad et al 1995).

Bacteraemia is diagnosed by culturing blood in the laboratory. At least 10 ml of blood must be inoculated into each of the culture bottles, one of which is incubated under anaerobic conditions, the other aerobically (see p. 28). To confirm the IV device as the source of infection, two sets of blood cultures should be taken, one from a peripheral vein and the second through the catheter. If the same organism is isolated from both sources, particularly if more organisms are obtained from the catheter specimen, this is suggestive of a catheter-related infection, although it is difficult to distinguish whether bacteria recovered from the central vascular catheter (CVC) are only colonizing it rather than causing the clinical signs of sepsis. New methods of measuring the concentration of micro-organisms in the catheter have been developed, by comparing the difference in time to positivity of blood specimens taken from the CVC and peripherally. A catheter-related BSI is indicated if the CVC specimen becomes positive at least 2 h before the peripheral specimen (Mermel et al 2001). This system enables catheter-related BSI to be reliably diagnosed by taking blood samples from the lumen without removing the catheter. However, more work on the efficacy of these methods is required (Farr 1999).

Studies on IV catheters are difficult to interpret because of the variety of diagnostic methods available. The low incidence of infection also means that differences are unlikely to be significant unless at least 1500 patients are included in the study (Widner 1997).

FACTORS THAT INFLUENCE THE RISK OF INFECTION

Type of catheter

There are several different types of intravascular catheter and each is associated with different risks of infection, influenced by the risk of mechanical complications, phlebitis and density of local skin flora (O'Grady et al 2002) (Table 9.2).

Peripheral catheters
Peripheral venous catheters are associated with very few infections, affecting less than 1% of catheters. About one-third of patients develop phlebitis, although the risk of phlebitis is reduced if a vein in the hand is used (Maki et al 1991a). Peripheral arterial catheters are used to measure intra-arterial pressure and oxygenation and frequent manipulation increases the risk of catheter-related BSI in these devices.

Central vascular catheters
These are inserted into the subclavian, internal jugular or femoral vein. In adults, the subclavian vein is considered to be the preferred site in terms of minimizing the risk of catheter-related BSI. However, they are more difficult to insert and are therefore preferable for patients in intensive care who require prolonged venous access (O'Grady et al 2002). Catheters inserted into the jugular vein are more likely to become colonized and are associated with a higher

Table 9.2   Approximate incidence of IV device-related bloodstream infection based on a combination of published data (reproduced with permission from Maki & Mermel 1998)

Type of device	Incidence (%)	Range (%)
Peripheral		
Venous	<0.2	0–1
Arterial	1	0.56–4.6
Central venous		
General purpose (multilumen)	3	1–7
Pulmonary artery	1	0–5
Haemodialysis	10	3–18
Long-term access		
Peripherally inserted central vascular catheter	0.2	
Cuffed (Hickman, Broviac)	0.2	0.1–0.5
Subcutaneous port	0.04	0.2–0.1

risk of BSI. This increased risk is probably related to the proximity to oropharyngeal secretions, the mechanical effects of head movement and the difficulty of fixing and dressing the insertion site (Mermel et al 1991). Femoral catheters are sited where the density of skin flora is high and in adults are associated with a similar risk of BSI to those inserted in the jugular vein (Goetz et al 1998). In children, femoral catheters have few mechanical complications and are associated with a lower risk of BSI (Goldstein et al 1997).

Studies have suggested that multilumen catheters increase the risk of catheter-related BSI (Weightman et al 1988). However, differences in risk are difficult to assess because triple-lumen catheters are more likely to be used for treatment of the seriously ill (Farkas et al 1992, Pearson 1996).

Pulmonary arterial catheters (Swan–Ganz)
These balloon-tipped catheters are inserted over the heart valves and are used to manage critically ill patients who are haemodynamically unstable. The trauma they cause to the valves and endocardium increases the risk of endocarditis. The risk of catheter-related BSI is around 1% but increases significantly with duration of catheterization (Mermel et al 1991).

Pressure monitoring systems
Where arterial catheters are used for pressure monitoring, the risk of catheter-related BSI is increased (Thomas et al 1993). Micro-organisms may be introduced into the fluid-filled system by unsterile

transducers, calibrating catheters or infusate or from the hands of the operator when the catheter is manipulated (Pearson 1996). Stopcocks may also become contaminated. Once in the system, micro-organisms can multiply in the fluid and move from the pressure monitoring system into the patient's bloodstream via the IV catheter. Several outbreaks associated with inadequate decontamination of reusable transducers have been reported. Infections have even occurred when the fluid in the monitoring system is isolated from the patient by a sterile disposable membrane as a result of contamination during manipulation (Beck-Sague et al 1990, Hekker et al 1990).

Tunnelled and totally implanted central venous catheters

These types of catheter (e.g. Hickman, Broviac, Porta-Cath) are indicated for use where prolonged venous access of more than 30 days is required, for example for chemotherapy. The catheter is inserted into the subclavian vein and either tunnelled under the skin to exit on the chest wall or totally implanted under the skin and accessed by inserting a needle through the skin into a subcutaneous self-sealing port. These types of catheter minimize the migration of micro-organisms along the outside of the catheter and there is evidence that they are associated with a lower risk of BSI compared to conventional venous catheters. The lowest rates of catheter-related BSI are associated with totally implanted catheters (Pratt et al 2001) (see p. 209).

Peripherally inserted central vascular catheters (PICCs)

These are used for medium- to long-term access, especially for outpatient treatment. The risk of BSI is lower than with non-tunnelled CVCs and similar to that associated with fully implanted catheters (Ryder 1995). Insertion is associated with fewer mechanical problems and does not require a surgical procedure (Graham et al 1991). However, as with other peripherally sited catheters, PICCs are associated with phlebitis, although to a lesser extent than other peripheral catheters (Raad et al 1993b).

Umbilical catheters

The umbilical vessels are commonly used for vascular access in newborn infants because they are easily cannulated and can be used to both measure haemodynamic status and take blood. The umbilical stump is heavily colonized with micro-organisms and catheter-related BSI will occur in approximately 5% of umbilical catheters. Tebbs et al (1996) found that over 30% of umbilical catheters were contaminated within 72 hours of placement and they should not be left in place for more than 5 days (O'Grady et al 2002).

Haemodialysis catheters

Patients dialysed using an IV catheter rather than an arteriovenous fistula or graft have a sevenfold increased risk of BSI (Hoen et al 1998). The use of central venous catheters for dialysis should therefore be avoided and if temporary access is required then cuffed devices are the preferred option (O'Grady et al 2002).

Duration of catheterization

The length of time for which a catheter is in place probably has most effect on the risk of infection. The longer a catheter is in place, the more opportunities for infection via the device will occur (Elliot 1988). To take account of this, many studies report infections related to the number of days of catheterization. For example, if 100 catheters are under study and each is in place for 10 days, the total number of days of catheterization is 1000. If two become infected, then the rate of infection is two per 1000 catheter-days. In peripheral IV devices, the risk of catheter colonization and phlebitis, both of which increase the risk of BSI, appears to rise 72–96 h after the device has been inserted (Lai 1998, Pratt et al 2001). With central vascular catheters, the daily risk of infection appears to be constant and most studies suggest that there is no difference in rate of catheter-related BSI whether they are changed routinely or left in place for the duration of catheterization (Cobb et al 1992). The duration of catheterization is particularly important for arterial catheters. Raad et al (1993b) found that for peripheral arterial catheters, the risk of catheter-related BSI was between 3% and 5% for each day of catheterization and by 21 days the risk of catheter-related BSI was 60%. In pulmonary arterial catheters, the risk of catheter-related BSI is substantially increased after 5 days; after 14 days the risk is 80%. These catheters should therefore be changed every 5 days and removed as soon as possible (Pearson 1996).

Catheter material

Common pathogens that cause catheter-related BSI, such as *S. epidermidis*, readily colonize catheters that have irregular surfaces. The smooth surface of Teflon and polyurethane catheters is therefore the most resistant to bacterial adherence.

Most short-term catheters are made of polyurethane, whereas long-term catheters are usually silicone (Pratt et al 2001). Some materials are also more throm-bogenic than others. Polyurethane catheters are less likely to cause phlebitis than Teflon catheters (Raad et al 1993a).

Catheters coated with antibacterial substances such as silver sulfadiazine and chlorhexidine have been developed recently. They have been shown significantly to reduce catheter colonization and catheter-related bloodstream infections and are probably cost-effective in high-risk patients (Maki et al 1997, Veenstra et al 1999a, b). Catheters coated with two antimicrobial agents, minocycline and rifampicin, have been found to be even more effective (Darouiche et al 1999). Although there is a risk that micro-organisms resistant to these antimicrobials may emerge, they are probably still of benefit in high-risk patients because of the reduction in use of other agents, such as vancomycin, if bloodstream infections are prevented (Mermel 2000, Pratt et al 2001).

PREVENTING INFECTION IN INTRAVASCULAR CATHETERS

Most bloodstream infections associated with IV catheters can be prevented by careful management of the catheter (Maki & Mermel 1998). Clear guidelines for the insertion, management and removal of catheters should be established and adhered to, especially in units where patients commonly require a central vascular catheter and where the risks of catheter-related BSI are relatively high. Of key importance is the use of strict aseptic technique for handling IV catheters and handwashing before and after contact with the catheter (Pratt et al 2001, Ward et al 1997). Education and training are an essential part of this process and several studies have demonstrated a substantial reduction in the numbers of infections where IV catheters have been maintained by specially trained personnel (Boulamiery-Verry et al 2004).

Insertion of the catheter

The catheterization procedure may introduce bacteria from the skin into the vein. These bacteria may be derived either from the patient or from the hands of the person inserting it. The catheter site has been described as 'not unlike an open wound containing a foreign body' (Maki et al 1973) and insertion should therefore be considered a minor surgical procedure carried out with a high standard of asepsis and preceded by thorough handwashing. Asepsis is particularly important for the insertion of central catheters, which is a more invasive procedure associated with a greater risk of infection. Raad et al (1994) showed that high levels of barrier precautions used for insertion were more important than the place of insertion (operating theatre or ward). Swan–Ganz

catheters inserted in the ICU using high-level barrier precautions (sterile gloves, gowns, masks, large drapes) were much less likely to become infected than those inserted in the operating theatre with a lesser level of barrier precautions. This was despite the fact that catheters inserted in ICU stayed in place for longer and were used more frequently for parenteral nutrition. Pratt et al (2001) recommend maximal barrier precautions without the use of facemask or cap.

The catheter should be firmly anchored to prevent movement, which may both carry micro-organisms from the skin into the wound and increase the risk of mechanical phlebitis (Maki et al 1973). Tape has been implicated as a source of infection and tape that is in direct contact with the insertion site should be sterile (Sheldon & Johnson 1979).

Skin preparation

Studies suggest that cleaning the site with chlorhexidine before insertion of a central or arterial catheter is associated with a lower rate of infection than 10% povidone-iodine or 70% alcohol (Garland et al 1995, Maki et al 1991a, Mimoz et al 1996). These studies used aqueous chlorhexidine but alcoholic preparations of chlorhexidine are likely to be at least if not more effective and have the additional advantage of rapid action and evaporation (Pratt et al 2001). To ensure maximum disinfection of the skin, the disinfectant should be applied for about 30 s and allowed to dry before starting the procedure.

Effective skin preparation will remove bacteria from hair as well as skin. Shaving around the insertion

---

Guidelines for practice: insertion of an intravenous catheter

- Wash hands before insertion
- Use chlorhexidine to clean skin and allow to dry before insertion
- Avoid shaving the site of insertion
- Secure catheter but do not cover the insertion site with non-sterile tape

For central vascular catheters:

- Use a single-lumen catheter where possible
- If access is required for more than 30 days use a tunnelled or implantable device
- Consider using an antimicrobial impregnated device for adults at high risk of catheter-related BSI
- Use an optimal aseptic technique for insertion including sterile gloves, gowns and large sterile drape

site causes microabrasions that encourage bacterial colonization and should therefore be avoided. See practice guidelines for the insertion of a catheter.

Catheter replacement

A marked increase in the incidence of phlebitis and catheter colonization has been reported when peripheral catheters are left in place for more than 72 h (Band & Maki 1980). Routine replacement of peripheral catheter every 48–72 h has therefore been recommended (Pearson 1996). However, other studies have shown no difference in rates of phlebitis when peripheral catheters were left in for 96 h (Lai 1998).

With central vascular catheters the situation is more complex. Although the risk of BSI associated with CVCs increases with duration of catheterization, the daily risk of infection appears to remain constant and the rate of catheter colonization and BSI is not reduced by routine replacement (Cobb et al 1992). With pulmonary artery catheters, the risk of BSI increases after 3 days of catheterization and these should be replaced at least every 5 days (Pearson 1996).

If the patient develops a BSI, central vascular catheters should be removed and a new catheter inserted at a different site. If a central catheter requires replacement because of malfunction, it can be exchanged over a guidewire rather than be removed completely; however, this should be avoided if there is evidence of infection at the insertion site (Cook et al 1997, Pearson 1996). If infection is suspected, the catheter tip should be cultured and, if the result is positive, a new catheter inserted at a different site (Pratt et al 2001).

Care of the insertion site

The conventional method of protecting the insertion site is with a dressing but there is considerable controversy about which type of dressing is most effective. Gauze dressings do not protect the site from moisture and do not allow the insertion site to be visualized easily. Transparent film dressings enable the insertion site to be viewed easily to detect early signs of phlebitis or infection and allow the patient to bathe, and they require less frequent attention. An accumulation of bacteria on the skin under transparent film dressings has been reported, although most studies have not demonstrated an increased risk of catheter-related infection. In a major study comparing transparent dressings and gauze used on peripheral catheters, Maki & Ringer (1987) found no significant difference in the rate of catheter colonization or phlebitis between the two types of dressing. There was also no increase in risk if transparent dressings were

left on for the lifetime of the catheter. Ricard et al (1985) also found no difference in skin colonization or catheter-related infection between films left on for 7 days and gauze changed every 2–3 days.

Studies on central vascular catheters have reported an increased rate of site infections and bacteraemia associated with transparent films (Conly et al 1989). However, a meta-analysis by Hoffman et al (1992) indicated that, although transparent films were associated with an increase in catheter tip colonization, there was no significant increase in catheter-related BSI. This finding was confirmed by Maki et al (1994) in a study on pulmonary arterial catheters in which gauze dressings (changed every 2 days) were compared with polyurethane transparent film (changed every 5 days). Other studies on pulmonary arterial catheters have shown a large increase in BSI when transparent films are used. This may be related to the collection of blood at the insertion site, which provides a rich medium for bacterial growth (Maki & Will 1984). One explanation for the conflicting information is the variation in moisture vapour permeability of dressings made by different manufacturers. New transparent films with a high vapour permeability may reduce skin colonization by allowing moisture to escape (Fletcher & Bodenham 1999, Maki et al 1991b).

Skin disinfectants used to clean the skin when the dressing is changed may reduce the rate of infection associated with central venous and arterial catheters, for example an aqueous solution of chlorhexidine, which has a residual antibacterial effect on the skin for several hours after application (Maki & Ringer 1987, Maki et al 1991a). See practice guidelines for care of the insertion site.

In short-term CVCs, chlorhexidine-impregnated dressings have been shown to significantly reduce the

---

Guidelines for practice: care of the insertion site

- Wash hands before contact with insertion site
- Use sterile gauze or transparent film to cover the insertion site
- Change dressing when no longer intact, when moisture collects at the site and at least every 7 days
- Clean central venous or arterial insertion sites with aqueous chlorhexidine each time the dressing is changed. Peripheral catheters are unlikely to benefit from cleaning with antiseptic
- Inspect the site every 2–3 days for signs of infection (e.g. inflammation, pain, pus)

risk of catheter-related BSI with no evidence of resistance to chlorhexidine emerging (Crnich & Maki 2002).

Topical antimicrobial agents applied to insertion sites have been recommended but are prone to encourage the growth of fungi such as candida or other resistant micro-organisms. They should therefore not be used routinely (Maki & Mermel 1998). Povidone-iodine ointment applied to subclavian haemodialysis catheters has been shown to reduce the incidence of catheter-related BSI (Levin et al 1991). A chlorhexidine-impregnated disc pressed on to the skin at the insertion site has also been reported to reduce catheter-related BSI significantly in central vascular catheters (non-tunnelled), PICC and arterial catheters for short- or medium-term use. The effect is not apparent for long-term catheters where the intralumen route is an important source of infections (Maki et al 2000).

Management of catheters and fluid administration sets

The aseptic management of the catheter hub, connection ports and administration sets is essential to prevent contamination of the system and subsequent infection.

Contamination of stopcocks used to administer drugs or infusates is common, although a causal relationship between colonization and subsequent infection is difficult to demonstrate (Cheeseborough & Finch 1985, Pearson 1996, Tebbs et al 1996). Hub contamination is increased by prolonged catheterization and frequent manipulation (Mermel 2000). The number of access points and catheter lumens should be kept to a minimum and access points should be disinfected with alcohol, chlorhexidine or povidone-iodine before use (Maki et al 1997, Pearson 1996, Pratt et al 2001).

Piggy-back systems, where a needle is inserted into a rubber membrane, may be beneficial and needle-less connections appear to be less prone to contamination (Casey et al 2002, Inoue et al 1992). However, needle-less systems may increase the incidence of catheter-related BSI where high-risk fluids such as parenteral nutrition are being administered (Danzig et al 1995).

Bacteria may also be introduced in the infusion fluid. Some bacteria, notably klebsiella and enterobacter, are able to grow even in simple IV solutions, such as 5% dextrose (Centers for Disease Control 1971). A number of outbreaks of infection in the 1970s were caused by IV fluids contaminated during manufacture but improvements in quality control methods have now made this an unlikely source of infection.

Infusion fluids may also become contaminated during use when drugs are added or when infusion fluids or administration sets are changed. Units of blood or platelets may contain bacteria, which can contaminate the infusion set (Walsh et al 1993). Curran et al (2000) reported a significant association between peripheral phlebitis and the use of infusion pumps, especially where the infusion fluid is made up at ward level. They suggest this may be caused by increased levels of particulates as well as the multiplication of micro-organisms in prolonged infusions and recommend that filters should be used to minimize the risk.

The extent to which fluids are accessed affects the risk of infection (Table 9.3). Administration sets in intensive care units, where lines are frequently manipulated for haemodynamic monitoring and drug administration, are more likely to become contaminated (Maki et al 1987, Mermel et al 1991). Bacteria introduced from contaminated infusate or during manipulation of the line will multiply over time and to prevent this, administration sets should be changed regularly (Maki et al 1987, Syndman et al 1987). Several studies have shown that replacing administration sets every 72 h is safe. However, they should be replaced more frequently if used to administer fluids that readily support the growth of bacteria, such as parenteral nutrition, lipid emulsions, blood and blood products (Pratt et al 2001).

Hands should be washed thoroughly before manipulating IV catheters or fluid administration sets. In most circumstances gloves are unnecessary but it may be preferable to use sterile gloves to attach new bags of parenteral nutrition fluid because of the high risk of infection (see p. 208).

Where systems are used for pressure monitoring, the tubing, flush catheter and transducer should be replaced every 96 h. Disposable transducers and closed flush systems are preferable. Dextrose should not be used in a pressure monitoring system because it supports the growth of micro-organisms and the

Table 9.3 Contamination of infusion fluids (reproduced with permission from Maki et al 1987)

Type or location of IV device	Infusions contaminated (%)
Peripheral	0.6
Central venous	1.5
Central – total parenteral nutrition	3.6
Devices on the intensive care unit	2.5
Devices on general wards	0.9

system should not be used for obtaining blood samples as this will increase the risk of contamination (Pearson 1996).

Flush solutions

The use of anticoagulants to flush IV catheters is intended to maintain patency, prevent bacteria from adhering to the catheter and reduce the risk of thrombosis. Current evidence suggests that in peripheral catheters, heparin flushes were no more beneficial than saline in maintaining patency and preventing infection. In central venous and arterial catheters, routine flushing with heparin reduces thrombus formation and may prevent catheter-related BSI (Pratt et al 2001, Randolph et al 1998). Glyceryl trinitrate applied on the skin near to the insertion site encourages vasodilation and reduces the incidence of phlebitis (O'Brien et al 1990).

IV filters

A filter placed between the catheter and the fluid administration set may reduce the incidence of phlebitis and can be used to prevent bacteria and endotoxins in the fluid from gaining access to the bloodstream. Filters may be cost effective with administration sets that are frequently accessed or where infusions prepared at ward level are being delivered by pump (Curran et al 2000, Spencer 1990). Filters cannot be used on Swan–Ganz catheters or where blood, blood products, lipid emulsion or amphotericin are being infused (Quercia et al 1986).

There is no evidence that wrapping hub joints with gauze soaked in antiseptic prevents infections and alcohol-based solutions may damage the catheter material (Medical Devices Directorate 1993). See practice guidelines for the care of administration sets.

Parenteral nutrition

The administration of elemental nutrients into a vein is used to feed patients who are unable to meet their nutritional requirements by oral or nasogastric feeding. Conventionally, parenteral nutrition is administered via a central venous catheter where the high blood flow reduces the thrombophlebotic effects of glucose. Bacteria can multiply easily in parenteral nutrition (PN) fluid and infection is a frequent complication of PN therapy, with a rate of around 14% (Mughal 1989). Particular care must therefore be taken to avoid contamination of the fluids and catheters used to administer PN. Fluids are usually prepared in the pharmacy using strict asepsis and under laminar flow ventilation to minimize the risk of contamination. A single catheter should be designated for administering PN and this should not be used to take blood or give drugs (Pratt et al 2001). Triple-lumen catheters should

---

Guidelines for practice: care of the administration set

- Wash hands before accessing IV catheters. Do not touch IV line connections or allow them to come into contact with non-sterile surfaces. Sterile gloves are not usually necessary provided sterile connections are not touched by hand
- Keep the number of access points on an intravenous line to a minimum. If a tap or stopcock is not in use then remove it
- Use single-lumen central vascular catheters if possible
- Administer IV drugs through the latex membrane on peripheral lines to avoid the use of ports
- Change administration sets every 72 h (24–48 h if accessed frequently) and always after the infusion of blood products
- Consider use of IV filters where lines are accessed frequently
- Remove catheter as soon as clinically indicated

Guidelines for practice: management of parenteral nutrition

The risks of infection associated with the infusion of parenteral nutrition are much greater than with other fluids and extreme care must be taken to avoid contamination.

- The catheter should be inserted under maximal aseptic conditions in the theatre or treatment room by an experienced doctor
- Designate the catheter for PN only (avoid using multilumen catheters). Do not add drugs or withdraw blood from the line
- Do not connect ports, stopcocks or taps
- Change the PN fluid and administration set every 24 h using sterile gloves and a no-touch technique
- Inspect the insertion site daily for signs of infection and clean with chlorhexidine when dressing is changed
- Record temperature and pulse 4 hourly to detect early signs of sepsis
- Take blood cultures through the line and from a peripheral vein if the patient becomes pyrexial

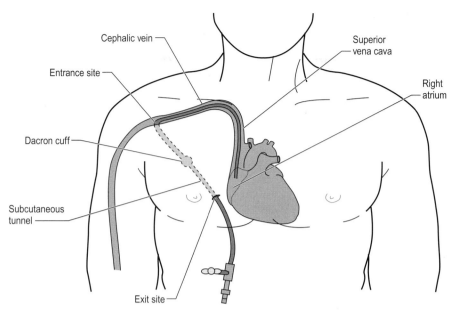

Figure 9.2   A tunnelled right atrial catheter.

not be used for PN, because the risk of sepsis has been reported to be four times that of single-lumen catheters. A high level of asepsis should be used for manipulating the administration set and fluids (see practice guidelines).

Peripherally inserted central catheters have been used successfully for short-term feeding using a lower concentration of glucose and are associated with a lower risk of infection (Hansell 1989). The use of glyceryl trinitrate patches may prolong the life of peripheral catheters used for PN (Khawaja et al 1988).

Hickman and subcutaneous lines

Intravenous catheters made from an inert material, silicone elastomer, were pioneered by Broviac and developed by Hickman. These catheters are inserted into a central vein and tunnelled under the skin to exit on the chest wall (Fig. 9.2). Tissue grows into a Dacron cuff positioned in the skin tunnel and this stabilizes the catheter so that a securing suture is not necessary and prevents bacteria migrating from the skin into the vein. Cuffs added to conventional central catheters reduce the incidence of infection (Flowers et al 1989).

Hickman catheters are used extensively in the management of patients requiring prolonged venous access, particularly for chemotherapy. They are associated with low rates of infection considering the length of time they are in the vein. The incidence of infection is estimated at 1.4 infections per 1000 catheter-

days, compared with more than three infections per 1000 catheter-days with non-tunnelled central vascular catheters (Widner 1997). Neutropenia or other forms of immunosuppression increase the risk of catheter-related BSI related to tunnelled catheters (Howell et al 1995, Raviglione et al 1989).

Initially, insertion site care should be the same as for other central catheters but approximately 10 days after insertion, the Dacron cuff has been secured by tissue ingrowth and the exit site suture can be removed. Some then recommend leaving the site exposed without a dressing but transparent dressings left in place for 5–7 days have also been used with no increase in risk of BSI (Johnstone 1982, Shivnan et al 1991). In common with other central catheters, provided that a good no-touch technique is used, gloves are not necessary to manipulate the administration set or to administer intravenous drugs, except perhaps where PN is being infused and the risk of introducing infection through line manipulation is much greater.

Totally implanted or subcutaneous central venous catheters (e.g. Port-a-Cath) with a self-sealing septum are being used increasingly, particularly for patients cared for in their own home. These catheters have the lowest risk of infection (approximately 0.2 infections per 1000 catheter-days; Groeger et al 1993).

Infection of the exit site or tunnel may occur and both may result in bloodstream infection. Bacteraemia associated with these long-term catheters occurs frequently but is usually asymptomatic and caused by coagulase-negative staphylococci. It is important to establish that micro-organisms recovered from the blood are a true catheter-related BSI, rather than skin contaminants or from another site. To avoid removing the catheter, bacterial infections can sometimes be managed by instilling antimicrobials into the catheter provided the BSI is not complicated by endocarditis, tunnel infection or another septic focus (Mermel et al 2001).

IV therapy teams

The impact of high-quality IV catheter care has been demonstrated by a number of studies in which trained IV therapy teams have been used to insert catheters and provide follow-up care; this approach is associated with substantially lower rates of catheter-related BSI (Boulamiery-Verry et al 2004). Others have used intensive education of staff and catheter care protocols to achieve reductions (Lange et al 1997, Parras et al 1994). As with many aspects of infection control, the provision of a high standard of IV catheter care is dependent on patient–nurse ratios and understaffing in the ICU can have a major impact on the risk of catheter-related BSI (Fridkin et al 1996).

Surveillance of catheter-related BSI in high-risk units such as the ICU, neonatal intensive care and haematology can provide essential information with which to evaluate practice, motivate change and encourage adherence to local protocols (Stonehouse & Butcher 1996). In the USA, hospitals that participate in the national surveillance system have achieved reductions in the incidence of BSI during the past decade (MMWR 2000).

Management of IV catheters in the home

It is often difficult to translate the care of IV catheters in hospital to the environment of the home, where the patient may be responsible for most of the care and the facilities and equipment available are less sophisticated. The risks of introducing infection may be lower because cross-infection from other patients is unlikely to occur. However, patients are still at risk of endogenous infection from their own skin flora. Thorough training of the patient or carers on the management of the catheter, in particular the importance of asepsis, is therefore essential (RCN 2003). The plan of care should be as simple as possible, although considerable distress can be caused by forcing patients to adopt unfamiliar procedures, which is unnecessary provided the general principles of infection control are adhered to.

Written instructions are preferable as detailed information may not be retained after discharge. Advice given by healthcare workers involved in care must be consistent.

References

Band JD, Maki DG (1980) Steel needles used for intravenous therapy. Morbidity in patients with hematologic malignancy. *Arch. Intern. Med.*, **140**: 31–4.

Beck-Sague CM, Jarvis WR (1993) Secular trends in the epidemiology of nosocomial fungal infections in the United States, 1980–1990. *J. Infect. Dis.*, **167**: 1247–51.

Beck-Sague CM, Jarvis WR, Brook JH et al (1990) Epidemic bacteremia due to *Acinetobacter baumannii* in five intensive care units. *Am. J. Epidemiol.*, **132**: 723–33.

Boulamiery-Verry A, Mercier C, Duffand F et al (2004) Totally implantable intravascular devices – related complications: effectiveness of insertion by a trained team. *J. Hosp. Infect.*, **56**(3): 248–9.

Casey A, Spare MK, Worthington T et al (2002) Needleless connectors – the way forward in the prevention of catheter-related infections? *J. Hosp. Infect.*, **50**: 77–9.

Centers for Disease Control (1971) Nosocomial bacteremias associated with intravenous fluid therapy. *MMWR*, **20** (suppl. 9): 1–2.

Cercenardo E, Ena J, Rodriguez-Creixems M et al (1990) A conservative procedure for the diagnosis of catheter-related infections. *Arch. Intern. Med.*, **150**: 1417–20.

Cheeseborough JS, Catlow R (1999) Contamination of intravenous heparin infusions. *J. Hosp. Infect.*, **43**(3): 248–9.

Cheeseborough JS, Finch RG (1985) Studies on the microbiological safety of the valved side-port of the 'Venflon' cannula. *J. Hosp. Infect.*, **6**: 201–8.

Cobb DK, High KP, Sawyer RG et al (1992) A controlled trial of scheduled replacement of central venous and pulmonary artery catheters. *N. Engl. J. Med.*, **327**: 1062–8.

Coello R, Charlett A, Ward V et al (2003) Device-related sources of bacteraemia in English hospitals – opportunities for the prevention of hospital-acquired bacteraemia. *J. Hosp. Infect.*, **53**: 46–57.

Conly JM, Grieves K, Peters B (1989) A prospective randomised study comparing transparent and dry gauze dressings for central venous catheters. *J. Infect. Dis.*, **159**: 310–19.

Cook D, Randolph A, Kemerman P et al (1997) Central venous catheter replacement strategies: a systematic review of the literature. *Crit. Care Med.*, **25**(8): 1417–24.

Crnich CJ, Maki DG (2002) The promise of novel technology for the prevention of intravascular device-related bloodstream infections 1. Pathogenesis and short term devices. *Clin. Infect. Dis.*, **34**: 1232–42.

Curran ET, Coia JE, Gilmour H et al (2000) Multicentre research surveillance project to reduce infections and phlebitis associated with peripheral vascular catheters. *J. Hosp. Infect.*, **46**: 194–202.

Danzig LE, Short L, Collins K et al (1995) Bloodstream infections associated with a needleless intravenous infusion system and total parenteral nutrition. *JAMA*, **273**: 1862–4.

Darouiche RO, Raad I, Heard SO et al (1999) A comparison of two antimicrobial-impregnated central venous catheters. *N. Engl. J. Med.*, **340**: 1–8.

Daschner FD, Frank U (1989) Intravenous catheter and device-related infection. *Curr. Opin. Infect. Dis.*, **2**: 663–7.

Donlan RM (2001) Biofilms and device-associated infections. *Emerg. Infect. Dis.*, **7**(2): 277–81.

Eggiman P, Harbarth S, Constantin MN et al (2000) Impact of a prevention strategy targeted at vascular-access care on incidence of infection in intensive care. *Lancet*, **355**: 1864–8.

Elliot TSJ (1988) Intravascular device infections. *J. Med. Microbiol.*, **27**: 161–7.

Elliot TSJ (1993) Line-associated bacteraemias. *Commun. Dis. Rep.*, **3**(7): R91–5.

Emmerson AM, Enstone JE, Griffin M et al (1996) The second national prevalence survey of infection in hospitals – overview of the results. *J. Hosp. Infect.*, **32**: 175–90.

Fang G, Keys TF, Gentry LO et al (1993) Prosthetic valve endocarditis resulting from nosocomial bacteremia: a prospective, multicenter study. *Ann. Intern. Med.*, **111**: 560–7.

Farkas JK, Liu N, Bleriot JP et al (1992) Single versus triple-lumen central catheter-related sepsis: a prospective randomized study in a critically ill population. *Am. J. Med.*, **93**: 277–82.

Farr BM (1999) Accuracy and cost-effectiveness of new tests for diagnosis of catheter-related bloodstream infections. *Lancet*, **354**: 1487–8.

Fletcher SJ, Bodenham AR (1999) Catheter-related sepsis: an overview. Part 1. *Br. J. Int. Care*, **9**(2): 46–53.

Flowers RH, Schwezer KJ, Kopel RJ et al (1989) Efficacy of an attachable subcutaneous cuff for the prevention of intravascular catheter-related infection. *JAMA*, **261**: 878–83.

Fridkin SK, Pear SM, Williamson J et al (1996) The role of understaffing in central venous catheter-associated bloodstream infections. *Infect. Contr. Hosp. Epidemiol.*, **17**: 150–8.

Garland JS, Buck RK, Maloney P (1995) Comparison of 10% povidone iodine and 0.5% chlorhexidine gluconate for the prevention of peripheral IV catheter colonization in neonates: a prospective trial. *Pediatr. Infect. Dis. J.*, **14**: 510–16.

Glynn A, Ward V, Wilson J et al (1997) *Hospital-acquired Infection: Surveillance, Policies and Practice.* Public Health Laboratory Service, London.

Goetz A, Wagener M, Miller J et al (1998) Risk of infection due to central venous catheters: effect of site of placement of catheter type. *Infect. Contr. Hosp. Epidemiol.*, **19**(11): 842–5.

Goldstein AM, Weber JM, Sheridan RL (1997) Femoral access is safe in burned children: an analysis of 224 catheters. *J. Paediatr.*, **130**: 442–6.

Graham DR, Keldermans MM, Klemm LW et al (1991) Infectious complications among patients receiving home intravenous therapy with peripheral, central or peripherally placed central venous catheters. *Am. J. Med.*, **91** (suppl. B): 95S–101S.

Groeger JS, Lucas AB, Thaler HT et al (1993) Infectious morbidity associated with long-term use of venous access devices in patients with cancer. *Ann. Intern. Med.*, **119**: 1168–74.

Hammond JS, Varas R, Ward CG (1988) Suppurative thrombophlebitis: a new look at a continuing problem. *South. Med. J.*, **81**: 969–71.

Hansell DT (1989) Intravenous nutrition: the central or peripheral route? *Intravenous Ther. Clin. Monitor.*, **July**: 184–90.

Health Protection Agency (2003) *Surveillance of Hospital-acquired Bacteraemia in English Hospitals, 1997–2002.* Health Protection Agency, London. Available online at: www.hpa.org.uk.

Hekker TA, van Overhagen W, Schneider AJ (1990) Pressure transducers: an overlooked source of sepsis in the intensive care unit. *Intens. Care Med.*, **16**: 511–12.

Hoen B, Paul-Dauphin A, Hestin D et al (1998) EPIBACDIAL: a multi-center prospective study of risk factors for bacteremia in chronic hemodialysis patients. *J. Am. Soc. Nephrol.*, **9**: 869–76.

Hoffman KK, Weber DJ, Samsa GP et al (1992) Transparent polyurethane film as an intravenous catheter dressing: a meta-analysis of the infection risks. *JAMA*, **267**: 2072–6.

Hospitals in Europe Link for Infection Control through Surveillance (HELICS) (2004) Protocol for the surveillance of nosocomial infections in intensive care units. Version 6.1. Available online at: http://helics.univ-lyon1.fr/

Howell PB, Walter PE, Doncwitz GR et al (1995) Risk factors for infection of adult patients with cancer who have tunnelled central venous catheters. *Cancer*, **75**: 1367–75.

Inoue Y, Nezu R, Matsuda H et al (1992) Prevention of catheter-related sepsis during parenteral nutrition: effect of a new connection device. *J. Parenter. Enteral Nutr.*, **16**: 581–5.

Johnstone JD (1982) Infrequent infections associated with Hickman catheters. *Cancer Nursing*, **April**: 125–9.

Khawaja HT, Campbell MJ, Weaver PC (1988) Effect of transdermal glyceryl trinitrate on the survival of peripheral intravenous infusions: a double-blind prospective clinical study. *Br. J. Surg.*, **75**: 1212–15.

Lai KK (1998) Safety of prolonging peripheral cannula and IV tubing use from 72 hours to 96 hours. *Am. J. Infect. Contr.*, **26**: 66–70.

Lange BJ, Weiman M, Feuer EJ et al (1997) Impact of changes in catheter management on infectious complication among children with central venous catheters. *Infect. Contr. Hosp. Epidemiol.*, **18**: 326–32.

Levin A, Mason AJ, Jindal KK et al (1991) Prevention of hemodialysis subclavian vein catheter infections by topical povidone-iodine. *Kidney Int.*, **40**: 934–8.

Linares J, Sitges-Serra A, Garau J et al (1985) Pathogenesis of catheter sepsis: a prospective study with quantitative and semiquantitative cultures of catheter hub and segments. *J. Clin. Microbiol.*, **21**: 357–60.

Maki DG, Mermel LA (1998) Infections due to infusion therapy. In: Bennett JV, Brachman PX (eds) *Hospital Infections*, 4th edn. Lippincott-Raven, Philadelphia.

Maki DG, Ringer M (1987) Evaluation of dressing regimens for prevention of infection with peripheral intravenous catheters, gauze, a transparent polyurethane dressing and an iodophor-transparent dressing. *JAMA*, **258**: 2396–403.

Maki DG, Will L (1984) Colonization and infection associated with transparent dressings for central venous, arterial and Hickman catheters: a comparative trial. Paper presented at the 24th Interscience Conference on Antimicrobial Agents and Chemotherapy. Abstract 991. American Society for Microbiology, Washington DC.

Maki DG, Goldman DA, Rhame FS (1973) Infection control in intravenous therapy. *Ann. Intern. Med.*, **79**: 867–87.

Maki DG, Hassemer C, Sarafini HW (1977) A semi-quantitative culture method for identifying intravenous catheter-related infection. *N. Engl. J. Med.*, **296**: 1305–9.

Maki DG, Botticelli JT, Le Roy ML et al (1987) Prospective study of replacing administration sets for intravenous therapy at 48 hour versus 72 hour intervals. 72 hours is safe and cost-effective. *JAMA*, **258**: 1777–81.

Maki DG, Ringer M, Alvarado CJ (1991a) Prospective randomised trial of povidone-iodine, alcohol and chlorhexidine for prevention of infection associated with central venous and arterial catheters. *Lancet*, **338**: 339–43.

Maki DG, Stolz S, Wheeler S (1991b) A prospective, randomised, three-way clinical comparison of a novel, highly impermeable, polyurethane dressing with 206 Swan–Ganz pulmonary artery catheters: Opsite IV3000 vs Tegaderm v gauze and tape. I. Cutaneous colonization under the dressing, catheter-related infection. Paper presented at Improving Catheter Site Care symposium, Series 179, pp. 61–6. Royal Society of Medicine Services, London.

Maki DG, Stolz SS, Wheeler S et al (1994) A prospective, randomised trial of gauze and two polyurethane dressings for site care of pulmonary artery catheters: implications for catheter management. *Crit. Care Med.*, **32**: 1729–37.

Maki DG, Stolz SS, Wheeler S et al (1997) Prevention of central venous catheter-related bloodstream infection by use of an antiseptic-impregnated catheter. A randomized controlled trial. *Ann. Intern. Med.*, **127**: 257–66.

Maki DG, Narans LL, Knasinski V et al (2000) Prospective, randomized, investigator-masked trial of a novel chlorhexidine-impregnated disk (Biopatch) on central venous and arterial catheters. *Infect. Contr. Hosp. Epidemiol.*, **21**(2): 96.

Medical Devices Directorate (1993) *Degradation of Silicone Tubing by Alcohol-based Antiseptics*. HN(93) 7. Department of Health, Wetherby, UK.

Mermel LA (2000) Prevention of intravascular catheter-related infections. *Ann. Intern. Med.*, **132**(5): 391–402.

Mermel LA, Stolz S, Maki DG (1991) Epidemiology and pathogenesis of infection with Swan–Ganz catheters. A prospective study using molecular epidemiology. *Am. J. Med.*, **91**(3b): 197.

Mermel LA, Farr BM, Sherertz RJ et al (2001) Guidelines for the management of intravascular catheter-related infections. *Infect. Contr. Hosp. Epidemiol.*, **22**(4): 222–42.

Mimoz O, Pieroni L, Lawrence C et al (1996) Prospective, randomized trial of two antiseptic solutions for prevention of central venous or arterial catheter colonization and infection in intensive care unit patients. *Crit. Care Med.*, **11**: 1818–23.

Morbidity and Mortality Weekly Report (2000) Monitoring hospital-acquired infections to promote patient safety – United States, 1990–1999. *MMWR*, **49**(8): 149–52.

Mughal MM (1989) Complications of intravenous feeding catheters. *Br. J. Surg.*, **76**: 15–21.

O'Brien BJ, Buxton MJ, Khawaja HT (1990) An economic evaluation of transdermal glyceryl trinitrate in the prevention of intravenous infusion failure. *J. Clin. Epidemiol.*, **43**: 757–63.

O'Grady NP, Alexander M, Dellinger EP et al (2002) Guideline for the prevention of intravascular catheter-related infections. *MMWR*, **51**: RR10.

Parras F, Ena J, Bouza E et al (1994) Impact of an educational program for the prevention of colonization of intravascular catheter. *Infect. Contr. Hosp. Epidemiol.*, **15**: 335–7.

Pearson ML (1996) Guideline for prevention of intravascular device-related infections. *Am. J. Infect. Contr.*, **24**: 262–93.

Pittet D, Wenzel RP (1995) Nosocomial bloodstream infections. Secular trends in rates, mortality and contribution to total hospital deaths. *Arch. Intern. Med.*, **155**: 1177–84.

Pittet D, Tarara D, Wenzel RP (1994) Nosocomial bloodstream infections in critically ill patients: excess length of stay, extra costs and attributable mortality. *JAMA*, **271**: 1598–607.

Plowman R, Graves N, Griffin M et al (2001) The rate and cost of hospital-acquired infections occurring in patients admitted to selected specialties of a district general hospital in England and the national burden imposed. *J. Hosp. Infect.*, **47**: 198–209.

Pratt RA, Pellowe CM, Loveday HP et al (2001) The Epic project: developing national evidence-based guidelines for preventing healthcare associated infections. *J. Hosp. Infect.*, **47** (suppl. A).

Public Health Laboratory Service (1998) *Protocol for Surveillance of Hospital-acquired Bacteraemia*. Nosocomial Infection National Surveillance Scheme, Public Health Laboratory Service, London. Available online at: www.hpa.org.uk.

Quercia RA, Hills SW, Klimek JJ et al (1986) Bacteriologic contamination of intravenous infusion delivery systems in an intensive care unit. *Am. J. Med.*, **80**: 364–8.

Raad II, Davies S, Becker M et al (1993a) Low infection rate and long durability of nontunnelled silastic catheters. A safe cost-effective alternative for long-term venous access. *Arch. Intern. Med.*, **153**: 1791–6.

Raad II, Umphrey J, Khan A et al (1993b) The duration of placement as a predictor of peripheral and pulmonary arterial catheter infections. *J. Hosp. Infect.*, **23**: 17–26.

Raad II, Hohn DC, Gilbreath BJ et al (1994) Prevention of central venous catheter-related infections by using maximal sterile barrier precautions during insertion. *Infect. Contr. Hosp. Epidemiol.*, **15**: 231–8.

Raad II, Baba M, Bodey GP (1995) Diagnosis of catheter-related infections: the role of surveillance and targeted quantitative skin cultures. *Clin. Infect. Dis.*, **20**: 593–7.

Randolph AG, Cook DJ, Gonzales CA et al (1998) Benefit of heparin use in central venous and pulmonary artery catheters: a meta-analysis of randomized controlled trials. *Chest*, **113**: 165–71.

Raviglione MC, Battan R, Pablos-Mendez A et al (1989) Infections associated with Hickman catheters in patients with acquired immune deficiency syndrome. *Am. J. Med.*, **86**: 780–6.

Ricard P, Martin R, Marcoux JA (1985) Protection of indwelling vascular catheters; incidence of bacterial contamination and catheter-related sepsis. *Crit. Care Med.*, **13**: 541–3.

Richet H, Hubert B, Nitemberg G et al (1990) Prospective multicenter study of vascular catheter-related complications and risk factors for positive central-catheter cultures in intensive care unit patients. *J. Clin. Microbiol.*, **28**: 2520–5.

Royal College of Nursing (2003) *Administration of IV Therapy to Children in the Community Setting. Guidance for Nursing Staff*, 3rd edn. Royal College of Nursing: London. Available online at: www.rcn.org.uk.

Ryder MA (1995) Peripheral access. *Opin. Oncol. Clin. North Am.*, **4**: 395–427.

Sheldon DL, Johnson WC (1979) Cutaneous mucomycosis: two documented cases of suspected nosocomial infection. *JAMA*, **241**: 1032–3.

Shivnan JC, McGuire D, Freeman S et al (1991) Comparison of transparent adherent and dry sterile gauze dressings for long-term central catheters in patients undergoing bone marrow transplant. *Oncol. Nurse Forum*, **18**: 1349–56.

Spencer RC (1990) Use of in-line filters for intravenous infusions in intensive care units. *J. Hosp. Infect.*, **16**: 281.

Stonehouse J, Butcher J (1996) Phlebitis associated with peripheral cannulae. *Prof. Nurse*, **12**(1): 51–4.

Syndman DR, Donnelly-Reidy M, Perry WC et al (1987) Intravenous tubing containing burettes can be safely changed at 72-hour intervals. *Infect. Contr.*, **8**: 113–16.

Tebbs SE, Chose A, Elliot TSJ (1996) Microbial contamination of intravenous and arterial catheters. *Int. Care Med.*, **22**(3): 272–3.

Thomas A, Lalitha MK, Jesudason MV et al (1993) Transducer related *Enterobacter cloacae* sepsis in post-operative cardiothoracic patients. *J. Hosp. Infect.*, **25**: 211–14.

Veenstra DL, Saint S, Saha S et al (1999a) Efficacy of antiseptic-impregnated central venous catheter in preventing catheter-related bloodstream infection: a meta-analysis. *JAMA*, **281**(3): 261–6.

Veenstra DL, Saint S, Sullivan S (1999b) Cost-effectiveness of antiseptic-impregnated central venous catheter for the prevention of catheter-related bloodstream infection. *JAMA*, **282**(6): 554–60.

Walsh R, Gurevich R, Cunha SA (1993) *Listeria*: a potential cause of febrile transfusion reactions. *J. Hosp. Infect.*, **24**: 81–2.

Ward V, Wilson J, Taylor L et al (1997) *Preventing Hospital-acquired Infection. Clinical Guidelines*. Public Health Laboratory Service, London.

Weightman NC, Simpson EM, Speller DCE et al (1988) Bacteraemia related to indwelling central venous catheters: prevention, diagnosis and treatment. *Eur. J. Clin. Microbiol. Infect. Dis.*, **7**(2): 125–9.

Widner AF (1997) Intravenous-related infections. In: Wenzel RP (ed.) *Prevention and Control of Nosocomial Infections*, 3rd edn. Williams and Wilkins, Baltimore, MD.

Further Reading

Pittet D, Hugonnet S, Harbarth S et al (2000) Effectiveness of a hospital-wide programme to improve compliance with hand hygiene. *Lancet*, **356**: 1307–12.

Chapter **10**

Preventing infection associated with urethral catheters

INTRODUCTION

Urinary tract infections (UTIs) are the most common infection acquired in hospital, affecting approximately 2.5% of patients admitted to hospital and accounting for over 20% of all such infections (Emmerson et al 1996, Glynn et al 1997, Plowman et al 2001).

The normal bladder has a number of defences against infection: the urethra is difficult for micro-organisms to pass along, the epithelial cells lining the bladder are resistant to bacterial adherence and the process of urination ensures that bacteria that do manage to gain access to the bladder are diluted by fresh urine and removed by the next urination. The presence of a urethral catheter interferes with these defences and as a result it is a major predisposing factor for healthcare-associated UTIs, three-quarters of which are related to indwelling urethral catheters. UTI is also a major problem in nursing homes and rehabilitation centres where the elderly, debilitated and others catheterized for prolonged periods are at greater risk of acquiring recurrent UTIs and of developing the long-term complications associated with the infection (Warren et al 1994).

SYMPTOMS, DIAGNOSIS AND TREATMENT OF URINARY TRACT INFECTION

In a non-catheterized individual the diagnosis of a UTI is usually based on clinical symptoms: frequency of micturition, pain on micturition (dysuria), fever and sometimes loin or suprapubic pain. These symptoms reflect an inflammatory process in the bladder or kidneys caused by the invasion of the tissues by micro-organisms. In the catheterized patient diagnosis of UTI is more complex; frequency and dysuria will not be apparent unless the catheter is removed and other symptoms may be absent, particularly in elderly or confused patients (Warren et al 1987).

The diagnosis of UTI may be confirmed in the microbiology laboratory by culturing a specimen of urine. Where bacteria are found to be present in urine, this is termed bacteriuria. In the non-catheterized patient, the specimen is readily contaminated by micro-organisms colonizing the periurethral area and therefore only the isolation of a single micro-organism in high concentration (more than 10^5 organisms per ml) is considered indicative of infection. In catheterized patients urine samples should be taken from the sampling sleeve on the catheter or drainage system (see p. 25). These specimens are less prone to contamination and a lower concentration of micro-organisms (10^2 per ml) may be considered significant, as they are likely to reach a much higher concentration within a few days (Saint & Lipsky 1999). In the catheterized patient bacteriuria is commonly asymptomatic and in these circumstances treatment is not usually indicated. The presence of white blood cells (pyuria) in the urine of bacteriuric patients is usually suggestive of host infection, although the cells may equally represent a response to the catheter or to urological surgery (Stamm 1983). Box 10.1 provides an example of a precise definition of urinary tract infection, which may be useful for monitoring infection rates or undertaking studies of catheter-associated UTI.

The micro-organisms that commonly cause UTI are found colonizing the periurethral area. In the non-catheterized patient virulent strains of *Escherichia coli* cause the most serious infections. These carry genes coding for fimbriae, adhesins and haemolysin that enable them to adhere to uroepithelial cells, invade and damage tissue (Johnson 1991). In catheterized patients in whom normal host defences are compromised, these strains rarely cause infection; instead, a wide range of species are responsible. Mostly these are Gram-negative bacilli but yeasts are an increasingly frequent cause of catheter-associated UTI, especially when the patient has received antimicrobial agents (Bronsema et al 1993).

If more than one type of bacterium is found in the urine of a non-catheterized patient, this is often attributed to contamination of the specimen by bacteria from the skin or perineum. In the catheterized patient, two or more types of bacteria are frequently identified. The longer the catheter is in situ, the greater the variety of bacteria isolated from the urine (Warren 2001).

Treatment of urinary tract infection

Bacteriuria in catheterized patients is generally asymptomatic with no evidence of bacteria invading

---

Box 10.1   Definition of catheter–associated urinary tract infection (Health Protection Agency 2000)

Urinary tract infection is considered to be catheter associated if the patient has an indwelling catheter in situ at the time of onset of UTI or has had an indwelling catheter removed within 3 days prior to the onset of UTI. A urinary tract infection must meet one of the following criteria.

Criterion 1 Patient without an indwelling urethral catheter
(a) Has $\geq 10^5$ micro-organisms per ml from a midstream specimen and one or more of the following with no other recognized cause: urgency, frequency, dysuria, loin pain, loin or suprapubic tenderness, fever (>38°C skin temperature) or pyuria ($\geq 10^4$ WBC per ml)

or

(b) Physician diagnoses UTI, institutes appropriate antimicrobial therapy and the patient has two or more of the following with no other recognized cause: urgency, frequency, dysuria, loin pain, loin or suprapubic tenderness, fever (>38°C skin temperature) or pyuria ($\geq 10^4$ WBC per ml)

Criterion 2 Patient has an indwelling urethral catheter in situ *and*
(a) 10^4 micro-organisms per ml from a catheter specimen of urine and one or more of the following with no other recognized cause: loin pain, loin or suprapubic tenderness, fever (>38°C skin temperature) or pyuria ($\geq 10^4$ WBC per ml)

or

(b) Physician diagnoses UTI, institutes appropriate antimicrobial therapy and the patient has two or more of the following with no other recognized cause: loin pain, loin or suprapubic tenderness, fever (>38°C skin temperature) or pyuria ($\geq 10^4$ WBC per ml)

---

the bladder tissues, ureters or kidneys. However, in up to 30% of catheterized patients with bacteriuria, the bacteria invade the tissues and the patient develops symptoms of UTI such as fever, flank pain and haematuria (Garibaldi et al 1982).

Asymptomatic bacteriuria does not usually require treatment unless the patient is at high risk of renal infection or bacteraemia (e.g. neutropenia, pregnancy or urological disorder) or is undergoing urological

Box 10.2   Biofilms

Micro-organisms commonly coat the surfaces of foreign materials inserted into the body by forming biofilms. These are sheets of micro-organisms that adhere to the surface by secreting an extracellular substance called glycocalyx. On urinary catheters biofilms form on the inner surface; they incorporate urinary proteins and salts and accumulate crystals of struvite and apatite. Eventually the biofilm, or 'encrustation', becomes so thick that it obstructs the flow of urine. The presence of some bacteria, e.g. *Proteus mirabilis*, in the urine is associated with rapid encrustation because they produce an enzyme called urease which converts urea to ammonia. This increases the pH of the urine and causes struvite and apatite to crystallize (Choong et al 2001).

surgery. In the catheterized patient, antibiotic therapy has no effect on the bacteriuria or incidence of febrile episodes while the catheter is in situ and is likely to encourage antibiotic-resistant strains to emerge (Nicolle 1997, Warren et al 1982).

Symptoms of infection usually resolve spontaneously if the catheter is removed and may be treated after removal if they persist (Stamm 1998). As bacteria embedded in the biofilm (see Box 10.2) on the surface of the catheter may be protected from antimicrobials, the catheter should be changed if treatment is commenced (Kumon et al 2002).

Sequalae associated with urinary tract infections

Patients with long-term catheters have approximately one episode of unexplained fever every 100 days and UTIs are responsible for two-thirds of these febrile episodes. Most of these fevers are low grade, resolve rapidly without antibiotic treatment and do not appear to increase the mortality rate (Peterson & Roth 1989, Warren et al 1987). However, although UTIs are usually easily treated at relatively low cost, they are associated with an increased hospital stay and nearly double the cost of care. The high frequency with which they occur makes their overall costs high in comparison with other hospital-acquired infections (Plowman et al 2001).

A study by Platt et al (1982) demonstrated that catheterized patients who acquired a UTI in hospital were three times more likely to die than those who did not, even if other factors such as age, duration of catheterization and the severity of the illness were taken into account. This increased mortality rate is probably related to subsequent infections such as bacteraemia or damage to the urinary tract.

Bacteraemia
The invasion of the bloodstream by bacteria colonizing the urinary tract is the most serious outcome of bacteriuria. Bacteraemia develops in approximately 5% of catheter-associated UTIs (Krieger et al 1983). As approximately 10% of patients admitted to hospital are catheterized, the urinary tract is an important source of hospital-acquired bacteraemia, responsible for approximately 9% of these infections (Coello et al 2003). Infections caused by Gram-negative bacilli, the most common uropathogen, are often severe and are associated with a high mortality.

Bacteraemia probably goes unrecognized in many catheterized patients. It is particularly likely to occur during catheterization, when trauma to the mucosa during the procedure enables bacteria to enter the bloodstream.

Secondary infections
Bacteria originating from the urinary tract may also circulate around the body to cause secondary infections at other sites, for example wounds and central venous cannulae (Garibaldi 1993).

Damage to the urinary tract
Evidence from autopsies suggests that chronic inflammation of the kidneys occurs in more than one-third of patients who have been catheterized for a prolonged period. These patients are also at risk of developing urinary tract stones and other periurethral infections such as urethritis and prostatitis (Bryan & Reynolds 1984, Warren et al 1988).

FACTORS THAT AFFECT THE ACQUISITION OF URINARY TRACT INFECTION

Bacteria enter the bladder of the catheterized patient in one of three ways: first, they may be introduced with the catheter at the time of insertion; second, they may travel along the outside of the catheter; and third, they may travel along the inside lumen of the catheter (Fig. 10.1). There are important differences between men and women in the significance of each route of infection. The perineum is frequently colonized by potential uropathogens from the intestinal tract, especially Gram-negative bacilli. In women the vagina can also be an important source of uropathogens. If the lactobacilli that normally live in the vagina are eliminated by antibiotic therapy or changes in vaginal pH, faecal flora may establish and subsequently invade

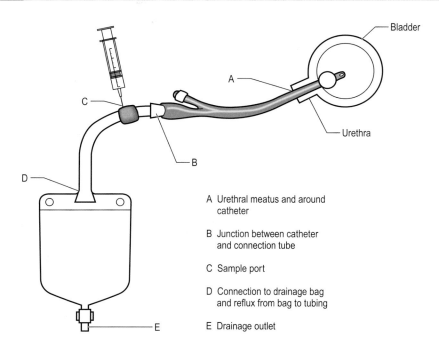

Figure 10.1 Potential points of entry of micro-organisms into the bladder of a catheterized patient.

A Urethral meatus and around catheter

B Junction between catheter and connection tube

C Sample port

D Connection to drainage bag and reflux from bag to tubing

E Drainage outlet

the urinary tract. In postmenopausal women vaginal pH is affected by the decline in oestrogen production which contributes to the increased incidence of UTI in this group (Nicolle 1997).

In women, the relatively short urethra enables bacteria from the perineum to reach the bladder more easily than in men. Garibaldi et al (1974) demonstrated that the risk of bacteriuria increased fourfold in women and twofold in men 72 h after meatal colonization was established. Kass & Schneiderman (1959) demonstrated that in the presence of a catheter, *Serratia marcescens* inoculated on to the urethral meatus travelled along the outside of the catheter and could be recovered in urine from the bladder a few days later. This route probably accounts for a significant proportion of UTI in catheterized women (Daifuku & Stamm 1984). Elderly institutionalized populations are particularly vulnerable to perineal colonization and asymptomatic bacteriuria is prevalent in up to 35% of men and 50% of women (Nicolle 1987, 1997).

In men, infection from perineal flora is less important because the urethra is longer and further away from the rectum. Generally, bacteria gain access to the bladder via the lumen of the catheter, frequently as a result of cross-infection from enteric bacteria carried on the hands of staff which enter the urine system when it is emptied, disconnected or handled (Daifuku & Stamm 1984). Bacteria introduced into the drainage bag take only a few days to reach the bladder via the drainage tubing. Some 15–20% of patients with

bacteriuria have the same micro-organism in their drainage bag before it reaches the bladder (Garibaldi et al 1974).

Nickel et al (1985) suggested that, in the patient catheterized for less than 7 days, most bacteria enter the drainage system from the drainage tap or following disconnection of the system. As the duration of catheterization increases, bacteria are more likely to enter the bladder alongside the catheter.

The duration of catheterization

Garibaldi et al (1974) demonstrated the strong relationship between the length of time the catheter was in place and the risk of UTI. They found that the risk of acquiring infection increased by 5% for each additional day of catheterization and that after 10 days, 50% of patients have bacteria in the urine. It is therefore not surprising that virtually all chronically catheterized patients have bacteria in their urine. This illustrates the importance of early catheter removal as a means of preventing catheter-associated UTI. Although indwelling catheters are no longer in common use as a means of managing incontinence, they are used in the management of surgical procedures and for the measurement of urine output. Glynn et al (1997), in a study of 19 hospitals in England and Wales, found considerable variation between hospitals in the proportion of patients catheterized. This suggests that there is potential to reduce catheter-associated

Table 10.1   Urinary catheter use by specialty in 19 hospitals in England and Wales

Specialty	Patients catheterized (%)		Duration of catheterization (days)	
Medicine	11.6	(5–7)	5	(3–9)
Surgery	34.4	(16–50)	3.5	(2–5)
Gynaecology	40.4	(21–72)	2	(0–3)
Orthopaedics	17.3	(10–26)	6	(3–11)
Overall rate	26.3	(12–35)	3	(2–4)

Values are median with range in parentheses.

UTI by reducing catheter insertion and duration of use (Table 10.1).

Patients who require a permanent or long-term catheter will inevitably acquire bacteria in the urine. Catheter management should therefore be focused on preventing both the introduction of new uropathogens and cross-infection to other patients. Treatment of bacteriuria in these patients is usually not indicated unless accompanied by symptoms such as fever.

Disruption of host defences

In addition to enhancing the passage of micro-organisms from the perineum to the bladder via the urethra, the presence of an indwelling urine catheter has important effects on other defences against infection. The presence of a foreign body in the bladder diminishes the activity of white blood cells, damages the mucosa and interferes with mechanisms that prevent adherence of bacteria to uroepithelial cells (Daifuku & Stamm 1986). Micro-organisms may accumulate on the surface of the catheter, protected from urine flow, host defences and antibiotics by the formation of a biofilm (see Box 10.2). Finally, the residual volume of urine that forms below the level of the drainage channels enables micro-organisms to multiply in the bladder.

MEASURES TO PREVENT INFECTION IN THE CATHETERIZED PATIENT

As the urethral catheter has become a routine feature of medical care, it is easy to forget the importance of prevention of infection in its management. The impact of good catheter management has been demonstrated by the reduction in catheter-associated UTI achieved over the last few decades through improvements in catheter design. In the 1960s urethral catheters drained into open buckets or bottles and more than 90% of catheterized patients developed bacteriuria. In the 1970s, the system of closed drainage system into a plastic bag was introduced and the rate dropped to

Table 10.2   Device-day rates of urinary tract infection in catheterized patients by specialty in 19 hospitals

Specialty	Infections per 1000 device–days	
Medicine	2.8	(0–9)
Surgery	3.9	(0–9.6)
Gynaecology	16.7	(1.4–33.4)
Orthopaedics	3.5	(0.8–10.3)
Overall rate	5.0	(2.5–11)

Values are median with range in parentheses.

25%. In the 1980s and 1990s even lower rates of around 10% were reported, reflecting improved infection control and decreasing duration of catheterization (Stamm 1991).

The key practices for preventing catheter-associated infection are minimizing the duration of catheterization and ensuring that the closed drainage system remains closed. Glynn et al (1997) demonstrated that the rates of UTI associated with urinary catheters varied considerably between different specialties and different hospitals, even when the duration of device use was taken into account by calculating the rate per 1000 device-days (Table 10.2). This suggests that the incidence of catheter-associated UTI could be reduced further by improvements in the management of urinary catheters.

Practices to prevent infection, based on research evidence, should be applied to the insertion of the catheter, the management of the urine drainage system and the care of the urethral meatus. Recommended practices are summarized in the guidelines for practice below and are discussed in more detail in the following sections.

Insertion of the catheter

The risk of developing bacteriuria after a single insertion and removal of a catheter ranges from 0.5% to

30% in the severely debilitated (Garibaldi 1993). The risk of infection then increases with each additional day for which the catheter remains in place. Indwelling urinary catheters should therefore only be used once all possible alternative methods have been considered (Pellowe et al 2003). The need for catheterization should also be reviewed regularly to ensure that the catheter is removed as soon as possible. Evidence suggests that in many cases this does not happen (Glynn et al 1997).

To minimize the risk of infection, the catheter should be inserted directly into the urethra without touching other parts of the perineum, which may be heavily colonized with bacteria. This probably explains why catheters inserted in the operating theatre, where the procedure is more easily performed, are associated with fewer infections (Castle & Osterhout 1974). It is impossible to remove the perineal flora completely prior to the procedure but cleansing before insertion may reduce the number of bacteria. Whilst cleansing with soap and water or saline is recommended, there is some evidence that prior cleansing with an antiseptic solution reduces the risk of bacteriuria (Panknin & Althaus 2001, Pratt et al 2001). A thorough explanation to the patient is likely to improve compliance and reduce the risk of contaminating the catheter or causing trauma to the urethra. The healthcare worker performing the procedure should be properly trained and competent. Trauma and discomfort are also likely to be reduced if a sterile single-use lubricant is applied to the urethra (Pratt et al 2001).

Securing the catheter to the patient's thigh has been recommended to prevent it moving in the urethra (Jenner 1983). There is no evidence that this reduces the infection rate but for some patients it may reduce discomfort.

Guidelines for practice: insertion of a urethral catheter

- Wash hands and use sterile gloves
- Prepare the patient and position comfortably
- Instil anaesthetic lubricating gel into the urethra
- Clean perineum and external meatus with saline, water or soap and water
- Use sterile equipment
- Insert catheter directly into urethra
- Select catheter appropriately
- Inflate balloon with correct amount of sterile water
- Remove the catheter as soon as possible

Intermittent catheterization In patients who need long-term catheterization, periodic emptying of the bladder by the insertion of a sterile or clean catheter every few hours has been shown to be effective in reducing the risk of infection (Perkush & Giroux 1993). Although patients managed in this way still usually become bacteriuric after 2–3 weeks, they have a reduced risk of developing bacteraemia, fever, stone formation and renal deterioration (Wyndaele & Maes 1990). The patient can be taught to self-catheterize safely using a clean reusable catheter washed between each use and stored in a clean covered container (Pellowe et al 2003, Warren 2001). Self-catheterization is an accepted form of management for many patients with spinal injury, enabling them to lead a more normal life in the community. If hospitalized, these patients should be helped to manage their catheterization using the technique with which they are familiar. The use of intermittent catheterization in other groups of patients has been recommended and may be a useful approach for managing problems with postoperative urinary drainage or retention (Pellowe et al 2003).

Suprapubic catheterization The risk of bacteria entering the bladder along the outside of the catheter may be avoided by insertion of a catheter directly into the bladder through the abdominal wall. The catheters are inserted under local or general anaesthesia and may be self-retaining or stitched to the abdominal wall. There is some evidence to suggest that suprapubic catheters are associated with lower rates of bacteriuria and may be cost-effective for long-term catheterization (Pellowe et al 2003, Saint & Lipsky 1999, Sheriff et al 1998). Intraurethral catheters are devices placed inside the urethra to relieve urinary retention associated with an enlarged prostate gland and may be left in place for months with a reduced risk of infection (Neilsen et al 1990).

Penile sheaths Drainage of urine into a penile sheath attached to a drainage bag reduces the risk of bacteria entering the bladder alongside the catheter and these devices have been associated with reduced rates of bacteriuria (Ouslander et al 1987). However, they should be changed frequently to prevent uropathogens colonizing the skin beneath the condom, causing local skin infection and providing a reservoir for the spread of hospital pathogens (Fierer & Ekstrom 1981).

Catheter valves These enable patients to control bladder emptying and may be preferable for patients with the mental acuity and physical dexterity to manage them as they reduce the risk of bacteria gaining access to the drainage system via the bag (Pellowe et al 2003, Roe 1990a).

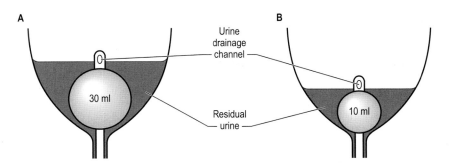

Figure 10.2   The urinary catheter retention balloon. (A) A 30 ml balloon. (B) A 10 ml balloon.

Type of catheter

Urinary catheters are available in a wide range of sizes and materials. Appropriate selection is essential to minimize trauma to the delicate mucosa of the bladder and urethra (Pomfret 1996).

Catheter size

The diameter of a catheter is measured in charrière: 8–10 Ch for paediatric catheters and 12–30 Ch for adult catheters. The lumen of even the smallest catheter is sufficient to cope with the volume of urine produced and the larger catheters are indicated only where the lumen may become blocked by an unusual amount of debris (e.g. following bladder or prostate gland surgery). To minimize trauma to the urethra, only 12 and 14 Ch catheters should be used for routine catheterization in adults, unless the urine contains a considerable amount of debris. Whistle-tip catheters have large drainage holes to accommodate clots and debris. The Conformacath catheter is designed to conform to the slit-like shape of the normal urethra to reduce discomfort and trauma to the mucosa. Pomfret (1992) found it offered a useful alternative method of catheterization for patients who could not tolerate a conventional catheter.

Catheters are now also available in a shorter length for female patients. Male length catheters used in female patients result in a considerable amount of excess tubing, which is more likely to kink and cannot be easily concealed under skirts when used with leg bags.

The most common sizes of retention balloon are 10 and 30 ml. Large balloons irritate the bladder mucosa, causing pain and discomfort to the patient (Roe & Brocklehurst 1987). They also increase the volume of urine remaining in the bladder, providing nutrients in which bacteria can multiply (Fig. 10.2). The 30 ml balloon is therefore usually indicated only after prostate surgery where its size and weight may reduce bleeding from the prostatic bed. All other catheters

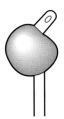

Figure 10.3   An underinflated retention balloon. The distorted balloon is more likely to damage the bladder mucosa.

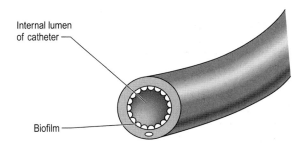

Figure 10.4   Biofilm formation inside a urethral catheter.

should be retained in the bladder with a 10 ml balloon. It is also essential to inflate the balloon with the correct amount of sterile water. Balloons that are underinflated or overinflated become misshapen and increase the risk that the bladder mucosa will be traumatized (Fig. 10.3).

Catheter material

Bacteria attach to the internal surface of the catheter, forming a biofilm (see Box 10.2). This biofilm, commonly referred to as encrustation, builds up over time and may eventually obstruct the lumen of the catheter, preventing the flow of urine (Fig. 10.4). Patients who are expected to have a catheter in place

Table 10.3   Selection of urinary catheters

Catheter material	Indication	Comments
Plastic	Very short-term use only; avoid if possible	Rigid material, irritates mucosa and causes trauma
Latex (thin silicone coat)	Short-term use, up to 14 days	Prone to encrustation, associated with trauma and strictures
Latex coated with Teflon	Short-term use, up to 28 days	Reduced mucosal irritation, resistant to encrustation
Latex with bonded silicone coating	Long-term use, up to 12 weeks	Minimal mucosal irritation, resistant to encrustation
Latex with hydrogel coating	Long-term use, up to 12 weeks	Minimal mucosal irritation, resistant to encrustation
All silicone	Long-term use, up to 12 weeks	Minimal mucosal irritation, resistant to encrustation

Note: examine the packaging carefully for a description of the catheter material.

for more than 3 weeks require one that will be resistant to encrustation and cause the minimum of irritation (Pomfret 1996) (Table 10.3).

Urinary catheters are made of plastic, latex coated with inert materials such as silicone or Teflon, or all-silicone. The bladder mucosa tolerates these materials to a variable extent and the material also influences the rate at which biofilms develop. Plastic catheters are associated with bladder spasm, urethral pain and leakage and their use should be avoided (Blannin & Hobden 1980). Silicone is a very inert material, causes minimal irritation and is fairly resistant to bacterial adherence and encrustation (Kumon et al 2002). Latex is a highly irritant material but when coated with a more inert material, such as silicone, can be tolerated for longer. Hydrogel coating absorbs liquid to become soft and slippery and therefore causes minimal damage to the urethral mucosa. It is also reasonably resistant to bacterial adherence and encrustation (Kumon et al 2002).

Various types of antimicrobial-impregnated catheters have been tried. Silver has generated the most interest as silver ions are antibacterial, non-toxic and do not encourage the emergence of antibiotic-resistant strains. Early studies on silver oxide-coated catheters did not demonstrate any benefit. However, more recently silver alloy-coated catheters have been shown to reduce the incidence of bacteriuria (Leidberg & Lindeberg 1990). Saint et al (2000) estimated that for the short-term catheterized, the effect of silver alloy catheters on the incidence of symptomatic UTI and bacteriuria would

be sufficient to generate considerable cost savings over standard catheters.

Frequency of catheter replacement
A transient bacteraemia may occur during recatheterization and long-term catheters should therefore not be changed unless necessary (Bryan & Reynolds 1984). Antimicrobial prophylaxis should be considered for patients at risk of endocarditis or previous history of bacteriuria in association with catheter replacement (Pellowe et al 2003). Provided the most appropriate size and type of catheter has been selected, the main indication for catheter change is blockage of the lumen by debris or encrustation. At least 50% of long-term catheterized patients will experience problems with encrustation and blockage (Pellowe et al 2003). The rate at which the catheter encrusts depends on the catheter material and the urine. An alkaline urine which contains high concentrations of proteins and calcium salts causes biofilms to develop more rapidly (Kunin et al 1987). The presence of certain types of bacteria in the urine, especially proteus and pseudomonas, also encourages the formation of biofilms. Some solutions are recommended for regular instillations into the bladder to prevent biofilm formation but the efficacy of these solutions has not been demonstrated (Pellowe et al 2003).

Blockage by encrustation may cause urine to leak around the side of the catheter. Bladder spasm caused by irritation of the mucosa may also force urine out of the bladder around the catheter. Large catheters are particularly associated with irritation and leakage and, where possible, should be replaced by a smaller size (Blannin & Hobden 1980).

Catheter insertion and changes should be accurately documented to enable care to be reviewed and planned appropriately. In the long-term catheterized, catheter-changing regimens should be designed to prevent blockage and based on individual patient assessment (Getliffe 1994).

Reducing colonization of the perineum

A considerable amount of advice about the management of urinary catheters relates to preventing bacteria that colonize the perineum from gaining access to the bladder from the urethral opening. Regular cleansing with an antiseptic solution used to be common practice (Crow et al 1988). However, the controlled trial by Burke et al (1981) found that catheterized patients who received no meatal cleansing had the lowest infection rate and that cleansing with soap was associated with fewer infections than with povidone-iodine. The conclusion to be drawn from this study is that bacteria are more likely to be introduced to the urethra during the cleaning procedure and a specific meatal cleansing procedure should be avoided. There is little evidence that bathing increases the incidence of UTI in catheterized patients. Degroot (1979), in a study on 10 catheterized patients, used a dye in the bathwater to indicate that the water did not pass into the bladder during bathing. Meatal care using soap and water and clean wipes should therefore be based on the usual hygiene requirements of individual patients and washing the meatus with soap and water during routine bathing or showering is all that is required (Pellowe et al 2003, Saint & Lipsky 1999).

Management of the drainage system

Bacteria enter the drainage system in the drainage bag or at the junction between the catheter and the

drainage bag. These bacteria reach the bladder along the tubing after a few days (Garibaldi et al 1974).

The significance of a closed system of urinary drainage to the prevention of UTI was not really appreciated until the 1960s. Before this, catheter urine had commonly flowed into an open container and infection rates as high as 95% within 24 h of catheterization were common. The plastic, drainable, urine drainage bags with which we are now familiar were introduced in the early 1970s and have had a significant impact on reducing the rate of UTI (Thornton & Andriole 1970).

Breaks in the closed system have been reported to occur frequently (Burke et al 1986). Crow et al (1988) found that the catheter–drainage bag junction was disconnected in 42% of patients and in 52% the bag was not properly positioned to ensure downward flow of urine.

The importance of not opening the drainage system was demonstrated in a 1983 study by Platt et al, who used catheters that had been presealed to a drainage bag. The seals could be removed and the bag disconnected but, nonetheless, a 17% reduction in disconnection was recorded. The control group of patients whose catheters were not sealed had three times more UTIs than the group with sealed catheters. These studies highlight deficiencies in the management of urine drainage systems which, if prevented, may reduce the incidence of bacteriuria in the short-term catheterized.

The drainage system should not be opened to take specimens, which should instead be obtained aseptically from the sampling port with a needle. The drainage bag should be emptied when necessary to avoid reflux of urine. A clean pair of gloves should be worn for emptying the drainage bag and discarded on completion of the procedure. When the bag is emptied, care should be taken to ensure that micro-organisms are not introduced on to the tap by contact with a contaminated container or other surface. Containers should be decontaminated in a bedpan washer or autoclaved after each use. Observational studies have shown that urine collection containers are commonly not decontaminated properly between uses (Glynn et al 1997).

Bacteria easily gain access to the drainage bag from the tap and multiply very rapidly in urine at room temperature (Bradley et al 1986). Bacteria remaining in the bag after it is emptied inoculate fresh urine entering the bag. The bacterial biofilm that adheres and spreads over the surface of the catheter and drainage bag enables bacteria in the bag to travel through non-return valves in the bag and along the lumen of the catheter into the bladder (Nickel et al

---

Guidelines for practice: perineal cleansing

- Routine bathing or showering as part of daily hygiene is sufficient
- The perineum should be cleaned after an episode of faecal incontinence
- Clean underneath the prepuce
- Use soap and water and clean wipes
- Wash hands before and after the procedure
- Antimicrobial creams are not necessary

1985). Flutter valves, drip chambers or airlocks are of no value in preventing bacteriuria.

Incorrect positioning of the drainage bag can assist the transfer of bacteria to the bladder. Roberts et al (1965) found that bacteria could be transported distances of 0.9–1.2 m in rising air bubbles, often generated when the tubing is kinked and columns of urine are formed. Drainage bags should therefore be positioned so that backflow is avoided and on a stand that prevents contact with the floor. If downward flow of urine cannot be maintained, the tubing should be clamped for a short period until the correct drainage can be resumed (Pratt et al 2001).

Bacteria grow less readily in dilute urine which has scarce nutrients (Asscher et al 1966). Encouraging the catheterized patient to drink plenty of fluid has the practical value of maintaining a constant downward flow of urine and reducing bacterial multiplication in the drainage bag. Some fluids (e.g. cranberry juice) are considered to reduce the number of bacteria in the urine by changing its acidity (Rogers 1991).

Cross-infection between catheterized patients

This has been frequently reported but the extent of the problem is probably underestimated. Schaberg et al (1980) showed that a significant proportion of nosocomial UTIs occur in clusters, particularly those caused by serratia and pseudomonas. Bacteria contaminating the drainage bag and the junction between catheter and bag are easily transferred to the hands when the bag is emptied or the drainage system is handled. The design of the tap influences the extent to which urine contaminates the hands during the emptying of the bag (Glenister 1987). Inadequately cleaned collection containers may also transmit infection between catheterized patients. Antibiotic-resistant strains of bacteria, which often have an ability to survive and transmit easily in the hospital environment, are commonly associated with outbreaks of infection amongst catheterized patients. The insertion of antiseptic solutions into urine drainage bags, although probably not effective or practical for routine use, may have a role in preventing transmission of nosocomial pathogens, for example in outbreaks of antibiotic-resistant strains, by reducing their con-centration in the bag urine (Thompson et al 1984, Warren 1997).

Catheter valves

These have been proposed as a method of preventing bacteria from gaining access to the bladder via the drainage bag. They enable the bladder to fill and to be emptied intermittently without the use of a drainage system. They may benefit the catheterized patient by reducing the incidence of infection, restoring bladder tone and improving the quality of life (Roe 1990a).

Bladder instillations

The administration of a bladder instillation involves disconnection of the closed drainage system which, as illustrated above, has been clearly demonstrated to increase the incidence of UTI. Such instillations should therefore be used only if a clear benefit can be demonstrated.

There is some evidence that antiseptics instilled in the bladder may prevent infection in patients who have had urological surgery but they are ineffective in treating established infections (Slade & Gillespie 1985). There is no evidence that they are of benefit in preventing bacteriuria in the long-term catheterized and extensive use of these solutions has been associated with the emergence of resistant bacteria (Stickler 1990).

Instillation of antiseptic solutions such as chlorhex-idine and noxythiolin should therefore not be used as part of routine management of the catheterized patient. A catheter blocked with debris should be flushed with saline, taking great care not to contaminate the connections (Pomfret 1996).

Other bladder instillations containing weak acids are intended to remove or control crystal formation

---

Guidelines for practice: maintenance of the drainage system

- Use a bag with an integral measuring chamber if monitoring of urine output is required
- Do not change the bag routinely
- Do not disconnect the catheter from the drainage bag unless absolutely necessary
- Empty the bag as infrequently as possible
- Wash hands before and after handling the drainage system
- Use clean gloves to handle the drainage system and discard afterwards
- Empty urine into a clean container and disinfect after use
- Take urine specimens from the sample port, not the drainage bag
- Ensure urine always flows downwards
- Avoid kinks in tubing
- Hang bag evenly on stand
- Do not change leg bags at night but connect to an overnight drainage bag
- Avoid use of bladder instillations

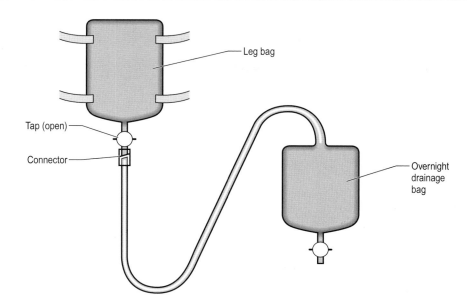

Figure 10.5   Overnight drainage system for a leg drainage bag.

Leg bag

Tap (open)

Connector

Overnight drainage bag

(e.g. Suby-G). These are indicated only for patients who have particular problems with rapidly encrusting catheters where they may remove or prevent encrustation and may reduce the need for frequent recatheterization (Roe 1990c).

Leg drainage bags

In the past patients using a bag attached to the leg for collecting urine changed it for a larger overnight drainage bag, which could contain the volume of urine produced at night but required frequent disconnection of the drainage system. Leg bag systems that enable an overnight drainage bag to be connected directly to the leg bag without incurring a break in the closed system

(Fig. 10.5) are preferred to minimize disconnection and reduce the risk of introducing micro-organisms. The overnight bag should be discarded after each use.

Patient education

In hospital, encouraging patients to care for their own urinary catheters can minimize the risk of cross-infection. The long-term catheterized patient in the community can benefit from education on how to manage the catheter and minimize the risk of introducing bacteria. Instructions should include advice on careful hand hygiene, perineal cleansing, positioning of the drainage bag and recognizing symptoms of infection (Roe 1990b).

References

Asscher AW, Sussman M, Waters WE et al (1966) Urine as a medium for bacterial growth. *Lancet*, **1**: 1039–41.

Blannin JP, Hobden J (1980) The catheter of choice. *Nursing Times*, **76**: 2092–3.

Bradley C, Babb J, Davies J et al (1986) Taking precautions. *Nursing Times*, **5 March**: 70–3.

Bronsema D, Adams J, Pallares R et al (1993) Secular trends in rates and etiology of nosocomial urinary tract infections at a university hospital. *J. Urol.*, **150**: 414–16.

Bryan CS, Reynolds KL (1984) Hospital-acquired bacteremic urinary tract infection. Epidemiology and outcome. *J. Urol.*, **132**: 494–8.

Burke JP, Garibaldi RA, Britt MR et al (1981) Prevention of catheter-associated urinary tract infections – efficacy of daily meatal care regimes. *Am. J. Med.*, **70**: 655–8.

Burke JP, Larsen RA, Stevens LE (1986) Nosocomial bacteriuria: estimating the potential for prevention by closed sterile urinary drainage. *Infect. Contr.*, **7**: 96–9.

Castle M, Osterhout S (1974) Urinary tract catheterisation and associated infection. *Nurs. Res.*, **23**: 170–4.

Choong S, Wood S, Fry C (2001) Catheter-associated urinary tract infections and encrustation. *Int. J. Antimicr. Ag.*, **17**(4): 305–10.

Coello R, Charlett A, Ward V et al (2003) Device-related sources of bacteraemia in English hospitals – opportunities for the prevention of hospital-acquired bacteraemia. *J. Hosp. Infect.*, **53**: 46–57.

Crow RA, Mulhall A, Chapman RG (1988) Indwelling catheterisation and related nursing practice. *J. Adv. Nurs.*, **13**: 489–95.

Daifuku R, Stamm W (1984) Association of rectal and urethral colonisation with urinary tract infection in patients with indwelling urethral catheters. *JAMA*, **252**: 2028–30.

Daifuku R, Stamm W (1986) Bacterial adhesion to bladder uroepithelial cells in catheter-associated urinary tract infection. *N. Engl. J. Med.*, **3145**: 1208–13.

Degroot JE (1979) Entrance of water into the bladder during Sitz bath in elderly catheterised and non-catheterised females. *Invest. Urol.*, **117**: 207–8.

Emmerson AM, Enstone JE, Griffin M et al (1996) The second national prevalence survey of infection in hospitals – overview of the results. *J. Hosp. Infect.*, **32**: 175–90.

Fierer J, Ekstrom M (1981) An outbreak of *Providencia stuartii* urinary tract infection. Patients with condom catheters are a reservoir of the bacteria. *JAMA*, **245**: 1553–5.

Garibaldi RA (1993) Hospital-acquired urinary infections. In: Wenzel RP (ed.) *Prevention and Control of Nosocomial Infections*, 2nd edn. Williams and Wilkins, Baltimore, MD.

Garibaldi RA, Burke JP, Dickman ML et al (1974) Factors predisposing to bacteriuria during indwelling urethral catheterisation. *N. Engl. J. Med.*, **291**: 215–19.

Garibaldi RA, Mooney BR, Epstein BJ et al (1982) An evaluation of daily bacteriologic monitoring to identify preventable episodes of catheter-associated urinary tract infection. *Infect. Contr.*, **3**: 466–70.

Getliffe K (1994) The characteristics and management of patients with recurrent blockage of long-term urinary catheters. *J. Adv. Nurs.*, **20**: 140–9.

Glenister H (1987) The passage of infection. *Nursing Times*, **83**(22): 68–73.

Glynn A, Ward V, Wilson J et al (1997) *Hospital-acquired Infection. Surveillance, Policies and Practice*. Public Health Laboratory Service, London.

Health Protection Agency (2000) *Protocol for Surveillance of Hospital-acquired Catheter-associated Urinary Tract Infection*. Health Protection Agency, London.

Jenner EA (1983) Prevention of catheter associated urinary tract infection. *Nursing*, **2**(13) (suppl.): 1–3.

Johnson JR (1991) Virulence factors in *Escherichia coli* urinary tract infection. *Clin. Microbiol. Rev.*, **4**: 80.

Kass EH, Schneiderman LJ (1959) Entry of bacteria into the urinary tract of patients with inlying catheters. *N. Engl. J. Med.*, **256**: 556–7.

Krieger JN, Kaiser DL, Wenzel RP (1983) Nosocomial urinary tract infections: secular trends, treatment and economics in a university hospital. *J. Urol.*, **130**: 102–6.

Kumon MH, Hashimoto M, Nishimurak K et al (2002) Catheter-associated urinary tract infection: impact of catheter materials on their management. *Int. J. Antimicr. Ag.*, **17**(4): 311–16.

Kunin CM, Chin QF, Chambers S (1987) Formation of encrustations on indwelling urinary catheters in the elderly: a comparison of different types of catheter materials in blockers and non-blockers. *J. Urol.*, **138**: 899–902.

Leidberg LP, Lindeberg T (1990) Silver alloy coated catheters reduce catheter-associated bacteriuria. *Br. J. Urol.*, **65**: 379–81.

Neilsen KK, Klarskov P, Nordling J et al (1990) The intraprostatic spiral. New treatment for urinary retention. *Br. J. Urol.*, **65**: 500–3.

Nickel JC, Grant SK, Costerton JW (1985) Catheter-associated bacteriuria: an experimental study. *Urology*, **36**: 369–75.

Nicolle LE (1987) Urinary tract infections in long-term care facilities. *Infect. Contr. Hosp. Epidemiol.*, **14**: 220–5.

Nicolle LE (1997) Asymptomatic bacteriuria in the elderly. *Infect. Dis. Clin. North Am.*, **11**(3): 647–63.

Ouslander J, Grengold B, Chen S (1987) External catheter use and the urinary tract infection among incontinent male nursing home patients. *J. Am. Geriatr. Soc.*, **35**: 1063–70.

Panknin H-T, Althaus A (2001) Guidelines for preventing infections associated with the insertion and maintenance of short-term indwelling urethral catheters in acute care. *J. Hosp. Infect.*, **49**(2): 146–7.

Pellowe CM, Pratt RJ, Harper P et al (2003) Evidence-based guidelines for preventing healthcare-associated infections in primary and community care in England. *J. Hosp. Infect.*, **55** (suppl. 2): S61–85.

Perkush I, Giroux J (1993) Clean intermittent catheterisation in spinal cord injury patients. A follow-up study. *J. Urol.*, **149**(5): 1068–71.

Peterson JR, Roth EJ (1989) Fever, bacteriuria and pyuria in spinal cord injured patients with indwelling urethral catheters. *Arch. Phys. Med. Rehabil.*, **70**: 839–41.

Platt R, Polk BF, Murdock B et al (1982) Mortality associated with nosocomial urinary tract infection. *N. Engl. J. Med.*, **307**: 939–43.

Platt R, Murdock B, Polk BF (1983) Reduction of mortality associated with nosocomial urinary tract infection. *Lancet*, **i**: 1893–7.

Plowman R, Graves N, Griffin M et al (2001) The rate and cost of hospital-acquired infections occurring in patients admitted to selected specialties of a district general hospital in England and the national burden imposed. *J. Hosp. Infect.*, **47**: 198–209.

Pomfret IJ (1992) Conformacath update. *J. Commun. Nurse*, **6**(8): 14–16.

Pomfret IJ (1996) Continence clinic catheters: design, selection and management. *Br. J. Nurs.*, **5**: 245–51.

Pratt RA, Pellowe CM, Loveday HP et al (2001) The Epic project: developing national evidence-based guidelines for preventing healthcare associated infections. *J. Hosp. Infect.*, **47** (suppl. A).

Roberts JMB, Linton KB, Pollard BR et al (1965) Long term catheter drainage in the male. *Br. J. Urol.*, **37**: 63–72.

Roe B (1990a) Do we need to clamp catheters? *Nursing Times*, **86**(43): 66–7.

Roe B (1990b) Study of the effects of education on the management of urine drainage systems by patients and carers. *J. Adv. Nurs.*, **15**: 223–31.

Roe B (1990c) Bladder instillations. *Nursing Standard*, **4**(51): 25–7.

Roe B, Brocklehurst JC (1987) Study of patients with indwelling catheters. *J. Adv. Nurs.*, **12**: 713–18.

Rogers J (1991) Pass the cranberry juice. *Nursing Times*, **87**: 36–7.

Saint S, Lipsky BA (1999) Preventing catheter-related bacteriuria. Should we? Can we? How? *Arch. Int. Med.*, **159**(8): 800–8.

Saint S, Elmore JG, Sullivan SD et al (1998) The efficacy of silver alloy-coated urinary catheters in preventing urinary tract infection: a meta-analysis. *Am. J. Med.*, **105**: 236–41.

Saint S, Veesha DL, Sullivan SD et al (2000) The potential clinical and economic benefits of silver alloy urinary catheters in preventing urinary tract infection. *Arch. Int. Med.*, **160**(17): 2670–5.

Schaberg DR, Haley RW, Highsmith AK et al (1980) Nosocomial bacteriuria: a prospective study of case clustering and antimicrobial resistance. *Ann. Intern. Med.*, **93**: 420–4.

Sheriff NM, Foley S, McFarlane J et al (1998) Long-term suprapubic catheterisation: clinical outcome and satisfaction survey. *Spinal Cord*, **36**: 171–6.

Slade N, Gillespie WA (1985) *The Urinary Tract and the Catheter: Infection and Other Problems*. John Wiley, Chichester.

Stamm WE (1983) Measurement of pyuria and its relation to bacteriuria. *Am. J. Med.*, **75** (suppl.): 53.

Stamm WE (1991) Catheter-associated urinary tract infections: epidemiology, pathogenesis and prevention. *Am. J. Med.*, **91** (suppl. 3B): 65S–71S.

Stamm WE (1998) Urinary tract infection. In: Bennett JV, Brachman PS (eds) *Hospital Infections*, 4th edn. Lippincott-Raven, Philadelphia.

Stickler DJ (1990) Antiseptics in bladder catheterization. *J. Hosp. Infect.*, **16**: 89–108.

Thompson RL, Haley CE, Searcy MA et al (1984) Catheter-associated bacteriuria. Failure to reduce attack rates using periodic instillations of a disinfectant into urinary drainage systems. *JAMA*, **251**: 747–51.

Thornton GF, Andriole VT (1970) Bacteriuria during indwelling catheter drainage II: effect of a closed sterile drainage system. *JAMA*, **214**: 339–42.

Warren JW (1997) Catheter-associated urinary tract infections. *Infect. Dis. Clin. North Am.*, **11**(3): 609–17.

Warren J (2001) Catheter-associated urinary tract infections. *Int. J. Antimicrob. Ag.*, **17**(4): 299–303.

Warren JW, Antony WC, Hoopes JM et al (1982) Cephalexin for susceptible bacteriuria in afebrile, long-term catheterised patients. *JAMA*, **248**: 454–8.

Warren JW, Damron D, Tenney JH (1987) Fever, bacteraemia and death as complications of bacteriuria in women with long-term urethral catheters. *J. Infect. Dis.*, **155**: 1151–8.

Warren JW, Muncie HL, Hall-Craggs M (1988) Acute pyelonephritis associated with bacteriuria during long-term catheterisation: a prospective clinicopathological study. *J. Infect. Dis.*, **158**: 1341–6.

Warren JW, Muncie HL Jnr, Hebel JR et al (1994) Long-term urethral catheterisation increases risk of chronic pyelonephritis and renal inflammation. *J. Am. Geriatr. Soc.*, **42**: 1286–90.

Wyndaele J-J, Maes D (1990) Clean intermittent self-catheterisation: a 12-year followup. *J. Urol.*, **143**: 906–8.

Further Reading

Berman P, Hogan DB, Fox RA (1987) The atypical presentation of infection in old age. *Age Ageing*, **16**: 201–7.

Cowan T (1997) Catheters designed for intermittent use. *Prof. Nurse*, **12**(4): 297–302.

Logan K (2003) Indwelling catheters: developing an integrated care pathway package. *Nursing Times*, **99**(44): 49–51

Vinder A (1990) Intermittent self-catheterisation. *Nursing Times*, **86**(43): 63–4.

Chapter **11**

Preventing infection of the respiratory tract

INTRODUCTION

The respiratory tract is divided into the upper part, from the nostrils to the larynx, and the lower part, from the larynx to the alveoli (Fig. 11.1). The respiratory tract is protected from micro-organisms carried on particles of dust or droplets of moisture in the air by hairs in the nose which filter larger particles as they are breathed in. In addition, ciliated cells covered with sticky mucus line most of the respiratory tract. The mucus traps small particles, preventing micro-organisms from reaching the lungs. The cilia, which are hair-like structures, beat rhythmically in a co-ordinated fashion, propelling mucus upwards towards the larynx from the lower respiratory tract and downwards from the nasal passages towards the larynx. When the mucus reaches the pharynx it is swallowed or coughed out of the respiratory system. If very small particles reach the alveoli they are engulfed by phagocytic cells of the immune system. The cough reflex is stimulated by larger particles on the larynx or trachea and is an important mechanism for the expulsion of micro-organisms.

Infections of the upper respiratory tract are usually minor; most are caused by viruses and are commonly acquired in the community (e.g. influenza, respiratory syncytial virus), although cross-infection between staff and patients may sometimes occur. Occasionally upper respiratory tract infections may progress to more serious infection of the lower respiratory tract, particularly in the very young or the elderly (Breuer & Jeffries 1990).

Infections of the lower respiratory tract, in particular pneumonia, are more serious and often life threatening. Primary pneumonia may develop in healthy people in the community, although most commonly it affects those with pre-existing pulmonary disease, the

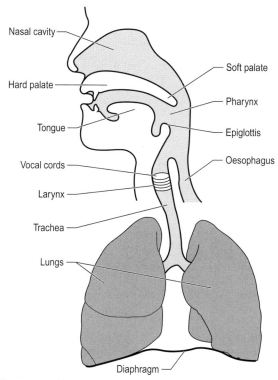

Figure 11.1 The respiratory tract.

Labels: Nasal cavity, Hard palate, Tongue, Vocal cords, Larynx, Trachea, Lungs, Soft palate, Pharynx, Epiglottis, Oesophagus, Diaphragm

immunocompromised or immobile, young children and the elderly. Whilst aspiration of micro-organisms colonizing the oropharynx is the most common cause of pneumonia, some cases result from the inhalation of micro-organisms from the environment (e.g. legionella, aspergillus) or from other people with infection (e.g. respiratory viruses).

Micro-organisms enter the lower respiratory tract from the oropharynx or on minute inhaled particles. When they reach the lungs, an inflammatory response is initiated. This causes the mucous membranes lining the alveoli and bronchi to swell and pus to collect in the alveoli, interfering with ventilation and gas exchange in the lungs. The accumulation of pus in the alveoli that occurs in pneumonia is termed 'consolidation'.

Pneumonia is the second most common hospital-acquired infection, accounting for 23% of such infections, and is associated with considerable mortality, particularly in the seriously ill (Emmerson et al 1996). The elderly are more vulnerable to pneumonia and patients over 65 years now account for half the hospital inpatient population. In intensive care units, the prevalence of hospital-acquired pnuemonia is over 20% (Kelsey et al 2000). Up to 50% of patients who

acquire pneumonia die and in nearly one-third of cases death is directly attributable to the pneumonia (Fagon et al 1993). Similarly, 50% of deaths in patients undergoing bone marrow transplantation are due to pneumonia (Pannuti et al 1992). The costs associated with hospital-acquired pneumonia are also high, with estimates of more than £2000 per patient and an increased length of stay in hospital of 12 days (Plowman et al 1999).

DIAGNOSIS OF PNEUMONIA

Amongst patients who are not critically ill, the diagnosis of pneumonia is based on fever, purulent respiratory secretions and the identification of new lung infiltrates by radiography. In the critically ill, the diagnosis is more complex and less precise. It may be difficult to establish the cause of a fever; purulent respiratory secretions are common and not a definitive indication of pneumonia; the significance of positive microbiology may be difficult to establish, especially in intubated patients; and other underlying conditions such as oedema may cause infiltrates seen by radiography (Centers for Disease Control 2002). Sampling the respiratory tract by means of fibreoptic bronchoscopy or bronchial lavage, although more invasive, is a more reliable method of obtaining microbiological specimens. A recent study by Fagon et al (2000) suggested that improvements in treatment and outcome associated with these invasive methods outweigh the risk of complications.

FACTORS THAT PREDISPOSE TO HEALTHCARE–ASSOCIATED PNEUMONIA

The risk of a patient developing pneumonia depends on the number of bacteria that enter the respiratory tract, the susceptibility of the patient to infection and the virulence of the organism. Circumstances that facilitate colonization of the oropharynx by pathogens or promote the aspiration of oropharyngeal secretions markedly increase the risk of pneumonia in hospitalized patients. These factors are summarized in Figure 11.2 and discussed in more detail in the following sections.

Colonization of the oropharynx

The most common cause of bacterial pneumonia is the aspiration of pathogens colonizing the surface of the oropharyngeal mucosa (Pugliese & Lichtenberg 1987). Some 45% of healthy people aspirate secretions from the oropharynx whilst they are asleep; however, the natural defences are usually able to remove bacteria introduced to the respiratory system in this way (Huxley et al 1978).

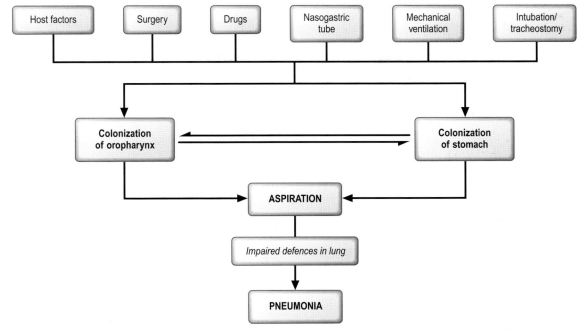

Figure 11.2   Factors that influence the acquisition of hospital-acquired pneumonia.

The risk of aspiration is increased in patients with abnormal swallowing, for example those with reduced consciousness, recent abdominal or thoracic surgery and where the normal defences are bypassed by instrumentation such as endotracheal and tracheostomy tubes and mechanically assisted ventilation (Craven et al 1986). Subsequent infection will be caused by the micro-organisms that are colonizing the oropharynx (Richards et al 1999).

In healthy people the oropharynx is often colonized by *Moraxella catarrhalis*, *Strep. pneumoniae* and *Haemophilus influenzae* and these organisms are responsible for most pneumonia acquired in the community.

Underlying illness such as pulmonary disease, coma, diabetes or hypotension, instrumentation of the respiratory tract or exposure to antimicrobial therapy promote oropharyngeal colonization by Gram-negative bacilli and these replace the normal flora of the oropharynx soon after admission to hospital (Torres et al 1993). Pneumonia that develops in the first 4 days after admission to hospital is considered as early-onset pneumonia and these cases are more likely to be caused by those pathogens normally associated with community-acquired infections. The pathogens responsible for pneumonias that develop after 4 days (late-onset pneumonia) reflect this change in oropharyngeal colonization. Thus, more than half of healthcare-associated pneumonia cases are caused by

Table 11.1   Pathogens found in healthcare-associated pneumonia in adult medical intensive care patients (reproduced with permission from Richards et al 1999)

Pathogen	% pneumonias
Pseudomonas aeruginosa	21
Staphylococcus aureus	20
Enterobacter	9
Klebsiella pneumoniae	8
Acinetobacter	6
Candida albicans	5
Escherichia coli	4
Serratia marcescens	4

Gram-negative bacilli, especially *Pseudomonas aeruginosa* and 20% by *S. aureus* (Koeman et al 2001, Richards et al 1999) (Table 11.1).

In order to colonize the oropharynx, micro-organisms must be able to adhere to the epithelial cells. After operation or during severe illness, levels of fibronectin, a protein that prevents bacteria from adhering to cells in the oropharynx, appear to be depleted. In the absence of fibronectin, Gram-negative bacteria are able to establish. Virulence factors such as fimbriae, capsules or enzymes produced by micro-organisms may also be important determinants of colonization. The level of colonization is particularly high in critically ill patients and is strongly associated with the development of pneumonia (Tablan et al 2004).

Various approaches have been tried to prevent Gram-negative micro-organisms from colonizing the oropharynx. Aerosolized antimicrobial agents eradicate the pathogens but the risks of infection with other more resistant micro-organisms have discouraged the use of this method. Selective decontamination of the digestive tract (SDD) in mechanically ventilated patients has also been recommended, using a paste of non-absorbable antimicrobial agents applied to the oropharynx several times a day. This aims to eliminate Gram-negative bacilli and candida from the oropharynx and stomach without affecting the normal flora. However, currently, there is insufficient evidence to demonstrate a clear benefit in terms of reduction of nosocomial pneumonia and there are concerns about the potential to promote antimicrobial resistance (Koeman et al 2001, Tablan et al 2004).

Colonization of the stomach

In healthy people the stomach is normally sterile because the hydrochloric acid destroys micro-organisms entering with ingested food. If the acidity is reduced to a pH of around 4, the stomach rapidly becomes colonized by large numbers of Gram-negative bacilli which subsequently colonize the oropharynx and cause pneumonia (Craven et al 1986). Bacterial colonization of the stomach is also more likely to occur in the elderly or malnourished and in those with gastrointestinal disease. Once in the stomach, bacteria may ascend the oesophagus to colonize the oropharynx and subsequently cause pneumonia (Torres et al 1993).

Drugs such as antacids and H_2 blockers are used to reduce gastric pH and prevent the formation of stress ulcers in critically ill or postoperative patients. Their use has been associated with high levels of micro-organisms colonizing the stomach (Prodham et al 1994). Sucralfate, a cryoprotective agent that has minimal effect on gastric pH, has been recommended as an alternative but clear benefits have yet to be demonstrated (Messori et al 2000, Tablan et al 2004).

Placing patients in a semirecumbent rather than supine position has been shown to reduce the risk of aspiration and gastro-oesophageal reflux, reducing the risk of pneumonia by a third in patients requiring mechanically assisted ventilation (Drakulovic et al 1999).

Nasogastric intubation

The presence of a nasogastric tube is associated with an increased risk of pneumonia, particularly when used for enteral feeding (Craven et al 1991, Drakulovic et al 1999). The nasogastric tube may favour reflux of gastric contents or enable micro-organisms to migrate along the tube to the upper airway. Enteral feeding may increase microbial colonization of the stomach by raising the pH or by introducing micro-organisms in feed solutions contaminated during handling and may also increase reflux from the stomach (Jacobs et al 1990).

Mechanical ventilation and respiratory equipment

The major risk factor for healthcare-associated pneumonia is mechanically assisted ventilation. The risk of acquiring ventilator-associated pneumonia (VAP) has been estimated at between two and 15 cases per 1000 days of ventilation, depending on the severity of underlying illness of patients requiring ventilation (National Nosocomial Infection Surveillance System 2002). Several factors combine to increase the risk of pneumonia significantly in these patients, including an increase in oropharyngeal colonization, impairment of the mechanisms that normally clear the airway and inhalation of contaminated aerosols (Garibaldi et al 1981).

Non-invasive positive pressure ventilation can be used for some patients with acute respiratory failure and has been associated with a reduced risk of pneumonia and shorter ICU stay (Keenan 2000).

Intubated patients are more likely to acquire pneumonia than those without such a device. The endotracheal and tracheostomy tubes cause irritation and injury to the mucosa, enhancing the ability of Gram-negative bacilli to colonize the oropharynx. They also bypass the nose filter and allow respiratory secretions to pool in the trachea above the tube cuff. These heavily contaminated secretions may leak around the cuff, particularly when it is deflated, or enter the bronchi during suctioning procedures (Fig. 11.3). Like other types of invasive tubing, endotracheal tubes are susceptible to the formation of biofilms, a sheet of bacteria and proteins that adheres to the surface of the tube and contaminates the airway (Koerner 1997). Orotracheal intubation has been associated with a lower risk of VAP and is therefore preferred to nasopharyngeal intubation (Tablan et al 2004).

Respiratory therapy equipment may become contaminated and deliver bacteria directly into the lungs. This is a particular problem when gases are mixed with aerosolized water from nebulizers or humidifiers because bacteria, particularly Gram-negative bacilli such as pseudomonas, are able to

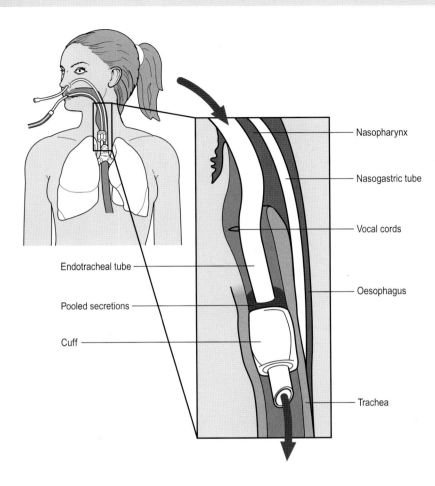

Figure 11.3   An endotracheal tube.

Endotracheal tube

Pooled secretions

Cuff

Nasopharynx

Nasogastric tube

Vocal cords

Oesophagus

Trachea

survive and multiply in the moist environment (Figs 11.4, 11.5).

Epidemics of hospital-acquired pneumonia related to contaminated nebulizers have been reported since the introduction of respiratory therapy equipment in the 1950s (Reinarz et al 1965). *Legionella* spp. thrive in water and are relatively resistant to heat. Outbreaks of infection associated with humidifiers and nebulizers, related to the use of tap water to fill or rinse the chamber or inadequate decontamination measures, have been reported (Arnow et al 1982, Mastro et al 1991). Nebulizers are especially hazardous as they create an aerosol of small droplets, 1–2 µm in diameter, that can be inhaled into the lower respiratory tract. If nebulizers in the inspiratory circuit of mechanical ventilators become contaminated with condensate in the tubing, they can result in contaminated aerosols being directed into the respiratory tract (Craven et al 1984a).

The large-volume nebulizers used in intermittent positive pressure breathing (IPPB) machines present the greatest risk because of the quantity of aerosol generated. Contamination of small-volume medication nebulizers has also been reported and has been associated with increased oropharyngeal colonization (Botman & de Krieger 1987, Hamill et al 1995).

Humidifiers increase the amount of water vapour in the inhaled gas but, unlike nebulizers, should not produce an aerosol of water droplets. Therefore, although the humidification reservoir may become contaminated with bacteria, the organisms are not as likely to be inhaled into the respiratory tract. Nonetheless, humidified circuits are prone to cause the condensation of water in the breathing tubing. Bacteria from the patient may colonize and multiply in this moisture and if the tubing is inadvertently raised, the condensate will drain into the patient's trachea and increase the risk of pneumonia (Craven et al 1984b). Stucke & Thompson (1980) found that 45% of ventilator tubing was contaminated before the same organism appeared in the tracheal aspirates,

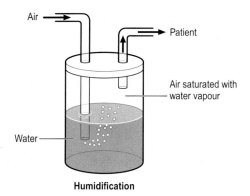

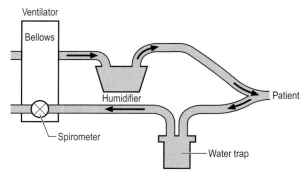

Figure 11.5 Ventilator tubing with a heated-water humidifier.

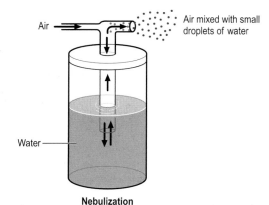

Figure 11.4 Humidification and nebulization.

implicating cross-infection as the source of contamination of the tubing.

Heat–moisture exchange (HME) filters, which recycle the moisture in exhaled air, eliminate the need for a humidifier and have the additional advantage of avoiding the collection of condensate in the tubing. There is some evidence that HMEs reduce the risk of VAP, although they have the disadvantages of increasing resistance to breathing and drying of the patients' secretions. New HMEs with an active humidifier have been designed to overcome these problems but their effect on pneumonia has yet to be tested (Cook et al 1998, Thomachot et al 2002).

Surgery

Three-quarters of cases of healthcare-associated pneumonia have been found to occur in patients who have undergone surgery. The risk is especially high in those who have had abdominal or thoracic procedures

(Haley et al 1985). This increased risk is related to several factors. The defences of the respiratory tract can be impaired by endotracheal intubation, the surgical procedure and anaesthetic gases. Aspiration is more likely to occur during anaesthesia and oropharyngeal colonization with Gram-negative bacilli commonly establishes within 48 h of major surgery (Johanson et al 1980). Coughing is often difficult and painful after an operation, especially procedures involving the abdominal or thoracic cavity, and respiration may be depressed by the use of sedatives and narcotic drugs for pain control.

Studies on interventions to reduce the risk of postoperative pneumonia have mostly focused on increasing lung expansion and removing secretions using a variety of approaches such as incentive spirometry, physiotherapy, breathing exercises and effective pain control (Chimillas et al 1998).

Arozullah et al (2001) have identified significant risk factors for predicting postoperative pneumonia in general surgical patients. These are listed in Box 11.1.

PREVENTION OF HEALTHCARE-ASSOCIATED PNEUMONIA

Management of the patient

Positioning of vulnerable patients is a simple measure that can have an important effect on the aspiration of oropharyngeal secretions. Torres et al (1993) demonstrated that intensive care patients positioned semirecumbently (45° angle) were 10 times less likely to aspirate oropharyngeal secretions. Positioning is also important to minimize the risk of fluid reflux from the stomach of patients with nasogastric tubes, especially those receiving enteral feeding. For patients at risk of developing pneumonia after operation (see

Box 11.1   Risk factors for postoperative pneumonia (reproduced with permission from Arozullah et al 2001)

- Type of surgery (e.g. abdominal aortic aneurysm repair, thoracic surgery, upper abdominal)
- Emergency surgery
- General anaesthetic
- Transfusion of more than 4 blood units
- Totally dependent functional status
- Age greater than 60 years
- Impaired sensorium
- History of chronic obstructive airways disease
- History of cerebrovascular accident
- Recent history of alcohol use
- Smoking within 1 year of surgery
- Greater than 10% weight loss
- Steroid use for chronic conditions
- Low or high blood urea nitrogen

Box 11.1), a programme of breathing exercises to encourage lung expansion and coughing should be implemented before operation. Lung expansion will also be helped by early ambulation. Some patients may need postural drainage and percussion after surgery to assist expectoration of sputum. Incentive spirometry and IPPB may also be of value, especially for patients with abnormal lung function (Chimillas et al 1998, Tablan et al 2004). Pain that interferes with deep breathing or coughing should be controlled with analgesics together with appropriate wound support (Wasylak et al 1990).

If oxygen therapy is required, it should always be humidified to prevent drying of respiratory secretions and subsequent impairment of the normal clearance mechanisms.

Oropharyngeal cleaning
Reducing oropharyngeal colonization by rigorous oral hygiene for patients at risk of pneumonia has been recommended (Tablan et al 2004, Yoneyama et al 1999). DiRiso et al (1996) reported a significant reduction in respiratory tract infection in ICU patients treated with an oral chlorhexidine mouth rinse twice daily.

Enteral feeding
The use of intermittent feeding regimens and acidifying feeds has been recommended as a means of decreasing gastric pH and reducing the risk of gut organisms colonizing the oropharynx. However, the impact of these approaches on the incidence of pneumonia has not been fully evaluated (Koeman et al 2001).

Management of respiratory therapy equipment

Contaminated respiratory equipment has frequently been incriminated in outbreaks of respiratory tract infection and an effective and organized approach to its decontamination is essential (Cefai et al 1990, Gorman et al 1993). Devices used for respiratory therapy can act as both a reservoir and vehicle of transmission for pathogenic micro-organisms. Since most of this equipment has direct or indirect contact with mucous membranes, it requires thorough cleaning followed by high-level disinfection. This can be achieved by autoclave, automated washing machine or, when these are unavailable, by chemical disinfectants (see Ch. 13). Tap water can be used to rinse off chemical disinfectants, provided the equipment can be dried completely to prevent the growth of any bacteria remaining after cleaning. This may not be possible for tubing or some types of nebulizer. Equipment should always be stored clean and dry to prevent microbial contamination.

Mechanical ventilators
The ventilator itself is not an important source of micro-organisms and filters placed between the breathing circuit and the machine can be used to protect it. Routine disinfection or sterilization of ventilators is not usually necessary (Hoffman et al 2004). Condensate that collects in the breathing circuits of humidified systems rapidly becomes colonized with bacteria from the patient's oropharynx (Craven et al 1984b). This may be directed into the patient's upper respiratory tract when the tubing is moved and should therefore be drained periodically, although not into the humidification reservoir or the patient's trachea. Staff handling the breathing circuit readily acquire the contaminating bacteria on their hands and can transfer them to other patients. Hands should therefore always be washed after the tubing is handled (Gorman et al 1993).

Anaesthetic breathing circuits can be protected with HME filters fitted on the inspiratory tubing, and humidification is not required; condensate does not collect in the tubing and only the exchange filter needs to be changed every 48 h. The internal tubing of anaesthetic machines may also be protected with HME filters.

Conventional advice is that breathing circuits used with mechanically assisted ventilation should be changed every 48 h unless used with an HME (Hoffman et al 2004). However, recent studies suggest that if breathing circuits are left unchanged for the duration of mechanical ventilation, the risk of VAP is not increased, whereas repeated change of breathing circuits probably does increase the risk of pneumonia (Fink et al 1998, Kollef et al 1995). Tablan et al (2004) advise that breathing circuits should only be changed between patients and if grossly contaminated.

The use of HME filters prevents condensate accumulating in the tubing and therefore minimizes the risk of bacterial contamination. There is some evidence that they reduce the risk of VAP (Kirton et al 1997) but their use has to be balanced against the possible adverse effects on respiratory function.

Ideally, breathing circuits should be disposable. If decontamination is required, this should be undertaken in a washer-disinfector designed to both wash and dry tubing (Das & Fraise 1997). An outbreak reported by Gray et al (1999) illustrates the hazards associated with the decontamination of ventilator circuits. Six preterm neonates acquired *Bacillus cereus* respiratory tract infection when circuits were contaminated by the organism in a washing machine. Although subsequently subjected to low-temperature steam, these spore-forming bacteria were able to survive this disinfection process and inadequate drying afterwards enabled them to multiply inside the tubing.

Spirometers and rebreathe bags have been associated with the transmission of infection and should be changed with the ventilator circuits (Irwin et al 1980, Weber et al 1990, Weems 1993, Woo et al 1986). Rebreathe bags may be protected from contamination by the use of a filter. Alternatively they should be autoclaved, preferably in a sterile supply department where porous-load autoclaving will ensure decontamination of the inside of the bag.

Nebulizers and humidifiers

Nebulizers and humidifiers should be decontaminated every 48 h, preferably in an automated washer-disinfector that holds items at a minimum temperature of 71°C for 3 min (Hoffman et al 2004). Some humidifiers can also be decontaminated by increasing the water temperature to 70°C or more. They should always be filled with sterile water to prevent colonization by legionella or other bacteria that will withstand the temperature of the water. Nebulizers and humidifiers should always be changed between patients and stored clean and dry when not in use.

Large-volume room air humidifiers or nebulizers (e.g. IPPB machines and ultrasonic room humidifiers) should be filled only with sterile water and decontaminated daily using high-level disinfection.

Medication nebulizers are readily contaminated and should be heat disinfected or cleaned with detergent and thoroughly dried after each use (Tablan et al 2004). Since it may be difficult to dry the internal surfaces, rinsing with alcohol after cleaning is recommended (Hoffman et al 2004). Effective decontamination is also important for patients receiving respiratory therapy in their own home (Pitchford et al 1987). Wall humidifiers can probably be used safely between patients provided the manufacturer's instructions are followed (Golar et al 1993).

Disposable humidification systems have not been shown to reduce the incidence of pneumonia but are a useful alternative when access to autoclaving facilities is not possible (Daschner et al 1988).

Respiratory suction

Bacteria colonizing the oropharynx accumulate in secretions and regular oropharyngeal suction in patients requiring mechanically assisted ventilation appears to reduce the risk of pneumonia (Schedler et al 2002). In addition, drainage of subglottic secretions that accumulate above the cuff using an endotracheal tube with a separate dorsal lumen for secretion removal has been reported to reduce the risk of VAP and may be cost-effective (Shorr & O'Malley 2001).

Bacteria colonizing the oropharynx are easily acquired on the hands and catheter during suctioning. To minimize the risk of cross-infection, a sterile suction catheter should be used, inserted directly into the trachea or pharynx and discarded after each use. Hands should be washed thoroughly before and after the procedure but clean gloves should also be worn to protect hands from contamination. There is no evidence that bacteria in suction canisters can reach the suction catheter, although a filter should be used on the canister to prevent release of bacteria into the environment. Canisters and the tubing between the canister and the patient should be changed between patients in units where they are in regular use. Multi-use closed-suction catheter systems are now available in which the catheter is contained inside a sterile sheath and incorporated into the ventilator circuit. This reduces the risk of introducing bacteria with the suction catheter and prevents condensate and tracheal secretions from contaminating the environment (Blackwood & Webb 1998, Cobbley et al 1991). However, although they do not appear to influence the risk of acquiring pneumonia, these systems have been associated with extensive hand contamination and difficulties with secretion removal (Blackwood & Webb 1998, Tablan et al 2004). Studies comparing multi-use closed-suction systems with the conventional single-use suction catheter system suggest that there is little difference in risk of pneumonia between the two (Deppe et al 1990).

Cross-infection

Bacteria that colonize the oropharynx of one patient may easily be transferred on the hands of staff to other patients. This is a particular problem in intensive care or neonatal units where contact with respiratory excretions is extensive and where colonization of the oropharynx with Gram-negative bacteria is very common. In one study, the hands of staff were found to be contaminated with Gram-negative bacilli after changing ventilator tubing and were rarely washed before new tubing was attached (Cadwallader et al 1990).

The routine use of gloves in intensive care units for contact with respiratory secretions has been associated with a decreased incidence of hospital-acquired pneumonia (Green et al 1987). However, gloves and plastic aprons must be discarded and hands washed after contact with respiratory secretions. The same protective clothing should never be worn for contact with other patients because of the risk of transferring micro-organisms. Patterson et al (1991) report an outbreak of acinetobacter in an ICU related to staff not changing gloves between caring for different patients.

Alcohol handrubs provide a rapid and effective means of removing transient flora from the hands and are particularly useful in intensive care settings where frequent handwashing is required.

Often outbreaks of infection are caused by bacteria resistant to a number of antibiotics. Controlling their spread usually requires isolation of colonized patients and rigorous use of protective clothing and handwashing to interrupt spread (Sakata et al 1989).

The infection control procedures required to prevent healthcare-associated pneumonia are summarized in the guidelines for practice.

Monitoring the incidence of hospital-acquired pneumonia

Awareness of the problem of hospital-acquired pneumonia and the need to consider its prevention when planning postoperative care and the management of respiratory therapy can significantly reduce the incidence of infection. Regular feedback of information to clinical staff on the incidence of hospital-acquired pneumonia in their ward has been shown to reduce the infection rate considerably (Haley et al 1985).

Kelleghan et al (1993) achieved a 57% reduction in the incidence of ventilator-associated pneumonia as a result of a continuous quality improvement programme focused on surveillance, feedback of pneumonia rates and increased awareness of infection prevention and control procedures.

OTHER CAUSES OF HEALTHCARE-ASSOCIATED PNEUMONIA

Most cases of hospital-acquired pneumonia are caused by bacteria and are not transmitted by an airborne route. However, airborne transmission is of significance in the spread of respiratory viruses, tuberculosis and, on rare occasions, legionella. Severely immunocompromised patients may be susceptible to a range of unusual respiratory pathogens, notably aspergillus and atypical mycobacterium, which may be associated with outbreaks of hospital-acquired infection in certain circumstances (see Ch. 6). Tuberculosis is transmitted by the inhalation of airborne droplets expelled from the lungs of an infected person but prolonged, close contact is usually necessary for transmission to occur (see p. 125).

Respiratory viruses

Viral respiratory infections commonly remain undiagnosed because clinical staff often do not request the laboratory techniques that such diagnosis requires. However, viruses have been found to be responsible for 20% of lower respiratory tract infections acquired in hospital (Valenti et al 1981). They often reflect the prevalence of the virus in the community and, in contrast to bacterial infections, most are acquired exogenously from other patients, staff or visitors. Viral respiratory infections are not particularly associated with debilitated patients, although they may result in serious disease in this group.

A large proportion of healthcare-associated viral pneumonias are caused by adenovirus, respiratory syncytial virus (RSV), influenza and parainfluenza viruses (Tablan et al 2004). RSV commonly affects children and community epidemics occur regularly in winter (Hall 2000). Children admitted to hospital with the infection act as a source of infection to other patients in the ward (Thorburn et al 2004). Outbreaks of nosocomial influenza usually occur when the infection is epidemic in the community. Secondary bacterial pneumonia may develop as a result of severe influenza, especially in the very young, elderly, immunocompromised or people with underlying heart or lung disease. Elderly residents of nursing homes are particularly vulnerable and annual vaccination of people at high risk of developing severe infection is recommended (Communicable Disease Report 1998, DoH 1996).

These respiratory viruses are spread by droplets expelled from the respiratory tract and deposited on to the eyes, nose or mouth (Hall 1983). However, virus may also be acquired on the hands either directly from respiratory secretions or indirectly via contaminated surfaces or equipment (Sattar et al 2002). In addition, influenza may be spread by small droplet aerosols and the virus may be shed for up to 7 days after the onset of symptoms (Breese-Hall et al 1980, Tablan et al 2004).

To prevent transmission, patients admitted with suspected viral respiratory infection should be nursed in a single room with isolation precautions or cohorted with other affected patients (see Ch. 14). Masks are not usually necessary as they are unlikely to protect the wearer. The greatest risk is from direct contact with secretions from the mouth and nose; gloves and aprons should be used to handle respiratory secretions, changed between patients and hands decontaminated after removal. Hands should always be washed after contact with the patient or their respiratory secretions. In units caring for immunocompromised or cardiac patients, additional measures are required to ensure early identification and isolation of infected patients. Contact with visitors under 12 years of age should also be restricted (Garcia et al 1997, Madge et al 1992).

Staff with respiratory infections also present a risk to patients and they should not care for patients who could develop serious illness if they acquired the infection.

Legionnaire's disease

Legionella pneumophila is commonly found in natural sources of water and in water supply systems. Under some conditions it multiplies in water systems and can be transmitted by an aerosol or spray of water from water cooling towers, whirlpool spas or humidifiers. Infection is acquired through the inhalation of small water droplets contaminated with the organism (Communicable Disease Report 2000, Joseph et al 1994).

L. pneumophila has been responsible for a number of outbreaks of nosocomial pneumonia, principally affecting the elderly or immunosuppressed. The mortality associated with legionella pneumonia is around 10% but in patients who acquire the infection in hospital, it is much higher at over 30% (Joseph et al 1994). A large outbreak at Stafford hospital in 1985 highlighted the importance of air conditioning design and maintenance. Since then guidance on the

prevention and control of legionellosis has been issued and focuses on the design, management and maintenance of water supply and air conditioning systems (Health and Safety Commission 2000). A designated person should have responsibility for assessing the risks of legionella in water systems and ensuring that systems for implementing and monitoring control measures are in place.

The risk from legionella infection can be minimized by chlorination of the water supply. However, the organisms can accumulate in biofilms on pipework and in storage tanks where they will be protected from biocides. Regular cleaning of the system and prevention of water stagnation in pipework, e.g. designing out dead-end pipes, is therefore essential for effective legionella control. Legionella can build up in infrequently used water outlets, e.g. shower heads, and care should be taken to ensure that these are either removed or flushed through regularly with water (Cooke 2004).

The thermal range in which legionella can multiply is 20–45°C. Water supply systems should therefore maintain temperatures at which the organism cannot multiply (less than 20°C or more than 60°C). Unfortunately, this means that the temperature of the hot water supply in hospitals must not fall below 50°C and therefore care must be taken to avoid scalds to patients or staff.

Respiratory therapy equipment has also been implicated in hospital-acquired legionellosis. Humidifiers or nebulizers contaminated with tap water can result in inhalation of aerosolized legionella (Arnow et al 1982). Other studies have implicated rebreathe bags attached to ventilators as a source of legionella, if rinsed with tap water (Woo et al 1986), and ice-making machines (Medical Services Directorate 1993).

There is no evidence that legionella can be transmitted from person to person and therefore isolation of infected patients is not necessary.

Severe acute respiratory syndrome (SARS)

This severe pneumonic disease is caused by a coronavirus (SAR-CoV). It was first recognized in November 2002 in Guangdong province in China and by July the following year had spread to 32 countries and affected more than 8000 people. The virus had been found in a number of wild animals sold for human consumption in markets in southern China and it is possible that contact with these animals was the origin of infection in humans.

The infection is associated with considerable morbidity and an average case:fatality ratio of 15%, although the risk of death is highest in the elderly

Guidelines for practice: prevention of hospital-acquired pneumonia

Handwashing and gloves

- Wear clean gloves for all contact with respiratory tract secretions (including oral hygiene) and discard after each procedure
- Wash hands after every contact with an intubated patient even if gloves are worn

Maintenance of respiratory therapy equipment

- Replace ventilator breathing circuits between patients or if grossly contaminated
- Protect breathing circuit with an HME filter if possible
- Do not allow condensate in tubing to drain towards patient
- Wear gloves to discard condensate and wash hands after the procedure
- Fill nebulizers and humidifiers with sterile water
- Replace all opened fluid containers daily
- Decontaminate humidifiers and nebulizers every 48 h (unless disposable)
- Clean and dry medication nebulizers between each treatment and discard between patients
- Change oxygen masks and tubing between patients and more frequently if soiled

Suctioning

- Use clean gloves and wash hands before and after procedures
- Use sterile suction catheters and sterile fluid to flush catheters
- Insert the catheter directly into the airway and discard after each use
- Change suction collection canisters between patients (or daily in short-term care units)
- Change suction tubing between patients

Postoperative care

- Implement breathing exercises before operation
- Early ambulation following surgery
- Control pain with analgesia
- Support wound to aid coughing

and those with co-morbidities. Children are rarely affected.

The primary mode of transmission appears to be direct contact between infectious respiratory secretions and mucous membranes (eyes, mouth, nose), although the virus is also present in other body fluids (faeces, urine, tears, saliva). Transmission may occur through contact with these body fluids and contaminated fomites but evidence for the role of these routes in transmission is limited.

The incubation period of SARS is 4–6 days and patients are most infectious approximately 10 days after the onset of illness. Transmission is most likely to occur from patients who are seriously ill. The virus seems to be less transmissible than other respiratory viruses and is spread by exposure to larger respiratory droplets that travel only a few metres, rather than smaller droplet nuclei that can be carried long distances.

In the 2002–3 outbreak of SARS, 20% of cases occurred in healthcare workers. Infection was frequently associated with exposure during high-risk procedures that cause aerosolization of respiratory secretions, e.g. intubation, suctioning. However, transmission to healthcare workers primarily occurred where cases were unrecognized and infection control precautions had not been implemented. Transmission in healthcare settings can be prevented by isolating patients, preferably in negative-pressure ventilation, and strictly applying respiratory isolation precautions (see Ch. 14) (Health Protection Agency 2004, WHO 2003).

Early identification of cases, isolation, vigorous contact tracing and home quarantine of close contacts during the incubation period are important in preventing and controlling outbreaks of SARS (Chow et al 2003).

Aspergillosis

Aspergillus is a fungus commonly found in soil, water and decaying vegetation. Inhalation of airborne spores may result in pneumonia in the severely immuno-compromised, e.g. organ transplant patients, advanced HIV disease, or people with pre-existing lung disease such as cystic fibrosis. Once established in the lung tissue, the fungus can disseminate via the bloodstream to other organs. The mortality associated with invasive pulmonary aspergillosis is extremely high (over 90%) (Tablan et al 2004).

The use of high-efficiency particulate air (HEPA) filters for incoming air and positive pressure ventilation in rooms are recommended for the most vulnerable patients, e.g. those undergoing allogenic bone marrow transplant. Regular monitoring of air pressure is essential to ensure correct pressure differentials are maintained (Humphries 2004). Patients who are severely immunocompromised should avoid leaving their rooms.

Aspergillus spore counts in the air are likely to be particularly high when the soil is disturbed, for example during construction work. Precautions against aspergillus should therefore be reviewed if construction or demolition work is planned. If a case of invasive aspergillosis occurs, an assessment should be made to establish when the infection was acquired in hospital and any potential source of the infection identified and eliminated. The environment should be kept as dust free as possible, using daily damp dusting and HEPA-filtered vacuum cleaners. Any water leaks should also be identified and resolved to prevent fungal growth in damp areas (Centers for Disease Control 2003). There is evidence that potted plants can act as a reservoir for aspergillus and flowers and plants should not be kept in the rooms of severely immunocompromised patients (Lass-flörl et al 2000).

Cystic fibrosis

Cystic fibrosis (CF) is caused by a defect in a gene that controls the regulation of salt and water movement across cell membranes. It results in a build-up of mucous secretions that obstruct many organs of the body, including the lungs. The abnormally thick secretions in the lungs impair the activity of the ciliary escalator and obstruct the bronchioles. As a result, the lungs become colonized and infected with a range of pathogenic bacteria. *Staphylococcus aureus* is a common cause of infection, especially in infants (Branger et al 1994). By 10 years of age, most patients will have *Pseudomonas aeruginosa* in their sputum. This organism has a range of toxic effects on the lung tissue but is rarely transmitted between patients and can usually be treated with aerosol or oral antimicrobial therapy (Pitt 2000).

Recently, another Gram-negative bacterium, *Burkholderia cepacia*, has been isolated from the lungs of patients with CF. In many patients colonization is asymptomatic but in 15–20% it results in a fatal fulminant pneumonia and septicaemia. Some strains of *B. cepacia* are transmissible and outbreaks of infection have been reported, although the outcome of acquisition of an outbreak strain appears to be mediated by host factors. Patients colonized with *B. cepacia* should take precautions to minimize the risk of spread to others. These include covering the nose and mouth when coughing, immediate disposal of tissues, keeping sputum pots covered, not sharing nebulizers or eating utensils, not sleeping in the same room as other patients with CF and frequent and thorough handwashing (Pitt 2000).

References

Arnow P, Chou T, Weil D (1982) Nosocomial Legionnaire's disease caused by aerosolised tap water from respiratory devices. *J. Infect. Dis.*, **146**: 460–7.

Arozullah AM, Khuri SF, Henderson WG et al (2001) Development and validation of a multifactorial risk index for predicting postoperative pneumonia after major noncardiac surgery. *Ann. Intern. Med.*, **135**(10): 847–57.

Blackwood B, Webb CH (1998) Closed tracheal suctioning systems and infection control in the intensive care unit. *J. Hosp. Infect.*, **39**(4): 315–22.

Botman MJ, de Krieger RA (1987) Contamination of small volume medication nebulisers and its association with oropharyngeal colonization. *J. Hosp. Infect.*, **10**: 204–8.

Branger C, Fournier JM, Loulergue J et al (1994) Epidemiology of *Staphylococcus aureus* in patients with cystic fibrosis. *Epidemiol. Infect.*, **112**: 489–500.

Breese-Hall C, Douglas RG, Gelman JM (1980) Possible transmission by fomites of respiratory syncytial virus. *J. Infect. Dis.*, **141**: 98–102.

Breuer J, Jeffries DJ (1990) Control of viral infections in hospital. *J. Hosp. Infect.*, **16**: 191–221.

Cadwallader HL, Bradley CR, Ayliffe GAJ (1990) Bacterial contamination and frequency of changing ventilator circuitry. *J. Hosp. Infect.*, **15**: 65–72.

Cefai C, Richards J, Gould FK et al (1990) An outbreak of *Acinetobacter* respiratory tract infection resulting from incomplete disinfection of ventilatory equipment. *J. Hosp. Infect.*, **15**: 177–82.

Centers for Disease Control (2002) *NNIS Criteria for Determining Nosocomial Pneumonia*. Department of Health and Human Services. Centers for Disease Control, Atlanta, GA.

Centers for Disease Control (2003) Guidelines for environmental control in healthcare facilities. *MMWR*, **52**: RR10

Chimillas S, Ponce JL, Delgado F et al (1998) Prevention of post-operative pulmonary complications through respiratory rehabilitation: a controlled clinical study. *Arch. Phys. Med. Rehab.*, **79**(1): 5–9.

Chow JY, Anderson SR, Delpech V et al (2003) SARS: UK public health response – past, present and future. *Comm. Dis. Public Health*, **6**(3): 209–15.

Cobbley M, Atkins M, Jones PL (1991) Environmental contamination during tracheal suctioning. *Anaesthesia*, **44**: 957–61.

Communicable Disease Report (1998) An outbreak of influenza in four nursing homes in Sheffield. *CDR Weekly*, **8**(16): 139.

Communicable Disease Report (2000) Legionella from guests of Welsh hotel indistinguishable from humidifier isolates. *CDR Weekly*, **10**(16): 141.

Cook D, de Jonghe B, Brochard L et al (1998) Influence of airway management on ventilator-associated pneumonia: evidence from randomised trials. *JAMA*, **279**(10): 781–7.

Cooke RPD (2004) Hazards of water. *J. Hosp. Infect.*, **57**: 290–3.

Craven DE, Lichtenberg DA, Goularte TA (1984a) Contaminated medication nebulisers in mechanical ventilatory circuits: a source of bacterial aerosols. *Am. J. Med.*, **77**: 834–8.

Craven DE, Goularte TA, Make BJ (1984b) Contaminated condensate in mechanical ventilator circuits: a risk factor for nosocomial pneumonia? *Am. Rev. Respir. Dis.*, **129**: 625–8.

Craven DE, Kunches LM, Kilinsky V et al (1986) Risk factors for pneumonia and fatality in patients receiving continuous mechanical ventilation. *Am. Rev. Respir. Dis.*, **133**: 792–6.

Craven DE, Steiger KA, Barber TW (1991) Preventing nosocomial pneumonia: state of the art and perspectives for the 1990s. *Am. J. Med.*, **91** (suppl. 3B): 44S–53S.

Das I, Fraise AP (1997) How useful are microbial filters in respiratory apparatus? *J. Hosp. Infect.*, **37**(4): 263–72.

Daschner FD, Kappstein I, Schuster F et al (1988) Influence of disposable ('Conchapak') and reusable humidifying systems on the incidence of ventilation pneumonia. *J. Hosp. Infect.*, **11**: 161–8.

Department of Health (1996) *Immunisation Against Infectious Disease.* HMSO, London.

Deppe SA, Kelly JW, Thoi LL et al (1990) Incidence of colonization, nosocomial pneumonia and mortality in critically ill patients using TrachCare closed suction system versus open suction system: prospective randomised study. *Crit. Care Med.*, **18**: 1389–93.

DiRiso AJ, Ladowski JS, Dillon AT et al (1996) Chlorhexidine gluconate 0.12% oral rinse reduces the incidence of total nosocomial respiratory infection and nonprophylactic systemic antibiotic use in patients undergoing heart surgery. *Chest*, **109**: 1556–61.

Drakulovic MB, Torres A, Bauer TT et al (1999) Supine body position as a risk factor for nosocomial pneumonia in ventilated patients: a randomised controlled trial. *Lancet*, **354**: 1851–8.

Emmerson AM, Enstone JE, Griffin M et al (1996) The second national prevalence survey of infection in hospitals – overview of the results. *J. Hosp. Infect.*, **32**: 175–90.

Fagon JY, Chastre J, Hance AJ et al (1993) Nosocomial pneumonia in ventilated patients: a cohort study evaluating attributable mortality and hospital stay. *Am. J. Med.*, **94**(3): 281–8.

Fagon JY, Chastre J, Wolffe M et al (2000) Invasive and noninvasive strategies for management of suspected ventilator-associated pneumonia in ventilated patients. A randomised trial.. *Ann. Intern. Med.*, **132**(8): 621–30.

Fink JB, Kause SA, Barrett L et al (1998) Extending ventilator circuit change interval beyond 2 days reduces the likelihood of ventilator-associated pneumonia. *Chest*, **113**(2): 405–11.

Garcia R, Raad I, Abi-Said D et al (1997) Nosocomial respiratory syncytial virus infections: prevention and control in bone marrow transplant patients. *Infect. Contr. Hosp. Epidemiol.*, **18**: 412–16.

Garibaldi RA, Britt MR, Coleman ML et al (1981) Risk factors for post-operative pneumonias. *Am. J. Med.*, **70**: 677–80.

Golar SD, Sutherland LLA, Ford GT (1993) Multi-patient use of pre-filled disposable oxygen humidifiers for up to 30 days: patient safety and cost analysis. *Respir. Care*, **38**: 343–7.

Gorman LJ, Sanai L, Notman W et al (1993) Cross-infection in an intensive care unit by *Klebsiella pneumoniae* from ventilator condensate. *J. Hosp. Infect.*, **23**: 17–26.

Gray J, George RH, Durbin GM et al (1999) An outbreak of *Bacillus cereus* respiratory tract infection on a neonatal unit due to contaminated ventilator circuits. *J. Hosp. Infect.*, **41**: 19–22.

Green SL, Overton S, Procter C (1987) The effect of glove wearing on the ICU nosocomial infection rates. 14th Annual APIC Educational Conference. Abstract 1.

Haley RW, Culver DH, White JW et al (1985) The efficacy of infection surveillance and control programs in preventing nosocomial infections in US hospitals. *Am. J. Epidemiol.*, **121**: 182.

Hall CB (1983) The nosocomial spread of respiratory syncytial viral infections. *Annu. Rev. Med.*, **34**: 311–19.

Hall CB (2000) Nosocomial viral respiratory infections: the 'cold war' has not ended. *Clin. Infect. Dis.*, **31**(2): 590.

Hamill RJ, Houton ED, Georghiou PK et al (1995) An outbreak of *Burkholderia cepacia* (formerly pseudomonas) respiratory tract colonization and infection associated with nebulised albuterol therapy. *Ann. Intern. Med.*, **122**(10): 762–6.

Health and Safety Commission (2000) *Legionnaire's Disease: The Control of Legionella Bacteria in Water Systems. Approved Code of Practice and Guidance.* HSE Books, Sudbury, Suffolk.

Health Protection Agency (2004) *SARS – Hospital Infection Control Guidance.* Available online at: www.hpa.org.uk/infections/topics_az/SARS.

Hoffman P, Bradley C, Ayliffe G (2004) *Disinfection in Healthcare*, 3rd edn. Blackwell Publishing, Oxford.

Humphries H (2004) Positive pressure isolation and the prevention of invasive aspergillosis. What is the evidence? *J. Hosp. Infect.*, **56**: 93–100.

Huxley EJ, Viroslav J, Gray WR et al (1978) Pharyngeal aspiration in normal adults and patients with depressed consciousness. *Am. J. Med.*, **64**: 564–8.

Irwin RS, Demars RR, Pratter MR et al (1980) An outbreak of *Acinetobacter* infection associated with the use of a ventilator spirometer. *Respir. Care*, **25**: 232–7.

Jacobs S, Chang RWS, Lee B et al (1990) Continuous enteral feeding: a major cause of pneumonia among ventilated intensive care unit patients. *J. Parenter. Enteral Nutr.*, **14**: 353–86.

Johanson WG, Higuchi JG, Chaudhuri TR et al (1980) Bacterial adherence to epithelial cells in bacillary colonization of the respiratory tract. *Am. Rev. Respir. Dis.*, **121**: 55–63.

Joseph CA, Watson JM, Harrison TG et al (1994) Nosocomial legionnaire's disease in England and Wales, 1980–1992. *Epidemiol. Infect.*, **112**: 329–45.

Keenan SP (2000) Noninvasive positive pressure ventilation in acute respiratory failure. *JAMA,* **284**(18): 2376–8.

Kelleghan SI, Salemi C, Padillo S et al (1993) An effective continuous quality improvement approach to the prevention of ventilator-associated pneumonia. *Am. J. Infect. Contr.,* **21**(6): 322–30.

Kelsey MC, Mitchell CA, Griffin M et al (2000) Prevalence of lower respiratory tract infection in hospitalised patients from the United Kingdom and Eire: results from the Second National Prevalence Survey. *J. Hosp. Infect.,* **46**: 12–22.

Kirton OC, DeHaven B, Morgan J et al (1997) A prospective, randomised comparison of an in-line heat moisture exchange filter and heated wire humidifiers. Rates of ventilator-associated early-onset (community-acquired) pneumonia or late-onset (hospital-acquired) pneumonia and incidence of endotracheal tube occlusion. *Chest,* **112**: 1055–9.

Koeman M, Vander Ven A, Ramsay G et al (2001) Ventilator-associated pneumonia: recent issues on pathogenesis, prevention and diagnosis. *J. Hosp. Infect.,* **49**(3): 185–62.

Koerner RJ (1997) Contribution of endotracheal tubes to the pathogenesis of ventilator-associated pneumonia. *J. Hosp. Infect.,* **35**(7): 83–9.

Kollef MH, Shapiro SD, Fraser VJ et al (1995) Mechanical ventilation with or without 7-day circuit changes: a randomised controlled trial. *Ann. Intern. Med.,* **123**: 168–74.

Lass-flörl C, Rak P, Niederwieser D et al (2000) *Aspergillus terreus* infection in haematological malignancies: molecular epidemiology suggests an association with in-hospital plants. *J. Hosp. Infect.,* **46**: 31–5.

Madge P, Payton JY, McColl JH et al (1992) Prospective controlled study of four infection control procedures to prevent nosocomial infection with respiratory syncytial virus. *Lancet,* **340**: 1079–83.

Mastro TD, Fields BS, Breiman RF et al (1991) Nosocomial legionnaire's disease and use of medication nebulisers. *J. Infect. Dis.,* **163**: 667–70.

Medical Services Directorate (1993) *Ice Cubes: Infection Caused by* Xanthomonas maltophila. HN(93)42. Department of Health, Wetherby, UK.

Messori A, Trippoli S, Vaiani M et al (2000) Bleeding and pneumonia in intensive care patients given ranitidine and sucralfate for prevention of stress ulcer: meta-analysis of randomised controlled trials. *BMJ,* **321**(7269): 1103–6.

National Nosocomial Infection Surveillance (NNIS) System Report (2002) Data summary from January 1992 to June 2002, issued August 2002. *Am. J. Infect. Contr.,* **30**: 458–75.

Pannuti C, Gingrich R, Pfaller MA et al (1992) Nosocomial pneumonia in patients having bone marrow transplant: attributable mortality and risk factors. *Cancer,* **69**(11): 2653–62.

Patterson JE, Vecchio J, Pantelick EL et al (1991) Association of contaminated gloves with the transmission of *Acinetobacter calcoaceticus var. anitratus* in an intensive care unit. *Am. J. Med.,* **91**(5): 479–83.

Pitchford KC, Corey M, Highsmith AK et al (1987) *Pseudomonas* species contamination of cystic fibrosis patients' home inhalation equipment. *J. Pediatr.,* **111**: 212–16.

Pitt TL (2000) *Burkholderia cepacia* in cystic fibrosis. *Br. J. Infect. Contr.,* **1**(3): 5–7.

Plowman R, Graves N, Griffin M et al (1999) *The Socio-economic Burden of Hospital-acquired Infection.* Public Health Laboratory Service, London.

Prodham G, Leuenberger P, Koerfer J et al (1994) Nosocomial pneumonia in mechanically ventilated patients receiving antacid, ranitidine, or sucralfate as prophylaxis for stress ulcer. A randomised controlled trial. *Ann. Intern. Med.,* **120**(8): 653–62.

Pugliese G, Lichtenberg DA (1987) Nosocomial bacterial pneumonia: an overview. *Am. J. Infect. Contr.,* **15**: 249–65.

Reinarz JA, Pierce AK, Mays BB et al (1965) The potential role of inhalation therapy equipment in nosocomial pulmonary infections. *J. Clin. Invest.,* **44**: 831–9.

Richards MJ, Edwards JR, Culver DH, Gaynes RP (1999) Nosocomial infections in medical intensive care units in the United States. National Nosocomial Surveillance system. *Crit. Care Med.,* **27**(5): 853–4.

Sakata H, Fujita K, Maruyama S et al (1989) *Acinetobacter calcoaceticus* biovar *anitratus* septicaemia in a neonatal intensive care unit: epidemiology and control. *J. Hosp. Infect.,* **14**: 15–22.

Sattar SA, Springthorpe VS, Tetro J et al (2002) Hygienic hand antiseptics: should they not have activity and label claims against viruses? *Am. J. Infect. Contr.,* **30**: 355–72.

Schedler B, Stott K, Lloyd RC (2002) The effect of a comprehensive oral care protocol on patients at risk for ventilator-associated pneumonia. *J. Advocate Health Care,* **4**: 27–30.

Shorr AF, O'Malley PG (2001) Continuous subglottic suctioning for the prevention of ventilator-associated pneumonia: potential economic implications. *Chest,* **119**(1): 228–35.

Stucke VA, Thompson REM (1980) Infection transfer by respiratory condensate during positive pressure respiration. *Nursing Times,* **76**(9): 3–4.

Tablan OC, Anderson LJ, Besser R et al (2004) Guidelines for preventing health-care-associated pneumonia, 2003: recommendations of CDC and the Healthcare Infection Control Practices Advisory Committee**.** *MMWR,* **26** (RR-3): 1–36.

Thomachot L, Vivand X, Broyadjiev I et al (2002) The combination of a heat and moisture exchanger and a booster: a clinical and bacteriologic evaluation over 96 hours. *Int. Care Med.,* **28**(2): 147–53.

Thorburn K, Kerr S, Taylor N et al (2004) Respiratory syncytial virus outbreak in a paediatric intensive care unit. *J. Hosp. Infect.,* **57**: 194–201.

Torres A, el-Ebiary M, Gonzales J et al (1993) Gastric and pharyngeal flora in nosocomial pneumonia acquired during mechanical ventilation. *Am. Rev. Respir. Dis.,* **148**(2): 352–7.

Valenti WM, Hall CB, Douglas RG et al (1981) Nosocomial viral infections I: epidemiology and significance. *Infect. Contr.*, **1**: 33–7.

Wasylak TJC, Abbott FV, English MJM et al (1990) Reduction of postoperative morbidity following patient-controlled morphine. *Can. J. Anaesth.*, **37**: 726–31.

Weber DJ, Wilson MB, Rutala WA et al (1990) Manual ventilation bags as a source for bacterial colonization of intubated patients. *Am. Rev. Respir. Dis.*, **142**: 892–4.

Weems JJ (1993) Nosocomial outbreak of *Pseudomonas cepacia* associated with contamination of reusable electronic ventilator temperature probes. *Infect. Contr. Hosp. Epidemiol.*, **14**: 583–6.

Woo AH, Yu VL, Goetz A et al (1986) Potential in-hospital modes of transmission of *Legionella pneumophila*. Demonstration experiments for dissemination by showers, humidifiers and rinsing of ventilation bag apparatus. *Am. J. Med.*, **80**: 567–73.

World Health Organization (2003) *Consensus Document on the Epidemiology of Severe Acute Respiratory Syndrome*. World Health Organization, Geneva.

Yoneyama T, Yoshida M, Matsui T et al (1999) Oral care and pneumonia. *Lancet*, **354**: 515.

Further Reading

Lee JV, Joseph C, for the PHLS Atypical Pneumonia Working Group (2002) Guidelines for investigating single cases of legionnaire's disease. *Comm. Dis. Public Health*, **5**(2): 157–62.

Taylor D, Littlewood S (1998) Respiratory system part 1: pneumonia. *Nursing Times*, **94**(7): 48–51.

Chapter **12**

Preventing gastrointestinal infection

INTRODUCTION

Gastrointestinal infections can be acquired directly, through the ingestion of contaminated food or water, or may be spread from person to person through contact with infected body fluids such as faeces or vomit. Hospital patients may be particularly susceptible to such infections, because illness or old age can reduce the production of gastric acid which normally prevents bacteria passing through the stomach. In addition, the very young, the elderly or the debilitated are likely to develop more serious disease and the infection may cause or accelerate their death (Cowden et al 1995).

Poor personal hygiene or food-handling practices in the kitchens of a hospital or nursing home can cause outbreaks of infection affecting large numbers of patients and staff. Measures to prevent cross-infection are also particularly important as contact with body fluids and the movement of staff and equipment between patients may greatly facilitate the transmission of gastrointestinal infections.

This chapter focuses on micro-organisms that cause foodborne infection and how the principles of food hygiene should be used to prevent infection. It also considers other gastrointestinal pathogens associated with outbreaks of infection in hospitals and the infection control precautions required to prevent their transmission.

FOODBORNE INFECTION

Food is an important source of infection. Around 90 000 cases of food poisoning are reported in England and Wales every year and there has been a marked increase in notifications during the past few decades (Wall et al 1996a) (Fig. 12.1). Some of these cases are sporadic, isolated infections most of which

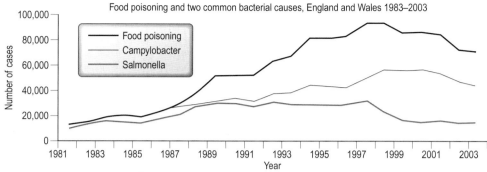

Figure 12.1 Food poisoning notifications (and those due to campylobacter and salmonella) in England and Wales, 1983–2003 (reproduced with permission from Mayon-White 2005).

are probably related to domestic food contamination. Campylobacter, in particular, causes disease after the ingestion of only a small number of organisms and cross-contamination of raw and cooked food in domestic kitchens is probably responsible for many campylobacter infections, most of which occur sporadically. However, several hundred outbreaks of foodborne illness also occur every year. Most of these outbreaks (43%) are associated with commercial food production in restaurants, pubs, etc. but 17% occur as a result of domestic food preparation and 13% are associated with catering in hospitals or residential institutions (Cowden et al 1995).

There has been a marked increase in the number of reported cases of foodborne illness since the 1990s, a pattern seen in many European countries and in North America. The reasons for this increase are not entirely clear but factors such as changes in food consumption, increasing use of restaurants, availability of convenience foods, travel abroad and changes in farming methods have probably all played a part (Mayon-White 2005). In addition, improvements in laboratory techniques for identifying faecal pathogens, e.g. norovirus, campylobacter, and enhanced systems for reporting and collating data mean that a proportion of the increase is probably also related to improved recognition of cases (Wall et al 1996a).

In the UK, there was a sharp upward trend in reported cases of foodborne illness in the 1980s. This was largely due to a dramatic increase in reported cases of salmonella and campylobacter, both commonly associated with poultry. With the introduction of intensive farming methods for rearing and processing chickens and producing eggs, poultry were becoming increasingly popular as a cheap, low-fat food.

Salmonella enteritidis suddenly emerged as an important cause of salmonella food poisoning and was found to have colonized the oviducts of large numbers of the chicken population, resulting in widespread contamination of eggs. If eaten raw or lightly cooked, these eggs could cause salmonella poisoning. Since the late 1990s vaccination of poultry flocks against *S. enteritidis* has addressed the problem and reports of the infection have declined rapidly (Cogan & Humphrey 2003, Kessel et al 2001).

Although many people affected by a gastrointestinal illness have a mild, self-limiting disease, a proportion of cases require hospitalization and some die as a result. The case–fatality rate is highest for *Escherichia coli* O157, which can cause thrombocytopenia and haemolytic uraemic syndrome with up to a third of symptomatic cases requiring hospitalization (Coia 1998, Evans et al 1998). A small number of deaths associated with outbreaks of salmonella are also reported, particularly in association with residential homes (Hansell et al 1998).

Table 12.1 illustrates the pathogens most commonly responsible for foodborne infections in the UK, the sources of infection and associated symptoms. In healthcare facilities, less than 2% of outbreaks of infection caused by intestinal pathogens are foodborne while 87% of hospital-based outbreaks are due to person-to-person spread and most are caused by norovirus (54%) and *Clostridium difficile* (13%) (Meakins et al 2003) (see Table 12.2).

The Food Safety Act 1990

This Act governs the production of food and drink from preparation to the point of sale and provides local authorities with the necessary powers to register food premises, enforce their compliance with

Table 12.1 Pathogens that cause foodborne illness

Micro-organism	Source of infection	Route of transmission	Symptoms
Aeromonas	Aquatic environments	Ingestion of contaminated water, shellfish or raw foods washed in contaminated water	Vomiting, diarrhoea
Bacillus *B. cereus* *B. subtilis*	Commonly found in the environment Contaminated cereals, dried food Contaminated dairy and meat products, especially pastries	Spores not always destroyed by cooking, germinate and release toxin if food stored in warm temperatures for prolonged periods	Emetic toxin causes rapid onset of vomiting (within 5 h). *B. cereus* also produces a diarrhoeal toxin which causes abdominal pain and diarrhoea 8–16 h after ingestion
Campylobacter	Gastrointestinal tract of birds (poultry), cattle, other animals	Undercooked poultry and meat; contaminated water; unpasteurized milk; cross-contamination of cooked and raw food. Infective dose low. Person-to-person spread possible but unusual	Severe abdominal pain, profuse diarrhoea, 2–5 days after ingestion
Clostridium perfringens	Gastrointestinal tract of animals	Spores on contaminated meat not destroyed by cooking and germinate if food kept warm and not reheated thoroughly. Symptoms caused by toxin produced in the gut during sporulation	Diarrhoea and abdominal pain, usually 12–18 h after ingestion
Escherichia coli Verocytotoxin producing (VTEC) Serotype O157 most common in UK	Gastrointestinal tract of animals, especially cattle	Undercooked beef and beef products, milk and vegetables. Also acquired by direct contact with infected animals and people	Bloody diarrhoea, abdominal pain 1–6 days after ingestion; 5% of patients develop haemolytic uraemic syndrome (HUS)
Enterotoxigenic (ETEC)	Gastrointestinal tract of animals and humans	Major cause of traveller's diarrhoea, acquired through ingestion of contaminated food and water	Diarrhoea, 12–72 h after exposure
Salmonella typhi/paratyphi	Gastrointestinal tract of humans	Food washed in sewage-contaminated water or contaminated by infected food handler. Person-to-person spread uncommon	Fever, malaise, nausea. Constipation followed by diarrhoea 1–3 weeks after infection
Other species	Gastrointestinal tract of animals, birds (poultry) and occasionally humans	Undercooked meat, especially poultry; eggs; dairy products. Close contacts may spread infection from person to person	Diarrhoea, vomiting, fever, 12–72 h after infection
Shigella	Gastrointestinal tract of humans	Occasionally spread by contaminated water or raw foods washed in contaminated water. Most cases spread by faecal–oral contact	Bloody diarrhoea caused by a toxin occurs 1–7 days after infection
Staphylococcus aureus	Infected or colonized skin lesions, fingers or nose of food handlers	Cooked food (e.g. meat, poultry, fish) and dairy products, handled and stored at warm temperatures for several hours before eating. Symptoms caused by an ingested toxin	Vomiting and abdominal pain, usually within 4 h of ingestion
Viruses (e.g. norovirus)	Gastrointestinal tract of humans	Contaminated water and food, especially shellfish; cold foods, e.g. sandwiches, contaminated by a food handler. Very low infective dose. Most cases spread from person to person by contact with faeces or vomit	Vomiting, diarrhoea, fever is 48 h after exposure
Yersinia enterocolitica	Gastrointestinal tract of animals and birds	Infection particularly associated with pork, but milk and milk products also implicated. Will grow at 4°C and may withstand pasteurization. Person-to-person spread may occur	Watery diarrhoea, abdominal pain, fever and arthritis 3–7 days after ingestion

Table 12.2 Intestinal pathogens causing healthcare-associated infection

Micro-organism	Route of infection	Symptoms
Norovirus (previously called Norwalk-like virus or small round structured virus)	Although may be foodborne, most transmission is person to person through contact with faeces or vomit. Associated with widespread contamination of the environment with virus particles carried in aerosols	Vomiting (often projectile) is the predominant symptom, with mild diarrhoea, headache, fever. Duration of illness 12–60 h, incubation period 15–48 h
Rotavirus	Spread by contact with infected faeces/vomit. Mostly affects children, usually acquired by age of 3 years, but outbreaks also occur among the elderly	Vomiting, fever, watery diarrhoea 24–72 h after exposure, symptomatic for 4–6 days
Clostridium difficile (toxogenic strains)	Pathogenic strains colonize the gut of susceptible people (elderly, impaired colon flora). Evidence for person-to-person spread via contaminated fomites or environment	Profuse, foul-smelling diarrhoea, fever, abdominal pain, pseudomembranous colitis (diagnosed by biopsy)

regulations and deal with unsafe food. Any premises involved in the production, supply or storage of food must be registered with the local authority. Environmental health officers employed by the local authority have the right to inspect premises, check their records and take samples of food. They can issue warnings: *improvement notices*, which specify remedial action to be taken within a given period, or *prohibition notices*, which require the immediate closure of the premises. They may also prosecute those responsible where breaches in the food legislation are identified.

The General Food Hygiene Regulations came into force in 1995 and aim to ensure that common food hygiene rules are applied across the European Community. There are also a range of product-specific regulations covering, for example, poultry, meat, fishery and dairy products. The General Food Hygiene Regulations apply to anyone who sells food, whether for profit or fundraising, publicly or privately, and requires those preparing, transporting or selling food to identify and control food safety risks systematically and to ensure that premises are hygienic. They also specify the mandatory training of people who handle food. The Food Safety (Temperature Control) Regulations 1995 provide specific guidance on temperatures at which certain foods must be kept. Specific guidance on food handling in healthcare establishments can be found in *Hospital Catering: Delivering a Good Service* (NHS Executive 1996a) and HSG(96)20 (NHS Executive 1996b).

In 1999 the Food Standards Agency was established to protect the interests of consumers in relation to health risks from food. This agency develops policies and provides advice on food safety as well as monitoring the enforcement of legislation.

PRINCIPLES OF FOOD HYGIENE

As food in its raw state is frequently contaminated with bacteria, great care must be taken to ensure that it is prepared, cooked and stored properly. There are many ways in which poor practice can result in food poisoning; the most common are listed in Box 12.1.

Box 12.1   The 10 most common causes of food poisoning (Roberts 1982)

1. Food prepared too far in advance
2. Food stored at room temperature
3. Food cooled too slowly before refrigeration
4. Food not reheated to a sufficiently high temperature to destroy food-poisoning bacteria
5. Cooked food contaminated with food-poisoning bacteria
6. Meat and meat products undercooked
7. Frozen meat and poultry not thawed completely
8. Cross-contamination from raw to cooked foods
9. Hot food stored below 63°C
10. Food handlers with gastrointestinal infection

Barrie (1996) points out that:

Food hygiene is more than cleanliness. It is the use of policies, practices and procedures to protect food from contamination, prevent multiplication of bacteria to numbers capable of causing food poisoning or food spoilage and ensure the destruction of disease-producing micro-organisms by thorough cooking.

The food-handling responsibilities of nurses vary enormously with different healthcare systems and with the type of food delivery. In a large general hospital nurses may be involved only with distribution of pre-prepared meals on trays, although they may be expected to make decisions about storing and reheating meals at ward level. In small hospitals, specialist units or nursing homes, nurses may participate in all stages of food production. As a large proportion of food poisoning occurs in the home, where knowledge of food hygiene may be limited, nurses may be required to advise and educate vulnerable patients on the prevention of gastrointestinal illness in their own homes. An understanding of the principles of food hygiene and infection control is therefore essential if appropriate advice is to be offered.

In the following section, safe handling of food is considered under the headings of preparation, cooking and storage.

Food preparation

Raw food is frequently contaminated with pathogens such as campylobacter, *Clostridium perfringens*, salmonella and toxogenic strains of *Escherichia coli* derived from the intestines of animals. It has been estimated that 30% of raw chicken carcases are contaminated with salmonella and 75% with campylobacter (Atabay & Corry 1997, Kessel et al 2001). Red meat, in particular minced beef, is susceptible to contamination by toxogenic strains of *E. coli* (Wall et al 1996b). *Bacillus cereus* and *C. perfringens* are widely found in the environment and may therefore contaminate a variety of produce, including rice and vegetables, but are also a common cause of food poisoning related to the consumption of red meat and poultry (Kessel et al 2001, Snerdon et al 2001). Milk and dairy products are readily contaminated during collection or processing.

Most intestinal pathogens must be ingested in very large numbers (at least several hundred in each gram of food) to overcome the acid in the stomach and establish infection in the gut. Thorough cooking will destroy most bacteria in food and the few that remain should be insufficient to cause infection. However, if

---

Guidelines for practice: preparation of food

- Always wash hands before and after handling food and after using the toilet
- Use separate, colour-coded utensils for raw and cooked food; clean thoroughly with detergent and water after each use
- Clean preparation surfaces thoroughly, using disposable cloths and detergent and water after each use
- Blenders, mixers and slicing machines must be dismantled and cleaned thoroughly with detergent and water after each use
- Wash all salads, fruit and vegetables in running water
- Do not store raw and cooked food together
- Keep food in the refrigerator covered to prevent inadvertent contamination

---

raw food is brought into contact with cooked food, for example by contact with or dripping on to cold meats in the refrigerator or on equipment such as chopping boards and knives, cross-contamination is likely to occur. The bacteria will then multiply on the cooked food and will not be killed by further cooking before ingestion. Campylobacter is particularly likely to be transmitted in this way. Although this organism is readily destroyed by cooking, infection can follow the ingestion of only a few hundred organisms as they multiply rapidly in the gut (Eley 1992).

One of the essential principles of safe food handling is to ensure that cooked food is never contaminated by uncooked food. Bacteria can be transferred from raw to cooked food on hands and equipment such as knives and chopping boards. A colour-coding system can be used to readily distinguish equipment used to prepare raw food from those used for ready-to-eat food (Food Standards Agency 2002a). Such equipment must always be washed with hot water and detergent after each use and have smooth surfaces to enable easy cleaning. Cloths used to clean surfaces or equipment will become contaminated rapidly and should be discarded or washed frequently.

Food that is eaten raw is not decontaminated by heat and must be washed under running water to remove micro-organisms. Salads or vegetables are reported as the source of infection in approximately 5% of outbreaks of food poisoning, associated in particular with salmonella, campylobacter and shigella (Long et al 2002). Salads prepared in hospitals have been found to be contaminated with various Gram-negative bacilli, which, although unlikely to cause infection in healthy people, may be harmful to an immunocompromised patient (Houang et al 1991). Gastrointestinal viruses, such as norovirus, require a very low dose to transmit infection. Outbreaks are frequently associated with salads, sandwiches or desserts prepared by affected food handlers (Long et al 2002). It is essential that hands are washed thoroughly before food handling and that those recovering from gastrointestinal illness should not be involved in handling food.

The important guidelines for practice when preparing food are summarized on page 249.

Cooking food

Inadequate cooking or reheating of food is a contributory factor in 50% of outbreaks of foodborne illness (Evans et al 1998). The destruction of bacteria in food by cooking depends on exposing them to heat for a sufficient period of time. However, there is a balance between eliminating bacteria and spoiling the taste and nutrient value of food by overcooking. Most bacteria are killed at temperatures of around 60°C but prolonged heating may be required to ensure that these temperatures are achieved throughout the food. It can take some time for heat to penetrate the centre of the food, particularly if the food is dense (e.g. mashed potato, raw meat) or is still frozen in the middle. Standard cooking times are based on the heating of food from room temperature and, if applied to food that is incompletely defrosted, may result in undercooking. This is particularly dangerous with some types of food, such as poultry, because salmonella and campylobacter can be present deep in the muscle tissue of poultry carcases and will survive incomplete cooking (Kessel et al 2001). Outbreaks of infection caused by *E. coli* O157 are often associated with the consumption of undercooked mince beef, e.g. beefburgers (Wall et al 1996b).

The same principles should be applied to reheating food before consumption. Different foods take different times to reheat and it can therefore be difficult to estimate the reheating time. For example, the gravy in a stew will heat more rapidly than the meat and a bubbling gravy does not mean that the meat has been reheated to the correct temperature. A thermometer should be used to check that the centre of the food is at 70°C before it is safe to serve.

Microwave ovens

Microwave ovens heat food from the inside outwards and vegetative bacteria are unlikely to survive provided that all parts of the food reach 70°C. Unfortunately, heating in microwave ovens tends to

---

Guidelines for practice: cooking food safely

- Defrost meat thoroughly before cooking
- Adhere to standard or recommended cooking times
- Use a thermometer to check the temperature in the centre of the food
- Reheat food thoroughly and use a thermometer to check the temperature

---

be uneven so that some parts of the food may become extremely hot whilst other parts remain cool (Knutson et al 1987). Food should therefore be allowed to stand for 5 min after heating to ensure that the heat is evenly distributed by conduction (Lund et al 1989). Precooked chilled foods should be reheated in the manner specified by the manufacturer. The time necessary to heat other foods is extremely difficult to estimate and a thermometer should be used to ensure that the food has been heated throughout.

Food storage

Raw food is not sterile and the micro-organisms present will multiply over time at ambient temperature. Inadequate storage of food is a contributory factor in 45% of outbreaks of foodborne illness (Evans et al 1998). Bacteria can multiply in most foods provided there is moisture present and the temperature is between 20° and 40°C (e.g. room temperature). At refrigeration temperatures of 5–10°C multiplication occurs extremely slowly so that food can be stored for a few days without spoiling. Below 0°C food can be stored for prolonged periods as most bacteria are unable to multiply at these temperatures. *Listeria monocytogenes* presents particular problems as it can multiply in the refrigerator. It is transmitted by food and, although rare, may cause serious infection in the immunocompromised, elderly and unborn child or neonate. It can survive drying, freezing and even cooking.

Bacteria may multiply in food eaten raw; for example, salmonella from eggs can contaminate mayonnaise or mousses (Lewis et al 1995) and some bacteria, notably *C. perfringens* and *B. cereus*, may survive the cooking process and multiply during subsequent storage. *C. perfringens* is found in the intestines of animals and in soil and may contaminate both meat and vegetables. It forms spores when the food is cooked, some of which may survive prolonged boiling. Unless the food is cooled rapidly, the spores will germinate and the bacteria may multiply rapidly in a warm kitchen. If large numbers of the vegetative cells are present in the food when ingested, they release a toxin as they form spores in the intestine, causing profuse diarrhoea and abdominal pain. Outbreaks of *C. perfringens* associated with storing presliced turkey in gravy are commonly reported around Christmas time (Kessel et al 2001). *B. cereus* is also able to survive cooking by forming spores. Outbreaks of infection have been associated particularly with prolonged storage of cooked rice at room temperature (Nickel et al 1999). Bacteria remaining after cooking multiply in the rice, sporulate and release a heat-resistant toxin that is not destroyed by subsequent reheating.

Storage temperature

To avoid these hazards food should always be stored at temperatures below 8°C or above 63°C. If food is not to be consumed immediately after preparation, it must be cooled quickly and stored in the refrigerator. Hot food should not be put in the fridge as it may raise the temperature inside the fridge.

Listeria can be isolated from freshly cut salads, paté and soft cheeses (Lund et al 1989). Outbreaks of infection associated with coleslaw, milk and cook-chill chicken have also been reported (Jones 1990). These foods should not be stored in the refrigerator for more than 3 days.

Eggs may contain salmonella both inside and outside the shell. Dishes prepared with raw eggs are a common cause of outbreaks of salmonella poisoning (Ejidokun et al 2000). Ideally eggs should be stored in the fridge, apart from other foods and used before becoming out of date. Hands should always be washed and dried after handling them (Food Standards Agency 2002b). The Food Standards Agency (FSA) advises caterers to use pasteurized eggs in any food that will not be cooked or only lightly cooked, e.g. mayonnaise. Raw shell eggs should not be used in catering for hospital patients.

Dry foods should be protected from moisture; whilst dry they are unable to support the growth of bacteria.

The standards for temperature control during the storage, processing and distribution of food are described in the Food Safety (Temperature Controls) Regulations 1995.

Meal delivery

The method of delivering meals to wards must ensure that the food is kept either hot or cold. Heated trolleys should maintain a temperature of at least 63°C and should incorporate a refrigerated compartment for cold desserts and salads. The meals should be served as rapidly as possible to reduce the risk of bacterial multiplication.

Meals should not be saved for more than 1 h if a patient is not on the ward at mealtimes. Bacteria may multiply in the food and subsequent reheating may not be sufficient to destroy them. Catering departments must offer a flexible service for patients who have missed meals to avoid the need for reheating at ward level (NHS Executive 1999). Particular care should be taken with the storage and reheating of ready-to-eat chilled meals to minimize the risk of contamination and to ensure micro-organisms are destroyed during reheating.

Separation of raw and ready-to-eat food

Foods that have already been cooked, e.g. cold meats, or are ready to eat, e.g. salads, are vulnerable to contamination by micro-organisms from raw foods. Ideally raw and ready-to-eat foods should be stored in separate cold stores or refrigerators and food should always be covered in sealed containers. If these foods cannot be stored separately then raw meat should be kept at the bottom of the fridge so that it cannot touch or drip onto ready-to-eat foods (Food Standards Agency 2002a).

Ward kitchens

These are subject to the Food Hygiene Regulations (see p. 248) and may be inspected during visits by the environmental health officer. The ward manager is responsible for ensuring that the regulations are complied with. The fittings should be designed to be cleaned easily, with smooth surfaces to prevent the collection of dirt or grease. A handwash basin with soap and hand towels must be available.

Refrigerators

Food stored in the refrigerator should be dated and discarded after it has reached its use-by date.

The refrigerator must be checked daily to ensure that food is covered, labelled and discarded when appropriate. Drugs, blood or specimens should never be kept in the food refrigerator. Refrigerators should be maintained at a temperature between 1° and 4°C and a thermometer inside should be used to check the temperature regularly. They should not be overloaded as this may interfere with the circulation of cool air and should be sited away from a heat source and out of direct sunlight.

Goldthorpe et al (1991) found that very few ward fridges maintained an adequate temperature and recommended the use of commercial larder fridges in place of the domestic fridge.

Ice machines

Ice-making machines are prone to contamination, especially if ice is removed by hand. Outbreaks of infection by Gram-negative bacteria and cryptosporidium associated with ice-making machines have been reported (King 2001, Medical Devices Agency 1993). They should be properly connected and cleaned and maintained regularly. A designated receptacle should be used to remove the ice and washed with detergent and water after each use (Barrie 1996, Medical Devices Agency 1993).

Cleaning of kitchen areas

To minimize the risk of cross-contamination, separate colour-coded mops, buckets and cloths should be used to clean kitchen areas and should not be confused with equipment used to clean other areas. Patients and their relatives should be discouraged from bringing food into the hospital because it is not possible to assess how safely it has been prepared.

Crockery and cutlery

Bacteria are easily removed from crockery and cutlery by washing in hot water and detergent. This is best done in a central wash-up area where dishes can be washed in an automatic machine at very high temperature. If items have to be washed at ward level, use clean hot water and detergent, rinse and leave to drain rather than dry with a cloth which may easily become contaminated with potential pathogens. If dishcloths are necessary, they should be disposable.

Personal hygiene

Food is easily contaminated by bacteria carried on the hands. Pathogens, such as salmonella or campylobacter, may be acquired by handling raw food and transferred to other food or equipment. *Staphylococcus aureus*, a pathogen carried on the skin of many people, can also cause gastrointestinal illness if transferred to food. Particular care should be taken when handling food eaten cold (e.g. sandwiches, desserts) as any contamination will not be removed by subsequent cooking.

People suffering from a gastrointestinal infection may excrete a large number of micro-organisms in their faeces. Some bacteria (e.g. salmonella, *E. coli*) may continue to be excreted in faeces for many months. Infected food handlers may be the primary cause of some outbreaks of food poisoning, especially those caused by salads or vegetables (Long et al 2002). Staff who develop gastrointestinal infection must be particularly scrupulous about hand hygiene before handling food and should seek advice from the occupational health department before returning to work.

In ward areas, staff should put on a clean apron and wash their hands before distributing food. Cold or cooked food such as salads and cold meats should be handled with gloves or utensils.

Meal delivery systems in hospitals

Safe food handling and delivery systems are of paramount importance in hospitals where many vulnerable patients and staff are at risk of food poisoning if the systems break down. In 1984 an outbreak of food poisoning at the Stanley Royd Hospital for the mentally ill affected 355 residents and resulted in the deaths of 19 (Fig. 12.2). The subsequent enquiry found standards in the handling, storage and preparation of food in the hospital kitchens to be very poor. This incident highlighted the vulnerability of hospital patients to food poisoning and resulted in the removal of Crown Immunity, which until 1987 had protected hospitals from prosecution by environmental health officers.

In large hospitals, meals may need to travel considerable distances between the kitchens and ward areas. The delivery system must therefore ensure that hot food is kept above 63°C and that cold food is refrigerated. Many institutions use cook-chill or cook-freeze catering systems, where the meals are prepared in the usual way but are then either rapidly cooled to a temperature of 0–3°C or frozen to −8°C. Cook-chill meals can be kept for up to 5 days, frozen meals for up to 8 weeks.

Cook-chill or cook-freeze meals are delivered to wards in chilled cabinets and reheated in the cabinet at a set temperature for a predetermined period of time. These delivery systems are an effective means of large-scale catering and are safe provided the correct controls are in place, especially in relation to the temperature used during preparation, storage and plating (Barrie 1996, NHS Executive 1996b).

The *Controls Assurance Standard: Catering and Food Hygiene* (NHS Executive 1999) required that all food storage, preparation and handling in NHS premises comply with current food safety legislation as well as providing for the nutritional requirements of patients. There must also be systems in place for monitoring the food safety management system at trust board level. Any member of staff involved in handling food must receive relevant training and, as a minimum, must have a basic knowledge of the principles of food hygiene (NHS Executive 1999).

Hazard analysis critical control points (HACCP)

A systematic approach is essential in monitoring standards of food safety and hygiene. A concept called hazard analysis critical control points (HACCP) is now widely used in the food industry and catering establishments and systematic hazard analysis is also expected in NHS catering services

PUBLIC INQUIRY INTO SALMONELLA OUTBREAK

SOCIAL SERVICES SECRETARY Norman Fowler has set up a full-scale public inquiry into the outbreak of food poisoning which has killed 27 patients at the Stanley Royd psychiatric hospital in Wakefield.

Announcing his decision last week, Mr Fowler said there was a need to establish 'the full facts surrounding the outbreak', although priority had been to bring it under control. Eight patients were still suffering from salmonella symptoms and three of them were seriously ill as *NT* went to press, but no new cases had been reported for 48 hours.

Investigation into the infection has shown that cold roast beef left out for 10 hours on a warm day had caused the rapid spread of the bacteria, according to Wakefield health authority, although the actual source of the infection is still not known.

District medical officer Dr Geoffrey Ireland said last week that the meat had been taken out of the refrigerator in the morning to be sliced and been left out until it was served later that afternoon. This has been denied by the hospital's kitchen staff. NUPE branch secretary George Rusling told *NT* the meat had been left out of the refrigerator no longer than four hours.

Figure 12.2   Press report of an outbreak of food poisoning at Stanley Royd Hospital.

(NHS Executive 1999). HACCP involves the identification of possible hazards in the production process and specification of the critical controls required to ensure safety (critical control points). Each control point is then monitored using defined criteria (e.g. a specific temperature or other check) (Box 12.2). Microbiological testing of food is usually not necessary, except where an outbreak of food poisoning is suspected.

Box 12.2   Steps in a hazard analysis critical control point (adapted from Anderton 1994)

- Assemble a HACCP team
- Define the process
- Identify and assess the hazards and risks:
  - characteristics
  - micro-organisms
  - severity and frequency
- Identify the critical control points, i.e. points where control must be achieved
- Specify monitoring and control procedures:
  - when action is taken
  - what action is taken
  - who takes action
  - limits requiring further action
- Implement control at critical points
- Verify HACCP periodically

HACCP can also be applied to other aspects of food provision such as the handling of expressed breast milk and enteral feeding (see below) (Anderton 1994, Hunter 1991).

Enteral feeds

Feeding via a nasogastric or percutaneous endoscopic gastrostomy (PEG) tube is increasingly used as an alternative to parenteral nutrition when patients are unable to feed themselves. However, there are significant microbiological hazards associated with supplying nutrition via these routes (Anderton 1985, 1993, Howell 2002). Many types of bacteria, including salmonella, klebsiella, enterobacter, *E. coli* and *S. aureus*, have been found in high concentrations in enteral feeds. These may cause gastroenteritis and, through colonization of the gut, may also result in septicaemia and pneumonia (Thurn et al 1990).

The liquid nutrients provide a favourable medium in which bacteria can grow and are easily contaminated during assembly and manipulation of the administration sets. Once the administration reservoir or tubing is contaminated, the bacteria can multiply rapidly in the feed at room temperature. If feeds are administered over several hours, bacteria may multiply to considerable numbers. The standards used in the preparation and handling of enteral feeds must therefore be even higher than with conventional meals. The important principles for the management of enteral feeding are summarized in the Guidelines for practice.

Guidelines for practice: the management of enteral feeds

- Use commercially prepared feeds in prefilled administration reservoirs where possible
- Pay scrupulous attention to principles of food hygiene if feeds are mixed on the ward
- Blenders used to prepare feed must be dismantled, thoroughly washed with detergent and dried after each use
- Wash hands before handling enteral feeding systems
- Avoid disconnecting the feed delivery system
- Do not allow the administration set connections to come into contact with any non-sterile object
- Administer feed over as short a time as possible
- Store opened feeds in the refrigerator and discard after 24 h
- Replace administration sets and reservoirs every 24 h. Do not wash out and reuse
- Flush tubing with plenty of tap water before and after aspiration of the tube, administering feeds or drugs

---

Preparation of enteral feeds

Contamination of enteral feeds occurs frequently, despite strict protocols for their management. Crocker et al (1986) found that the onset of contamination is delayed if the feed is supplied in prefilled, ready-to-use administration reservoirs. Where feeds were transferred to an administration reservoir, the rate of contamination was much higher and, if the mixture had to be reconstituted before adding to the reservoir, 75% were contaminated after 12 h and 100% after 24 h in use. There is considerable potential for feeds prepared in a hospital kitchen or ward to become contaminated through contact with equipment such as blenders, mixers or liquidizers. Feeds must therefore be prepared under controlled conditions, preferably in the dietary department, using an extremely high standard of hygiene (Thurn et al 1990). Once a container of feed has been opened, it must be stored in the refrigerator and discarded after 24 h.

Administration of feeds

Manipulation of enteral feeding systems increases the risk of feed contamination (Pellowe et al 2003). Administration sets should be designed to require minimal manipulation and recessed connections may help to reduce the risk of contamination (McKinley et al 2001). Hands must be washed before handling enteral feeds or the feed administration systems and a rigorous no-touch technique must be used when assembling the administration sets and handling the feed. The use of clean, disposable gloves has been recommended to minimize the risk of contamination (Anderton & Aidoo 1991). Commercially prepared feeds in ready-to-use administration reservoirs are preferable as they are supplied as sterile liquids. However, if the connection between nutrient container and administration set is contaminated during assembly, large numbers of micro-organisms may be recovered from the feed after 24 h (Beattie & Anderton 1999).

Sterile ready-to-use feeds should be administered over a maximum of 24 h. Non-sterile, reconstituted feeds should be administered within 4 h. The feeding tube should be flushed with fresh tap water before and after aspiration, feed changing or drug administration to minimize the risk of micro-organisms adhering to the internal surface and the administration reservoir and tubing should be discarded after a maximum of 24 h in use (Pellowe et al 2003, Ward et al 1997). Similarly, syringes used to flush feeding tubes should be treated as single-use items and discarded after each use (Medical Devices Agency 2000).

Attempts to decontaminate containers with detergent and water or disinfectants are unlikely to be successful. Tubing experimentally inoculated with klebsiella could be decontaminated only after flushing with soapy water for 10 min followed by immersion in 125 ppm hypochlorite for 7 h (Anderton & Nwoguh 1991).

Enteral feeds prepared by patients at home are also susceptible to contamination and these patients should be prepared with a rigorous education programme before discharge (Anderton et al 1993). In the home, syringes used to check the position of the nasogastric tube or to flush tubing with water between feeds can be used more than once provided they are supplied by the manufacturer for this purpose and are not packaged as single-use disposable items.

Application of hazard analysis critical control points
Anderton (1994, 2000) has recommended the application of HACCP to enteral tube feeding. A team of key staff should be involved, such as a dietician, representative ward/unit nurses and doctors, pharmacist, infection control nurse and microbiologist. This team should then define the process and identify the key hazards (see Box 12.2). Control measures can then be defined for each of the hazards identified, for example selecting well-designed feed administration systems, protocols for handling feeds, systems for recording the time feeds are left at ward temperature and a system to audit the controls established.

Percutaneous endoscopic gastrostomy tubes
Gastrostomy tubes may also be vulnerable to infection at the entry site. After insertion, the site should be inspected daily for signs of inflammation and for the first few days cleaned to remove exudate. The tube should also be rotated daily for a month to prevent the formation of scar tissue. Once the site has healed the patient can bathe normally and a dressing is not required (Howell 2002).

Milk feeds and milk banks

The potential for contamination during preparation and handling also applies to milk feeds and expressed breast milk. Most milk feeds can be supplied safely in commercial sterile, prefilled bottles. When special milk diets are required, the milk should be prepared using an extremely high standard of hygiene (Burnett et al 1989).

Rowan & Anderson (1998) highlighted the problem of contamination of dietary food supplements such as 'build-up' by *Bacillus cereus*. This spore-forming organism may contaminate pasteurized milk and be present in low numbers in powdered food supplements. When the powdered supplement is reconstituted with the milk and stored above 5°C, the presence of glucose in the milk enables *B. cereus* to multiply and enterotoxin to be produced by toxogenic strains of *B. cereus*.

Breast milk expressed by the mother for subsequent feeding to a baby unable to breastfeed, or for donation to a milk bank, is vulnerable to contamination by potential pathogens such as staphylococci, streptococci or coliforms. Outbreaks of infection associated with contaminated expressed breast milk (EBM) have been reported, including bacteraemia and fatal cases of necrotizing enterocolitis (Graham et al 1999). Breast pumps can be difficult to decontaminate and increase the bacterial contamination of the milk (Boo et al 2001). Although pasteurization of EBM for milk banking eliminates potential pathogens, contamination after pasteurization has also been reported (Brown et al 2000).

Careful controls are required to ensure that EBM is stored and handled safely and a HACCP approach has been recommended (Balmer et al 1997, Hunter 1991). Mothers should be advised to wash their hands and clean their skin around the nipples prior to expressing and to collect milk into disinfected containers. Pumps used to express milk must be scrupulously cleaned and decontaminated after each use.

Milk donated to a milk bank should be microbiologically tested and pasteurized prior to storage and heavily contaminated samples should be discarded (Balmer & Wharton 1992).

PREVENTING THE SPREAD OF GASTROINTESTINAL INFECTION

More than 50% of outbreaks of gastrointestinal disease reported to the Health Protection Agency occur in hospitals or residential homes. Over half are caused by norovirus and a further 13% by *Clostridium difficile* (Table 12.3). Unlike community settings, person-to-person spread is the predominant mode of transmission. The risk of mortality in association with gastrointestinal disease is also significantly increased in outbreaks that occur in hospitals (Meakins et al 2003). Preventing and controlling these outbreaks is therefore an important priority.

Spread of gastrointestinal infections occurs particularly easily amongst children or other groups of patients or clients who have a poor understanding of hand hygiene and where staff may have considerable contact with excreta. Inadequate decontamination of hands after contact with faeces or vomit is responsible for most transmission. However, in the case of gastrointestinal viruses environmental contamination and aerosols from vomit may also be an important factor (Patterson et al 1997). The routine use of standard precautions for handling body fluids should prevent the transmission of gastrointestinal illness in most healthcare settings (see Ch. 7). Wearing disposable gloves and aprons for contact with excreta or vomit and scrupulous handwashing after contact with affected patients are particularly important control measures (see Guidelines for practice).

Staff may acquire infection from patients with gastrointestinal infection. In the case of norovirus, the attack rate in staff is similar to that of patients (Lopman et al 2003). Although gastrointestinal pathogens may be excreted for several days or weeks after the infection,

Table 12.3   Main pathogens associated with outbreaks of gastrointestinal disease in hospitals in England and Wales, 1992–2000 (Meakins et al 2003)

Pathogen	No. outbreaks (%)
Norovirus	754 (54)
Clostridium difficile	176 (13)
Salmonella	51 (4)
Rotavirus	39 (3)
Clostridium perfringens	13 (1)

provided personal hygiene is good (e.g. handwashing after using the toilet) the risk of transmission is minimal once the symptoms have resolved. However, advice should be sought from the occupational health department before affected staff return to clinical duties.

Norovirus

Norovirus generally causes a relatively mild and short-lived disease characterized by severe vomiting but often accompanied by nausea, abdominal cramps, headache and fever. Cases occur both sporadically and as small outbreaks in the community. The virus can be spread by contact with faeces, exposure to aerosols in vomit, food and water. Oysters grown in sewage-contaminated water can be a vehicle for norovirus infection but other ready-to-eat foods, e.g. salads, that become contaminated by an infected food handler are also a common foodborne source of norovirus (Lopman et al 2003).

Eighty per cent of reported outbreaks of norovirus occur in hospitals or residential care facilities. The virus may be initially introduced by any of the above routes but then spreads rapidly from person to person. Hospitals are particularly prone to outbreaks during the winter, possibly because of the increase in admissions with respiratory illness and transfers of patients between hospitals and residential homes (Lopman et al 2003).

Although little can be done to prevent norovirus being introduced to healthcare facilities, prompt identification of possible cases may help to limit spread (Box 12.3). However, the onset of illness is very rapid, with no prodrome.

In an outbreak it may not be feasible to place all affected patients in a single room. Where possible, they should be cohorted in one part of the ward such as a bay and isolation precautions applied to the whole bay. Virus is excreted for up to 10 days with maximum excretion occurring 24–72 h after exposure

---

Guidelines for practice: preventing the spread of gastrointestinal infections

- Nurse the patient in a single room whilst symptomatic
- Wear gloves and apron for direct contact with faeces/vomit and discard after use
- Wash hands after any contact with the patient
- Remove spills of body fluid promptly and clean the area thoroughly
- Instruct the patient to wash hands thoroughly after using the toilet
- Place bedpans directly into bedpan washer/macerator without emptying the contents first

> **Box 12.3   Criteria for suspecting an outbreak of norovirus (Chadwick et al 2000)**
>
> - Vomiting (often projectile) in more than 50% of cases
> - Duration of illness 12–60 h
> - Incubation period of 15–48 h
> - Both staff and patients affected

(Chadwick et al 2000). Gloves and aprons should be worn for all contact with affected patients or their environment and hands washed when protective clothing is removed and before leaving the affected area. Environmental contamination has been implicated in the spread of norovirus which has been found to survive for 12 days on contaminated carpets (Cheeseborough et al 1997). Spillages of faeces or vomit must be cleaned up promptly using detergent and water, followed by disinfection with 0.1% hypochlorite solution. Seventy-two hours after the last case, all affected areas should be thoroughly cleaned and disinfected.

When an outbreak begins on one ward, rapid, stringent action is necessary to prevent a hospital-wide outbreak. The ward should be closed to new admissions and transfers of both staff and patients to other wards should be avoided. Staff affected should not return to work until 48 h after their symptoms have resolved. Patients in affected wards should not be transferred to residential homes during the outbreak unless they have had the infection and fully recovered.

Rotavirus

Rotavirus is a very common cause of diarrhoea in children and extensive outbreaks of infection amongst susceptible groups of patients such as children and the elderly have been reported although these are rarely foodborne (Lewis et al 1989). During the acute stage of the illness millions of virus particles are excreted in the stools and virus continues to be shed for several days following recovery. Transmission of the infection on hands following contact with excreta, bedding or nappies can therefore occur extremely easily (Breuer & Jeffries 1990).

Clostridium difficile

Outbreaks of toxin-producing strains of *C. difficile* are an increasing problem in hospitals. Whilst *C. difficile* may be carried asymptomatically, pathogenic strains cause pseudomembranous colitis, which can be fatal. Patients often develop infection following alteration of the normal gut flora by antimicrobial therapy but toxogenic strains may also be transmitted between patients. The elderly and those whose normal bowel flora may have been affected by antimicrobial therapy, abdominal surgery, cancer or tube feeding are most vulnerable (National *Clostridium difficile* Standards Group 2004).

Symptomatic patients who have toxin-producing strains of *C. difficile* should be isolated whilst they have diarrhoea. Cohorting of affected patients and the staff caring for them should be considered if there is evidence of spread between patients. The environment may become heavily contaminated with *C. difficile* spores, particularly when epidemic strains are prevalent. Although evidence for its role in transmission is limited, it has been implicated in the spread of infection (Fawley & Wilcox 2001, Sanmore et al 1996).

The use of protective clothing when handling excreta and rigorous attention to hand hygiene after contact with symptomatic patients or their environment are required to prevent spread and control outbreaks. Alcohol handrubs will not reliably remove spores from the hands and soap and water should be used instead.

The floors and surfaces in the rooms of patients should be regularly cleaned to prevent the build-up of spores (DoH 1994). Evidence for the relative value of detergent or disinfectant for cleaning is conflicting (Dettenkofer et al 2004, Wilcox & Fawley 2000). Skoutelis et al (1993) found that carpeted floors were significantly more likely than other surfaces to become contaminated with *C. difficile* and remained contaminated for longer periods. However, they did not find evidence of increased risk of transmission of *C. difficile* in association with carpeted floors.

OUTBREAKS OF GASTROINTESTINAL ILLNESS

A sudden increase in diarrhoea or vomiting among patients or staff may indicate an outbreak of infection. Outbreaks may be foodborne or occur as a result of person-to-person transmission. Specimens of faeces should be taken from all symptomatic patients as soon as possible and examined in the laboratory for both bacteria and viral pathogens. The specimens can provide crucial evidence to indicate the source of the infection. Patients whose symptoms have resolved may still excrete the organism and specimens should be sent to the laboratory to identify the causative organism.

Control of outbreaks of gastrointestinal illness requires prompt notification of the infection control team, who will then investigate the source and advise

---

Box 12.4   Key steps in the control of suspected outbreaks of gastrointestinal infection

When more than one patient or member of staff is affected by unexplained diarrhoea or vomiting, the following actions should be taken.

In a hospital
- Inform the doctor in charge of the patients
- Inform the infection control doctor or nurse
- Ensure sufficient supplies of gloves and aprons
- Collect stool specimens from affected patients for viral and bacterial culture
- Wash hands after contact with affected patients
- Use protective clothing for handling body fluids
- Change gloves and wash hands between patients
- Transfer affected patients to single rooms and follow isolation precautions
- Ensure affected staff attend the occupational health department

In a nursing home
- Inform the general practitioner responsible for affected patients
- Inform the consultant for communicable disease control (CCDC)
- Ensure sufficient supplies of gloves and aprons
- Collect stool specimens from affected patients for viral and bacterial culture
- Wash hands after contact with affected patients
- Use protective clothing for handling body fluids
- Change gloves and wash hands between patients
- Ensure affected staff consult their general practitioner

---

on the management of patients to minimize the risk of further spread (Box 12.4). The infection control team may involve the consultant for communicable disease control (CCDC) or director of public health and local environmental health officers in measures to control outbreaks of gastrointestinal illness in hospitals. In community settings the CCDC (based in the local health protection unit) will take responsibility for providing advice, investigating and monitoring outbreaks.

References

Anderton A (1985) Growth of bacteria in enteral feeding solutions. *J. Med. Microbiol.*, **20**: 63–8.

Anderton A (1993) Bacterial contamination of enteral feeds and feeding systems. *Clin. Nutr.*, **12** (suppl. 1): 16–32.

Anderton A (1994) What is the HACCP (hazard critical control point) approach and how can it be applied to enteral tube feeding? *J. Hum. Nutr. Diet.*, **7**: 53–60.

Anderton A (2000) Microbial contamination of enteral tube feeds – how can we reduce the risks? *Penlines*, **16**: 2–6. Available online at: www.peng.org.uk.

Anderton A, Aidoo KE (1991) The effect of handling procedures on microbial contamination of enteral feeds – a comparison of the use of sterile vs non-sterile gloves. *J. Hosp. Infect.*, **17**(4): 297–301.

Anderton A, Nwoguh CE (1991) Re-use of enteral feeding tubes – a potential hazard to the patient? A study of the efficacy of a representative range of cleaning and disinfection procedures. *J. Hosp. Infect.*, **18**: 131–8.

Anderton A, Nwoguh CE, McCune I et al (1993) A comparative study of the numbers of bacteria present in enteral feed prepared and administered in hospital and the home. *J. Hosp. Infect.*, **23**: 43–9.

Atabay HI, Corry JEL (1997) The prevalence of campylobacters and arcobacters in broiler chickens. *J. Appl. Microbiol.*, **83**: 619–26.

Balmer SE, Wharton BA (1992) Human milk banking at Sorrento Maternity Hospital, Birmingham. *Arch. Dis. Child*, **67**: 556–9.

Balmer SE, Nicoll A, Weaver GA et al (1997) *Guidelines for the Collection, Storage and Handling of Mother's Breast Milk to be Fed to Her Own Baby on a Neonatal Unit*. Queen Charlotte and Chelsea Hospitals, London.

Barrie D (1996) The provision of food and catering services in hospital. *J. Hosp. Infect.*, **33**: 13–33.

Beattie TC, Anderton A (1999) Microbiological evaluation of four enteral feeding systems which have been deliberately subjected to faulty handling procedures. *J. Hosp. Infect.*, **42**(1): 11–20.

Boo NY, Nordiah AJ, Alfizah H et al (2001) Contamination of breast milk obtained by manual expression and breast pumps in mothers of very low birthweight infants. *J. Hosp. Infect.*, **49**(4): 274–81.

Breuer J, Jeffries DJ (1990) Control of viral infections in hospital. *J. Hosp. Infect.*, **16**: 191–221.

Brown NM, Arbon J, Redpath C (2000) Contamination of milk bank samples with *Pseudomonas aeruginosa* during pasteurisation by penetration of organism through the screw lid during cooling. *J. Hosp. Infect.*, **46**(4): 321–2.

Burnett IA, Wardley BL, Magee GS (1989) The milk kitchen, Sheffield children's hospital, before and after a review. *J. Hosp. Infect.*, **13**: 179–86.

Chadwick PR, Beards G, Brown D et al (2000) Management of hospital outbreaks of gastro-enteritis due to small round structured viruses. *J. Hosp. Infect.*, **45**: 1–10.

Cheeseborough JS, Barkess-Jones L, Brown DW (1997) Possible prolonged environmental survival of small round structured viruses. *J. Hosp. Infect.*, **35**: 325–6.

Cogan AT, Humphrey TJ (2003) The rise and fall of *Salmonella enteritidis* in the UK. *J. Appl. Microbiol.*, **94**: 1145–95.

Coia JE (1998) Nosocomial and laboratory acquired infections with *Escherichia coli* O157. *J. Hosp. Infect.*, **40**(2): 107–14.

Cowden JM, Wall PG, Adak G et al (1995) Outbreaks of foodborne infectious intestinal disease in England and Wales: 1992–1993. *CDR Rev.*, **5**(8): R109–24.

Crocker KS, Krey SH, Markovic M et al (1986) Microbial growth in clinically used enteral delivery systems. *Am. J. Infect. Contr.*, **14**: 250–6.

Department of Health (1994) Clostridium difficile *Infection: Prevention and Management*. PHLS Joint Working Group Report. Public Health Laboratory Service, London.

Dettenkofer M, Hauer T, Daschner FD (2004) Detergent versus hypochlorite cleaning and *Clostridium difficile* infection. *J. Hosp. Infect.*, **56**(1): 78–9.

Ejidokun OO, Killalea D, Cooper M et al (2000) Four linked outbreaks of *Salmonella enteritidis* phage type 4 infection – the continuing egg threat. *Commun. Dis. Public Health*, **3**(2): 95–100.

Eley AR (ed.) (1992) *Microbial Food Poisoning*. Chapman and Hall, London.

Evans HS, Madden P, Douglas C et al (1998) General outbreaks of infectious intestinal disease in England and Wales: 1995 and 1996. *Commun. Dis. Public Health*, **1**: 165–71.

Fawley WN, Wilcox MH (2001) Molecular epidemiology of endemic *Clostridium difficile* infection. *Epidemiol. Infect.*, **126**: 343–50.

Food Standards Agency (2002a) *Guide to Food Hygiene*. Food Standards Agency, London. Available online at: www.fsa.org.uk.

Food Standards Agency (2002b) *Eggs – What Caterers Need to Know*. Food Standards Agency, London. Available online at: www.fsa.org.uk.

Goldthorpe G, Kerry P, Drabu YJ (1991) Refrigerated food storage in hospital ward areas. *J. Hosp. Infect.*, **18**: 63–6.

Graham JC, Morgan S, Ford M et al (1999) Sepsis and ECMO: beware the breast milk. *J. Hosp. Infect.*, **43**: 75–6.

Hansell AL, Sen S, Sufi F et al (1998) An outbreak of *Salmonella enteritidis* phage type 5a infection in a residential home for elderly people. *Commun. Dis. Public Health*, **1**(3): 172–5.

Houang E, Bodnarak P, Ahmet Z (1991) Hospital green salads and the effects of washing them. *J. Hosp. Infect.*, **17**: 125–31.

Howell M (2002) Do nurses know enough about percutaneous endoscopic gastrostomy? *Nursing Times*, **98**(17): 40–2.

Hunter PR (1991) Application of Hazard Analysis Critical Control Point (HACCP) to the handling of expressed breast milk on a neonatal unit. *J. Hosp. Infect.*, **17**: 139–46.

Jones D (1990) Foodborne listeriosis. *Lancet*, **336**: 1171–4.

Kessel AS, Gillespie IA, O'Brien SJ et al (2001) General outbreaks of infectious intestinal disease linked with poultry, England and Wales 1992–1999. *Commun. Dis. Public Health*, **3**: 171–7.

King D (2001) Ice machines – an audit of their use in clinical practice. *Commun. Dis. Public Health*, **4**(1): 48–9.

Knutson KM, Marth EH, Wagner MK (1987) Microwave heating of food. *Food Sci. Technol.*, **20**: 101–10.

Lewis DA, Paramathasan R, White DE et al (1995) Marshmallows cause an outbreak of infection with *Salmonella enteritidis* phage type 4. *CDR Rev.*, **6**(13): R183–5.

Lewis DC, Lightfoot NF, Cubitt WD et al (1989) Outbreaks of astrovirus type 1 and rotavirus gastroenteritis in geriatric inpatient populations. *J. Hosp. Infect.*, **14**: 9–14.

Long SM, Adak GK, O'Brien SJ et al (2002) General outbreaks of infectious intestinal disease linked with salad vegetables and fruit, England and Wales 1992–2000. *Commun. Dis. Public Health*, **5**(2): 101–5.

Lopman BA, Adak GK, Reacher MH et al (2003) Two epidemiologic patterns of Norovirus outbreaks: surveillance in England and Wales, 1992–2000. *Emerg. Infect. Dis.*, **9**(1): 71–7.

Lund BM, Knox MR, Cole MB (1989) Destruction of *Listeria monocytogenes* during microwave cooking. *Lancet*, **i**: 218.

Mayon-White R (2005) Re-emerging infections. Part 3: Gastrointestinal and foodborne infections. *Br. J. Infect. Contr.* **6**(1): 11–14.

McKinley J, Wildgoose A, Wood W et al (2001) The effect of system design on bacterial contamination of enteral feeding tube feeds. *J. Hosp. Infect.*, **47**: 138–42.

Meakins SM, Adak GK, Lopman BA et al (2003) General outbreaks of infectious intestinal disease (IID) in hospitals, England and Wales, 1992–2000. *J. Hosp. Infect.*, **53**: 1–5.

Medical Devices Agency (1993) *Ice Cubes: Infection Caused by* Xanthomonas maltophilia. HN(93)42. Department of Health, London.

Medical Devices Agency (2000) *Enteral Feeding Systems*. Medical Devices Agency, London.

National *Clostridium difficile* Standards Working Group (2004) Report to Department of Health. *J. Hosp. Infect.*, **56** (suppl. 1): 1–38.

NHS Executive (1996a) *Hospital Catering: Delivering a Quality Service*. Department of Health, Wetherby, UK.

NHS Executive (1996b) *Management of Food Hygiene and Food Services in the National Health Service.* HSG(96)20. Department of Health, Wetherby, UK.

NHS Executive (1999) *Control Assurance Standard: Catering and Food Hygiene.* Department of Health, Wetherby, UK.

Nickel GL, Little CL, Mithani V et al (1999) The microbiological quality of cooked rice from restaurants and take-away premises in the United Kingdom. *J. Food. Prot.,* **62**(8): 877–82.

Patterson W, Haswell P, Fryers PT et al (1997) Outbreak of small round structured virus gastro-enteritis arose after kitchen assistant vomited. *CDR Rev.,* **7**(7): R101–3.

Pellowe CM, Pratt RJ, Harper P et al (2003) Evidence-based guidelines for preventing healthcare-associated infections in primary and community care in England. *J. Hosp. Infect.,* **55** (suppl. 2): S61–85.

Roberts D (1982) Factors contributing to outbreaks of food poisoning in England and Wales 1970–79. *J. Hyg.,* **89**: 491–8.

Rowan NJ, Anderson JG (1998) Growth and enterotoxin production by diarrhoeagenic *Bacillus cereus* in dietary supplements prepared for hospitalised HIV patients. *J. Hosp. Infect.,* **38**: 139–46.

Sanmore MH, Venkataraman L, DeGirolami PC et al (1996) Clinical and molecular epidemiology of sporadic and clustered cases of nosocomial *Clostridium difficile* diarrhoea. *Am. J. Med.,* **100**: 32–40.

Skoutelis AT, Westenfelder GO, Beckerdite M et al (1993) Hospital carpeting and epidemiology of *Clostridium difficile. Am. J. Inf. Contr.,* **22**: 212–7.

Snerdon WJ, Adak GK, O'Brien SJ et al (2001) General outbreaks of infectious intestinal disease linked with red meat, England and Wales, 1992–1999. *Commun. Dis. Public Health,* **4**(4): 259–67.

Thurn J, Crossley K, Gerdts A et al (1990) Enteral hyperalimentation as a source of nosocomial infection. *J. Hosp. Infect.,* **15**: 203–18.

Wall PG, de Louvois J, Gilbert RJ et al (1996a) Food poisoning: notifications, laboratory reports and outbreaks – where do the statistics come from and what do they mean? *CDR Rev.,* **6**(7): R93–9.

Wall PG, McDonnell RJ, Adak GK et al (1996b) General outbreaks of vero cytotoxin producing *Escherichia coli* O157 in England and Wales from 1992 to 1994. *CDR Rev.,* **6**(2): R26–33.

Ward V, Wilson J, Taylor L et al (1997) *Preventing Hospital-acquired Infection. Clinical Guidelines.* Public Health Laboratory Service, London.

Wilcox MH, Fawley WN (2000) Hospital disinfectants and spore formation by *Clostridium difficile. Lancet,* **356**: 1324.

Further Reading

Department of Health (1990) *Management of Food Services and Food Hygiene in the National Health Service.* NHS Management Executive. HMSO, London.

Department of Health, Public Health Medicine Environmental Group (1996) *Guidelines on the Control of Infection in Residential and Nursing Homes.* Department of Health, Wetherby, UK.

Department of Health and Social Security (1986) *Report of the Committee of Inquiry into an Outbreak of Food Poisoning at Stanley Royd Hospital.* HMSO, London.

Hobbs BC, Roberts D (1993) *Food Poisoning and Food Hygiene,* 6th edn. Edward Arnold, London.

Chapter 13

Cleaning, disinfection and sterilization

INTRODUCTION

The transmission of infection in association with equipment has been recognized as a problem since micro-organisms were first perceived as the cause of infection. Inadequate decontamination has frequently been responsible for outbreaks of infection in hospital (Cefai et al 1990, Kolmos et al 1993). The emergence of new human pathogens, such as HIV and variant CJD, has focused attention on the potential of medical equipment to transmit infection. Safe decontamination of equipment between patients is an essential part of routine infection control (see Ch. 7). The method of decontamination selected should consider the risk of the item acting as a source or vehicle of infection and the processes that it will tolerate.

The environment is commonly perceived as a more important source of infection than evidence suggests. Microbes cannot multiply in dry environments and most die fairly rapidly on surfaces or in the air. The few that remain are unlikely to be present in sufficient numbers to initiate infection even if they could reach a susceptible site on the patient. The environment does provide a more important microbiological hazard where moisture is present, for example in food, solutions or equipment containing water. Here, bacteria may multiply rapidly to create a source of infection, provided that a suitable vehicle transfers them to a susceptible site on the patient.

LEVELS OF DECONTAMINATION

There are three levels of decontamination which are defined in Table 13.1. Cleaning involves the use of detergent to remove visible contamination from equipment but also removes a large proportion of the micro-organisms. Cleaning alone is an adequate

Table 13.1   Levels of decontamination

Method	Process
Sterilization	Removes or destroys all micro-organisms, including spores
Disinfection	Reduces the number of micro-organisms to a level at which they are not harmful. Spores are not usually destroyed
Cleaning	Physical removal of contamination (blood, faeces, etc.) and many micro-organisms with detergent

method of decontamination for a wide range of equipment. Cleaning, by removing organic material and reducing the number of micro-organisms present, is an essential preparation for most equipment undergoing sterilization or disinfection. Disinfection and sterilization can be achieved by physical methods, such as heat, or by chemicals. Chemical disinfectants exhibit a wide variation in their effect on different micro-organisms and are susceptible to inactivation by organic material and instability. Decontamination by heat is the preferred method as it is more efficient and easier to regulate.

When equipment is exposed to heat or chemical agents, there is a delay in effect on micro-organisms whilst the agent penetrates the cells. The penetration time is extended if organic material is present. Micro-organisms are then steadily destroyed, rapidly by some methods, more slowly by others. If the process destroys all micro-organisms including spores, it is described as *sterilization*. Physical processes, such as steam sterilization, are the most effective method of sterilization, although a few chemicals, used in a specific way, can be used to sterilize. Other processes will not destroy all micro-organisms, particularly bacterial spores, and are described as *disinfection*. The terms sterilization and disinfection are often used incorrectly. For example, it is not correct to refer to the immersion of baby bottles in hypochlorite solution as sterilization. In fact, this is a disinfection procedure which destroys some, but not all, micro-organisms present.

Selecting the level of decontamination

The decision to clean, disinfect or sterilize depends on the risk of the equipment transmitting infection or acting as a source of infection (Table 13.2).

This risk depends on how the item is used. If the skin is penetrated, normally sterile body areas are entered or there is contact with broken mucous membranes, then the risk of introducing infection is high and the items used must be sterile. Items that have contact with less susceptible sites, such as mucous membranes, or which may be contaminated by micro-organisms that are easily transmitted to others are in a medium-risk category. Disinfection is usually adequate for these items, although sterilization is preferable as it reliably removes contamination. Equipment used on intact skin presents a low risk, is unlikely to transmit infection and may be decontaminated by cleaning.

The level of decontamination selected for routine use must be adequate to destroy any pathogens likely to be present. It should not be necessary to use a higher level of decontamination for a patient known to have an infection, although special procedures are indicated for some instruments used on patients with *Mycobacterium tuberculosis* or Creutzfeldt–Jakob disease (see p. 276).

As a general rule, methods of sterilization or disinfection employing heat, such as autoclaves and

Table 13.2   Categories of decontamination

Category	Indication	Examples	Level of contamination	Methods
High risk	Items that penetrate skin or mucous membranes or that enter sterile body areas	Surgical instruments, needles, syringes	Sterilize	Autoclave and use sterile Sterile single-use disposable
Medium risk	Items that have contact with mucous membranes or are contaminated by microbes that are easily transmitted	Vaginal speculum, endoscopes, bedpans, crockery	Disinfect or sterilize	Autoclave (not in packs) Chemically disinfect Pasteurize
Low risk	Items used on intact skin	Washbowls, mattresses	Clean	Wash with detergent and hot water and dry

bedpan washers, are more reliable than chemicals and should be used wherever feasible.

Quality control is more easily achieved in centralized sterile supply departments (SSD) where healthcare equipment can be decontaminated under highly controlled conditions using automated processes. Such departments will process equipment from hospital and community facilities and will be able to decontaminate a range of heat-sensitive equipment. The Medical Devices Directive (MDD 93/42/EEC) specifies standards for decontamination services. In the future SSDs will be expected to comply with these standards and services are likely to become concentrated in large centres serving several hospitals and other healthcare facilities.

Traceability

The emergence of variant Creutzfeldt–Jakob disease (vCJD) in the UK has raised concerns about identifying and quarantining instruments used on patients subsequently found to have this prion disease. Thus, there is a requirement for all invasive surgical instruments and endoscopes to be traceable and a record kept of their identity, procedures used for decontamination and patients they have been used on (DoH 1999).

Decontamination policy

Confusion often surrounds the decontamination of equipment used in healthcare. To prevent unsafe or unnecessary decontamination, hospitals should have a decontamination policy. This will provide guidance on the method of decontamination for instruments, equipment and the environment. The policy should be developed by those with expertise in decontamination, including the infection control nurse, consultant microbiologist, pharmacist and sterile supplies department manager. An example of advice contained in a decontamination policy is shown in Table 13.3.

The decontamination of reusable equipment should be considered at the time of purchase and, where necessary, advice from the manufacturer, infection control specialist or SSD sought to ensure an appropriate reprocessing system is established. Key questions that should be considered are listed in Box 13.1.

Medical equipment is also used in primary care and a range of invasive procedures are now commonly performed in general practice surgeries by practice nurses, general practitioners and other healthcare professionals. These staff also need guidelines on safe decontamination procedures (Cooper et al 2003, Finn & Crook 1998). Useful advice for the primary healthcare team can be found in *Infection Control in the*

Box 13.1   Key questions for reprocessing equipment
• Is the item intended for reuse?
• How will the item be used and what level of decontamination will be required?
• What is the manufacturer's recommended method of decontamination and is this available?
• Is the item heat tolerant and fully immersible?
• Can the item be processed by SSD?
• Does it have to be disassembled for cleaning?

Community (Lawrence & May 2003) and can also be obtained from the local infection control team.

Decontamination of equipment before service or repair

Equipment that has been in contact with patients or their body fluids may transmit infection to those required to service or repair it. Such equipment must be made safe to handle by ensuring it is thoroughly cleaned and decontaminated before it is inspected and a certificate documenting the method of decontamination should accompany the item (Medicines and Healthcare Products Regulatory Agency 2003, NHS Management Executive 1993). This also applies to equipment that is returned to the manufacturer. An example of a decontamination certificate is shown in Figure 13.1.

The method used to decontaminate the equipment depends on how it has been used (see Table 13.2). Equipment that is not contaminated with body fluids can generally be cleaned with detergent. If equipment cannot be decontaminated without being dismantled, it must be clearly marked with a biohazard label and advice on the protective measures required communicated to the relevant engineer.

Reuse of single–use equipment

The reuse of equipment intended for single use sometimes occurs within healthcare facilities in the name of economy. Although it may seem wasteful to discard expensive items, their decontamination and reuse raise a number of issues.

First, the decontamination process may cost more in staff time and materials than the item itself. Second, the decontamination procedure may damage the item and cause it to malfunction on subsequent uses. For example, plastics may lose flexibility or crack. Third, the manufacturer's warranty for the product is likely to be voided by reprocessing and the person who reprocesses it may take on liability should it cause injury to a patient. Finally, reprocessing may not completely remove micro-

Table 13.3 A policy for the decontamination of equipment

Item	Method	Frequency
Ambu-bags	Protect with filter Autoclave	Change filter after each patient After each patient
Anaesthetic masks	Washer-disinfector or SSD	After each patient
Aural speculum	Single-use, or return to SSD Clean and autoclave	After each use After each use
Baby bottles	Use presterilized feeds if possible Clean, immerse in hypochlorite (125 ppm av. Cl) for 1 h or boil for 5 min	After each use
Baby scales	Clean	After each use
Baths	Clean If patient has large open wounds or bathwater contaminated by body fluid, wipe with hypochlorite (1000 ppm av. Cl) after cleaning	After each use
Bath hoists	Clean	After each use
Bedpans	Washer-disinfector Disposables – macerate, clean bedpan carriers	After each use
Bowls (washing)	Clean, dry and store inverted	After each use
Breast pump	Use filter to protect machine Individual tubing for each patient Dishwasher (65°C)	After each use
Commodes	Clean	When visibly soiled
Doppler probe	Clean and dry	After each use

Duvets
   PVC covered
   Fabric
   Duvet cover
	
	Clean
	Launder
	Launder
		
		After each patient
		Every three months
		After each patient and when soiled

Humidifiers	Clean, store dry	Every 48 h Refill with sterile water Maintain at at least 50°C while in use
Incubators	Clean	After each patient
Instruments	Autoclave or hot air oven	After each use
Jugs	Washer–disinfector, or clean and dry, or SSD	After each use
Laryngeal masks	Return to SSD	After each use

Laryngoscopes
   Blades
   Handles
	
	Clean and autoclave or washer–disinfector
	Clean
		
		After each use
		After each use

Mattresses	Clean, allow to dry before turning Ensure cover intact	After each patient and when visibly soiled
Mops	Launder	Daily
Nailbrushes (operating department)	Use sterile, send to SSD or discard	After each use
Nebulizers (medicine)	Clean and dry Discard	After each use After each patient

Table 13.3   A policy for the decontamination of equipment (*cont'd*)

Item	Method	Frequency
Peak flow meter	Clean	Discard mouthpiece after each patient
Pillows	Clean Ensure cover intact	After each patient and when visibly contaminated
Razors Electric	Brush out hairs; immerse head in alcohol for 10 min	After each use
Specula Vaginal	Single-use disposable, or clean autoclave Use sterile speculum for IUD insertion	After each use
Spirometer	Change mouthpiece	After each patient
Stethoscope	Alcohol wipe	After each use

Suction
  Bottles
  Tubing
  Filter
	Clean or autoclave (SSD) if possible, or use disposable liners
	Single-use
		After each use, discard liners when full
		Change between patients
		Change when discoloured and every 3 months

Temperature probes	Use a plastic sleeve Clean, wipe with alcohol, store dry	For each use After each patient
Thermometers	Wipe with alcohol or use a plastic sleeve Clean, immerse in alcohol for 10 min and store dry	For each use After each patient
Thermometer holders	Clean	After each patient
Tonometer prisms	Clean, immerse in hypochlorite (500 ppm av. Cl) for 10 min, rinse and dry	After each use

Toys
  Hard
  Soft
	Clean
	Launder
		When soiled

Tracheostomy tubes (silver)	Autoclave	After each patient
Trolleys Dressing	Clean	Daily
Urinals	Washer–disinfector Macerate disposables	After each use

Ventilators
  Machine
  Tubing
	Protect with filter on expiratory circuit
	Protect with filter at patient end of circuit
		Change filter every 48 h
		Change filter every 48 h
		Discard single use/heat disinfect reusable tubing after each patient

Clean = wash with detergent and water, then dry.

organisms, in particular prions or other harmful substances such as endotoxins (Medical Devices Agency 2000a). The report by Yardy & Cox (2001) of infections (one ultimately fatal) transmitted to patients after the reuse of single-use equipment used for urodynamic studies clearly illustrates these dangers. The Medicines and Healthcare Products Regulatory Agency (previously the Medical Devices Agency) advises that devices designed for single use must not be reused under any circumstances (Medical Devices Agency 2000b).

METHODS OF DECONTAMINATION

Cleaning

Cleaning is important for two reasons: in its own right as a method of decontaminating low-risk items and as preparation for disinfection or sterilization. Many pieces of equipment classed as low risk can be decontaminated safely between patients by cleaning, for example washing bowls, cots, beds and commodes.

Cleaning involves the use of detergent and water to remove organic material and with it micro-organisms. Detergent is essential for effective cleaning. It breaks up grease and dirt and improves the ability of water to remove soil. Approximately 80% of micro-organisms are removed during the cleaning procedure (Ayliffe et al 1967). However, drying the equipment after it has been cleaned is also extremely important to prevent any bacteria that remain from multiplying. The importance of thoroughly drying equipment before storage was demonstrated in a study by Greaves (1985) in which 34% of washing bowls were not dried completely before storage and more than 50% of these damp bowls were found to be contaminated with large numbers of Gram-negative bacilli. These bacteria could be transmitted readily to another patient when the bowl was next used.

Cloths used for cleaning also become heavily contaminated with bacteria, which are readily transferred to hands and equipment (Scott & Bloomfield 1990) and they should be discarded after each use. Gram-negative bacilli can survive in solutions of detergent and items should not be left to soak for prolonged periods in bowls of detergent (Werry et al 1988).

DECONTAMINATION CERTIFICATE

For issue prior to inspection, service or repair of any medical or laboratory equipment.

TO (Works dept/Manufacturer): ....

Description of equipment ....

Serial No. .... Unit .... Date ....

Tick box A if applicable, otherwise complete sections B and C.

A. ☐ This equipment has not been in contact with blood, body fluid, respired gases or pathological specimens.

B. Has this equipment been exposed to hazardous material?

Blood, body fluids, respired gases or pathological specimens   Yes/No

Chemicals or substances hazardous to health   Yes/No

Other hazards   Yes/No

Provide details of contamination: ....

C. Has this equipment been cleaned and decontaminated?

Yes/No   Method ....

If No, state why ....

Note: equipment which has not been decontaminated must not be returned/presented without prior agreement of recipient.

I declare that I have taken all reasonable steps to ensure the accuracy of the above information.

Signature .... Name .... Position ....

Figure 13.1 Example of a decontamination certificate.

Blood and body fluids must be completely removed from instruments before they are subjected to a disinfection or sterilization process. Thorough cleaning with detergent and water removes a significant proportion of the micro-organisms and increases the efficiency of disinfection. Organic material such as blood is coagulated, or fixed, by heat or chemicals and consequently difficult to remove after sterilization. Hollow tubing is particularly difficult to clean effectively and requires the use of special brushes or high-powered water jets. Most tubing is single use and disinfection of this type of item should not be attempted because of the difficulty of ensuring complete decontamination and the risk of subsequent cross-infection (Anderton & Nwoguh 1991).

Automated washing machines provide a highly efficient means of cleaning. They enable contaminated instruments to be decontaminated safely without direct handling by staff. Ultrasonic cleaning machines are also useful for removing body fluids from delicate instruments, with intricate surfaces. Cleaning will not be successful if blood and body fluids are fixed onto the surface by prior heating or if blood has been allowed to dry onto the surface.

Decontamination by heat

Heat is the best method of decontamination for medical equipment. Its effects are predictable and it is easily controlled. The process is most efficient in the presence of water because the heat will be conducted evenly to all parts of an object.

The number of micro-organisms destroyed depends on the temperature and the period of exposure: the higher the temperature, the shorter the period of exposure. Additional time should be allowed for all parts of the item to reach the selected temperature.

There are a number of decontamination methods based on the use of heat; those used most commonly are described below.

Pasteurization

In this process items are heated to temperatures between 65° and 80°C at which many micro-organisms are destroyed provided they are exposed for a sufficient length of time. The higher the temperature, the shorter the exposure period required. Pasteurization is used to disinfect a variety of medium-risk equipment but cannot be used to sterilize.

Examples of pasteurization used in a clinical setting are: bedpan washers which disinfect at a temperature of 80°C for at least 1 min; the disinfection of linen at 71°C for not less than 3 min during the wash cycle (NHS Executive 1995); and automatic dishwashers.

Automated washer-disinfectors may be useful for cleaning and disinfecting instruments with hot water before sterilization and enable blood and body fluid to be removed without the need to handle the instruments. Cleaning is achieved using water sprays or ultrasonic vibration. An initial low temperature wash removes protein from the equipment; this is followed by washing in detergent in hot water and a final thermal disinfection rinse (71°C or greater). Washer-disinfectors are routinely used to clean instruments in SSDs but bench-top ultrasonic and washer-disinfectors are also available. They must be properly operated and maintained and meet the specification described in HTM 2030 (NHS Estates 1994).

Boiling

Although not commonly employed in hospitals in developed countries, boiling can be used to disinfect medium-risk equipment. Most bacteria and viruses are destroyed by boiling for a few minutes; however, sterilization by this method is not possible as some bacterial spores will not be destroyed.

Boiling is relatively easily controlled visually. Instruments should be completely immersed in boiling water and the 5-min disinfection period timed from when the water returns to boiling point. Additional instruments should not be added during this time.

Water boilers have been used in some general practice surgeries for the decontamination of vaginal specula, ear syringes, etc. However, they must not be used to decontaminate surgical instruments or other equipment used for high-risk procedures. Small autoclaves provide a more practical option and are now widely available (Medical Devices Agency 1997).

Steam under pressure (autoclave)

This is the most reliable method of sterilizing equipment. At atmospheric pressure water boils at 100°C but while this temperature is sufficient to destroy vegetative bacteria, much higher temperatures are required for the destruction of spores.

If water is heated inside a closed container at increased pressure, it boils at a higher temperature. For example, at a pressure of 1.03 bar (15 lb per inch^2) it boils at 121°C; at 2.2 bar (32 lb per inch^2) it boils at 134°C. The steam produced at these higher temperatures will destroy any micro-organisms present on items inside the container, by condensing on to their surface and releasing energy in the form of heat. The higher the temperature of the steam, the more rapidly spores will be destroyed. At 121°C this takes 15 min, at 134°C 3 min. As a mixture of air and steam inside the chamber reduces the temperature inside and prevents steam from penetrating

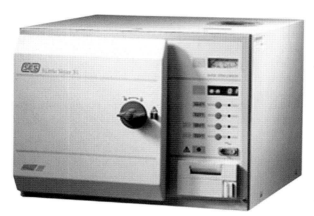

Figure 13.2 A bench-top autoclave.

completely, the efficiency of sterilization is improved if air is removed.

Autoclaves are the most common method of sterilization for high- and medium-risk equipment. Instruments used for medium-risk procedures require pathogens from one patient to be removed before use on another and can be used again in a clean, but not necessarily sterile, condition. They should be stored in a clean, covered container after autoclaving (e.g. vaginal specula). Instruments used in high-risk procedures *must* be sterile at the point of use. To prevent contamination of these instruments on removal from the autoclave, they must either be autoclaved inside a sealed packet or autoclaved immediately before use. Equipment must be cleaned prior to autoclaving as blood and body fluids will prevent steam condensing on the surfaces and once proteins have been fixed by exposure to heat, they are very difficult to remove.

There are two main types of autoclave: vacuum assisted (porous load) and non-vacuum assisted (e.g. some bench-top autoclaves).

Porous-load autoclaves These use pumps to remove the air from the chamber before steam is introduced. The vacuum created inside the chamber allows steam to penetrate all parts of the load, including lumens and porous materials such as paper or linen. This enables prewrapped instruments to be sterilized. The drying cycle, which completes the process, ensures that packs removed from the autoclave are dry. Packed instruments will remain sterile indefinitely provided the wrapping remains intact and does not become wet. Porous-load autoclaves are generally large industrial machines used in SSDs to process large volumes of surgical instruments and other equipment supplied in packs. However, bench-top vacuum-assisted autoclaves are now available for processing prepacked instruments or hollow equipment in clinics and surgeries. To ensure effective sterilization, packs should be placed on trays or baskets that enable steam to circulate freely. Indicator tape should be placed on

each pack to show it has been put through an autoclave cycle and instruments should also be labelled to ensure they can be readily tracked.

Non–vacuum assisted autoclaves These simpler autoclaves (Fig. 13.2) do not have a prevacuum stage in the process. They can therefore not be used to sterilize equipment that requires penetration of steam, such as wrapped instruments, porous materials (e.g. dressings) or hollow items. The chamber should not be overloaded so that steam is able to condense easily on all surfaces. Although wrapped instruments must not be sterilized in these autoclaves instruments can be protected from recontamination by covering with sterile paper or storing in a sterile container after sterilization. A process indicator should be included on the tray and instruments labelled to enable them to be tracked (see Guidelines for practice: using small autoclaves).

Purchase and maintenance of bench–top autoclaves Wherever possible, sterilized instruments should be obtained from a SSD to ensure that the process is high quality, properly controlled and the instruments can be readily tracked. However, bench-top steam sterilizers are available and frequently used in surgeries, clinics and dental practices. Where such autoclaves are in use, it is essential to select the correct type of sterilizer for the equipment intended for processing and to ensure that guidance on monitoring the efficacy of the process is followed and that the sterilizer is properly maintained. Information about selecting, using and maintaining bench-top sterilizers can be found in device bulletins published by the Medical Devices Agency (DB 6905 1997; DB 9804 1998; DB 2000(05) 2000(a)). New sterilizers must be validated by a trained person before they are first used. Vacuum-assisted sterilizers must have a facility to undertake daily steam penetration tests to ensure that the cycle is effectively sterilizing packed instruments (Medical Devices Agency 2002a).

An autoclave that is not functioning correctly may not sterilize instruments. Autoclave tape that changes colour on exposure to specific temperatures indicates that an item has been through an autoclave but is not a guarantee of sterility. Internal controls on the machine should indicate when the process has failed and these should be closely monitored. For more detailed information see Babb & Lowe (2003).

All autoclaves require regular, skilled maintenance to ensure their safety and reliability. There should be a planned and documented testing and maintenance programme carried out by specialist technicians (British Standards Institution 1994, Medical Devices Agency 1998). Advice on installing, testing and maintaining autoclaves should be obtained from a qualified, authorized person, registered with the Institute of Healthcare Engineers and Estates Management.

Hot air ovens

Hot air can also be used to sterilize but higher temperatures and longer exposure times are necessary because air does not conduct heat as efficiently as steam. Sterilization can be achieved by holding at a temperature of 170°C for 1 h; however, instruments must reach the required temperature before commencing timing and must be allowed to cool before removal. This limits their use to instruments that can withstand high temperatures and to situations where a rapid turnround of equipment is not essential (UK Health Departments 1994).

Instruments must be cleaned thoroughly before sterilization because organic matter will be baked on to the surface and become very difficult to remove. The sterilizer must have an automatic controller and not be possible to open part-way through a cycle. They also need to undergo regular testing to ensure sterilization is effective (Medical Devices Agency 2002b).

Ethylene oxide

Equipment easily damaged by heat cannot be sterilized in an autoclave or hot air oven and, for these items, a lower temperature can be used in combination with ethylene oxide gas.

Ethylene oxide is not corrosive but it is irritant, toxic, explosive and possibly mutagenic. It is absorbed into many materials and will then gradually leach out, causing harm to patients and staff in contact with the equipment. Items must therefore be completely aired after the process to remove all traces of the chemical. This can take up to 7 days.

Ethylene oxide is flammable and can be explosive when mixed with air in certain concentrations. It is harmful at far lower concentrations than can be detected by smell and the gas must be safely vented from the area. Ethylene oxide sterilization requires the use of specialist facilities and the process must be closely controlled by trained operators. Ethylene oxide facilities are not available in most hospitals but it is used by industry for the sterilization of medical devices and drugs. Gas plasma sterilization using hydrogen peroxide vapour is a possible alternative to ethylene oxide.

Irradiation

This method is not used in hospitals but is widely employed commercially for the sterilization of plastic disposable items such as syringes and cannulae. The process may alter plastic materials and resterilization of disposable equipment should not be attempted. Ultraviolet light radiation can be used to kill micro-organisms but it is not reliable and will not destroy spores.

Decontamination by chemicals

A variety of chemicals is used for the decontamination of skin, equipment and the environment. Most can be used only to disinfect, not to sterilize, equipment, as they are mostly not active against spores and have limited antimycobacterial activity. Some viruses with lipid membranes are easily destroyed, whereas those without are more resistant.

Chemical disinfection has considerable disadvantages (Box 13.2). Many disinfectants (or biocides) are corrosive and highly irritant and disposable gloves

---

Box 13.2   Disadvantages of chemical disinfectants

- Most are not active against all micro-organisms
- Mycobacteria and spores are not easily destroyed
- Variable ability to destroy viruses
- Poor penetration of blood, pus and other organic material
- May be inactivated by organic material, detergent, rubber or plastics
- May be unstable, particularly if diluted, and may support the growth of some micro-organisms
- Often corrosive, toxic or irritant
- Variable exposure time required to achieve disinfection

and aprons should be worn to handle them. After disinfection, equipment usually needs to be rinsed in water to remove traces of the irritant chemical. Disinfectants must be used at the correct dilution: too high a concentration may be corrosive, toxic and irritant, too low a concentration may be ineffective. Diluted disinfectants are often unstable and lose activity, enabling some bacteria, particularly pseudomonas, to grow in the solution. Some microorganisms are known to be able to develop reduced susceptibility to disinfectants, especially Gram-negative bacteria such as pseudomonas, acinetobacter and *Escherichia coli,* and in some circumstances have been found to exhibit cross-resistance to antibiotics (Russell 2004). Whilst this is currently not a widespread problem, increasing use of biocides in household products may encourage such resistant pathogens to emerge. Unnecessary use of disinfectants should therefore be avoided (Russell 2004).

Effective disinfection cannot be achieved unless the solution is in contact with a surface for a reasonable period of time. Some solutions have a very rapid antimicrobial action, for example alcohols and hypochlorite disinfectants, and on clean surfaces kill microbes within a few minutes. Other disinfectants may take longer; for example, immersion in glutaraldehyde for several hours is required to destroy bacterial spores. The important principles for using chemical disinfectants are summarized in the Guidelines for practice. It is important to check with the hospital disinfection policy or infection control team to ensure the correct method of decontamination is selected.

Decontamination by heat, preferably in an SSD, is a considerably more reliable process and should be used in preference to chemicals wherever possible. This may mean purchasing additional instruments to enable high-quality processing or using single-use equipment.

COSHH regulations and the use of chemical disinfectants

The Control of Substances Hazardous to Health (COSHH) Regulations require employers to assess the risks presented by the use of hazardous substances in the workplace and to determine the control measures required to ensure that they are handled safely (Health & Safety Executive 2002). The COSHH Regulations first came into force in 1989. They incorporate Codes of Practice on general substances hazardous to health, carcinogenic substances and biological agents (see p. 155). Chemical disinfectants may be inflammable, toxic if inhaled or ingested and irritant to eyes or skin. Even detergent can damage the skin but may be used safely if the proper precautions are followed. Where possible, a hazardous chemical should be replaced by a less dangerous chemical or a different process. If this is not possible, equipment should be provided to protect against exposure (e.g. a covered container) and a safe system of work established for handling the chemical. Box 13.3 lists the factors that should be considered when assessing the risk of a chemical disinfectant.

Information about each chemical used in a department should be provided in the form of a risk assessment and a copy kept in a readily accessible place. This should specify how the chemical should be

---

Guidelines for practice: important principles of chemical disinfection

- Check the disinfection policy to ensure disinfection is necessary and which agent to use
- Check the appropriate COSHH assessment
- Wear protective clothing if indicated
- Clean equipment thoroughly with detergent to remove blood and body fluid
- Make up the correct dilution of the chemical
- Completely immerse equipment for the correct time
- Discard disinfectant after use, clean container and store dry

---

Box 13.3   Control of Substances Hazardous to Health: factors to be considered for risk assessment of chemical disinfectants

- Establish how the chemical is used (e.g. how often, what for, in what amounts)
- Determine potential harmful effects of the chemical
- Decide how to prevent or control exposure to the chemical:
  - use an alternative
  - restrict use
  - use an automated process
  - use covered containers and/or install ventilation
  - define a safe system of working with the chemical, including management of spillages
  - use protective clothing if exposure cannot be prevented by other means
- Inform and train users
- Health surveillance (if appropriate)

stored and handled, protective clothing required and how to manage spillages.

The pharmacy or supplies department can often help to draw up risk assessments. The risk of injury from disinfectants can be minimized provided the staff who use the chemicals are properly trained and follow the guidelines for use of the chemical described in the assessment.

Occupational exposure standards

The Health and Safety Executive also publishes occupational exposure limits to certain substances that may have serious effects on health if inhaled (Health & Safety Executive 2001). The Occupational Exposure Standards (OESs) are levels of exposure that scientific information suggests will not damage the health of workers regularly exposed to the substance. Maximum Exposure Limits (MELs) are applied to more hazardous substances, for which a safe level of exposure does not exist or cannot be practically achieved. This places a duty on the employer to reduce exposure to the substance below the MEL and to minimize the number of people exposed and the duration of exposure.

The Health and Safety Executive recommends an OES for a number of disinfectants, including phenol, iodine and alcohol, as these chemicals may irritate the eyes, skin or mucous membranes and should not be used in large quantities in poorly ventilated areas. Glutaraldehyde may cause more serious health effects, including asthma, and has been assigned a MEL.

Properties of common chemical disinfectants

Alcohol

Examples: ethanol (industrial methylated spirit, IMS), isopropanol, alcohol handrub, alcohol-impregnated wipes.

Alcohol rapidly destroys bacteria, including mycobacteria and fungi, but has no effect on bacterial spores. Both ethanol (70%) and isopropanol (60–70%) are effective against enveloped viruses but for non-enveloped viruses only 90% ethanol is effective. Alcohol does not penetrate protein-based organic matter and should be used only on clean surfaces. It damages some materials (e.g. lens cement in fibreoptic scopes) and is inflammable. It is not a suitable disinfectant for most equipment but its rapid action and volatility make it useful for skin disinfection and it is often used for this in combination with other chemicals such as chlorhexidine. Mixed with emollients, it is a highly effective hand disinfectant. Alcohol handrubs should not be used to attempt to decontaminate soiled equipment as they are unlikely to be effective (Van den Berg et al 2000).

Alcohol-impregnated wipes are widely used to disinfect surfaces but because of the short contact time, are unlikely to have much effect and their use is probably unnecessary (Thompson & Bullock 1992).

Chlorhexidine

Examples: handwash solution (Hibiscrub), Hibitane.

Gram-positive bacteria are more susceptible to chlorhexidine than Gram-negative organisms. It is fungicidal but has no effect on mycobacteria or spores and has limited activity against viruses. Chlorhexidine is recommended mainly as a skin disinfectant, combined either with a detergent in a handwash solution or with alcohol as a preoperative skin disinfectant or handrub. It has the advantage of being highly effective against the resident microbial flora of the skin, with an action persisting for several hours after the initial application. Although not an irritant to intact skin, some studies have suggested that chlorhexidine is toxic to fibroblasts and may interfere with the healing of wounds (Neidner & Schöpf 1986).

Its limited spectrum of activity, inactivation by organic matter and expense make chlorhexidine an unsuitable disinfectant for most equipment. Solutions used to immerse equipment may become contaminated by bacteria after time (Oie & Kamiya 1996). The main use of chlorhexidine is in surgical scrubs (see p. 158).

Glutaraldehyde

Glutaraldehyde has a wide range of antimicrobial activity. It kills bacteria, fungi and viruses rapidly, mycobacteria in 20–60 min and bacterial spores in 3–10 h, depending on the product. Glutaraldehyde does not corrode metal and is not seriously inactivated by organic material, although it penetrates such material only slowly. Protein material will be coagulated on to the surface; therefore blood or other organic material must be removed completely before immersion.

Once activated, alkaline solutions of glutaraldehyde remain active for 14–28 days (depending on the product), although they should be replaced if organic matter builds up and if the solution becomes cloudy.

Glutaraldehyde can be used for high-level decontamination of heat-sensitive equipment but it is highly irritant to skin and mucosa and extensive exposure has been associated with sensitization reactions, including dermatitis and asthma. It must therefore only be used in designated areas with appropriate exhaust ventilation and protective clothing to ensure that staff are not exposed to unsafe levels of the chemical (Health & Safety Executive 2001). As a result many hospitals have sought alternative agents for decontaminating heat-sensitive equipment such as flexible endoscopes.

Other aldehydes

Examples: orthophthaldehyde (e.g. Cidex OPA), succine dialdehyde (e.g. Gigasept).

Active against bacteria, including mycobacteria, viruses and fungi but not sporicidal. Not readily inactivated by organic material or damaging to metals and although they produce less vapour than glutaraldehyde, they may still be irritant and asthmagenic.

Hexachlorophane and triclosan

Examples: hexachlorophane (Ster-zac powder), triclosan (Manusept, Aquasept, Ster-zac bath concentrate).

Ster-zac powder is used on intact skin as a preoperative disinfectant and for reducing staphylococcal colonization to prevent infection on the umbilicus in the newborn. More active against Gram-positive than Gram-negative bacteria, triclosan (Irgasan) has similar properties and spectrum of activity as hexachlorophane.

Hydrogen peroxide

Examples: hydrogen peroxide, Virkon.

These solutions have a wide range of activity against bacteria, viruses and fungi but are readily inactivated by organic matter. Hydrogen peroxide has a low toxicity and irritancy but may be corrosive to some metals and should not be used to decontaminate equipment without seeking advice from the manufacturer. Concentrated solutions may irritate the skin and mucous membranes.

Peracetic acid

Examples: Nu-cidex, Steris, Persafe, Gigasept PA, Aperlan, Perascope.

This peroxygen compound kills bacteria, fungi and viruses rapidly and bacterial spores within 10 min. It is not readily inactivated by organic matter and buffered solutions containing corrosion inhibitors cause minimal corrosion, although they may damage rubber and brass after prolonged immersion (Haythorne 1998). Peracetic acid is useful for the high-level decontamination of heat-sensitive equipment such as endoscopes but has a strong smell and is irritant to skin and mucous membranes so should be used in an area with exhaust ventilation.

Hypochlorites (and other chlorine-based disinfectants)

Examples: hypochlorite (Milton, Chloros, Domestos), sodium dichloroisocyanurate (NaDCC – Presept, Haz-Tabs), chlorine dioxide (Tristel).

Hypochlorites are active against bacteria, viruses and fungi. At concentrations of 1000 ppm or more, they also destroy spores and mycobacteria. Although probably the best general-purpose disinfectant, hypochlorites have a number of disadvantages which make them unsuitable for the decontamination of instruments. Particular problems are the corrosive effect on some metals and ready inactivation by organic material.

To prevent corrosion of surfaces, hypochlorite should be washed off with detergent and water and should not be used on fabric or carpets because it will bleach out the colour. Hypochlorites should not be mixed with large volumes of acidic substances (e.g. urine) in confined spaces because this may result in the release of harmful chlorine gas (DoH 1990).

Dilute solutions of hypochlorite lose their activity quite rapidly and fresh solution should be made up daily. The concentration of hypochlorite solutions is often expressed as parts per million of available chlorine (ppm av. Cl). Domestos and other brands of thick bleaches contain between 10 000 and 50 000 ppm av. Cl and may need to be diluted before use.

In strong concentrations (e.g. 10 000 ppm av. Cl) the chlorine is less likely to be inactivated by the organic matter and can be used to decontaminate spills of body fluid (Table 13.4). A granular form of NaDCC is useful for decontamination of body fluid spills as the spill is absorbed and can be removed more easily (see p. 173 and Plate 24). Making the correct dilution of hypochlorite solutions can be difficult but the addition of NaDCC tablets to water provides the easiest method of making up solutions of the required strength.

Non-abrasive powders that contain hypochlorite are sometimes used to clean baths, although whether these powders have any advantage over detergent is debatable.

Chlorine dioxide is rapidly sporicidal (within 10 min) and is increasingly used as an alternative to

Table 13.4 Recommended uses of different strengths of hypochlorite (Hoffman et al 2004)

	% hypochlorite	ppm* available chlorine
Blood and body fluid spills	1	10 000
Laboratory discard jars	0.25	2500
Environmental disinfection	0.1	1000
Infant feeding bottles	0.0125	125

* parts per million.

glutaraldehyde for decontaminating heat-sensitive equipment such as endoscopes. It is irritant to skin and mucous membranes.

Phenolics

Examples: Hycolin, Clearsol, Stericol.

The phenolics are active against bacteria and fungi but have little effect on bacterial spores and a variable activity against viruses, particularly those without lipid envelopes. Although inexpensive, stable and not readily inactivated by organic material, phenolic disinfectants are no longer widely used for environmental disinfection. However, they have good activity against mycobacteria and are used in microbiology laboratories. Their spectrum of activity is not wide enough to enable them to be used to disinfect equipment. In addition, phenolics are absorbed by rubber and plastics and are irritants. They should therefore not be used to disinfect items used on skin or mucous membranes.

Superoxidized water

Example: Sterilox.

An electrolytic process is used to produce a solution that rapidly destroys bacteria (including mycobacteria), viruses and fungi and destroys spores within 10 min. It has low irritancy but is inactivated by organic matter and solutions are unstable so must be discarded after use. It is a useful agent for decontaminating heat-sensitive equipment such as fibreoptic endoscopes.

Quaternary ammonium compounds (QACs)

Examples: Cetavlon, Roccal.

These agents are more active against Gram-positive than Gram-negative bacteria, are fungicidal but have variable activity against mycobacteria and viruses. They are not sporicidal. Although they have good detergent properties, they are easily inactivated and may support the growth of bacteria in dilute solutions. They are not suitable for disinfecting equipment.

Decontamination of the environment

The complete removal of micro-organisms from the environment is neither practical nor desirable (Collins 1988). The majority of micro-organisms present in the environment are not harmful and not readily transferred to susceptible sites on the patient. In epidemics of infection, contamination of the environment with the epidemic strain is frequently reported; however, in most circumstances it is difficult to demonstrate that the environment is either the source of infection or responsible for transmission. Micro-organisms acquired on hands through direct contact

with an infected patient or body fluids is a more likely route of cross-infection in most situations (Marshall et al 2004). The termination of outbreaks of infection is sometimes associated with extensive cleaning programmes but it is often difficult to establish whether other factors, such as the removal of affected patients or staff, have had a more important effect (Noone & Griffiths 1971).

Nonetheless, some micro-organisms are particularly adept at surviving in the environment, notably those that withstand desiccation such as staphylococci, enterococci and acinetobacter, and those that form spores such as *Clostridium difficile* and *Bacillus cereus* (Neeley & Maley 2000). In some circumstances, high levels of environmental contamination with these organisms probably contribute to their spread, for example where patients with *C. difficile* or glycopeptide-resistant enterococci have diarrhoea (Gray & George 2000). The accumulation of dust in clinical areas has also been linked to the transmission of staphylococci (Rampling et al 2001). While disinfectants may help to reduce environmental contamination, their effect is short-lived (Ayliffe et al 1967). Most micro-organisms are present in visible dust and dirt, so the key to achieving minimal levels of microbial contamination is the regular removal of dust and the removal of dirt by cleaning with detergent. Disinfectants may sometimes have a place in the treatment of environmental contamination where it may be contributing to the spread of infection. For example, in outbreaks of norovirus environmental contamination appears to contribute to the spread of infection and disinfection is recommended (Chadwick et al 2000). Noble et al (1998) reported a case of vancomycin-resistant enterococci transmitted as a result of extensive flooding of a blocked toilet. Decontamination of the environment in this instance required the use of disinfectants in addition to thorough cleaning.

Whilst there is little direct evidence to demonstrate a link between cleanliness and hospital-acquired infection, high-quality cleaning is important because it ensures a pleasant environment for patients, implies good standards of care and minimizes the risk of the environment acting as a reservoir for micro-organisms. A comprehensive cleaning service with clearly defined routine cleaning programmes, well-trained staff and regularly monitored standards is therefore essential. The frequency and type of cleaning required will depend on the clinical area. High-risk areas such as ICU or operating departments will need more frequent cleaning than lower risk areas such as outpatient departments. Guidance on cleaning standards and methods for a range of clinical areas have been published (DoH 2004a). Effective cleaning requires teamwork between clinical and cleaning staff with clearly defined responsibilities and a commitment to facilitate cleaning by keeping clinical areas tidy. Ward housekeepers can play an important role in fostering teamwork and ensuring standards are monitored and maintained (DoH 2004b, Lack & Wraight 2002).

Furniture, floors and walls

Surfaces in clinical areas should be kept clean and dry to prevent the accumulation and growth of micro-organisms. Most of the micro-organisms found on floors and other horizontal surfaces are from dust particles that have settled (Collins 1988). Dust particles are largely composed of skin scales, respired droplets and fibres from clothing or linen, of which only a small proportion carry micro-organisms. The most important component of an effective cleaning programme is the regular removal of dust from these surfaces using either a vacuum cleaner or a dust control mop. Removal of dust by these methods is more effective than a damp mop which tends to redistribute bacteria rather than remove them (Ballemans et al 2003). The accumulation of large amounts of dust in areas that are less readily visible or more difficult to clean, such as behind radiators and under beds, has been associated with the transmission of some hospital pathogens such as methicillin-resistant *Staphylococcus aureus* and *Clostridium difficile* (Rampling et al 2001, Teare et al 1998). All fixtures and fittings must therefore be included in the routine cleaning schedule to prevent the build-up of dust.

Bacteria are rarely found on vertical surfaces such as walls and these require only spot cleaning to remove splashes or stains (Ayliffe et al 1967).

Mopping with detergent and water is of value for surfaces that are soiled or exposed to spillages. However, because the cleaning equipment is prone to become heavily contaminated with Gram-negative organisms, wet cleaning methods have been associated with the spread of pathogenic bacteria in high-risk clinical settings (Van Dessel et al 2002). Care should be taken to ensure that mopheads are laundered after each use and at least every day and stored dry. Chemical disinfection of mop heads should not be attempted as it is unlikely to be effective. Cleaning buckets must also be emptied, cleaned and left dry. Although the routine use of disinfectants has been recommended (Rutal & Weber 2001), there is little evidence that they affect either the level of contamination or rates of healthcare-associated infection (Danforth et al 1987, Ruden & Daschner 2002). Ayliffe et al (1967) demonstrated that, although disinfectants removed more bacteria from floors than detergent, recontamination of the floor occurred within 1 h of treatment. Disinfectant granules (e.g. sodium dichloroisocyanurate) can be used to remove spills of body fluids and to destroy micro-organisms present, reducing the risk of infection to the person clearing up the spillage (UK Health Departments 1998). These granules should not be used on urine spills, as irritant chlorine vapour may be released (DoH 1990). They should also not be used on fabric or carpet, as they will damage these materials.

Carpets

Although there is little evidence that carpets increase the risk of infection, they are associated with significantly higher levels of microbial contamination than hard floors (Skoutelis et al 1993). It is probably not advisable to fit carpets to areas where frequent contamination with body fluids or other spillages are anticipated or where patients vulnerable to gastro-intestinal illness such as *Clostridium difficile* or norovirus are likely to be cared for. If carpets are fitted they must be washable and the fibres should be short and water-repellent to enable spills to be dealt with more easily. They should be vacuum cleaned daily to remove bacteria in dust and spillage of body fluid should be removed with detergent and water, preferably using a cleaning machine.

Baths, washbasins and toilets

Bacteria are able to survive more easily in these moist environments; however, the routine use of disinfectants is not justified because they do not present a major source of micro-organisms (Levin et al 1984). Bacteria colonizing washbasins and taps are usually environmental organisms and unlikely to cause disease in humans even if transferred to vulnerable sites on patients (Ayliffe et al 1974, Orsi et al 1994). Toilet seats do not usually become heavily contaminated by faecal micro-organisms and are an unlikely route of cross-infection (Newsom 1972). Regular cleaning with detergent will remove pathogens and reduce the risk of cross-infection. Disinfectants are not necessary for routine use but may sometimes be indicated in outbreaks of gastroenteritis (Chadwick et al 2000).

Baths may become contaminated with pathogenic bacteria after use by a patient with a large open wound. An outbreak of group A streptococci in episiotomy wounds was associated with two baths that were not properly cleaned between patients. An important factor in this outbreak was the damaged surface on the baths, which prevented effective cleaning (Dowsett & Wilson 1981). Harsh scouring agents should not be used to clean baths as these may damage the enamel. Thorough cleaning with detergent after each patient is sufficient.

Whirlpool baths and birthing pools, which have channels where stagnant water may collect, have been associated with the transmission of infection and require maintenance and the use of disinfectants to prevent the multiplication of pathogenic Gram-negative bacilli (Hollyoak et al 1995, Kingsley et al 1999). Thorough cleaning with detergent between patients is sufficient. Bath hoists may become easily contaminated with bacteria and should be thoroughly cleaned with detergent after each use (Murdoch 1990). Washbowls have been associated with outbreaks of infection by Gram-negative bacilli when not washed and dried properly after use (Joynson 1978).

Beds and mattresses

Bedframes accumulate dust and should be cleaned regularly. Babies' incubators should be cleaned routinely with detergent and water. If disinfection is required, a dilute solution of hypochlorite (125 ppm av. Cl) is suitable but should be rinsed off. Some incubators have an integral humidifier which should be disinfected by raising the temperature of the water to at least 70°C for 10 min, or removed and autoclaved (Hoffman et al 2004).

Mattresses with an intact impermeable cover do not support the growth of bacteria if clean and dry. If contaminated with body fluid, they should be cleaned with detergent and water and the surface thoroughly dried. Some chemical disinfectants (e.g. phenol) can damage mattress covers and their use should be avoided (Loomes 1988). The mattress cover should be inspected carefully for signs of wear or loss of impermeability and should be turned over regularly to prolong its life (DoH 1991). Outbreaks of infection associated with damaged mattresses and caused by Gram-negative bacteria have been reported (Sherertz & Sullivan 1985).

SPECIAL DECONTAMINATION PROBLEMS

Fibreoptic endoscopes

Decontamination of flexible fibreoptic endoscopes presents particular problems as the narrow channels are difficult to clean and they will not withstand the high temperatures in an autoclave. Decontamination between patients must therefore rely on thorough cleaning followed by chemical disinfection.

A number of cases of pathogens transmitted between patients on endoscopes have been reported. These have included salmonella, Gram-negative bacilli and *Helicobacter pylori* associated with gastroscopy; hepatitis C associated with colonoscopy and *Mycobacterium tuberculosis* following bronchoscopy (Bronowicki et al 1997, Langenberg et al 1990, Spach

et al 1993). Endoscopic retrograde cholangiopancreatography (ERCP) is particularly associated with a risk of infection, usually due to pseudomonas and other Gram-negative bacteria (Earnshaw et al 1985). There is a small risk of transmission of vCJD associated with endoscopy because the prion is known to be present in lymphoid tissue which may be encountered in the gut. If endoscopy has to be undertaken in a patient with suspected or confirmed vCJD, a dedicated endoscope should be used (British Society of Gastroenterology 2003, Medicines and Healthcare Products Regulatory Agency 2002). Infections may also be acquired when waterborne micro-organisms, such as pseudomonas and mycobacteria, contaminate the rinse water in automatic washing machines (Medicines and Healthcare Products Regulatory Agency 2002).

Cross-infection following endoscopy is usually the result of a failure to follow decontamination procedures, for example inadequate manual cleaning, inadequate exposure of all the channels of the endoscope to disinfectant, the use of contaminated rinse water or inadequate drying of the endoscope (Cooke 2004). Careful adherence to decontamination procedures is therefore essential.

The risk of infection, and hence the level of decontamination required, depends on the invasiveness of the procedure. Endoscopes used in normally sterile body areas (e.g. laparoscopes, arthroscopes) are invasive and should be sterilized before and after use, preferably in an SSD. Most of these scopes are rigid and modern designs are usually fully autoclavable. However, if operative endoscopes are heat sensitive they should undergo high-level disinfection, such as low-temperature steam or thermal disinfection at 73°C for 3 min. They are unlikely to be contaminated with many spores provided they are thoroughly cleaned prior to disinfection (Ayliffe et al 2000, Hoffman et al 2004).

Endoscopes that have contact with mucous membranes but not sterile body cavities can be decontaminated by chemical disinfection after use. Biopsy forceps and other accessories that penetrate the tissues should be sterilized after each patient or be single use only (Medicines and Healthcare Products Regulatory Agency 2002). Filters can be used on sigmoidoscopes to prevent contamination of the inflation bulb and tubing.

The principles for processing all heat-sensitive endoscopes between patients are:

- an initial manual clean
- disinfection (preferably in an automated washer)
- rinsing with bacteria-free water to remove traces of the disinfecting chemical.

Endoscopes should be decontaminated before each session, between each patient and at the end of the session. A final flush with 70% alcohol at the end of the session can be used to dry the channels, reducing the risk that bacteria will multiply during overnight storage (British Society of Gastroenterology 2003).

Records should be kept of the endoscope serial number used in each patient so that future contact tracing is possible should a problem occur (Medicines and Healthcare Products Regulatory Agency 2002). Each scope should be processed with a designated set of brushes that can be traced with it.

Thorough manual cleaning of the external and internal surfaces of the endoscope with detergent and water is essential to maximize the efficacy of decontamination. All channels should be brushed and flushed with detergent and water, brushes should be the correct size and in good condition. Biopsy forceps and other accessories should be cleaned to ensure that all debris is removed prior to autoclaving. The decontamination process should then be completed in an automated endoscope reprocessor (AER) that thoroughly irrigates all the channels in a cycle that includes detergent, followed by immersion in disinfectant for an appropriate time and then rinsing with water. The manufacturer's instructions must be carefully followed to ensure that all channels are properly connected to the washing process (Medicines and Healthcare Products Regulatory Agency 2002). These machines not only significantly improve the quality of disinfection but also reduce exposure of staff to the disinfectant.

Until recently, glutaraldehyde was the standard disinfectant for processing flexible endoscopes. However, concerns about its safety have led to the use of alternative disinfectants such as peracetic acid, chlorine dioxide and superoxidized water. The recommended immersion times for these agents vary and advice should be sought from the manufacturers of the disinfectant, endoscope and AER on suitable agents and exposure times. The main infection risk associated with flexible bronchoscopes is the transmission of respiratory pathogens, particularly mycobacteria. *Mycobacterium avium intracellulare* is more resistant to chemical disinfectants and longer immersions times may be required to destroy it on scopes used on patients with known or suspected infection (British Thoracic Society 2001, Medicines and Healthcare Products Regulatory Agency 2002).

Endoscopes must be thoroughly rinsed after decontamination to ensure that all traces of the disinfectant are removed before reuse. Sterile or filtered water should be used to rinse the channels as tap water may contain mycobacteria which can contaminate the scope and cause misleading laboratory results from specimens. The water used for rinsing must be checked regularly to ensure it is not contaminated with bacteria (NHS Estates 1997, Working Party Report 2002). The AER must be properly cleaned and disinfected at the start of a day's list and tanks and pipelines should be drained when the machine is not in use to minimize the risk of microbial contamination in the water storage tank.

The greatest risk of infection from contaminated rinse water is with endoscopes used for ERCP and bronchoscopy. A number of such outbreaks of infection have been reported and have included some fatalities (Cooke 2004). The endoscope should be flushed with isopropyl alcohol prior to these procedures to ensure that the internal surfaces are thoroughly dried. Routine use of an alcohol flush at the end of the day is also advisable to ensure the endoscope is dry and prevent bacteria multiplying inside overnight.

The Health Technical Memorandum 2030 (NHS Estates 1997) provides guidance on appropriate AERs, including safety features such as vapour extraction and quality of water supply and the requirements for commissioning and performance testing.

Staff responsible for decontaminating endoscopes should wear appropriate protective clothing and must be trained to undertake the process. They are likely to be exposed to disinfectant vapours and irritant chemicals and should therefore receive regular health surveillance.

Prions

These proteins, which cause Creutzfeldt–Jakob disease (CJD), variant CJD (vCJD), bovine spongiform encephalopathy and scrapie, are particularly resistant to conventional methods of decontamination. They cannot be inactivated by most chemicals, including glutaraldehyde and formaldehyde, and are not reliably removed by autoclaving. Autoclaving at 134–137°C for six 18 min cycles and immersion in sodium hydroxide (2 M solution for 1 h) can destroy the infective material but these methods are only partially effective (Taylor 2003). Prions are destroyed by hypochlorite at 20 000 ppm for 1 h.

The main risk of transmission is related to surgery involving tissue where the concentration of the prion proteins is greatest. Tissues with high infectivity are the brain, spinal cord and posterior eye. Tissues with medium infectivity are the anterior eye and cornea, olfactory epithelium and, for vCJD, lymphoid tissue (e.g. tonsil, spleen, thymus, appendix). All other tissues have a low risk of infectivity, including blood and blood products (Advisory Committee on Dangerous Pathogens 2003).

Instruments and protective clothing used for invasive procedures involving high- or medium-risk tissues, on patients with definite or probable CJD or vCJD, or who have been identified as at risk of CJD (e.g. history of familial or iatrogenic CJD) should be destroyed by incineration after use. No attempt should be made to sterilize reusable instruments and, where possible, single-use items should be used. Instruments used on patients with possible CJD or vCJD should be quarantined until a definite diagnosis is made (Table 13.5) (Advisory Committee on Dangerous Pathogens 2003).

Viruses

The fragile structure of most viruses results in their destruction at temperatures of 70°C or higher, for example in washing machines, dishwashers and bedpan washers. They are also readily destroyed by autoclaving. Enveloped viruses (e.g. HIV) are susceptible to most disinfectants but non-enveloped viruses are more resistant to chemicals (Sattar et al 1989, 2002). Hepatitis B and C viruses are susceptible to chlorine-based agents, peracetic acid, glutaraldehyde and 70% ethanol (Deva et al 1996). Hypochlorite, glutaraldehyde and peracetic acid are effective against all viruses; alcohol is effective against some viruses but less so for those without lipid envelopes (Hanson et al 1989). Phenolics and quaternary ammonium compounds (e.g. Dettol, Savlon) are also not a reliable method of destroying viruses and are not recommended for routine disinfection (Hoffman et al 2004).

Bacterial spores

Some Gram-positive bacteria are able to enclose their cells in highly resistant casings called spores (see p. 6). Spores are resistant to a wide range of physical processes and chemical agents. They can be reliably destroyed by steam sterilization (e.g. 134°C for 3 min) but not by boiling at 100°C or pasteurization at a lower temperature. Some chemical agents will destroy spores, e.g. chlorine-based agents, glutaraldehyde, peracetic acid, but they are less reliable than steam.

In the clinical environment, *Clostridium difficile* is the most problematic spore-former in terms of infection control. Disinfection of the environment with chlorine-based agents has been recommended to control outbreaks but these agents can be corrosive and their use is controversial (Dettenkofer et al 2004). Alcohol handrubs will not destroy spores and thorough washing with soap and water is required to minimize the risk of cross-infection with *C. difficile*.

Table 13.5 Recommendations for handling instruments potentially contaminated with CJD or vCJD (Advisory Committee on Dangerous Pathogens 2003)

Likelihood patient has CJD or vCJD	Surgery involving high- or medium–risk tissue	Surgery involving low–risk tissue
Symptomatic patient with definite or probable diagnosis of CJD/vCJD*	Use single-use where possible Destroy instruments that are not single-use	No special reprocessing of instruments required
Symptomatic patient with possible CJD*	Quarantine instruments until definite diagnosis made (then destroy or reprocess accordingly)	No special reprocessing of instruments required
Asymptomatic patient with familial# or iatrogenic+ CJD/vCJD, or who has been identified by CJD incidents panel as at risk of vCJD	Use single-use where possible Destroy instruments that are not single-use	No special reprocessing of instruments required
Asymptomatic patient not in risk category	No special reprocessing of instruments required	No special reprocessing of instruments required

*Patient fulfils diagnostic criteria for CJD or vCJD.
Two or more blood relatives affected by prion disease; known to have (or blood relative known to have) a genetic mutation indicative of familial CJD.
+ Recipients of hormone derived from human pituitary glands (e.g. human growth hormone, gonadotrophin); recipients of a dura mater graft (e.g. if had an operation for a tumour or cyst of spine before August 1992).

References

Advisory Committee on Dangerous Pathogens, Spongiform Encephalopathy Advisory Committee (2003) *Transmissible Spongiform Encephalopathy Agents, Safe Working and the Prevention of Infection.* Department of Health, London.

Anderton A, Nwoguh CE (1991) Re-use of enteral feeding tubes – a potential hazard to the patient? A study of the efficacy of a representative range of cleaning and disinfection procedures. *J. Hosp. Infect.,* **18**: 131–8.

Ayliffe GAJ, Collins BJ, Lowbury EJ (1967) Ward floors and other surfaces as reservoirs of hospital infection. *J. Hyg. (Lond.),* **2**: 181.

Ayliffe GAJ, Babb JR, Collins BJ et al (1974) *Pseudomonas aeruginosa* in hospital sinks. *Lancet,* **ii**: 578–81.

Ayliffe GAJ, for the Minimal Access Therapy Decontamination Working Group (2000) Decontamination of minimally invasive surgical endoscopes and accessories. *J. Hosp. Infect.,* **45**: 263–77.

Babb J, Lowe S (2003) Cleaning, disinfection and sterilisation. In: Lawrence J, May D (eds) *Infection Control in the Community.* Churchill Livingstone, Edinburgh.

Ballemans CAJM, Blok HEM, Swennenhuis J et al (2003) Dry cleaning or wet mopping: a comparison of bacterial colony counts in the hospital environment. *J. Hosp. Infect.,* **53**: 150–8.

British Society of Gastroenterology (2003) *Guidelines for Decontamination of Equipment for Gastrointestinal Endoscopy.* British Society of Gastroenterology, London.

British Standards Institution (1994) *Bench Top Autoclaves. Specialist Technicians.* BS EN 554. British Standards Institution, London.

British Thoracic Society Bronchoscopy Guidelines Committee (2001) British Thoracic Society Guidelines on diagnostic flexible bronchoscopy. *Thorax,* **56** (suppl. 1): 1–21.

Bronowicki J-P, Venard V, Botté C et al (1997) Patient-to-patient transmission of hepatitis C virus during colonoscopy. *N. Engl. J. Med.,* **337**: 237–40.

Cefai C, Richards J, Gould FK et al (1990) An outbreak of *Acinetobacter* respiratory tract infection resulting from incomplete disinfection of ventilatory equipment. *J. Hosp. Infect.,* **15**: 177–82.

Chadwick PR, Beards G, Brown D et al (2000) Management of hospital outbreaks of gastro-enteritis due to small round structured viruses. *J. Hosp. Infect.,* **45**: 1–10.

Collins BJ (1988) The hospital environment: how clean should a hospital be? *J. Hosp. Infect.,* **11** (suppl. A): 53–6.

Cooke RPD (2004) Hazards of water. *J. Hosp. Infect.,* **57**: 290–3.

Cooper T, Tait J, Bingham P (2003) Decontamination in primary care: development and implementation of a quality improvement programme using audit. *Br. J. Infect. Contr.,* **4**(6): 15–19.

Danforth D, Nicolle LE, Hume K et al (1987) Nosocomial infection on nursing units with floors cleaned with a disinfectant compared with detergent. *J. Hosp. Infect.,* **10**: 229–35.

Department of Health (1990) *Spills of Urine: Potential Misuse of Chlorine-releasing Disinfecting Agents.* SAB59(90) 41. Medical Devices Agency, Department of Health, London.

Department of Health (1991) *Hospital Mattress Assemblies: Care and Cleaning.* Safety Action Bulletin SAB(91)65. Department of Health, Wetherby, UK.

Department of Health (1999) *Variant Creutzfeldt–Jakob Disease – Minimising the Risk of Transmission.* HSC1999/178. Department of Health, London.

Department of Health (2004) *Revised Guidance on Contracting for Cleaning.* NHS Estates. Department of Health, Wetherby, UK.

Department of Health (2004) *A Matron's Charter: An Action Plan for Cleaner Hospitals.* Department of Health, Wetherby, UK.

Dettenkofer M, Hauer T, Daschner FD (2004) Detergent versus hypochlorite cleaning and *Clostridium difficile* infection. *J. Hosp. Infect.,* **56**(1): 78–9.

Deva AK, Vickery K, Zou L et al (1996) Establishment of an in-use method for evaluating disinfection of surgical instruments using the duck hepatitis B model. *J. Hosp. Infect.,* **33**: 119–30.

Dowsett EG, Wilson PA (1981) An outbreak of *Streptococcus pyogenes* infection in a maternity unit. *CDR,* **81**(17): 3.

Earnshaw JJ, Clark AW, Thom BT (1985) Outbreak of *Pseudomonas aeruginosa* following endoscopic retrograde cholangiopancreatography. *J. Hosp. Infect.,* **6**: 95–7.

Finn L, Crook S (1998) Minor surgery in general practice – setting standards. *J. Public Health Med.,* **20**(2): 169–74.

Gray JW, George RH (2000) Experience of vancomycin-resistant enterococci in a children's hospital. *J. Hosp. Infect.,* **45**: 11–18.

Greaves A (1985) We'll just freshen you up, dear. *Nursing Times,* **March 6** (suppl.): 3–8.

Hanson PJV, Gor D, Jeffries DJ et al (1989) Chemical inactivation of HIV on surfaces. *BMJ,* **298**: 862–4.

Haythorne A (1998) Alert to alternatives. *Nursing Times,* **94**(37): 76.

Health and Safety Executive (2001) *Occupational Exposure Limits,* EH 40/02. HSE Books, London. Available online at: www.hsebooks.co.uk.

Health and Safety Executive (2002) *Control of Substances Hazardous to Health Regulations. Approved Code of Practice and Guidance,* 4th edn. HSE Books, London. Available online at: www.hsebooks.co.uk.

Hoffman P, Bradley C, Ayliffe G (2004) *Disinfection in Healthcare,* 3rd edn. Blackwell Publishing, Oxford.

Hollyoak V, Boyd P, Freeman R (1995) Whirlpool baths in nursing homes: use, maintenance and contamination with *Pseudomonas aeruginosa. CDR Rev.,* **5**(7): R102–4.

Joynson DHM (1978) Bowls and bacteria. *J. Hyg.,* **80**: 423–4.

Kingsley A, Hutter S, Green N et al (1999) Waterbirths: regional audit of infection control practices. *J. Hosp. Infect.,* **41**: 155–7.

Kolmos HJ, Thuesen B, Nielsen SV et al (1993) Outbreak of infection in a burns unit due to *Pseudomonas aeruginosa* originating from contaminated tubing used for irrigation of patients. *J. Hosp. Infect.,* **24**: 11–22.

Lack L, Wraight J (2002) Developing the new role of clinical housekeeper in a surgical ward. *Prof. Nurse*, **18**(4): 197–200.

Langenberg W, Rauws EAJ, Oudbier JH et al (1990) Patient-to-patient transmission of *Campylobacter pylori* infection by fibreoptic gastroduodenoscopy and biopsy. *J. Infect. Dis.*, **161**: 507–11.

Lawrence J, May D (eds) (2003) *Infection Control in the Community*. Churchill Livingstone, Edinburgh.

Levin MH, Olsen B, Nathan C et al (1984) Pseudomonas in the sinks of an intensive care unit: relation to patients. *J. Clin. Pathol.*, **37**: 424–7.

Loomes S (1988) Is it safe to lie down in hospital? *Nursing Times*, **84**(49): 63–5.

Marshall C, Wessellingh S, McDonald M, Spelman D (2004) Control of endemic MRSA – what is the evidence? A personal view. *J. Hosp. Infect.*, **56**: 253–68.

Medical Devices Agency (1997) *Purchase, Operation and Maintenance of Bench-top Steam Sterilisers*. Device Bulletin DB 6905. Department of Health, Wetherby, UK.

Medical Devices Agency (1998) *Validation and Periodic Testing of Bench-top Vacuum Steam Sterilisers*. Device Bulletin DB 9804. Department of Health, Wetherby, UK.

Medical Devices Agency (2000a) *Guidance on the Purchase, Operation and Maintenance of Vacuum Benchtop Steam Sterilisers*. Device Bulletin DB 2000(05). Department of Health, Wetherby, UK.

Medical Devices Agency (2000b) *Single Use Medical Devices: Implications and Consequences of Re-use*. Device Bulletin DB 2000 (04). Department of Health, Wetherby, UK.

Medical Devices Agency (2002a) *Steam Penetration Tests in Vacuum Benchtop Sterilisers*. Safety Notice SN 2002 (24). Department of Health, Wetherby, UK.

Medical Devices Agency (2002b) *Dry Heat (Hot Air) Sterilisers*. Safety Notice SN 2002 (02). Department of Health, Wetherby, UK.

Medicines and Healthcare Products Regulatory Agency (2002) *Decontamination of Endoscopes*. Device Bulletin DB 2002(05). Medicines and Healthcare Products Regulatory Agency, London.

Medicines and Healthcare Products Regulatory Agency (2003) *Management of Medical Devices Prior to Repair, Service or Investigation*. Device Bulletin DB 2003(05). Medicines and Healthcare Products Regulatory Agency, London.

Murdoch S (1990) Hazards in hoists. *Nursing Times*, **86**(49): 68–70.

Neely AN, Maley MP (2000) Survival of enterococci and staphylococci on hospital fabrics and plastics. *J. Clin. Microbiol.*, **38**(2): 724–6.

Neidner R, Schöpf R (1986) Inhibition of wound healing by antiseptics. *Br. J. Dermatol.*, **115**(S31): 41–4.

Newsom SWB (1972) Microbiology of hospital toilets. *Lancet*, **ii**: 700–3.

NHS Estates (1994) *Sterilisation*. Health Technical Memorandum 2010. Department of Health, Wetherby, UK.

NHS Estates (1997) *Washer-disinfectors*. Health Technical Memorandum 2030. Department of Health, Wetherby, UK.

NHS Executive (1995) *Hospital Laundry Arrangements for Used and Infected Linen*. HSG(95)18. Department of Health, Wetherby, UK.

NHS Management Executive (1993) *Decontamination of Equipment Prior to Inspection, Service or Repair*. HSG(93)26. HMSO, London.

Noble MA, Issac-Renton JL, Boyce DL et al (1998) The toilet as a transmission vector of vancomycin-resistant enterococci. *J. Hosp. Infect.*, **40**: 237–41.

Noone P, Griffiths RJ (1971) The effect on sepsis rates of closing and cleaning hospital wards. *J. Clin. Pathol.*, **24**: 721–5.

Oie S, Kamiya A (1996) Microbial contamination of antiseptics and disinfectants. *Am. J. Infect. Contr.*, **24**: 389–95.

Orsi GB, Mansi A, Tomao P et al (1994) Lack of association between clinical and environmental isolates of *Pseudomonas aeruginosa* in hospital wards. *J. Hosp. Infect.*, **27**: 49–60.

Rampling A, Wiseman S, Davis L et al (2001) Evidence that hospital hygiene is important in the control of methicillin-resistant *Staphylococcus aureus*. *J. Hosp. Infect.*, **49**: 109–16

Ruden H, Daschner F (2002) Should we routinely disinfect floors? *J. Hosp. Infect.*, **51**: 309–11.

Russell AD (2004) Bacterial adaptation and resistance to antiseptics, disinfectants and preservatives is not a new phenomenon. *J. Hosp. Infect.*, **57**: 97–104.

Rutal WA, Weber DJ (2001) Surface disinfection: should we do it? *J. Hosp. Infect.*, **48** (suppl.): S64–8.

Sattar SA, Springthorpe VS, Karim Y et al (1989) Chemical disinfection of non-porous inanimate surfaces experimentally contaminated with four human pathogenic viruses. *Epidemiol. Infect.*, **102**(3): 493–505.

Sattar SA, Springthorpe VS, Tetro J et al (2002) Hygienic hand antiseptics: should they not have activity and label claims against viruses? *Am. J. Infect. Contr.*, **30**: 355–72.

Scott E, Bloomfield SF (1990) The survival and transfer of microbial contamination via cloths, hands and utensils. *J. Appl. Bacteriol.*, **68**: 271–8.

Sherertz R, Sullivan M (1985) An outbreak of infections with *Acinetobacter calcoaceticus* in burn patients: contamination of patients' mattresses. *J. Infect. Dis.*, **151**: 252–8.

Skoutelis AT, Westenfelder GO, Beckerdite M et al (1993) Hospital carpeting and epidemiology of *Clostridium difficile*. *Am. J. Infect. Contr.*, **22**: 212–17.

Spach DH, Silverstein FE, Stamm WE (1993) Transmission of infection by gastrointestinal endoscopy and bronchoscopy. *Ann. Intern. Med.*, **118**: 117–28.

Taylor DM (2003) Transmissible degenerative encephalopathies: inactivation of the unconventional causal agents. In: Fraise AP, Lambert PA, Maillard J-Y (eds) *Principles and Practice of Disinfection, Preservation and Sterilisation*, 4th edn. Blackwell Science, Oxford.

Teare EL, Corless D, Peacock A (1998) *Clostridium difficile* in district general hospitals. *J. Hosp. Infect.*, **39**: 241–2.

Thompson G, Bullock D (1992) To clean or not to clean? *Nursing Times*, **88**(34): 66–8.

UK Health Departments (1994) *Dry Heat Sterilisers: Purchase, Maintenance and Use.* SAB (94)23. HMSO, London.

UK Health Departments (1998) *Guidance for Clinical Health Care Workers: Protection Against Infection with Blood-borne Viruses. Recommendations of the Expert Advisory Group on AIDS and the Advisory Group on Hepatitis.* Department of Health, Wetherby, UK.

Van den Berg RW, Claahsen HL, Niessen M et al (2000) *Enterobacter cloacae* outbreak in the NICU related to disinfected thermometers. *J. Hosp. Infect.*, **45**: 29–34.

Van Dessel H, Kamp-Hopmans TEM, Fruit AC et al (2002) Outbreak of a susceptible Acinetobacter species 13TU in an anaesthesiology intensive care unit. *J. Hosp. Infect.*, **52**: 89–95.

Werry C, Lawrence JM, Sanderson PJ (1988) Contamination of detergent cleaning solutions during hospital cleaning. *J. Hosp. Infect.*, **11**: 44–9.

Working Party Report (2002) Rinse water for heat labile endoscopy equipment. *J. Hosp. Infect.*, **51**: 7–16.

Yardy GW, Cox RA (2001) An outbreak of *Pseudomonas aeruginosa* infection associated with contaminated urodynamic equipment. *J. Hosp. Infect.*, **47**: 60–3.

Further Reading

Block SS (2001) *Disinfection, Sterilisation and Preservation*, 5th edn. Lippincott, Williams and Wilkins, Philadelphia.

Fraise AP, Lambert PA, Maillard J-Y (eds) (2003) *Principles and Practice of Disinfection, Preservation and Sterilisation*, 4th edn. Blackwell Science, Oxford.

Hoffman P, Bradley C, Ayliffe G (2004) *Disinfection in Healthcare*, 3rd edn. Blackwell Publishing, Oxford.

NHS Estates (2005) Infection A2Z decontamination website. Available online at: www.healthcareA2Z.org.

Chapter **14**

Management of the infectious patient

INTRODUCTION

Micro-organisms cause a wide variety of human infections, some of which are described in Chapter 6. For many of these pathogens, the simple precautions outlined in Chapter 7 are sufficient to prevent their spread from person to person. However, there are a few for which additional precautions are considered necessary to minimize the risk of transmission. Although such precautions are most relevant in hospitals where the frequency of contact with staff and the presence of other vulnerable patients may facilitate their spread, they may also be required in residential or nursing homes, where they should be adapted to local circumstances. In the past these precautions were referred to as 'barrier nursing' but are now more commonly known as isolation precautions.

The assessment of whether such measures are necessary is influenced by a number of factors including the ease with which the micro-organism is transmitted, the route of transmission, the epidemiological significance of the organism in the local setting and the extent to which other susceptible individuals may be exposed (Box 14.1). For example, isolation in a single room is recommended for a patient admitted to hospital with open tuberculosis because, although the risk of transmission is small, this infection is spread by an airborne route. However, the majority of infections encountered among hospital patients are spread by direct contact and the use of a single room therefore has no real part to play in preventing their transmission; rather, this depends on the application of standard precautions: using protective clothing for contact with body fluid and hand decontamination after contact with the patient (Lynch et al 1987).

Systems of isolation precautions have evolved in response to changes in healthcare provision and hospital pathogens. Most recently, the widespread adoption of routine precautions for contact with blood and body fluids has enabled many infections to be managed without additional isolation precautions. Some hospitals use the term 'source isolation' to indicate that the patient is the source of infection and to distinguish them from 'protective isolation', which may be required for patients at risk of infection (see Ch. 4).

Many isolation procedures in use today are based on tradition and there is a lack of empirical evidence regarding their efficacy in preventing the transmission of infectious diseases (Jackson & Lynch 1985, 1996). Examples of such practices include the use of separate cleaning equipment for isolation rooms and the use of masks. The persistent application of unnecessary

practice may relate to an underlying confusion about the processes involved in transmission and infection and is exacerbated by the difficulty of directly relating an outcome (infection) with a particular event (e.g. lack of handwashing). Since micro-organisms are invisible, misconceptions about them readily influence the way that healthcare workers both apply and do not apply infection control precautions (Jenner et al 1999, Prieto 2003). Knowledge of the principles of how different infections transmit from person to person (see Chs 6 and 7) is therefore essential to both understand and effectively implement rational isolation precautions.

HISTORICAL PERSPECTIVE

The fear of infectious disease was recorded long before microbes were identified as the cause of infection in the late 19th century. Isolation was an early remedy for infection and segregation of infected individuals has been practised for at least 4000 years. The oldest comprehensive isolation system is set out in the Bible, in the Book of Leviticus, and these principles applied throughout the Middle Ages, particularly for leprosy and plague (Selwyn 1991).

Isolation procedures were first introduced in hospitals in the early 20th century. To cope with the lack of single rooms or cubicles, two approaches were employed: barrier nursing and 'bed isolation'. Barrier nursing involved the use of special procedures to prevent the spread of micro-organisms, for example gloves and gowns as a barrier for patient contact. Bed isolation involved the segregation of the infected patient to one part of the ward. Frequently the bed was surrounded by a partition, wire screen or curtain soaked in disinfectant (Glenister 1991). The purpose of the screen was to keep the patient away from other patients and to remind the staff to take barrier precautions. Many workers, including Florence Nightingale in her concept of 'fever nursing' for the care of patients with infection, realized that infection was rarely transmitted by the air or from the environment but that contact with body fluids was usually responsible and transmission could be prevented by the use of barrier precautions. This was an early recognition of the importance of basing isolation precautions on the epidemiology of the infecting micro-organism; that is, how it spreads from person to person.

In the early 20th century patients with infectious diseases were commonly segregated in 'fever hospitals'. As the century progressed, improvements in public health and the introduction of antimicrobial agents had a marked effect on the incidence of infectious disease. Most patients could be treated in the community or as outpatients and the demand for fever hospitals declined. By the 1960s most fever hospitals had closed and patients with infectious diseases were admitted to general hospitals instead.

Categories of isolation

In the 1950s categories of isolation precautions were developed; these aimed to simplify the application of precautions in these general hospital settings (Bagshawe et al 1978). Infections were allocated to a particular category according to their principal route of transmission and a specific set of precautions was defined for each category. Commonly used categories were: strict isolation for highly infectious disease such as viral haemorrhagic fevers; respiratory isolation for tuberculosis and viral respiratory infections; wound and skin isolation for infected or colonized wounds; and enteric isolation for gastrointestinal pathogens such as salmonella (Control of Infection Group 1974, Garner & Simmons 1983).

The advantage of this type of system was that staff needed to learn only a few procedures and were less likely to make mistakes. The disadvantage was that it could not be tailored to particular patients or types of infection. As not all infections allocated to a category would be spread in exactly the same way, more precautions would often be applied than necessary.

Disease–specific isolation precautions

Categories of isolation were particularly difficult to apply to multidrug-resistant micro-organisms that could be spread by a variety of routes, depending on the micro-organism and the site of infection. As the problems with these organisms increased in the 1980s, the need for isolation precautions tailored to individual infections incorporating an element of local decision making was recognized and disease-specific isolation precautions were introduced (Garner & Simmons 1983). In this system, only the precautions needed to prevent transmission of a particular infection were used. For example, hepatitis A is a gastrointestinal infection that spreads by contact with faeces. The precautions necessary to prevent the spread of infection would be the use of protective clothing for direct contact with faeces and handwashing after contact with the patient.

This system had the advantage of eliminating unnecessary practices and could be adapted for individual patients. However, as staff were expected to make more decisions about what precautions were necessary, mistakes were likely to occur. In addition, the procedures were diagnosis driven; that is, they would be implemented only when a particular infection or disease was diagnosed. Frequently a patient may have

been infectious for several days before the clinical illness had become apparent or the micro-organisms detected. For example, a patient may carry methicillin-resistant *Staphylococcus aureus* (MRSA) for many days before a swab result indicates its presence.

Integrating routine and isolation precautions

By the end of the 1980s the routine use of precautions to minimize the transmission of bloodborne viruses in all healthcare settings, originally referred to as 'universal precautions', was advocated. These precautions were first recommended by the Centers for Disease Control in Atlanta, USA, in 1985 in response to growing concerns about the risk to healthcare workers from human immunodeficiency virus (HIV) (Centers for Disease Control 1987). Until then, special precautions had been taken only with body fluids from patients known or suspected to be infected with bloodborne viruses. HIV had highlighted the difficulty of identifying people who were incubating a disease and who were infectious but who had no outward signs of the infection. Universal precautions recognized that there were a few simple practices that could be used in the care of all patients that would minimize the risk of bloodborne viruses being transmitted to healthcare workers, for example the safe management of sharps and the use of protective clothing in situations where blood or body fluid was likely (see Ch. 7).

The change in emphasis towards regarding blood and body fluids from all patients as a potential major source of infection had important implications for isolation precautions. As body fluids are involved in the transmission of a wide range of pathogens, universal precautions could be used in routine care to prevent their transmission (Lynch et al 1987, 1990, Wilson & Breedon 1990). The routine precautions could adequately contain many infectious diseases without the need for isolation. For example, if gloves were worn routinely for contact with excreta, patients with infections spread through contact with excreta would not require additional isolation precautions.

However, if universal precautions were to be effective in preventing cross-infection between patients, as well as protecting staff from bloodborne viruses, it was important to ensure that protective clothing was both used and changed appropriately. By changing protective clothing after each procedure, micro-organisms acquired on gloves used for contact with body fluid would not be introduced to a susceptible site on the same or another patient.

In 1987, Lynch et al introduced a new system called 'body substance isolation' which recommended the use of universal precautions with all moist body substances as a means of preventing the transmission of hospital pathogens. Healthcare workers were required to use clean gloves for contact with moist body substances, mucous membranes and non-intact skin and to change them after each procedure. By ensuring that basic precautions were taken to prevent transmission from patients who are unknowingly incubating infection or colonized with pathogens, isolation procedures for patients known to have infectious disease could be simplified and focused on a smaller number of pathogens. Additional precautions (e.g. the use of masks) were recommended only for a few infections transmitted by airborne respiratory droplets (e.g. varicella, tuberculosis) (Jackson & Lynch 1985). This approach also helped to address the problem of preventing transmission of micro-organisms before a diagnosis being made.

Although the integration of routine and isolation precautions has caused some controversy, particularly in relation to the cost of protective clothing and the effect of lapses in routine use of precautions, it has now been incorporated into the latest advice on isolation precautions (Garner 1996, Garner & Hierholzer 1993). This adopts a simplified approach to isolation, recommending the routine use of standard precautions and three categories of additional isolation precautions (Box 14.3). Isolation is recommended for infections, such as MRSA, which can be transmitted through direct contact with patients or their environment (contact precautions); infections spread by respiratory secretions, such as meningococcal meningitis (respiratory droplet precautions); and infections such as tuberculosis that are transmitted via inhaled droplet nuclei (airborne precautions) (see Box 14.3).

Special isolation precautions are not necessary for bloodborne viruses or enteric infection where the risk of environmental contamination or person-to-person spread is low.

THE PRINCIPLES OF ISOLATION PRECAUTIONS

The objective of isolation is to minimize the risk of micro-organisms from the affected person being transferred to others. It is important to recognize that it is the micro-organisms rather than the person that require isolation and precautions should be specifically directed at the route of transmission of the micro-organisms concerned. Care should be planned for individual patients, avoiding the use of unnecessary precautions and taking the patient's needs into account (Box 14.2).

The advice contained in the following section is intended to provide some general principles of

---

Box 14.2   An example of isolation precautions

Mrs Jones has been admitted with gastroenteritis caused by salmonella. She has frequent diarrhoea and is receiving intravenous fluids but is mostly able to care for herself. To prevent the transmission of salmonella to other patients on the ward, gloves and a plastic apron should be worn by staff who have direct contact with faeces, commodes or bedpans. These should be removed and hands washed afterwards. For any other care, such as adjusting Mrs Jones' intravenous therapy or assisting her with daily hygiene, gloves and apron are not necessary. Staff should always wash their hands before leaving the room, although an alcohol handrub can be used if the hands are not soiled. Mrs Jones' visitors need not wear protective clothing but should be asked to wash their hands before leaving.

---

isolation precautions, when they may be required and the rationale behind their use. If standard infection control precautions are used routinely for contact with blood and body fluid from all patients (see Box 7.2), additional precautions will be necessary only for a limited number of infections (see Box 14.3). A guide to routes of transmission and recommended precautions for infections commonly encountered in hospitals in the UK is shown in Table 14.1.

The precautions should be used for patients who are either known or suspected to have an infectious disease or when a patient presents with significant signs or symptoms, such as vomiting or diarrhoea, skin rash or pyrexia of unknown origin.

Local policies should be consulted before placing a patient in isolation. The application of precautions may vary according to the type of ward or unit and the presence of other patients at particular risk of infection. The infection control team will be able to advise on appropriate precautions and identify unnecessary practices. A simple set of isolation procedures suitable for minimizing the risk of transmission of micro-organisms spread by direct contact or exposure to respiratory droplets is illustrated in Table 14.2.

Single-room accommodation

Physical separation from other patients is indicated where an infection is transmitted by airborne particles. This is particularly important for micro-organisms carried on droplet nuclei (e.g. measles, chickenpox, pulmonary tuberculosis). Droplet nuclei are minute particles expelled from the respiratory tract that may remain airborne for long periods, travel long distances

---

Box 14.3   Categories of isolation precautions and indications for their use

Standard infection control precautions should be used routinely for contact with blood and body fluid from all patients. Additional precautions are recommended for infections or micro-organisms transmitted by the following routes.

1. Airborne
Infections transmitted by the inhalation of micro-organisms on droplet nuclei. These minute particles are expelled from the respiratory tract and may remain suspended in air for a long time.
Examples: tuberculosis, varicella, measles.
Isolation precautions: single room (preferably with air-handling system); limit patient movement; masks recommended for some procedures; use gloves and plastic aprons for handling respiratory secretions; wash hands on leaving the room.

2. Respiratory droplets
Infections transmitted by contact with respiratory secretions, including particles produced during coughing and sneezing. These particles do not travel far or remain airborne. Many of these infections are also spread by direct contact with infective material.
Examples: meningococcal meningitis, mumps, pertussis, diphtheria, some respiratory viruses.
Isolation precautions: single room; limit patient movement; use gloves and plastic aprons for contact with infective material; wash hands on leaving the room.

3. Contact with patients or their environment
Infections transmitted by direct contact with patients (e.g. by touching their skin, lesions or nasal secretions). Some micro-organisms may also be able to survive in the immediate environment and be transferred by contact with surfaces or equipment.
Examples:
- enteric infection where prolonged survival in the environment may contribute to the transmission of infection (e.g. *Clostridium difficile*, enteroviruses)
- some respiratory viral infections such as respiratory syncytial virus, influenza
- skin infections such as impetigo, group A streptococcus
- antibiotic-resistant micro-organisms infecting or colonizing skin or other body sites (e.g. MRSA, vancomycin-resistant enterococcus).
Isolation precautions: single room preferable; limit patient movement; use gloves and plastic aprons for contact with infective material from patients or their immediate environment; wash hands on leaving the room.

(Adapted from Garner 1996)

---

in air currents and, if inhaled, may penetrate deep into the lung (see p. 40). As a minimum, patients with these infections must be placed in a well-ventilated single room with the door kept closed. Ideally, negative pressure ventilated isolation rooms should be used to ensure that droplet nuclei are diluted by extracting room air outside the building (Fig. 14.1).

Negative pressure isolation facilities are required for the management of patients with tuberculosis being cared for in areas where immunocompromised patients are present as they are particularly vulnerable to acquiring the infection, even after brief exposure (Breathnach et al 1998). Procedures that induce the patient to cough (e.g. bronchoscopy, sputum collection, administration of nebulized medication) should always take place in a room with adequate exhaust ventilation.

Since patients with HIV are more vulnerable to acquiring tuberculosis, Hannan et al (2000) also recommend the use of isolation facilities in outpatient departments for these patients, together with a comprehensive patient management system that aims to ensure that both patients known to have tuberculosis and new patients with signs and symptoms of the disease are effectively segregated in the outpatient setting. The recommended minimum infection control precautions required for patients with pulmonary tuberculosis are summarized in Table 14.3 (Inter-departmental Working Group on Tuberculosis 1998).

Some infections are transmitted by larger respiratory droplets (e.g. pertussis, meningococcal meningitis). Unlike droplet nuclei, these will not travel a great distance or remain airborne for prolonged periods; however, a single room is recommended to

Table 14.1   Routes of transmission and isolation precautions for common infections

This table provides a guide to the routes of transmission for infections that may be encountered in hospital patients and whether isolation precautions are indicated. *Routine infection control precautions should be used in the care of all patients.*
    ICT, infection control team; IDU, infectious diseases unit

Infection or disease	Route of transmission	Period of infectivity to others	Isolation precautions	Comments
AIDS: *see* Human immunodeficiency virus				
Amoebic dysentery: *Entamoeba histolytica*	Ingestion of faecally contaminated food or water	While cysts being excreted (may be years)	No	
Bronchiolitis (infants)	Respiratory droplets and direct contact with secretions	While symptomatic (5 days or longer)	Yes	Commonly caused by respiratory viruses (e.g. respiratory syncytial virus, parainfluenza)
Campylobacter	Usually foodborne, also contact with contaminated animals or meat. Person-to-person transmission unlikely	Excreted in faeces for several weeks	No	
Candidiasis	Contact with lesions and secretions	Duration of illness	No	Can be spread by hands or equipment
Cellulitis (e.g. group A streptococci)	Direct contact with lesion	Until culture negative or after completion of course of antibiotics	Yes	Organism may be difficult to eradicate from chronic wounds
Chickenpox: *Varicella zoster virus*	Inhalation or direct contact with vesicle fluid or respiratory secretions	1–2 days before rash and 5 days after lesions first appear (longer in immunosuppressed)	Yes (single room essential)	Staff attending patient must be immune
Chlamydia trachomatis		May be carried on mucous membranes for months		
Conjunctivitis	Sexual contact, contact with discharge from eye		No	
Genital	Sexual contact		No	
Respiratory	Infected mother to baby during birth		No	
Chlamydia pneumoniae	Not defined but probably airborne respiratory droplets and direct contact with secretions	Unknown, but prolonged outbreaks have been reported	No	Spread may occur among families, institutions e.g. military barracks
Chlamydia psittaci	*See psittacosis*			
Cholera	Ingestion of faecally contaminated food or water	During illness (although persistent, asymptomatic carriage may occur)	Yes	Case-to-case transmission can occur so routine precautions with excreta is essential
Clostridium perfringens Food poisoning	Contaminated food (usually inadequately heated meat)	Not transmitted from person to person	No	Heavy bacterial contamination of food required for transmission to occur

Table 14.1   Routes of transmission and isolation precautions for common infections (*cont'd*)

Infection or disease	Route of transmission	Period of infectivity to others	Isolation precautions	Comments
Gas gangrene	Traumatic wounds contaminated by soil; endogenous infection of surgical wounds	Not transmitted from person to person	No	Gangrene only develops in poorly perfused, necrotic wounds required for gangrene to develop
Clostridium difficile (pseudomembranous colitis)	Direct or indirect contact with faeces	Duration of diarrhoea	Yes (if symptomatic)	Disease only caused by toxigenic strains. Spores may survive in the environment for prolonged periods
Creutzfeldt–Jakob disease (CJD)	Unknown. Can be transmitted by grafts of human brain tissue, instruments, corneas or growth hormone derived from pituitary glands	Duration of illness	No	Variant CJD probably acquired through ingestion of meat contaminated with bovine spongiform encephalopathy agent
Crytococcosis: *Cryptococcus neoformans*	Found in pigeon faeces and soil	Not transmitted from person to person	No	Usually affects immunocompromised, causing chronic meningitis
Cytomegalovirus (CMV)	Intimate contact with mucous membranes. Fetus may be infected in utero, during delivery or by breast milk	Virus excreted in urine and saliva for months. May persist episodically for years	No	Severe disease more likely in immunosuppressed
Diphtheria: *Corynebacterium diphtheriae* (toxigenic strains)	Direct contact with oral or nasal secretions of infected person	Until throat swabs negative (usually 2 weeks)	Yes	Immunization in infancy protects against systemic disease; local nasopharyngeal infection may occur
Escherichia coli gastroenteritis				
Enterohaemorrhagic (O157, verotoxin)	Usually food or waterborne, may be transmitted by contact with animals and from person to person	Excreted in faeces for 1 week (longer in children)	Assess risk of transmission for individual patients	Associated with haemolytic–uraemic syndrome, usually in under 5 years
Enterotoxigenic	Foodborne (developing countries)	Prolonged excretion in faeces	No	Major cause of traveller's diarrhoea
Enteropathogenic	Foodborne (baby milk and weaning foods). Transmission via hands, especially in nurseries	Prolonged excretion in faeces	No	Causes severe prolonged diarrhoea in infants, especially in developing countries
Ebola virus: *see* Viral haemorrhagic fever				
Erysipelas: *see* Streptococci				
Giardiasis: *Giardia intestinalis*	Ingestion of contaminated drinking water; contact with faeces	Duration of infection (may be months)	Assess risk of transmission for individual patients	Often acquired abroad. Can be transmitted from person to person, especially among children

(cont'd)

Table 14.1 Routes of transmission and isolation precautions for common infections (*cont'd*)

Infection or disease	Route of transmission	Period of infectivity to others	Isolation precautions	Comments
Glandular fever (infectious mononucleosis): Epstein–Barr virus	Contact with saliva	Oropharyngeal carriage may persist for months or years	No	Infection may be transmitted on hands if contaminated with saliva
Gonorrhoea: *Neisseria gonorrhoeae*				
Genital infection	Sexual contact with infected mucous membranes of genital tract	Until organism eradicated by appropriate therapy	No	
Ophthalmia neonatorum	Infection acquired from infected birth canal during delivery	While discharge persists	Yes	Can be spread by contact with conjunctival discharge
Hepatitis A	Person-to-person spread by faecal–oral contact; food contaminated by infected handler; contaminated water	Maximum infectivity immediately before and for a few days after onset of jaundice	Assess risk of transmission for individual patients	Hepatitis A vaccine or immunoglobulin may be used to protect family contacts from infection
Hepatitis B	Sexually transmitted; blood inoculation through skin or on to mucous membranes; acquired transplacentally or intrapartum from infected mother	May persist indefinitely as carrier state	No (unless uncontrolled bleeding)	Main risk to healthcare workers is from contaminated sharps. All healthcare workers should be protected by vaccination; specific immunoglobulin available
Hepatitis C	Blood inoculation through skin Sexual transmission possible but less common	May persist indefinitely	No	
Hepatitis E	Faecal–oral route, mostly via contaminated water; person-to-person spread possible but uncommon	Virus persists in stools for at least 2 weeks after onset of jaundice	No	
Herpes simplex				
Cold sores, herpetic whitlow	Direct contact with lesion, exudate or saliva	Virus may be shed into saliva for several weeks after symptoms resolve	No	Staff may develop herpetic whitlow through contact with active cold sores. Staff with active lesions should avoid contact with immunosuppressed patients
Genital herpes	Sexually transmitted	Active lesions infectious for 7–12 days. Transient asymptomatic viral shedding common	No	
Neonatal herpes	Via infected birth canal; can be transmitted congenitally if mother acquires primary infection during pregnancy	Duration of illness	Yes	Separate infant from other neonates. Handle secretions from mother and baby using gloves and aprons

Table 14.1   Routes of transmission and isolation precautions for common infections (*cont'd*)

Infection or disease	Route of transmission	Period of infectivity to others	Isolation precautions	Comments
Herpes zoster virus: *see* Shingles				
Human immunodeficiency virus (HIV)	Sexually transmitted; inoculation of blood or body fluid through skin or on to mucous membranes; transmitted from mother to baby in utero during delivery, or in breast milk shortly after birth	Indefinitely	No	Main risk to healthcare workers is from contaminated sharps
Impetigo: *Staphylococcus aureus*, group A streptococcus	Direct contact with lesion	Duration of lesion (until culture negative or after completion of course of antibiotics)	Yes	Young children often highly susceptible
Influenza	Airborne respiratory droplets; contact with secretions	3–5 days from onset; longer in children	Yes	Vaccination of healthcare workers recommended when epidemics occur
Lassa fever: *see* Viral haemorrhagic fever				
Legionnaire's disease: *Legionella pneumophila*	Inhalation of contaminated aerosols. Not spread from person to person	Not transmitted from person to person	No	
Leptospirosis (Weil's disease)	Contact of abraded skin or mucous membranes with water, soil or vegetation contaminated by urine of animals	Not transmitted from person to person	No	Hazard to farmers, sewer workers, etc., watersports, bathers
Listeriosis: *Listeria monocytogenes*	Ingestion of contaminated food; from mother to baby in utero or during delivery	Shed in faeces for several months; shed in vaginal discharge for 7–10 days	Neonates	Outbreaks of infection in nurseries have been reported. Elderly, neonates and immunocompromised particularly susceptible
Lyme disease: *Borrelia burgdorferi*	Transmitted by tick bite	Not transmitted from person to person	No	
Malaria	Transmitted by mosquito bite; transfusion of blood from infected person	Not transmitted from person to person	No	Rare cases associated with blood transfusion
Marburg virus: *see* Viral haemorrhagic fever				
Measles	Airborne by respiratory droplets; direct contact with nose or throat secretions	From just before rash appears until 4 days after	Yes	Highly infectious. May cause severe illness in immunosuppressed children. Immunoglobulin available for susceptible people
Meningitis *Neisseria meningitidis* (meningococcal meningitis)	Direct contact with respiratory droplets, nasal or oral secretions	Until organism no longer present in nasal or oral secretions (after 24 h of antibiotics)	Yes	Most infections subclinical. Rifampicin antibiotic prophylaxis offered to close family contacts

(cont'd)

Table 14.1   Routes of transmission and isolation precautions for common infections (*cont'd*)

Infection or disease	Route of transmission	Period of infectivity to others	Isolation precautions	Comments
Haemophilus influenzae	Direct contact with respiratory droplets, nasal or oral secretions	Until organism no longer present in nasal or oral secretions (after 24–48 h of antibiotics)	Yes	Most common in children aged between 2 months and 5 years
Viral (e.g. enteroviruses, mumps)	Faecal–oral or respiratory spread (depends on agent)	Before and during acute illness	No	
MRSA: *see Staphylococcus aureus*				
Mumps	Transmitted by respiratory droplets and direct contact with saliva	7 days before symptoms appear and up to 9 days afterwards	Yes	Highly infectious. Previous infection confers lifelong immunity
Pneumonia (pneumococcal): *Streptococcus pneumoniae*	Respiratory droplets; direct contact with nasal or oral secretions	Until organisms no longer present in nasal or oral secretions (after 24–48 h of antibiotics)	No (unless antibiotic-resistant strain)	Susceptibility increased by underlying lung disease, immunosuppression, and very young/elderly
Poliomyelitis	Mainly by the faecal–oral route but transmission through direct contact with nasal or oral secretions also occurs	Most infectious for the few days before and after onset of symptoms. Virus persists in faeces for several weeks	Yes (IDU)	Live-attenuated vaccine strain of virus shed in faeces following immunization and may infect non-immune contacts
Psittacosis: *Chlamydia psittaci*	Inhalation of dust contaminated by bird droppings, secretions or feathers	Birds may shed organisms for weeks. Person-to-person spread unlikely	No	Parakeets and parrots are the main reservoir. Also reported in poultry, pigeons, seabirds
Rotavirus	Mainly by faecal–oral route but possibly also through contact with respiratory secretions	Virus shed in faeces for up to 8 days after onset of symptoms (longer in immunocompromised)	Yes	Outbreaks in elderly care and paediatric units reported
Respiratory syncytial virus (RSV)	By direct contact with respiratory secretions or droplets	While symptomatic	Yes	Highly transmissible on paediatric wards
Rubella	Direct contact with respiratory secretions or droplets. Also shed in urine of infants with congenital infection	7 days before and at least 4 days after onset of rash	Yes	Carers should be rubella-immune. In congenital rubella, babies excrete virus for months
Salmonella Enteric fever (*S. typhi* or *S. paratyphi*)	Usually foodborne but may be transmitted from person to person via hands	Excreted in faeces for several weeks (especially infants)	Assess risk of transmission for individual patients	Carriers may inadvertently infect food

Table 14.1   Routes of transmission and isolation precautions for common infections (cont'd)

Infection or disease	Route of transmission	Period of infectivity to others	Isolation precautions	Comments
Other species				
Scabies	Prolonged skin-to-skin contact	Until mite destroyed by treatment	No (unless Norwegian scabies)	Norwegian scabies occurs only in immunocompromised, but is highly contagious
Severe acute respiratory syndrome (SARS)	Probably mucous membrane contact with respiratory droplets or secretions; possibly contact with faeces	No reported transmission 10 days after fever resolved	Yes	Negative pressure isolation and use of respirator masks for cases
Scarlet fever: *see* Streptococci				
Shigella	Direct or indirect contact with faeces; can also be water- or foodborne	Infectious while organism present in faeces	Yes (until symptom-free and normal stool)	Highly infectious. Outbreaks in nurseries caused by transmission on hands
Shingles (herpes zoster)	Contact with lesion exudate	7 days after lesions first appear	Yes	Seronegative contacts develop chickenpox and should be excluded while patient is infectious
Staphylococcus aureus, methicillin-resistant infection (MRSA)	Direct contact with infected or colonized lesions or skin	While organism present in lesions, in nose or on skin	Yes (seek advice from ICT)	Epidemic strains may cause outbreaks. Build-up of organism in environment may contribute to spread
Streptococci (groups A, reported C and G)	Direct contact with lesions	Until culture negative (or after course of antibiotics completed)	Yes	Outbreaks of infection
Syphilis: *Treponema pallidum*	Direct contact with lesions during sexual contact; from infected mother to baby	During primary and secondary stages	No	Infectivity rapidly reduced by treatment. Wear gloves for contact with lesions
Tetanus: *Clostridium tetani*	Direct inoculation from contaminated source	Not transmitted from person to person	No	Booster immunization not required after five doses in childhood or as adult
Toxoplasmosis: *Toxoplasma gondii*	Ingestion of infective oocysts in dirt or tissue cysts in undercooked meat. Primary infection in early pregnancy may result in transplacental infection of fetus	Not transmitted from person to person	No	Most infections asymptomatic; immunity develops readily
Tuberculosis (pulmonary) *Mycobacterium tuberculosis*	Inhalation of airborne droplet nuclei	While viable bacilli in sputum	Yes (for first 14 days of antibiotics)	Prolonged exposure usually required to transmit infection. Infectivity reduced after 14 days of effective treatment Special precautions required for multidrug-resistant strains

(cont'd)

Table 14.1   Routes of transmission and isolation precautions for common infections (*cont'd*)

Infection or disease	Route of transmission	Period of infectivity to others	Isolation precautions	Comments
Viral haemorrhagic fever Lassa Ebola–Marburg Crimean–Congo (tickborne)	Person-to-person transmission by direct contact with blood, pharyngeal secretions or urine, and by sexual intercourse	Variable; depends on virus	Yes – transfer to regional IDU	Crimean–Congo fever is tickborne; Lassa fever transmitted by direct contact with rat urine. Reservoir of Ebola–Marburg unknown
Whooping cough: *Bordetella pertussis*	Direct contact with respiratory secretions and probably airborne droplets	Highly infectious in early stages; non-infectious 3 weeks after onset of paroxysms	Yes	Children under 5 years most susceptible

Adapted from Wilson J (2000) *Clinical Microbiology: A Guide for Healthcare Professionals*, 8th edn. Baillière Tindall, London.

Table 14.2   An isolation policy

Indication
Isolation is necessary when a patient has or is suspected to have a communicable infection.

Check the list of communicable infections (see Table 14.1) to find out whether isolation is necessary and what material from the patient is infectious.

Remember: *Standard precautions must be used with all patients including those in isolation.*

AIMS

To prevent the transmission of micro-organisms from an infected patient to others
To provide psychological support and reassurance to the patient while in isolation
To ensure that all staff are aware of the correct precautions to take and that unnecessary precautions are avoided

Equipment
Single room with a washbasin, preferably with shower and toilet
Remove excess equipment from the room before patient is isolated
Hand soap
Disposable gloves
Paper towels
Yellow waste bag
Plastic aprons
Alcohol handrub

Practice	Rationale
Patient: explain reason for isolation and provide reassurance	To reduce anxiety and gain patient's co-operation
Aprons: wear plastic apron for contact with body fluid and infectious material, discard **between procedures** and before leaving the room	To protect clothing from contamination and prevent cross-infection
Gloves: wear for contact with body fluids and infectious material. Discard **between procedures** and before leaving the room	To prevent contamination of hands and prevent cross-infection
Masks: not usually necessary	There is no evidence that they protect from respiratory infection

Table 14.2 An isolation policy (cont'd)

Practice	Rationale
Hands: always decontaminate hands when gloves are removed and before leaving the room	To prevent transfer of micro-organisms to other patients and between susceptible sites on the same patient
Faeces/urine/vomit: discard directly into bedpan washer/macerator	Prompt disposal essential to prevent transmission of micro-organisms
Linen: place in an alginate bag, then into a red nylon outer bag	To prevent dissemination of micro-organisms and protect laundry staff
Disposable items: discard used or soiled items into a yellow plastic bag	To ensure waste is incinerated
Equipment: clean/disinfect before removing from the room (see disinfection policy/contact ICN)	To prevent the spread of micro-organisms
Crockery: use normal utensils and return to main kitchens in usual way	Risk of cross-infection from crockery is minimal. Washing in hot water and detergent is sufficient
Visitors: instruct to decontaminate their hands before leaving the room. Children and susceptible visitors should be discouraged from visiting	For most infections the risk to visitors is minimal as they do not have contact with body fluids
Other departments: avoid visits to other departments. If necessary, the department should be notified in advance and the patient seen at the end of the list. Porters need not wear protective clothing but should be instructed to decontaminate their hands on completion of the journey	To keep contact with other patients to a minimum and enable the department to take appropriate precautions
Cleaning: inform domestic supervisor that the patient is being isolated. Use designated cleaning equipment for the room. Ask the domestic to wear gloves and apron to clean, discard them on leaving the room and decontaminate their hands	To maintain a clean environment and minimize risk of spread
In case of death: follow the usual last offices procedure. Body bags may be required for some infections	Body fluids leaking after death may present a risk to mortuary staff
Duration of isolation: refer to list of communicable infections or contact ICN	Isolation can be distressing for the patient and should not be continued for longer than necessary

Termination of isolation
See above for treatment of bedlinen, disposable items and equipment. It is not necessary to discard unused packets of disposable equipment.

Cleaning: all furniture and surfaces, including the mattress and bedframe, should be cleaned with detergent and water. Once cleaned, the room may be reused immediately.

Special points
Chickenpox, shingles (herpes zoster), measles
Patients with these infections must not be looked after by staff unable to give a definite history of the infection or appropriate vaccination.
Pulmonary tuberculosis (smear positive)
Visitors, apart from immediate family, should be discouraged for the first week of antituberculosis treatment.

minimize the risk of transmission to other patients likely to be in close proximity in an open ward.

Many of the infections encountered in healthcare settings are spread by contact rather than by an airborne route and hence the contribution that physical isolation of the patient makes to preventing the spread of infection is likely to be minimal. Placing the patient in a single room may help to prevent transmission by reducing the number of contacts between staff and patients or by increasing adherence to infection control precautions. These effects are frequently overlooked, with the result that the value of single rooms themselves as a measure to prevent transmission is overemphasized (Cooper et al 2003).

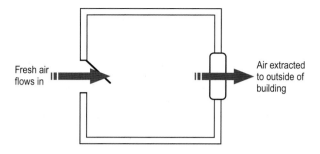

Fresh air flows in

Air extracted to outside of building

Figure 14.1 Negative pressure ventilation. Isolation rooms with negative pressure ventilation dilute the number of infectious airborne particles in the room and ensure that air flows from the room to the outside of the building, not to other patient areas. This is achieved by extracting air to create a lower pressure inside the room. Air from adjacent rooms will be drawn in through vents and around doors. The rate at which air is extracted must exceed the rate of supply. The continuous replacement of air within the room ensures that airborne infectious particles from the patient are diluted. Doors and windows must be kept shut to ensure that the pressure differential and direction of airflow are maintained. Newly commissioned negative pressure rooms should undergo thorough functional assessment to ensure the air flows are correct. Regular monitoring of the air pressure differentials is also essential since should the system fail, infectious airborne particles may flow into other patient areas. Staff should be trained in how to monitor systems and ideally an automatic indicating system should be located at ward level (Hannan et al 2000, Hoffman et al 2004).

Table 14.3 Summary of isolation precautions recommended for patients with *Mycobacterium tuberculosis*

Status of patient	Recommended infection control precautions	
	Patient in ward area with no immunocompromised patients	Patient in ward area with significantly immunocompromised patients
TB suspected	Isolate in single room	Isolate in single room with automatically monitored negative air pressure
	Encourage patient to cover mouth and nose when coughing	
TB confirmed and sputum smear positive	Isolate in single room	Isolate in single room with automatically monitored negative air pressure
	Encourage patient to cover mouth and nose when coughing	
	Respirator masks should be worn for aerosol-generating procedures, e.g. sputum induction	
	Discontinue isolation after 2 weeks of chemotherapy, provided there is clinical improvement, the patient can adhere to therapy and there are no multidrug-resistant mycobacterium in sputum	
TB confirmed or suspected but sputum smear negative	Isolation not necessary	Isolate in single room
Multidrug-resistant TB suspected or confirmed	Isolate in single room with negative air pressure	Isolate in single room with automatically monitored negative air pressure
	Encourage patient to cover mouth and nose when coughing	
	All persons entering the room should wear a high-efficiency filtration mask	
	Patient to wear a mask when being transported to other clinical areas	
	If multidrug-resistant TB is confirmed, isolation whilst in hospital should be continued until cultures are negative	

Source: Interdepartmental Working Party on Tuberculosis (1998).

Ayliffe et al (1971) studied the effect of single rooms on the acquisition of MRSA. They found the counts of airborne bacteria were higher in the open ward but no difference in the rate of nasal acquisition of the organism between patients managed in the open ward or in single rooms. Similarly, Preston et al (1981) found no change in colonization or infection rates when the structure of an intensive care unit was changed from an open unit to single rooms.

In some situations a private room is advisable because the patient's illness is particularly likely to result in contamination of the environment (e.g. profuse diarrhoea, vomiting or bleeding) or because the patient is unable to follow infection control measures, for instance young children or the psychologically disturbed. Some micro-organisms, notably *Clostridium difficile* and antibiotic-resistant bacteria such as glycopeptide-resistant enterococci, although mostly transmitted by direct contact, can also heavily contaminate and persist in the environment (National *Clostridium difficile* Standards Working Party 2004, Weber & Rutala 1997). Placing these patients in single rooms may therefore be required to limit the extent of environmental contamination and facilitate cleaning once the patient has been discharged or the isolation discontinued.

Notices at the entrance of the room or displayed by the patient's bed can indicate to visitors and staff, particularly those who may not work regularly on the ward, that special precautions are being observed (Fig. 14.2).

Usually patients with infections that are transmitted only by contact can be allowed to leave their rooms for treatment. This is particularly important for those who require physiotherapy or other forms of rehabilitation. Provided the infection is not transmitted by an airborne route, the door to the room can be kept open. This may help to minimize the psychological impact of isolation on the patient.

If more than one patient is infected or colonized with the same organism, they can be nursed together in the same ward or area rather than individual rooms. This is called cohorting and can be a useful approach for managing outbreaks of infection, as demonstrated in the study by Doherty et al (1998) on the management of respiratory syncytial virus amongst children. A few hospitals have specialist isolation facilities for the management of patients with infectious diseases. Regional infectious diseases units in London and Newcastle have high-level facilities with air-handling systems and bed isolators. Patients with viral haemorrhagic fevers must be transferred to these units (Advisory Committee on Dangerous Pathogens 1996).

In nursing or residential homes, the most commonly encountered infectious diseases are viral respiratory infections and gastroenteritis. These can often spread rapidly amongst the residents and the isolation of those affected either in a single room or by sharing with others who are affected may be necessary to prevent spread. The room should have a handwash basin to ensure that staff can easily wash their hands after contact in outbreaks of gastroenteritis. The designation of toilets for use by symptomatic residents may be a useful control measure (Public Health Medicine Environmental Group 1996, Whitlock & Lawrence 2003).

Protective clothing

Protective clothing should be used to minimize the risk of acquiring pathogens on hands or clothing and worn when contact with material likely to transmit the

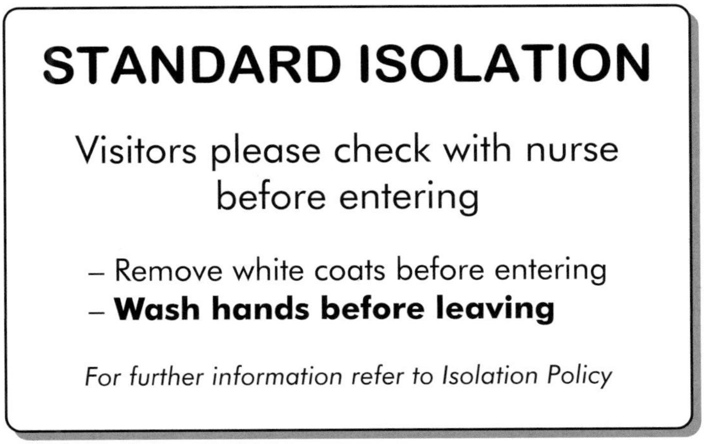

Figure 14.2   Example of an isolation notice.

STANDARD ISOLATION

Visitors please check with nurse before entering

— Remove white coats before entering
— **Wash hands before leaving**

For further information refer to Isolation Policy

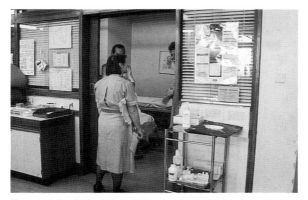

Figure 14.3 An isolation room.

infection is anticipated. It is not usually necessary to wear protective clothing every time the room is entered, as some activities are unlikely to result in contact with infective material, but it should be readily available both inside and outside the room (Fig. 14.3).

The infective material varies according to the type of infection (see Table 14.1). For example, if a patient has cellulitis the micro-organisms will be present on the affected area of skin. Gloves and plastic apron should be used for direct contact with the skin and for handling bedlinen. If a patient has shigella, the pathogen will be excreted in faeces. Gloves and apron should be worn for any direct contact with faeces or items contaminated with faeces. If protective clothing is worn routinely for contact with blood and body fluid, in many instances additional protective clothing will not be required for isolated patients because body fluids are the main source of infectious material.

The important principle is to ensure that protective clothing is discarded before contact with another patient. Usually this means removing protective clothing before leaving the room; however, it may sometimes be necessary to take equipment out of the room (e.g. to place a bedpan in the washer-disinfector). In this situation the gloves and apron should be removed once the procedure has been completed and hands washed.

In addition, it is important to recognize that, as with the care of any patient, protective clothing may also need to be changed during a particular episode of care to ensure that bacteria from an infected or colonized site on the patient are not transferred to a susceptible site such as a wound or urinary catheter. For example, gloves and aprons worn on entering an isolation room should be changed between handling a bedpan and emptying the urine drainage bag.

Gloves

Disposable gloves are worn to reduce the contamination of hands with micro-organisms and therefore minimize the risk of transferring infection to other patients. They should be worn for direct contact with infectious material and *changed between* procedures, as would be expected for the care of any other patient. However, several studies have shown that staff overlook the need to change gloves between procedures when caring for patients in isolation (Kim et al 2002, Prieto 2003). If gloves are not changed between procedures then pathogens from contaminated sites may be transferred to susceptible sites such as a wound or urinary catheter, causing subsequent infection in the isolated patient.

Gloves should be discarded before leaving the room or before initiating care on another patient. Hands are easily contaminated during the removal of gloves and should therefore be washed after gloves have been discarded (Olsen et al 1993).

Gloves need not be worn to enter the room if contact with infectious material is not anticipated. For example, where a patient is being isolated with pulmonary tuberculosis, gloves are only required for contact with sputum or respiratory secretions.

Gowns and aprons

Clothing may become contaminated while caring for patients, particularly during procedures involving heavily contaminated sites such as infected wounds and burns (Hambraeus 1973, Perry et al 2001, Speers et al 1969). The number of organisms actually transferred to the clothing is quite small and most will not survive there for very long periods. The front, the part that has most direct contact with patients and their immediate environment, is most likely to become contaminated (Babb et al 1983).

Micro-organisms can pass through fabric gowns, particularly when they are wet (Hoborn 1990). Plastic aprons are impermeable and therefore provide the most practical form of protection for the parts of the clothing most likely to become contaminated. They should be worn when contact with infectious material is anticipated and changed between procedures and before leaving the room. The reuse or disinfection of aprons is impractical and not cost-effective.

Masks

The Control of Substances Hazardous to Health Regulations 1999 require that all other control measures, such as room ventilation, should be taken before considering the use of personal protective clothing such as masks. In a well-ventilated isolation room, masks are probably of limited value (Fennelly & Nardell 1998).

Two types of facemask are available in healthcare settings: simple surgical masks or respirator masks. Surgical masks are designed to minimize the risk of large respiratory droplets being expelled from the mouth or nose during high-risk procedures, e.g. surgery, and protect these mucous membranes from contamination with body fluids in situations where splashing may occur. They are not designed to protect against infection by airborne pathogens. High-efficiency respirators are designed to protect against inhalation of airborne droplet nuclei (see p. 40) that are implicated in the transmission of tuberculosis or some respiratory viruses. These are recommended to filter particles of less than 1 μm in diameter with at least 95% efficiency. The European Standard (1991) EN 149 describes several filtering standards for respiratory protection, including FFP2 (filtering with 92% efficiency) and FFP3 (filtering with 98% efficiency). Respirator masks will not protect against airborne droplet nuclei unless they fit closely around the nose and mouth as air will be drawn in around the sides (Belken 1997). Staff required to use these masks should undergo face-fit testing and respirators must be discarded after each use.

There is limited scientific evidence to demonstrate the efficiency and cost-effectiveness of respirators in protecting against airborne infections (Adal et al 1994). However, they are currently recommended for the care of patients with suspected or known severe acute respiratory syndrome (SARS) and for aspects of care of patients with open tuberculosis that increase the exposure to infectious airborne particles, for example cough-inducing procedures, prolonged periods of care with highly dependent patients (Health Protection Agency 2005, Interdepartmental Working Group on Tuberculosis 1998).

Patients with infectious tuberculosis should be educated to minimize the release of tubercle bacilli into the air by coughing and sneezing into tissues, keeping their mouth covered. Provided the patient is able to co-operate with this practice, it is not usually necessary for them to wear a mask while being transported through other patient areas (Joint Tuberculosis Committee of the British Thoracic Society 2000). However, it is recommended that patients with multidrug-resistant tuberculosis wear masks when in transit to other departments to act as a physical barrier in case of inadvertent coughing (Interdepartmental Working Group on Tuberculosis 1996).

Immunization is a more effective means of protecting staff from infections transmitted by an airborne route. The BCG vaccine for tuberculosis confers 70–80% immunity lasting at least 15 years. Although it does not completely eliminate the risk of acquiring the infection, it does reduce it considerably (Joint Tuberculosis Committee of the British Thoracic Society 2000).

Immunity is also the most reliable factor protecting staff against acquiring chickenpox (varicella zoster virus) and measles. Varicella zoster virus (VZV) is highly transmissible. Most adults born in the UK acquire and develop immunity to the virus during childhood, although people born in some other countries, such as the West Indies and Hong Kong, are less likely to have been exposed. Staff who have no immunity to VZV are unlikely to be protected by the use of masks and should therefore avoid contact with the infected patient. VZV is a particular problem in wards or units that care for immunocompromised patients (e.g. haematology, renal or HIV units), as these patients are vulnerable to developing serious disease. Staff who work in these areas should have their immunity checked so that, if non-immune, they can be managed appropriately should they be exposed to the infection or an outbreak occur (Jones et al 1997). Measles usually occurs in children and vaccination is now offered routinely in the UK (UK Health Departments 1996).

Other respiratory infections expelled in larger respiratory droplets are more likely to be transmitted on hands than inhaled (Sattar et al 2002). However, surgical masks may help to reduce the risk of transmission during some procedures where there is close contact with respiratory secretions (e.g. bronchial suction, intubation) and they should be worn to protect staff when there is a risk of blood or body fluid splashing into the face.

Handwashing

Hands are probably the most important route by which micro-organisms are transmitted from patient to patient. Handwashing is therefore an essential component of preventing the spread of infection. In addition to the requirement to wash hands after contact with a patient under isolation precautions or their environment, the usual indications for handwashing during the care of the patient must still be applied (see Ch. 7).

Micro-organisms may be acquired on the hands by contact with the patient, equipment or the patient's immediate environment. Although the use of gloves to handle infective material will reduce the extent of contamination, gloves may become punctured during use and micro-organisms may be transferred to the skin as gloves are removed (Olsen et al 1993). Hands should therefore always be washed when protective clothing is removed and before leaving the room. As the micro-organisms are acquired transiently on the skin, most are easily removed by washing with soap and water. However, some antibiotic-resistant Gram-negative bacilli appear to be particularly resistant to removal by soap and water and antiseptic soap solutions may be recommended to prevent their spread (Pellowe et al 2003).

Alcohol handrubs provide a quicker alternative to soap and water for hands that are physically clean, for example for decontaminating hands after gloves have been removed or on leaving the room when there has been no direct contact with body fluids.

Excreta

Safe disposal of excreta from patients with infections transmitted by the faecal–oral route is particularly important, although excreta from all patients should be treated as potentially infectious and disposed of in the same way. Excreta from patients unable to use the toilet should be discarded into a bedpan washer or a macerator to avoid aerosolization of pathogens. Bedpans can be taken out of an isolation room wearing gloves and plastic apron and placed directly into the bedpan washer. Protective clothing can then be discarded into a yellow waste bag and hands washed. There is no risk of cross-infection if the healthcare worker has no direct contact with other patients until gloves and aprons have been removed and hands washed. The practice of attempting to remove intestinal pathogens from excreta with disinfectants is unnecessary because more pathogens enter the sewage system in domestic waste than from hospitals.

Pathogens on reusable bedpans are destroyed provided the bedpan washer achieves a temperature of 80°C for at least 1 min during the wash cycle. Most modern bedpan washers have a temperature display to enable the temperature to be checked.

Spillage of excreta should be cleaned up promptly, preferably with disposable wipes and using gloves and a plastic apron. Decontamination with disinfectants may be indicated where contamination affects a large area (see p. 273). Toilets splashed with excreta from patients with intestinal infections may in theory present a risk to others. This risk can be eliminated by regular cleaning of the toilet with detergent and ensuring that patients have access to handwashing facilities after using the toilet.

Waste material and linen

Waste generated during the care of an infected patient may be contaminated with infectious material and must be disposed of safely. Waste from an infectious patient does not require any special labelling but should be discarded into clinical waste bags (see p. 169). The outer surfaces of waste bags do not become significantly contaminated and there is no reason to enclose them inside a second bag before disposal (Maki et al 1986).

Linen may transmit infection to laundry workers who sort it before washing. To minimize this risk, it is recommended that linen used by patients with certain infectious diseases should not be sorted until it has been disinfected by washing. Linen used by patients with enteric infection, open tuberculosis and some other infections specified by the infection control team should be segregated by placing in a water-soluble bag with water-soluble stitching. This should then be sent to the laundry in a red outer bag. The alginate bag is placed directly into a washing machine and splits open when in contact with water. Micro-organisms on linen are removed by detergent and the dilution of the water and destroyed by the water temperature of at least 71°C during the wash cycle (NHS Executive 1995).

Equipment

In most situations routine decontamination procedures are sufficient to prevent cross-infection on equipment used by patients in isolation. These are discussed in Chapter 13.

Whilst micro-organisms can be isolated from low-risk equipment such as stethoscopes and sphygmomanometer cuffs, there is little evidence to suggest that they are associated with the transmission of infection since these items only come into contact with intact skin and this provides an effective barrier to micro-organisms (Rutala 1996).

Items, such as commodes, that are likely to become contaminated by infectious material should be cleaned with detergent after each use. It may, however, be more practical to allocate such equipment for sole use by the patient and to clean thoroughly when no longer required.

Items that do not become contaminated with infectious material do not require special cleaning and it is not usually necessary to discard unused disposable items in the room after the patient has been discharged or taken out of isolation.

Disposable crockery and cutlery for infectious patients is not necessary. Crockery and cutlery are unlikely to become contaminated with significant numbers of pathogens and bacteria will not be able to survive and multiply on the surface of clean, dry plates or cutlery. After use they should be washed in hot water and detergent, preferably in a dishwasher that has a rinse temperature of approximately

80°C, and allowed to dry before storage or reuse (Barrie 1996).

Cleaning

The environment is not a significant factor in the transmission of most infections because most micro-organisms are unable to survive for long on clean, dry surfaces. However, some bacteria can survive for prolonged periods in dust as they form spores or are extremely resistant to desiccation (Neely & Maley 2000). The accumulation of pathogens in the environment has been reported in association with high levels of dust and sometimes the control of outbreaks of infection has been correlated with increases in cleaning frequency (Rampling et al 2001). However, most of the evidence linking the environment with the transmission of infection is circumstantial: environmental contamination usually occurs concurrently with the presence of affected patients and cannot be conclusively established as the source of infection; many changes to clinical practice are usually implemented in order to control outbreaks of infection and it is therefore not possible to measure the specific contribution that the environment may make to transmission.

Widespread environmental contamination may occur when large numbers of micro-organisms are being dispersed, for example from patients with *Clostridium difficile* or glycopeptide-resistant enterococci who have diarrhoea (Boyce et al 1994, Hoffman 1993). Although the spores may be difficult to eliminate by routine cleaning, evidence for the value of disinfectants in removing them is conflicting (Dettenkofer et al 2004). The main risk presented by the contaminated environment is that healthcare workers will acquire pathogens on their hands or gloves by touching surfaces or equipment (Boyce et al 1997). However, provided gloves are removed and hands washed on leaving the room or isolation area, this risk can be minimized.

Contamination of the environment is not implicated in the spread of mycobacteria, as infection can be acquired only through the inhalation of droplet nuclei.

Equipment and surfaces should be kept free of dust and spills of body fluid to prevent micro-organisms accumulating. The room or bed area of the infected patient should be cleaned routinely in the same way as other areas. Disposable cleaning cloths should be used and discarded. Some hospitals designate a separate mop and bucket to clean the room. Disinfectants are generally only indicated if there is gross contamination of the environment (Noble et al 1998).

Domestic staff do not usually have direct contact with the patient and the risk of their acquiring infection from a patient is even less than that of nursing or medical staff. To reduce the risk to a minimum, they should be instructed to wear protective clothing to clean the room and to remove it and wash their hands before leaving. Careful reassurance is essential as they may be extremely concerned about acquiring infection from the isolated patient and the standard of cleaning may suffer as a result.

After an isolated patient has been discharged, the room should be cleaned before the next patient is admitted. A thorough clean to remove all dirt and dust is usually sufficient, using normal detergent-based cleaning agents. Afterwards the next patient can be admitted. Leaving isolation rooms for a period of time to air is unnecessary, as most infections are not spread by an airborne route and most harmful micro-organisms will have been removed by cleaning.

Transport of infected patients

Limiting visits to other departments reduces the opportunities for transmission. If transport to another department is necessary, infected lesions should be covered with a dressing and the patient asked to cover the mouth if coughing or sneezing. The personnel involved with the transport are unlikely to have contact with the infectious material and therefore do not need to wear protective clothing; however, they should be instructed to wash their hands afterwards. The receiving department should be informed in advance and advised of the precautions required.

Some infections present particular risk to mortuary staff (e.g. Creutzfeldt–Jakob disease, bloodborne viruses, tuberculosis, gastrointestinal infections). They should therefore be informed when a patient who has died had an infection so that the appropriate precautions can be taken when the body is handled. In some instances the body may need to be placed inside a plastic body bag (e.g. viral haemorrhagic fever, rabies, yellow fever) (Cutter 1999, Healing et al 1995).

Visitors

Visitors are unlikely to have contact with infectious material, such as faeces or respiratory secretions, and unlike staff, they will not usually be able to transmit infection through contact with other patients on the ward. Visitors should be advised to wash their hands before leaving the patient's room but there is usually no reason for them to wear protective clothing. Where appropriate, children and elderly visitors, who may be more susceptible to the infection, should be advised of the risks of visiting whilst the patient remains infectious (e.g. if the patient has chickenpox, respiratory syncytial virus).

For patients with tuberculosis, visiting should be restricted to close relatives for the first few days of treatment. They will already have been exposed to the infection before the patient's admission and will be followed up by the local Health Protection Unit to establish whether they have already acquired the infection.

Psychological effects of isolation

Isolation affects individual patients in different ways and, as social beings, humans generally do not like being isolated from others. The combination of isolation and fear of being infectious can be particularly stressful for some patients. Gammon (1998) measured four psychological constructs in a group of isolated patients and a control group of patients in hospital but not isolated. He found that the stressor of hospitalization was made worse by isolation. The isolated patients had significantly higher levels of anxiety and depression and lower self-esteem and sense of control. Anxiety may alter symptoms or induce secondary unrelated symptoms, affect the ability to listen and reduce the ability to cope. Carers must be sensitive to actions that increase anxiety, such as lack of communication, the use of excessive protective clothing or an inconsistency in the use of protective clothing, which can be confusing. A nurse who understands how the infection is transmitted can reassure and explain things to the patient.

The value of providing information to isolated patients was demonstrated in a second study by Lewis et al (1999). This showed that providing patients in isolation with information about their disease, its symptoms and treatment, the control measures and their rationale, together with advice about their responsibilities, significantly reduced their levels of anxiety and depression and increased their self-esteem and sense of control.

Psychological disorders have been reported in patients who have been isolated (e.g. anxiety, time disturbance, hallucinations) (Denton 1986). Some become extremely demanding, fussy or irritable and the nurse should recognize this behaviour as a response to isolation rather than that of a 'difficult' patient. Knowles (1993) studied eight patients in isolation. Many expressed feelings of loneliness, abandonment, inferiority and boredom (Table 14.4). Although the nurses often understood the patient's response to isolation, they did not take account of these problems and change the nursing care that they gave.

Patients with an infectious disease are often isolated for far longer than is necessary. The recommended

Table 14.4 Patient's response to isolation and nurses' perception of the situation. From Knowles (1993) with permission

Patient	Patient's response to isolation	Nurses' perception of patient's response
A	Feels 'browned off' and isolated Feels confined and frustrated by lack of progress Feels lonely, misses company of others No meaningful activities when alone	Is depressed, feels isolated Is neglected and stigmatized Dislikes being alone
B	Feels neglected and imprisoned Feels inferior, stigmatized	Gets forgotten by staff Feels cut off
C	Feels isolated and abandoned Feels physically separate from the ward Makes sleeping and pastimes easier	Feels isolated Appreciates quiet
D	Feels enclosed Makes pastimes more pleasurable Values own company, not lonely	Gets forgotten by staff Values quiet, facilitates pastimes
E	Feels neglected, shunned, inferior Feels shut in Lack of meaningful activity when alone Misses company of others	Feels neglected, isolated, lonely Feels shut in Easier access to television
F	Is bored Values privacy Feels isolated, enclosed, imprisoned, stigmatized, punished Lacks information and control, feels anxious as a result	Is bored Values privacy

period of isolation varies for each infection but usually precautions can be stopped once the symptoms have resolved, for example when diarrhoea has stopped, or for some infections after a short course of appropriate antimicrobial therapy (see Table 14.1).

For many infections, where transmission occurs only through direct contact with the infectious material, the stress of isolation can be relieved by allowing the patient out of the room. Isolation procedures should not interfere with rehabilitation, for example physiotherapy or occupational therapy.

Implementing isolation precautions and information for patients

At a clinical level isolation precautions can be difficult to implement; often there is confusion about how to apply the precautions and uncertainty about their effectiveness (Prieto 2003) (Box 14.4). Prieto & Clark (1999) point to the conflicting advice given in a variety of national guidelines in relation to the use of gloves and how the importance of changing gloves between procedures is frequently overlooked. They go on to describe how, in practice, staff tend to put on gloves when they enter an isolation room and remove them only on leaving the room. As a result they observed occasions when soiled gloves continued to be used for clean activities where cross-infection could have occurred. This highlights the importance of clear, simple and consistent policies that address the issues that most commonly lead to confusion and explain the rationale behind them. The infection control nurse has a major role to play in explaining isolation precautions and should be called upon for advice whenever necessary. The precautions must be applicable to all

> **Box 14.4   Nurses' concerns about isolation precautions (Prieto & Clark 1999)**
>
> - Confusion about the correct way to implement precautions, leading to inconsistencies in practice
> - Lack of information at ward level
> - Uncertainty about effectiveness of precautions
> - Lack of adherence to precautions
> - Inadequate isolation facilities
> - Detrimental effects of isolation on patients

members of the healthcare team. In general, they tend to be regarded as the sole responsibility of nurses, are often not addressed in medical textbooks and have little place in doctors' training.

Consistency is also important for the patient. Patients need to understand the rationale for the precautions themselves and be reassured that all staff with whom they have contact apply them similarly. When a patient is discharged, the same precautions may not be necessary in their home or if they are transferred to residential care. The reasons for this may require careful explanation and good communication between hospital, nursing home and community staff.

The nurse must also play an important role as health educator. For example, patients with *Salmonella typhi* may continue to excrete the organisms in their stool for several weeks after the symptoms have resolved. To ensure that the infection is not transmitted to other members of the patient's family, the importance of handwashing after using the toilet and before preparing any food should be discussed (see Ch. 12).

References

Adal KA, Anglim AM, Palumbo CL et al (1994) The use of high-efficiency particulate air-filter respirators to protect hospital workers from tuberculosis. *N. Engl. J. Med.,* **331**: 169–73.

Advisory Committee on Dangerous Pathogens (1996) *Management and Control of Viral Haemorrhagic Fevers.* HMSO, London.

Ayliffe GAJ, Collins BJ, Lowbury EJL et al (1971) Protective isolation in single-bed rooms: studies in a modified hospital ward. *J. Hyg. (Camb).,* **69**: 511–27.

Babb JR, Davies JG, Ayliffe GAJ (1983) Contamination of protective clothing and nurses' uniforms in an isolation ward. *J. Hosp. Infect.,* **4**: 49–57.

Bagshawe KD, Blowers R, Lidwell OM (1978) Isolating patients in hospital to control infection. Part IV: nursing procedures. *BMJ,* **ii**: 808–11.

Barrie D (1996) The provision of food and catering services in hospital. *J. Hosp. Infect.,* **33**: 13–33.

Belken NL (1997) The evolution of the surgical mask; filtering efficiency versus effectiveness. *Infect. Contr. Hosp. Epidemiol.,* **18**: 48–57.

Boyce JM, Opal SM, Chow JW et al (1994) Outbreak of multidrug resistant *Enterococcus faecium* with transferable vanB class vancomycin resistance. *J. Clin. Microbiol.,* **32**: 1148–53.

Boyce JM, Potter-Bynoe G, Chenevert C et al (1997) Environmental contamination due to methicillin-resistant *Staphylococcus aureus*: possible infection control implications. *Infect. Contr. Hosp. Epidemiol.,* **21**: 442–8.

Breathnach AS, de Ruiter A, Holdsworth GMC et al (1998) An outbreak of multidrug resistant tuberculosis in a London teaching hospital. *J. Hosp. Infect.,* **39**(2): 111–18.

Centers for Disease Control (1987) Recommendations for the prevention of transmission of HIV transmission in health care settings. *MMWR*, **36**: (2S).

Control of Infection Group, Northwick Park Hospital and Clinical Research Centre (1974) Isolation system for general hospitals. *BMJ*, **2**: 41–6.

Cooper BS, Stone SP, Kibbler CC et al (2003) Systematic review of isolation policies in the hospital management of methicillin-resistant *Staphylococcus aureus*: a review of the literature with epidemiological and economic modelling. *Health Technol. Assess.*, **7**(39): 1–97.

Cutter M (1999) In the bag? *Nursing Times*, **95**(20): 55–6.

Denton P (1986) Psychological and physiological effects of isolation. *Nursing*, **3**(3): 88–91.

Dettenkofer M, Hauer T, Daschner FD (2004) Detergent versus hypochlorite cleaning and *Clostridium difficile* infection. *J. Hosp. Infect.*, **56**: 78–9.

Doherty JA, Brookfield DS, Gray J et al (1998) Cohorting of infants with respiratory syncytial virus. *J. Hosp. Infect.*, **38**: 203–6.

European Standard (1991) *Specification for Filtering Half Masks to Protect Against Particles*. BS EN149. British Standards Institution, London.

Fennelly KP, Nardell EA (1998) The relative efficacy of respirators and room ventilation in preventing occupational tuberculosis. *Infect. Contr. Hosp. Epidemiol.*, **19**(10): 754–9.

Gammon J (1998) Analysis of the stressful effects of hospitalisation and source isolation on coping and psychological constructs. *Int. J. Nurs. Pract.*, **4**: 84–96.

Garner JS (1996) Guideline for isolation precautions in hospital. *Infect. Contr. Hosp. Epidemiol.*, **17**: 53–80.

Garner JS, Hierholzer WJ (1993) Controversies in isolation policies and practice. In: Wenzel RP (ed.) *Prevention and Control of Nosocomial Infections*, 2nd edn. Williams and Wilkins, Baltimore, MD.

Garner JS, Simmons BP (1983) Guideline for isolation precautions in hospitals. *Infect. Contr.*, **4**: 245–325.

Glenister H (1991) *Surveillance methods for hospital infection*. PhD thesis, Surrey University.

Hambraeus A (1973) Transfer of *Staphylococcus aureus* via nurses' uniforms. *J. Hyg. (Camb.)*, **71**: 799–814.

Hannan MM, Azadian BS, Gazzard BD et al (2000) Hospital infection control in an era of HIV infection and multi-drug resistant tuberculosis. *J. Hosp. Infect.*, **44**: 5–11.

Healing TD, Hoffman PN, Young SEJ (1995) The infection hazards of human cadavers. *CDR Rev.*, **5**(5): R61–8.

Health Protection Agency (2005) *Severe Acute Respiratory Syndrome: Hospital Infection Control Guidance*. Available online at: www.hpa.org.uk/infections/topics_az/ SARS/ pdfs/ hosp_infect_cont.pdf.

Hoborn J (1990) Wet strike through and transfer of bacteria through operating barrier fabrics. *Hyg. Med.*, **15**: 15–20.

Hoffman PN (1993) *Clostridium difficile* and the hospital environment. *PHLS Microbiol. Dig.*, **10**(2): 91–2.

Hoffman PN, Weinbren MJ, Stuart SA (2004) A practical lesson in negative-pressure isolation ventilation. *J. Hosp. Infect.*, **57**(4): 345–9.

Interdepartmental Working Group on Tuberculosis (1996) *The Prevention and Control of Tuberculosis in the United Kingdom: Recommendations for the Prevention and Control of Tuberculosis at a Local Level*. Department of Health, London.

Interdepartmental Working Group on Tuberculosis (1998) *The Prevention and Control of Tuberculosis in the United Kingdom: UK Guidance on the Prevention and Control of Transmission of 1. HIV Related Tuberculosis and 2. Drug-resistant, Including Multiple Drug-resistant, Tuberculosis*. Department of Health, London.

Jackson MM, Lynch P (1985) Isolation practices: a historical perspective. *Am. J. Infect. Contr.*, **13**(1): 21–31.

Jackson MM, Lynch PL (1996) Invited commentary: guideline for isolation precautions in hospitals, 1996. *Am J. Infect. Contr.*, **24**: 203–6.

Jenner EA, Mackintosh C, Scott GM (1999) Infection control evidence into practice. *J. Hosp. Infect.*, **42**: 91–104.

Joint Tuberculosis Committee of the British Thoracic Society (2000) Control and prevention of tuberculosis in the United Kingdom. Code of Practice 2000. *Thorax*, **55**: 887–901.

Jones EM, Barnett J, Perry C et al (1997) Control of varicella-zoster infection on renal and other specialist units. *J. Hosp. Infect.*, **36**(2): 133–40.

Kim PW, Roghmann MC, Perencevich EN et al (2002) Rates of hand disinfection associated with glove use, patient isolation and changes between exposure to various body sites. *Am. J. Infect. Contr.*, **31**: 97–103.

Knowles HE (1993) The experience of infectious patients in isolation. *Nursing Times*, **89**(30): 53–6.

Lewis AM, Gammon J, Hosein I (1999) The pros and cons of isolation and containment. *J. Hosp. Infect.*, **43**: 19–23.

Lynch P, Jackson MM, Cummings MJ et al (1987) Re-thinking the role of isolation practices in the prevention of nosocomial infections. *Ann. Intern. Med.*, **107**: 243–6.

Lynch P, Cummings MJ, Roberts PL et al (1990) Implementing and evaluating a system of generic infection precautions: body substance isolation. *Am. J. Infect. Contr.*, **18**: 1–12.

Maki DG, Alvarado C, Hassemer C (1986) Double bagging of items from isolation rooms is unnecessary as an infection control measure: a comparative study of surface contamination with single and double bagging. *Infect. Contr.*, **7**: 535–7.

National *Clostridium difficile* Standards Working Group (2004) Report to Department of Health. *J. Hosp. Infect.*, **56** (suppl. 1): 1–38.

Neely AN, Maley MP (2000) Survival of enterococci and staphylococci on hospital fabrics and plastic. *J. Clin. Microbiol.*, **38**(2): 724–6.

NHS Executive (1995) *Hospital Laundry Arrangements for Used and Infected Linen*. HSG(95) 18. Department of Health, Wetherby, UK.

Noble MA, Issac-Renton JL, Boyce DL et al (1998) The toilet as a transmission vector of vancomycin-resistant enterococci. *J. Hosp. Infect.*, **40**: 237–41.

Olsen RJ, Lynch P, Coyle MB et al (1993) Examination gloves as barriers to hand contamination in clinical practice. *JAMA*, **270**(3): 350–3.

Pellowe CM, Pratt RJ, Harper P et al (2003) Evidence-based guidelines for preventing healthcare-associated infections in primary and community care in England. *J. Hosp. Infect.*, **55** (suppl. 2): S1–S27.

Perry C, Marshall R, Jones E (2001) Bacterial contamination of uniforms. *J. Hosp. Infect.*, **48**: 238–41.

Preston GA, Larson EL, Stamm WE (1981) The effect of private isolation rooms on patient care practices, colonization and infection in an intensive care unit. *Am. J. Infect. Contr.*, **24**: 207–8.

Prieto JA (2003) *Influencing infection control practice: assessing the impact of a supportive intervention for nurses*. PhD Thesis, University of Southampton.

Prieto J, Clark J (1999) Dazed and confused. *Nursing Times*, **95**(28): 49–53.

Public Health Medicine Environmental Group (1996) *Guidelines on the Control of Infection in Residential and Nursing Homes*. Department of Health, Wetherby, UK.

Rampling A, Wiseman S, Lacey L et al (2001) Evidence that hospital hygiene is important in the control of methicillin-resistant *Staphylococcus aureus*. *J. Hosp. Infect.*, **49**: 109–16.

Rutala WA (1996) Disinfection and sterilisation of patient-care items. *Infect. Contr. Hosp. Epidemiol.*, **17**(6): 377–84.

Sattar SA, Springthorpe VS, Tetro J et al (2002) Hygienic hand antiseptics: should they not have activity and label claims against viruses? *Am. J. Infect. Contr.*, **30**: 355–72.

Selwyn S (1991) Hospital infection – the first 2500 years. *J. Hosp. Infect.*, **18** (suppl. A): 5–65.

Speers R, Shooter RA, Gaya H et al (1969) Contamination of nurses' uniforms with *Staphylococcus aureus*. *Lancet*, **ii**: 233–5.

UK Health Departments (1996) *Immunization Against Infectious Disease*. Stationery Office, London.

Weber DJ, Rutala WA (1997) Role of environmental contamination in the transmission of vancomycin-resistant enterococci. *Infect. Contr. Hosp. Epidemiol.*, **18**: 306–9.

Whitlock M, Lawrence J (2003) Residential and nursing homes. In: *Infection Control in the Community*. Churchill Livingstone, Edinburgh.

Wilson J, Breedon P (1990) Universal precautions. *Nursing Times*, **86**(37): 67–70.

Further Reading

Crummey V (1997) Major undertaking. Funeral directors' knowledge of infection risks. *Nursing Times*, **93**(11): 72–6.

Gammon J (1998) A review of the development of isolation precautions. *Br. J. Nurs.*, **7**(6): 307–10.

Gaskill D, Henderson A, Fraser M (1997) Exploring the everyday world of the patient in isolation. *Oncol. Nurs. Forum*, **24**(4): 695–700.

Oldman T (1998) Isolated cases. *Nursing Times*, **94**(11): 67–9.

Van Rijn RR, Kuijper EC, Kreis RW (1997) Seven-year experience with a 'quarantine and isolation unit' for patients with burns. A retrospective analysis. *Burns*, **23**(4): 345–8.

Chapter 15

Ectoparasitic infections and environmental infestations

INTRODUCTION

This chapter examines the problem of infections and infestations by arthropods and other animals. It begins with a review of parasites that can infect the human skin and then looks at the variety of pests that may infest the healthcare environment.

ECTOPARASITIC INFECTIONS

The prospect of a close encounter with lice or scabies usually induces alarm in most people. In reality, most of these infections can be eradicated easily and the risk of staff or other patients acquiring the parasite is slight. An understanding of how they are transmitted is essential if the treatment is to be carried out effectively and the affected individual approached sensitively. It is also important to consider education and treatment of other members of the family.

Lice (pediculosis)

Lice can be caught only by close contact; they cannot jump or fly but need to be close enough to walk on to another host. They feed from the host, usually taking blood about five times a day. An allergic reaction develops to the bites, causing them to itch. This allergic reaction can take up to 3 months to develop and carriers easily become desensitized and therefore no longer notice the bites. Lice found off the body on bedding, chairs, floors, etc. are either dead, dying or injured and are unable to crawl on to another host.

There are about 500 different species of lice but only three of these use humans as their host and each lives on a specific part of the body.

The head louse (Pediculus humanus capitis)
This species lives on head and eyebrow hair. It mostly affects children, although adults may also acquire the

infection. Estimates of the prevalence of infection amongst schoolchildren vary between 1% and 2%. However, if exposure over time is taken into account, an annual incidence approaching 40% has been reported. Infestation is far more common in girls than boys (Harris et al 2003). A study in southern England suggested that 10% of schoolchildren acquire lice in a year (Ibarra 1989, Maunder 1993).

The adult head louse is between 1 and 4 mm long (Plate 27). The female louse can produce over 50 eggs, laying about six each day and sticking them close to the base of hairs where it is warmest. The eggs hatch after 7–10 days, leaving the egg cases or nits so firmly stuck to the hair that they can remain attached until the hair falls out (Plate 28). The louse nymphs then moult three times, reaching adulthood after 6–12 days. Some 11–18 h after the last moult, they are ready to mate. Transmission to another host occurs when two heads are in direct contact and the louse moves on to a new head. They are able to climb rapidly in dry hair, although they move to a new head only when adult. They are sensitive to cold, preferring temperatures of at least 31°C. This keeps them close to the scalp and their source of food. Lice prefer a clean head of hair where they can move around easily. They are able to cling on tightly to hairs and are not removed by washing.

Head lice are invariably acquired from family members or close friends. The infection is difficult to detect in its early stages. Lice use a local anaesthetic to make the feeding process painless. Itching, although a common symptom, may not develop for weeks. A pruritic rash may appear at the back of the neck. They are best detected by using a fine-toothed comb in wet hair. The eggs are only the size of a grain of sugar and are difficult to see as their colour is matched to that of the skin.

Treatment and control The two main approaches to head lice eradication are chemical insecticides and physical removal by wet combing.

Several chemical insecticides are available for the treatment of lice, most of which can be obtained from the pharmacist without a prescription. The conventional treatments are based on the insecticides malathion, an organophosphate (e.g. Prioderm, Suleo-M and Derbac-M), carbaryl (e.g. Carylderm, Derbac-C and Suleo-C) and pyrethroid compounds (e.g. Lyclear, Full Marks). Two applications of lotion applied 7 days apart have been recommended for effective treatment (British National Formulary 2004), although for most products the manufacturers recommend only a single application. The lotion should be applied to dry hair and most formulations should be left on the scalp for 12 h to ensure as far as possible that both lice and eggs

are destroyed. A hair-dryer should not be used for alcohol-based products. After 12 h the hair should be washed. Shampoos are also available but, although they contain a higher concentration of insecticide, they are not as effective because they are not in contact with the hair for long enough and are unlikely to destroy eggs. Three separate treatments with shampoo are therefore required to eradicate the lice. Lyclear cream rinse leaves a residual pesticide in the hair and although this may continue to kill nymphs as they hatch from eggs, the reducing concentration of pesticide is likely to encourage resistance to emerge.

Although single, or infrequent, application of these pesticides is considered safe, some chemicals, especially carbaryl and to a lesser extent malathion, are readily absorbed through the skin and repeated use may be harmful (Communicable Disease Report 1997). Alcohol-based solutions are contraindicated in small children or asthmatics. Both local skin irritation and systemic effects such as headache, dizziness and general malaise have been reported (Antony et al 1997).

Repeated use of pediculicides has led to the emergence of pesticide-resistant lice (Burkhart 2004). Resistance to pediculicides is thought to be common and failure of treatment in up to a third of cases has been reported (Downs et al 1999).

Unconventional treatments for head lice are available (e.g. essential oils) but their efficacy is unproven and they may also exhibit toxicity (Figueroa et al 1998).

Eradication of head lice by systematic combing In recent years, concerns about the inadequacy and toxicity of pediculicides have led to the development of a mechanical method of eradicating infection. This method, called 'Bug Busting', involves combing the hair with a fine-tooth comb after shampooing and while it is still wet. Lice stop moving when hair is wet and the addition of conditioner lubricates the hair, enabling the lice to be removed easily with the comb. Once the hair has been thoroughly combed, the conditioner should be rinsed out of the hair. The process should then be repeated three more times at intervals of 4 days (Fig. 15.1). This will ensure that any nymphs hatching from eggs in the hair will be removed before they are fully grown and able to lay more eggs. Provided all adult lice are removed on the initial combing and new lice are not acquired, the affected person will not transmit lice. Eggs are not easily removed by a fine-tooth comb but as they hatch during the Bug Busting period, the nymphs will be removed by combing. This technique has been reported to be highly effective at eradicating infection

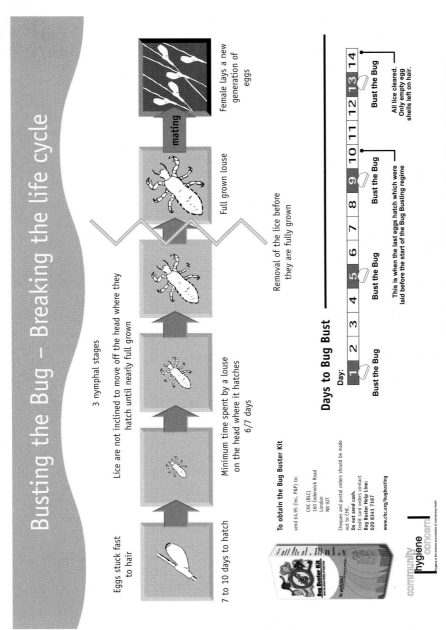

Figure 15.1 Bug Busting: the eradication of head lice by systematic combing. From the poster 'Busting the bug – breaking the life cycle. Produced by the charity Community Hygiene Concern.

in children and Bug Buster kits are available on prescription (Plastow et al 2001, Vander Stichele et al 2002). Although there has been controversy about the practicability of a mechanical method of lice eradication, a recent comparative study has established that the Bug Buster kit is four times more effective than pediculicides at eradicating head lice (Hill et al 2005).

Close family or friends who have had sufficient contact to enable transmission of lice should also be checked for infection. Head lice cannot be transmitted to others on clothing or linen and therefore no special precautions are necessary. Patients with head lice need not be isolated, except on paediatric wards where close contact between children may transmit the lice.

Crab (pubic) lice (Phthirus pubis)

The prevalence of infection with crab lice (phthiriasis) is unknown but probably common. These lice are much broader and flatter than head lice and have large claws on the second and third pairs of legs (Fig. 15.2) which enable them to move around in the less dense, coarse body hair. Pubic and perianal hair is most frequently affected but crab lice can infect all coarse body hair, including hair on the axilla, chest, arms, beard, eyebrows and eyelashes, and may also affect head hair. Although frequently considered a sexually transmitted disease, phthiriasis is transmitted by other close physical contact, particularly within families. Children may acquire crab lice through contact with axillary, chest and arm hair. Crab lice are not transmitted on clothing, bedlinen or other inanimate objects as, once off the body, they die rapidly.

The female louse lays several eggs on a single hair. These incubate for between 6 and 8 days and after hatching, the lice take 17 days to mature. It can take a minimum of 4–6 weeks for the host to react to the bite of the lice during which time they usually remain

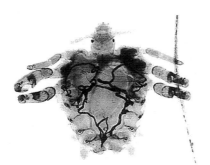

Figure 15.2 Adult crab (pubic) louse (reprinted with kind permission of Dr J Lane, London School of Hygiene and Tropical Medicine).

undetected, but once sensitized, the itching around the affected area is severe.

Treatment and control Crab lice can be treated with the same formulations recommended for head lice but aqueous-based solutions are recommended for use on genital hair and permethrin is not recommended as it causes irritation of the genitalia. The solution should be applied to all hairy parts of the body; a second treatment 7 days later is usually necessary to ensure eradication. A single application of shampoo or cream rinse formulation is unlikely to be effective.

If eyelashes or eyebrows are affected the lice can be eradicated by applying petroleum jelly twice a day for 10 days. This will kill the nymphs as they hatch (Figueroa et al 1998). The Bug Busting method described for the treatment of head lice can also be used to eradicate crab lice but is unlikely to be effective unless carried out with assistance.

Crab lice on clothing or bedding are not transmitted to other people and can be removed by washing. Isolation precautions are not necessary.

Body louse (Pediculus humanus humanus)

The body louse is very similar to, but slightly larger than, the head louse. It causes pediculosis corporis or infestation of clothing or bedding from where the lice visit the body to feed. It only affects people who are unable to change their clothes at regular intervals and nowadays is confined mostly to vagrants and people living on the streets. The louse lives in the clothing, laying its eggs in clusters on the fibres, especially the seams of underwear. Provided the clothing is worn continuously, nymphs hatch from the eggs after about 8 days but this will take longer if they are exposed to lower temperatures by removal of the clothing. The progress through nymphal moults varies according to the time in contact with the body. If clothing is worn continuously, the nymphs reach adulthood in approximately 8 days. If worn for only a few hours a day, this may take 3 weeks. Adult lice live for up to 30 days but will die of starvation after a few days if the clothes are removed and they are unable to feed. Although heavy infestation sometimes occurs, usually only 10–20 lice are present (Figueroa et al 1998). Bite marks usually occur along the seams of clothing, particularly underwear. They are often extremely itchy and may be accompanied by evidence of an inflammatory wheal around the bite.

Transmission occurs in overcrowded conditions by contact with infested clothing and bedding.

To survive, body lice depend on the same clothes being worn for prolonged periods, that are washed in cool water and then reworn immediately. They are therefore easy to eradicate as they will die if the clothing is not worn for 3 days and, provided the clothes are changed once a week, the young lice will not be able to feed when they hatch out of the eggs. Lice are also destroyed by washing clothes in hot water and hot tumble-drying destroys both lice and eggs.

The human body louse is responsible for the transmission of a number of serious infectious diseases. Trench fever (*Bartonella quintana*) can be transmitted by lice. *Borrelia recurrentis* causes relapsing fever which is characterized by bouts of fever lasting for several weeks. It is a spirochaete which multiplies in the body of the louse and is transmitted to human hosts when the lice feeds. Although not seen in Europe now, cases do occur in Africa and South America. Typhus, caused by *Rickettsia prowazeki*, is a severe fever associated with a death rate of 10–20% and is transmitted by louse faeces entering a cut on the skin. Epidemics of typhus and relapsing fever are associated with cold, lack of fuel, overcrowding, famine and war – conditions that are conducive to louse infestation.

Treatment and control   Clothing should be washed in hot water (60°C or more) and be changed at least once a week. Fifteen minutes in a hot tumble-dryer is sufficient to destroy both lice and eggs. No treatment of the skin or isolation precautions are necessary.

Scabies

Scabies is caused by a small mite, *Sarcoptes scabiei* (Fig. 15.3). It is a common infection and endemic in many developing countries. Epidemics are cyclical, with the prevalence of infection peaking every 10–30 years. In the UK reported cases of scabies increased in the 1990s with outbreaks affecting schools, residential homes and hospitals, especially units for patients with acquired immune deficiency syndrome (AIDS) or the elderly (Burgess 2003).

The mites live in the deeper layers of the epidermis. The female burrows through the stratum corneum, tunnelling up to 5 mm a day. The male mite moves between burrows searching for a mate. A fertilized female lives for approximately 4–6 weeks during which time she lays between 40 and 50 eggs. Eggs hatch after 3–4 days and the larvae establish a new tunnel off the maternal burrow. They moult several times before becoming adults, 10–15 days later. On average an affected person will harbour between 15 and 20 female adult mites.

Despite the conventional view of scabies as a highly infectious disease, it is not easily transmitted from person to person or easily spread by social contact. The mite moves extremely slowly and therefore prolonged contact is required for it to move on to another host. It can be transmitted between family members and sexual partners and in hospital is often seen in care of the elderly and psychiatric settings where holding hands may be more common.

The majority of mites are found on the hands and wrists, especially where the skin is thin (e.g. between the fingers). However, they may also occur on the elbows, axillae and nipple areas, groins, buttocks and genitalia. They do not commonly spread to the head and neck except in the elderly or immune-deficient patients and are unusual on the soles of the feet and palms of the hands, except in children (Taplin 1986).

The main symptoms of scabies infection are caused by an allergic response to the presence of the mite. Severe itching, especially at night, develops 2–6 weeks after the first infection. An allergic rash with erythematous papules, vesicles or itchy nodules appears, characteristically affecting the body symmetrically on the arms, trunk, waist, inner thighs and calves. The rash and itching are not necessarily related to the site of the mites (Maunder 1983). Sarcoptes also affect animals, for example causing mange in dogs. Whilst these mites are usually unable to establish on a human host, exposure to the mite faeces on the animal may cause sensitized individuals to develop a scabies-like allergic rash.

If the person has had a previous infection with the scabies mite, the immune response is rapid and itching develops within hours. The mite may then be killed before it can re-establish an infection.

The appearance of a generalized rash or itch may be diagnosed as scabies but because of the implications of

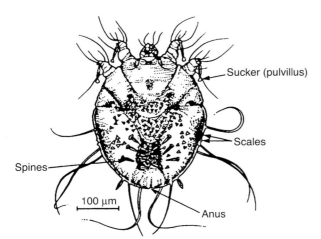

Figure 15.3   The scabies mite *Sarcoptes scabiei* (dorsal view of female) (redrawn with permission from Kettile DS (1990) *Medical and Veterinary Entomology*, CAB International; original drawing by HJ Hawthorne).

tracing and treatment of contacts, it is important to make a definite diagnosis. Burrows are not easily seen but may be visible as tiny white lines, 15–30 cm long and with a (0.5 mm) brown spot, the female mite, at one end. To an experienced eye these are diagnostic of scabies. However, the diagnosis can be confirmed by the examination of skin scrapings from a suspected burrow under the microscope to detect parasites, their eggs or faecal pellets. These are more easily obtained from the skin if a drop of mineral oil is applied before gently collecting scrapings with a needle or scalpel blade.

Norwegian (crusted) scabies

This form of scabies occurs when the scabies mite infects a person with a deficiency of their immune system, caused by either disease or immuno-suppressive therapy. In the absence of a normal immune system, the body cannot control the mite infection and the mite multiplies rapidly, causing many thousands of mites to spread all over the body, including the head. This widespread infection usually results in hyperkeratotic (crusted) lesions, particularly on the nailbeds, palms, soles, wrists, buttocks and penis, and is known as Norwegian scabies. Sometimes the presentation may be atypical, with no crusted lesions or itching, despite widespread infections with large numbers of mites. Crusted scabies may also be localized, affecting only the fingers, toes or head (Chosidow 2000). Skin scales and crusts are heavily contaminated with mites and affected individuals are highly infectious.

Outbreaks of scabies, from an unrecognized index case of Norwegian scabies, commonly spread through nursing homes or elderly care units and may result in many patients and staff becoming infected (Anderson et al 2000). Particular problems are associated with wards caring for a high proportion of patients with AIDS, where rapid spread may occur and several cases of Norwegian scabies may develop as a result (Sirera et al 1990). Contacts with a normal immune system may develop conventional scabies.

Treatment and control   There are two main forms of treatment for scabies: malathion (lotion) and permethrin (cream). These should be applied to the whole body and left on for up to 24 h. The lotion should be reapplied to the hands when they are washed. Benzylbenzoate can also be used but is not recommended for initial treatment as it does not destroy the mite eggs. Two applications of the treatment 7 days apart are recommended to eradicate the mite and its eggs (Burgess 2003). In cases of Norwegian scabies it may be necessary to apply several applications of treatment at intervals of 3 days (Burgess 2003). Treatment of pregnant women, nursing mothers or children should be under medical supervision. An oral drug, ivermectin, has been shown to be effective against scabies and may be useful in combination with topical treatments for the treatment of severe infections and for controlling outbreaks (Chosidow 2000, Hadfield-Law 2001).

Patients should be warned that itching persists for some time after treatment because it takes a few days for the allergic response to subside even though the mites have been killed. Retreatment is not indicated unless itching persists for longer than 1 week.

All close contacts of the affected person should be treated at the same time even if they are asymptomatic because of the long delay between infection and the development of symptoms.

Scabies mites are not readily transmitted by clothes or bedlinen and these items should be laundered normally using hot water and a dryer.

Patients with scabies do not require isolation as actual skin-to-skin contact is required to transmit infection. However, infection is more likely to be transmitted from patients with Norwegian scabies and isolation precautions are recommended until treatment has been completed. Linen and clothing can be decontaminated by washing and mites removed from the environment by regular cleaning.

Early identification of cases is essential to control spread and ensure effective treatment of affected patients and their contacts. Staff should be vigilant for cases of scabies in nursing and residential homes for the elderly or in units caring for immunocompromised patients. These should have established procedures for diagnosing and managing cases of scabies and for the identification and simultaneous treatment of contacts.

INFESTATION OF THE ENVIRONMENT

Healthcare premises provide an ideal environment in which pests can flourish. They are warm and full of people whose habits inevitably provide a constant source of food. Pests can be described as animals or insects that cause damage or annoyance or, in some cases, present a risk of infection.

Pests that most commonly infest hospitals are cockroaches, Pharaoh's ants, fleas, birds, rodents and cats. Although it is unlikely that all pests could be totally eradicated from hospitals or other centres of healthcare, an effective and continuous strategy to control their numbers is essential. Healthcare staff have a crucial role to play in the reporting of pests or signs of infestation and should be aware of the system of reporting and treating infestations that occur in their place of work. Pests frequently appear only at night and are not easily observed. Even small signs should be reported. The sighting of a single cockroach, egg case or mouse dropping is probably indicative of an infestation problem.

The Department of Health recommends that each hospital or unit of management should nominate a pest control officer (PCO) with responsibility for all aspects of pest control (NHS Management Executive 1992). These individuals should be trained in the recognition of pests and methods of controlling them, keep a record of pest sightings, investigate reports and ensure that appropriate action is taken. Most hospitals have a contract with a pest control servicing company that will treat infestations, provide a rapid response to sightings of pests and undertake regular inspections of the site. The PCO is responsible for liaison with the contractor and monitoring the contract. This may involve periodic inspections of the site at night when the activity of many pests is at its greatest. In large complex buildings, information on pest sightings from staff is particularly valuable.

Cockroaches

Cockroaches have existed for millions of years and there are over 3000 different species. The two most common species in the UK are the German (*Blattella germanica*) and oriental (*Blatta orientalis*) cockroach; American (*Periplaneta americana*) and brown banded cockroaches are only rarely seen. Any large building that is warm is prone to infestation.

Cockroaches feed on an enormous variety of meat and vegetable matter, including sewage and organic waste. They also need a supply of water and cavities in which to hide. They can live in tiny cracks and crevices and behind wall and floor tiles and, because they are strongly nocturnal, infestation often goes unnoticed until the population is very large. The life cycle of the cockroach includes three stages: the eggs are enclosed within a capsule; they hatch out as nymphs – smaller, wingless versions of the adult insect which after several moults mature into adults. Some species hide their eggs in cracks; German cockroaches carry them until nearly ready to hatch whereas oriental cockroaches abandon them. Both German and oriental adult cockroaches have wings but do not fly.

The German cockroach is the smallest, about 12 mm long, and accounts for about 10% of cockroach infestations. Its common name is the 'steamfly' as it prefers warm and humid conditions and is therefore most commonly found in kitchens. It is good at climbing and may be found in heated trolleys, vending machines, refrigerator motors and behind false ceilings. The oriental cockroach is larger, about 25 mm long, and accounts for about 90% of all cockroach infestations in heated buildings (Fig. 15.4A). However, it can tolerate cooler conditions and so may be found outside, around the perimeter of buildings and in drains and underground ducting. The American cockroach is the largest species found in the UK, about 35 mm long. It needs access to water and warm conditions of between 24° and 33°C and is usually found in large heated greenhouses and in ports and airports where it is introduced from abroad on ships or aeroplanes.

Many hundreds of cockroaches can live in gaps behind tiles, gaining access through breaks or cracks (Fig. 15.4B). Infestation in clinical areas can be discouraged by employing simple preventive measures

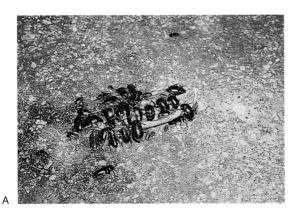
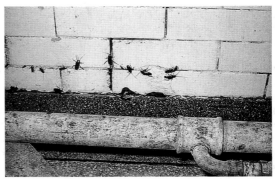

A   B

Figure 15.4   (A) Adults and nymphs of the oriental cockroach feeding on a courgette discarded in a kitchen yard. (B) Mixture of oriental and German cockroaches on a kitchen wall. Notice also the slugs! (Reproduced with kind permission of Mr L Baker.)

such as storing food in tight-fitting containers and secure cupboards, not leaving out prepared food, discarding waste food and refuse promptly and ensuring that leaking pipes and damaged surfaces are repaired (Smith 1988).

Many bacteria have been isolated from the bodies and faecal droppings of cockroaches, which they probably acquire through feeding on food, decaying matter and faeces. The microbes they carry reflect the microbial flora of the environment in which they live (Bennett 1993, Fotedar et al 1991). Although it is difficult to prove that cockroaches are responsible for particular cases of infection, they could in theory transmit infection if allowed to crawl over working surfaces or prepared food. Circumstantial evidence for transmission of infection by cockroaches was provided by Graffar & Mertens (1950) who reported an outbreak of *Salmonella typhimurium* in a Brussels children's ward. Cockroaches were observed running over the children and their bedclothing at night. *S. typhimurium* was isolated from one of the captured insects and the outbreak came to an end once the infestation had been eradicated. Cotton et al (2000) reported an outbreak of antibiotic-resistant *Klebsiella pneumoniae* in a neonatal unit infested with cockroaches. Although the outbreak micro-organism was found on cockroaches, there was no direct evidence that these were responsible for the transmission of infection; other factors such as overcrowding and understaffing were probably of greater significance.

Ants

Garden ants, attracted by food debris, may occasionally cause a minor problem in buildings but are easily controlled by treatment with insecticide. Far more serious problems can be caused by Pharaoh's ants, tiny insects 1–2 mm long which can invade equipment and contaminate food (Fig. 15.5). Originally introduced from tropical countries, they can survive easily in centrally heated buildings in temperate climates. Nest colonies each containing several thousand worker ants are sited in almost any concealed area, for example behind tiles, light fittings and in brickwork. Nests have been found in heated food trolleys, drink-vending machines and autoclave units. They eat both meat and vegetable matter but prefer meat and sweet substances. They can chew through plastic and have been found in intravenous fluid administration sets and sterile packs (Beatson 1973). They will also search out suppurative lesions and feed on the discharge from the wound.

Infestation in operating theatres or central sterile supply departments enables ants to invade sterile

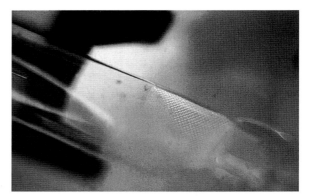

Figure 15.5 Pharoah's ants trapped in the filter of an administration set (reproduced with kind permission of Mr L Baker).

packs. Infestation in the laundry or other service departments results in ants being transferred throughout the hospital. They can also spread through ducting.

There is some evidence that these ants can transmit infection and indeed, they are more likely to be found in contact with patients and their equipment than more shy insects, such as cockroaches. A large range of bacteria, including pseudomonas, staphylococci and enterobacter, have been isolated from the surface of their bodies (Beatson 1972). Their affinity for moist areas such as sinks, toilets and sluices means they could acquire pathogenic bacteria on their bodies and transfer them on to food, sterile packs or patients' wounds.

Suspected infestation with Pharaoh's ants should be reported promptly to the PCO so that extensive treatment by a professional pest control company can be carried out without delay.

Fleas

There are more than 1000 species of flea and although they feed on any warm-blooded animal, they require a specific host on which to breed. Human fleas are now rarely encountered, although Thomas et al (2000) described an outbreak of human fleas that affected staff in a geriatric unit. They dislike the warm, dry environment of modern homes and are usually found only in association with vagrants or homeless people. They live in the environment, feeding infrequently from their hosts and should be treated by washing infested clothing and applying insecticide to the environment.

Cat and dog fleas (Fig. 15.6) are responsible for most flea bites on humans (Watkins & Wyatt 1989). They thrive in the warm, dry environment of the

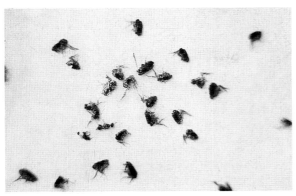

Figure 15.6 Mixture of cat and dog fleas caught in 1 h on sticky tape in a radiography department (reproduced with kind permission of Mr L Baker).

domestic home and live in furniture and carpets, jumping on to passing animals and humans for food. The bites are commonly seen on the ankles and lower legs, although many people become desensitized to them and do not develop an immune response to the bite. Infestations in hospitals may originate from colonies of feral cats or animals kept as pets and can be very troublesome. Feral cats living in ducting or basements may support a large population of fleas which may then gain access to the building. Cat flea infestations have even been responsible for the closure of an operating department and a laundry (Baker 1981). If infestation with fleas is suspected in a hospital department, the pest control officer should be contacted who will arrange for the source of the infestation to be identified and treated with insecticides.

Preventing flea infestations depends on control of feral cat populations by neutering. Pet animals should be regularly treated to ensure they are kept free of fleas. The environmental health department of the local authority or a company specializing in pest control can be called in to treat severe infestation with fleas in the home.

Birds

Birds, particularly pigeons and house sparrows, become pests when their population is large enough to cause a nuisance, by fouling, noise or secondary pests such as mites and fleas. Roosting can be deterred by nets, wires, spikes, etc. and they should be prevented from gaining access to buildings. To avoid attracting birds, refuse must be carefully sited, spillages cleared up promptly and deliberate feeding discouraged.

Rodents

The main rodent pests are rats and mice. They can cause damage to furnishings, spoil food and may also carry pathogenic bacteria. They are often detected by evidence of damage or droppings. Rodents can be discouraged by storing food in tightly closing containers or secure cupboards and discarding waste promptly. Waste for disposal should not be stored for prolonged periods and the storage area should be kept clean and tidy.

References

Anderson BM, Haugen H, Rasch M et al (2000) Outbreak of scabies in Norwegian nursing homes and home care patients: control and prevention. *J. Hosp. Infect,*. **45**: 160–4.

Antony H, Birtwhistle S, Eaton K et al (1997) *Environmental Medicine in Clinical Practice*. British Society for Allergy Environmental and Nutritional Medicine, Southampton.

Baker LF (1981) Pests in hospital. *J. Hosp. Infect.*, **2**: 5–9.

Beatson SH (1972) Pharaoh's ants as pathogen vectors in hospitals. *Lancet*, **i**: 425–7.

Beatson SH (1973) Pharaoh's ants enter giving sets. *Lancet*, **i**: 606.

Bennett G (1993) Cockroaches as carriers of bacteria. *Lancet*, **i**: 732.

British National Formulary (2004) British Medical Association and Royal Pharmaceutical Society of Great Britain, London.

Burgess I (2003) Understanding scabies. *Nursing Times*, **99**(7): 44–5.

Burkhart CG (2004) Relationship of treatment-resistant head lice to the safety and efficacy of pediculocides. *Mayo Clin. Proc.*, **79**: 661–6.

Chosidow O (2000) Scabies and pediculosis. *Lancet*, **355**: 819–26.

Communicable Disease Report (1997) Head lice. *CDR Weekly*, **7**(41): 365.

Cotton MF, Wasserman E, Pieper CH et al (2000) Invasive disease due to extended spectrum beta-lactamase-producing *Klebsiella pneumoniae* in a neonatal unit: the possible role of cockroaches. *J. Hosp. Infect.*, **44**: 13–17.

Downs AMR, Stafford KA, Harvey I et al (1999) Evidence for double resistance to permethrin and malathion in head lice. *Br. J. Dermatol.*, **141**: 508–11.

Figueroa J, Hall S, Ibarra J (eds) (1998) *Primary Health Care Guide to Common UK Parasitic Disease*. Community Hygiene Concern, London.

Fotedar R, Shrinivas U, Banerjee U et al (1991) Nosocomial infections: cockroaches as possible vectors of drug-resistant klebsiella. *J. Hosp. Infect.*, **18**: 155–9.

Graffar M, Mertens S (1950) Le role des blattes dans la transmission des salmonelloses. *Ann. Inst. Pasteur*, **79**: 654–60.

Hadfield-Law L (2001) Dealing with scabies. *Nursing Standard*, **15**(31): 37–42.

Harris J, Crawshaw JG, Millership S (2003) Incidence and prevalence of head lice in a district health authority. *Commun. Dis. Public Health*, **6**(3): 246–9.

Hill N, Moor G, Cameron MM et al (2005) Single-blind, randomised comparative study of the Bug Buster kit and over the counter pediculicide treatments against head lice in the United Kingdom. *BMJ*, **331**: 384–7.

Ibarra J (1989) Headlice in schools. *Health at* School, **4**: 147–51.

NHS Management Executive (1992) *Pest Control Management for the Health Service*. HSG(92)35. Department of Health, Wetherby, UK.

Maunder J (1983) The increase in scabies. *Postgrad. Doctor,* **6**: 198–202.

Maunder J (1993) An update on headlice. *Health Visitor,* **66**(9): 317–18.

Plastow L, Luthra M, Powell R et al (2001) Head lice infestation; bug busting versus traditional treatment. *J. Clin. Microbiol.,* **10**(6): 775–83.

Sirera G, Ruis F, Romeu J et al (1990) Hospital outbreak of scabies stemming from two AIDS patients with Norwegian scabies. *Lancet*, **335**: 1227.

Smith P (1988) An unpleasant case of cracked tiles. *Health Services J.,* **26 May** (S): 6.

Taplin D (1986) Cutaneous infestations. In: Vickers CFH (ed.) *Modern Management of Skin Diseases*. Churchill Livingstone, Edinburgh.

Thomas P, Cutter J, Joynson PHM (2000) An outbreak of human fleas infestation in a hospital. *J. Hosp. Infect.,* **45**: 330–5.

Vander Stichele RH, Gyssels L, Bracke C et al (2002) Wet combing for head lice: feasibility in mass screening, treatment preference and outcome. *J. Roy. Soc. Med.,* **95**: 348–52.

Watkins M, Wyatt T (1989) A ticklish problem; pest infestation in hospitals. *Prof. Nurse,* **May**: 369–92.

Further Reading

Community Hygiene Concern (2000) *Bug Buster Teaching Pack*. CHC, 160 Inderwick Road, London N8 9JT (tel: 020 8421 7167). Available online at: www.chc.org/bugbusting.

Figueroa J, Hall S, Ibarra J (eds) (1998) *Primary Health Care Guide to Common UK Parasitic Disease*. Community Hygiene Concern, London.

Public Health Medicine Environmental Group (1996) *Guidelines on the Control of Infection in Residential and Nursing Homes*. Department of Health, London.

Glossary

Abscess A localized collection of pus.

Active immunity Immunity that develops in response to a stimulus (e.g. infection or vaccine) and is dependent on the production of B and T lymphocytic memory cells.

Acute infection An infection that runs its course in a relatively short period.

Adenosine triphosphate A chemical compound that contains energy-rich bonds and serves as the main 'energy currency' of the cell. It breaks down into adenosine diphosphate and a phosphate ion, releasing energy.

Aerobe A microbe that grows in the presence of oxygen. A strict aerobe requires oxygen. *See* anaerobe.

Agar A polysaccharide made from seaweed and used to solidify bacteriological media.

Agglutinate To stick to one another, clump (of particles, red cells, etc.); the result is agglutination.

Algae Photosynthetic microbes; the blue-green algae are prokaryotes and the others are eukaryotes.

Allergic response An exaggerated immune response to an antigen resulting in histamine release, inflammation and tissue damage. The effects may be localized (e.g. hay fever, asthma) or systemic (e.g. anaphylactic shock).

Allergy An undesirable immune response due to hypersensitivity to an antigen.

Amino acid An organic acid, constituent of proteins. It has the structure R-C-COOH
|
NH$_2$

Amoeba A eukaryotic organism that lacks a rigid cell wall and moves by means of pseudopods.

Anaerobe A microbe that grows in the absence of oxygen. A strict anaerobe will not grow in the presence of oxygen; a facultative anaerobe can grow in the presence or absence of oxygen.

Anaphylaxis A hypersensitivity reaction.

Antagonism One drug interferes with another so that the sum of the effect is less than if either were given alone (e.g. penicillin and tetracycline).

Antibiotic A substance that is toxic to micro-organisms; the first antibiotics to be used were derived from other micro-organisms but many are now partly or wholly synthesized (= antimicrobial agent).

Antibody A protein produced by B lymphocytes which appears in the body fluids after contact with a foreign molecule ('antigen') and which combines specifically with that antigen.

Antigen *See* antibody.

Antimicrobial agent *See* antibiotic.

Antiseptic A chemical used to kill microbes on body surfaces.

Antiserum A serum that contains antibodies to a particular antigen.

Antitoxin A serum containing antibodies to a toxin, either as a result of natural infection or, more often, in response to injection of toxoid.

Arthropod An animal that has a hard outer 'skeleton' and jointed legs; examples are insects, ticks and lice.

Aseptic Free of micro-organisms.

ATP *See* adenosine triphosphate.

Attenuated A microbe that has lost its virulence and can be safely used as a vaccine.

Autoclave A machine in which materials are exposed to steam under pressure and therefore at a temperature higher than that of boiling water.

Autogenous From within the individual.

B

Bacillus Any rod-shaped bacterium; also the name of a genus of Gram-positive bacteria, often found in soil and dust.

Bacteraemia The presence of bacteria in the blood without clinical signs or symptoms of infection.

Bactericidal Capable of killing bacteria (e.g. penicillins).

Bacteriophage A virus that infects bacterial cells.

Bacteriostatic A drug that prevents bacteria from replicating; if the drug is withdrawn, bacteria can multiply again (e.g. tetracycline). (A drug that is bacteriostatic may in high concentration or in certain circumstances become bactericidal, e.g. fusidic acid.)

Bacteriuria The presence of micro-organisms in the bladder with no signs or symptoms of infection.

Basophil A white cell of the blood. It attracts lymphocytes to the site of an infection by releasing vasoactive chemicals that increase blood flow to the area.

BCG An attenuated strain of tubercle bacilli that is used as a vaccine against tuberculosis.

Binary fission Division of one cell into two daughter cells; the usual method of reproduction in bacteria.

Biofilm A film of proteins and micro-organisms that forms over the surface of foreign material when it is in contact with tissue.

B lymphocyte One of the two main cell types of the immune system, chiefly involved in the production of antibodies.

Broad spectrum Agents that work against many types of bacteria. Often used for initial treatment when the cause of an infection is unknown.

C

Capsid Protein coat of a virus made from polypeptide subunits.

Capsule A slimy substance, usually polysaccharides, that forms a protective layer around some bacterial cells.

Carbohydrate A compound of carbon, hydrogen and oxygen in a ratio of two hydrogen molecules to each oxygen and carbon molecules (e.g. glucose = $C_6H_{12}O_6$).

Carrier An individual who has a body surface colonized by a pathogen but without being affected by disease.

Catalyst A substance that increases the rate of a chemical reaction but is itself unchanged by the reaction.

Cell-mediated immunity The part of the immune response mediated by T lymphocytes and directed against intracellular pathogens (e.g. viruses, malignant cells).

Cell wall The rigid outer layer of most prokaryotic cells and of some eukaryotic cells.

Cellulose A carbohydrate composed of glucose molecules; an important constituent of plant cell walls.

Chemotaxis Movement of a cell in response to the presence of a chemical.

Chlorophyll A green pigment found in plants and some bacteria that absorbs light to provide energy for the synthesis of carbohydrates from water and carbon dioxide (photosynthesis).

Chromosome Contains the genetic information of the cell and is composed of long threads of DNA and associated proteins.

Clone A group of organisms descended from a single parent by asexual reproduction and therefore exact copies of it.

Coccobacillus A short oval rod, i.e. between a coccus and a bacillus in shape.

Coccus A spherical bacterium.

Colonization A microbe that establishes itself in a particular environment such as a body surface without producing disease is said to 'colonize' the site.

Colony When a bacterial cell (or a few cells) multiplies on a solid medium until the group is visible to the naked eye, the group is called a colony. A typical colony contains 10–100 million cells.

Commensal A commensal organism lives in association with another, without benefiting or harming it. Many members of the gut flora appear to be commensals. Commensals may be pathogenic if the host is immunocompromised.

Communicable A disease that can be transmitted from one person to another is communicable (*syn.* contagious, infectious).

Community-acquired infection An infection acquired in the community, not as a result of treatment in hospital.

Complement A complex of proteins in the blood that promote the activity of phagocytic cells; the sequential reactions between the component proteins are triggered by micro-organisms or an antigen–antibody complex.

Conjugation The transfer of genetic material from one bacterial cell to another by the formation of a small tube between them (sex pilus).

Conjugative plasmid A plasmid that carries the genes required to form a sex pilus and transfer plasmid DNA into another cell.

Contagious *See* communicable.

Counterstain A stain used to enhance contrast in a differential stain.

Culture A culture of microbes is the result of inoculating a medium with them and incubating it until large numbers are present.

Cystitis Infection of the bladder.

Cytokines Immunological proteins that act as chemical messengers for the immune system, e.g. interleukin.

Cytoplasm In a prokaryote, everything inside the cytoplasmic membrane; in a eukaryote, everything inside the cytoplasmic membrane, except the nucleus.

Cytoplasmic membrane The membrane that surrounds the cell and retains the cytoplasm.

D

Delayed(-type) hypersensitivity A hypersensitivity reaction that develops 24 h or more after exposure to an antigen.

Denaturation (a) Of proteins: the loss of folding brought about by heat or chemicals; associated with the loss of normal biological activity. (b) Of DNA: breaking the hydrogen bonds that hold two DNA strands together, resulting in their separation.

Deoxyribonucleic acid (DNA) The large molecule in which genetic information is encoded, the genetic material. The component nucleotides contain the sugar deoxyribose.

Dermatophyte A fungus that infects the skin, hair and nails without invading the deeper tissues.

Diffusion The process whereby random movement of molecules tends to equalize their concentration across areas of higher and lower concentration.

Diploid A diploid cell contains two copies of each chromosome. The body cells of most eukaryotic organisms are diploid.

Disinfection A process that reduces the number of micro-organisms to a level at which they are not harmful, but which does not usually destroy spores.

DNA *See* deoxyribonucleic acid.

Dysentery A severe form of infectious diarrhoea, characterized by blood and mucus in the stools.

E

Ectoparasite A parasite that lives on the outer surface of the host (e.g. a tick or louse).

Electron A negatively charged particle.

Electron microscope A microscope in which a beam of electrons is used instead of light rays to produce an image.

Electrophoresis The separation of molecules by subjecting them to an electric field in which they move at different rates.

ELISA (enzyme-linked immunosorbent assay) A technique for detecting antigens and antibodies, in which a coloured compound is formed by an enzyme linked to the detector antibody.

Encephalitis Inflammation of the brain.

Endemic If a disease is endemic, cases regularly occur in the population with little variation in incidence. *See* epidemic.

Endocarditis An inflammation, especially one due to infection, of the lining of the heart, including its valves.

Endogenous From within the body; an endogenous infection is caused by micro-organisms that are part of the normal flora.

Endoplasmic reticulum A complicated membrane system extending throughout the cytoplasm of the eukaryotic cell.

Endotoxin Lipopolysaccharides in outer membrane of Gram-negative cells. When cells are lysed, these are released and may cause severe systemic symptoms (endotoxic shock).

Envelope An outer membrane that surrounds the capsid of some viruses and may be derived partly or wholly from the host cell.

Enzyme A protein that catalyses a biochemical reaction.

Eosinophil A white cell of the blood whose main role is to attack large micro-organisms (e.g. protozoa).

Epidemic When the incidence of an endemic infection increases to an unusually high level or infections not usually seen in that population occur.

Epidemiology The study of the occurrence of diseases, how and when they occur, how and why they are transmitted.

Erythema A reddening of the skin caused by dilation of capillary blood vessels; often a sign of inflammation or infection.

ESBL Extended-spectrum β-lactamases. Enzymes that hydrolyse second and third generation cephalosporins.

Eukaryotic cell One of two types of living cells, in which the nucleus is delimited from the cytoplasm by a membrane.

Exogenous From outside the body; compare with 'endogenous'. Exogenous infections are caused by micro-organisms acquired from another person, animal or the environment.

Exotoxin Proteins secreted by bacteria that damage host tissues.

F

Facultative An organism that can adapt its metabolism; thus a facultative anaerobe can live in the absence or presence of oxygen.

Fermentation Production of energy from carbohydrates in the absence of oxygen. The electrons generated are passed to organic molecules.

Fibrin The final product of blood coagulation, formed by the action of the enzyme thrombin on the precursor fibrinogen. Makes a mesh that seals off damaged blood vessels (i.e. a clot).

Flagellum A hair-like appendage on the surface of the cell used for locomotion.

Fluorescent antibody technique A technique for detecting microbes in which the antibody is tagged with fluorescent dyes and thus rendered visible when viewed with a special microscope (fluorescence microscope) in which ultraviolet light is used.

Fomites Inanimate objects or material on which disease-producing agents may be conveyed (e.g.

patients' personal possessions such as bedding, clothes).

G

Gangrene Death of tissue or part of the body due to deficiency or cessation of the blood supply.

Gas gangrene Death of tissue or part of the body due to infection by *Clostridium perfringens*.

Gene A 'unit of heredity'; a segment of DNA that encodes the structure of a protein.

Genome The complete set of genes contained in the chromosomes.

Genus In biological nomenclature, the genus is the larger grouping and is written with a capital; the species is the smaller grouping. Both words are modern Latin and are printed in italics when the species name is given.

Glycocalyx A more or less diffuse layer outside the cell wall of prokaryotes; it consists of polysaccharide, polypeptide or both.

Glycogen A polysaccharide stored by animals and some bacteria.

Golgi complex An organelle present in the cytoplasm of eukaryotic cells; it is involved in the secretion of proteins from the cell.

Gram stain A staining procedure that distinguishes two types of prokaryote: Gram positive and Gram negative.

Granulocytes Phagocytic cells of the immune system that circulate in the blood. There are three types: neutrophils (the largest proportion), basophils and eosinophils.

GRE Glycopeptide-resistant enterococci. These enterococci are resistant to glycopeptide antibiotics (vancomycin and teicoplanin).

H

Haemolysin An enzyme that lyses red cells. Many bacteria produce haemolysins.

Haploid A haploid cell contains only one copy of each chromosome. The cells of prokaryotic organisms are haploid. Compare with 'diploid'.

Heat labile Easily destroyed by heat.

Helix, helical Spiral.

Herd immunity Protection of an entire population against a particular infection, through the induction of immunity in at least 60% of individuals.

Histamine A molecule released by mast cells; it causes increased permeability of blood vessels and is responsible for the signs of inflammation; excess is associated with hay fever, asthma, etc.

Histocompatibility antigens Cell surface antigens involved in many aspects of immunological recognition; they are the main antigens recognized in the rejection of grafts. In humans the chief group of such antigens is called the HLA system.

Hospital-acquired infection An infection acquired as a result of treatment in hospital = nosocomial infection.

Humoral immune system Antibody production by B lymphocytes.

Hypersensitivity An exaggerated or inappropriate immune response, leading to inflammation or tissue damage.

I

Icosahedron A solid figure with 12 (vertices) corners and 20 triangular faces.

Immunity Protection against infection by a particular microbe. Results from infection by or immunization against that microbe.

Immunization The process of artificially inducing immunity to infection by a microbe.

Immunocompromised Impaired immune response that renders the host particularly susceptible to infection.

Immunoglobulin An antibody.

Incidence The number of new cases occurring in a population over time.

Incubation period The interval between contact with the microbe and the development of the symptoms and signs of infection.

Infection Entry of a harmful microbe into the body and its multiplication in the tissues.

Inflammation A response to infection or other injury characterized by swelling, heat, redness and pain.

Inoculum Material (containing bacteria) added to a growth medium to initiate a culture; hence 'inoculate'.

Interferons A group of immunological proteins that carry signals between cells.

Interleukins Immunological proteins, messenger molecules released by cells of the immune system.

In vitro 'In glass', i.e. carried out in the test tube, in the laboratory.

In vivo 'In the living', i.e. in the animal (or patient).

L

Latent infection A condition in which the clinical signs of infection are absent and the causative organism may be temporarily undetectable; under certain conditions the infection may again become obvious.

Leucocyte *See* granulocytes.

Lipid A fat; a molecule made up of glycerol and fatty acids.

Lipopolysaccharide A constituent of the Gram-negative bacterial cell wall, in which chains of various sugars are linked to lipid A.

Lymphocytes Cells involved in the specific immune response. B lymphocytes produce antibodies; T lymphocytes attack intracellular pathogens and malignant cells and co-ordinate the activity of other immune system cells.

Lysis Destruction or decomposition of a cell under the influence of a specific agent.

Lysosome An intracellular organelle; contains enzymes that digest unwanted molecules.

Lysozyme An enzyme that can dissolve the cell walls of certain bacteria.

M

Macrophage A type of phagocyte mainly found in the tissues.

Malaise A general feeling of being unwell.

Mantoux test A tuberculin skin test.

Mast cell Mediator cells in the tissues that influence the response of the immune system by releasing vasoactive chemicals (e.g. histamine). Responsible for the inflammatory response and hypersensitivity reactions.

Meiosis A form of cell division, characteristic of eukaryotic cells; it results in haploid progeny cells (male and female gametes).

Messenger RNA The transcript of the DNA from which a polypeptide is synthesized by the ribosome.

Metabolism A general term for all the biochemical processes that occur in a living cell.

Metabolite Breakdown products of the process of metabolism.

Micro-organism A creature too small to be seen with the naked eye (or only just visible); the term includes bacteria, fungi, protozoa, some of the algae and the viruses.

Minimum inhibitory concentration (MIC) The lowest concentration of an antibiotic or other agent that will inhibit the growth of a micro-organism.

Mitochondrion An intracellular organelle that contains the energy-generating systems of eukaryotic cells.

Mitosis Division of a eukaryotic cell into two diploid daughter cells.

Monocyte A white cell of the blood, which develops into the tissue macrophage.

Mutation A change in the sequence of the bases in the DNA strand.

Myalgia Pain in the muscles, a feature of many viral infections.

Mycelium An intertwined mass of filaments (hyphae), typical of the growth of fungi.

Mycoses Infections caused by fungi; can be superficial (e.g. affecting the skin) or deep, invading tissue and causing systemic infection.

N

Narrow spectrum An antibiotic with activity against only one, or a limited range of, bacteria.

Natural killer cells Large lymphoid cells capable of killing cells with the appropriate receptors on the surface.

Neutrophil A phagocytic white cell of the blood. Accounts for the greatest proportion of white cells circulating in the blood.

Normal flora The community of microbes that colonize a body surface.

Nosocomial Acquired or occurring in a hospital; for example, a nosocomial infection = a hospital-acquired infection.

Nuclease An enzyme that catalyses the breakdown of nucleic acids.

Nucleic acid The organic acids DNA and RNA that carry the genetic code of the cell.

Nucleolus An area in the nucleus of a eukaryotic cell where RNA is synthesized.

Nucleotide The components of DNA or RNA, made up of a sugar, an organic base and a phosphate group.

Nucleus (a) The central part of an atom, made up of protons and neutrons; or (b) the part of the eukaryotic cell that contains the genetic material.

O

Objective lens The lens of a microscope that forms the primary image of the specimen.

Obligate An obligate organism is restricted to a particular way of life; for example, an obligate parasite cannot live free without a host; an obligate aerobe cannot live without oxygen.

Ocular lens The lens of a microscope that further magnifies the primary image formed by the objective lens.

Opportunistic organism One capable of causing infection when the immune system of the host is impaired.

Organelle A distinct structure within the cytoplasm of a eukaryotic cell that possesses a separate function (e.g. the mitochondria, Golgi complex).

Organic compound Contains carbon.

Osmosis The movement of a solvent (e.g. water) from a less concentrated to a more concentrated solution through a semipermeable membrane.

Oxidation The addition of oxygen to, or the removal of electrons from, a substance.

P

Pandemic A worldwide outbreak of an infectious disease.

Parasite An organism that lives in or on another creature and obtains food and shelter without benefiting the host. Hence 'parasitism'. *See* commensal, symbiosis.

Parenteral Administered by injection directly into the tissues (e.g. subcutaneously, intramuscularly, intravenously).

Passive immunity Immunity conferred on the host animal by antibodies made in another host.

Pathogen A microbe capable of causing disease.

Pathogenicity The ability of a microbe to invade and cause disease.

Peptide A chain of amino acids.

Peptidoglycan A major structural component of bacterial cell walls, consisting of chains of sugars crosslinked by peptides.

Peptones Short chains of amino acids derived from the breakdown of proteins.

pH The symbol denoting hydrogen ion concentration; the pH ranges between 0 and 14, and its value indicates the relative acidity or alkalinity of a solution.

Phage *See* bacteriophage.

Phagocyte A cell capable of phagocytosis.

Phagocytosis The ingestion of material by a cell either in order to destroy foreign matter or for its own nutrition.

Photosynthesis The use of solar energy by green plants and some bacteria to synthesize carbon compounds from carbon dioxide and water.

Plasma The fluid in which blood cells are suspended. It contains a high concentration of protein and inorganic salts (e.g. sodium, potassium, calcium).

Plasma cell A cell that develops from a B lymphocyte and that manufactures a specific antibody.

Plasmid A small circle of DNA that may be present in the cytoplasm of a microbial cell. Plasmids often carry genes for antibiotic resistance.

Polymer A molecule made up of similar subunits.

Polymorphonuclear leucocyte The blood contains three polymorphonuclear leucocytes: the neutrophil, the eosinophil and the basophil.

Polypeptide A chain of at least four, and usually more, amino acids.

Precipitate The result of a reaction between two soluble substances to form an insoluble material that 'falls' out of solution.

Precipitin reaction A reaction between antigen and antibody resulting in a visible precipitate.

Prevalence The number of cases occurring within a population at one particular time.

Primary response The production of antibody in response to the first contact with the antigen.

Probe A short single-stranded segment of DNA or RNA that is identical in base sequence to a part of a gene, plasmid, ribosome, etc. and which can be used to detect the presence of the gene or plasmid, and hence to identify the microbe of which it is a part.

Prokaryotic cell One of two chief types of living cells, in which the nucleus is not delimited from the cytoplasm by a membrane. In general, prokaryotic cells are smaller and of less complex structure than eukaryotic cells.

Prophylaxis Treatment intended to prevent disease rather than cure it (e.g. prophylactic antibiotic therapy).

Prostaglandin A group of hormones present in a wide variety of tissues and body fluids.

Protein A large molecule, one of the main constituents of living matter; it consists of one or more polypeptide chains.

Protozoa Microscopic single-celled eukaryotic microbes; some are free living, others are important parasites.

Pus An accumulation of fluid as a result of infection; it consists of living and dead microbes, phagocytes and tissue cells, together with the fluid that has accumulated in the tissue because of inflammation.

R

Reservoir (of infection) The site where a microorganism normally lives and the permanent source of infection; for example, foxes are a reservoir of rabies in western Europe.

Respiration The generation of energy by the conversion of organic compounds to carbon dioxide and water.

Restriction endonucleases Enzymes that cut DNA strands at specific base combinations.

Reverse transcriptase An enzyme that synthesizes DNA from an RNA template. The human immunodeficiency virus contains a reverse transcriptase.

Ribonucleic acid (RNA) A nucleic acid in which the component nucleotides contain the sugar ribose. The ribonucleic acids of cells are messenger RNA, transfer RNA and ribosomal RNA; in addition, the genome of some viruses consists of RNA.

Ribosome The protein-synthesizing 'factory' of the cytoplasm.

S

Saprophyte An organism that lives on dead organic matter.

Sensitivity The susceptibility of certain organisms to specific agents.

Septicaemia Bacteria present in the bloodstream and accompanied by symptoms and signs of infection with no other recognized cause.

Seroconversion The production of specific antibodies in response to an antigen.

Serotype A strain of a bacterial species that can be differentiated by the antigens present on its surface; these are detected by antibodies (serological methods).

Serum The liquid that separates from clotted blood. Similar composition to plasma, but without substances used in coagulation (e.g. fibrinogen).

Species *See* genus.

Spore A resistant casing that some bacteria use to enclose their cells in adverse environmental conditions. Spores germinate when conditions improve and the cell recommences multiplication.

Sterilization A process that removes or destroys all micro-organisms including spores.

Strain A group of bacteria with different properties to other bacteria of the same species. Strains are distinguished in the laboratory by specialist 'typing' techniques.

Subclinical infection An infection that produces no symptoms or signs of disease; said of the early stages or a very mild form of the disease.

Superinfection Acquisition of a more resistant strain of the organism already causing infection or replacement of normal flora by antibiotic-resistant organisms because of antibiotic use.

Surveillance The systematic observation of the occurrence of disease in a population with analysis and dissemination of the results.

Symbiosis An association between two species in which there is mutual benefit.

Syndrome A set of symptoms and signs that forms a distinctive clinical picture suggesting a particular disease.

Synergy When the effect of two antibiotics (or other drugs) given together is greater than can be accounted for by the effect of each acting alone.

Systemic Involving the whole body.

T

Teichoic acid A polymer of an alcohol, phosphate and other molecules found in Gram-positive cell walls.

Titre A measure of the concentration of an antibody in serum.

Topical A drug that is applied directly to the affected part (e.g. skin or eye) is applied topically.

Toxin Any poisonous substance produced by a living organism, especially a microbe.

Toxoid A microbial toxin treated (usually with dilute formaldehyde) so that its toxic activity is destroyed but it is still capable of stimulating the production of antibodies that recognize the microbial toxin.

Trace element A chemical element required for growth, but needed in only very small amounts.

Transcription Copying the sense strand of the DNA into messenger RNA.

Transduction The introduction of new genes into a bacterial cell, by a bacteriophage. The new genes are derived from the bacterium in which the phage previously replicated.

Transfer RNA Small RNA molecules that carry individual amino acids to the ribosome.

Transformation The introduction of new genes into a cell by the uptake of fragments of DNA from solution.

Translation Synthesis of a polypeptide chain from the messenger RNA template.

Transposon A 'jumping gene'; a segment of DNA that can move from one DNA molecule to another or from one site to another in the same DNA molecule.

Tuberculin test A skin test used to detect infection by mycobacteria.

U

Ultraviolet light Invisible light of wavelength shorter than the light at the violet end of the visible spectrum.

V

Vaccination The process of inducing immunity by administering a vaccine.

Vaccine A preparation of killed or inactivated microbes, inactivated microbial toxins or microbial antigens used to induce immunity.

Vector An animal, usually an arthropod (insect or tick), that transfers an infectious microbe from one host to another.

Virulence The ability of an organism to cause disease.

Virus A micro-organism capable of reproduction only inside living cells.

VISA/GISA *Staphylococcus aureus* that has intermediate resistance to vancomycin (VISA) or glycopeptides (teicoplanin and/or vancomycin) (GISA).

VRSA *Staphylococcus aureus* that is resistant to vancomycin.

Z

Zoonosis An infectious disease of animals that may be transmitted to humans. Brucellosis, rabies and toxoplasmosis are examples.

Index

NOTE:

Note: The glossary has not been included in the index.
Page numbers suffixed by 'f' refer to figures; those suffixed by 't' refer to tables